TRICHOSCOPY
A Text and Atlas

TRICHOSCOPY

A Text and Atlas

Second Edition

Editors

Subrata Malakar
MBBS MD(Dermatology) DCH
Director and Chief Dermatologist
Rita Skin Foundation
Kolkata, West Bengal, India

Surit Malakar
MBBS MD(Dermatology)
Medical Director and Consultant Dermatologist
Rita Skin Foundation
Kolkata, West Bengal, India

JAYPEE
JAYPEE BROTHERS MEDICAL PUBLISHERS
The Health Sciences Publisher
New Delhi | London

JAYPEE **Jaypee Brothers Medical Publishers (P) Ltd**

Headquarters
EMCA House
23/23-B, Ansari Road, Daryaganj
New Delhi 110 002, India
Landline: +91-11-23272143, +91-11-23272703
+91-11-23282021, +91-11-23245672
E-mail: jaypee@jaypeebrothers.com

Corporate Office
Jaypee Brothers Medical Publishers (P) Ltd.
4838/24, Ansari Road, Daryaganj
New Delhi 110 002, India
Phone: +91-11-43574357
Fax: +91-11-43574314
E-mail: jaypee@jaypeebrothers.com

Overseas Office
JP Medical Ltd.
83, Victoria Street, London
SW1H 0HW (UK)
Phone: +44-20 3170 8910
E-mail: info@jpmedpub.com

EU GPSR Authorised Representative
Logos Europe, 9 rue Nicolas Poussin
17000, La Rochelle, France
Phone: +33 (0) 6 67 93 73 78
E-mail: Contact@logoseurope.eu

Website: www.jaypeebrothers.com
Website: www.jaypeedigital.com

Inquiries for bulk sales may be solicited at: jaypee@jaypeebrothers.com

***Trichoscopy: A Text and Atlas* / Subrata Malakar, Surit Malakar**

First Edition: 2017

Second Edition: 2025, Reprint: **2026**

ISBN: 978-93-6616-424-3

Printed in India

Dedicated to

My Wife Late Dr Rita Shah Malakar

(Dr Subrata Malakar)

My Mother Late Dr Rita Shah Malakar

(Dr Surit Malakar)

Contributors

Barnali Chowdhury MD
(Dermatology, Venereology and Leprosy)
Consultant Dermatologist
Medica Superspecialty Hospital
Kolkata, West Bengal, India

BS Chandrashekar MD DNB
Chief Dermatologist and Medical Director
CUTIS Academy of Cutaneous Sciences
Bengaluru, Karnataka, India

Madura C MD FRGUHS
Medical Director
Consultant Dermatologist
Dermatosurgeon and Hair Transplant Surgeon
Department of Dermatology
CUTIS Academy of Cutaneous Sciences
Bengaluru, Karnataka, India

Priya Diwaker DDVL
Consultant
MediGenix Clinic
Raipur, Chhattisgarh, India

Purva Mehta Movdawalla DNB
Consultant Dermatologist
Trichologist and Aesthetician
Nucleus Eye & Skin Clinic
Mumbai, Maharashtra, India

Samipa S Mukherjee DDV DDVL
FRGUHS (Pediatric Dermatology)
Chief Dermatologist and Director
Dr Samipa's – The Skin Hair Nail Clinic
Bengaluru, Karnataka, India

Souvik Sardar MD
Consultant Dermatologist
Eleganz Skin & Hair Clinic
Kolkata, West Bengal, India

Subrata Malakar MBBS
MD(Dermatology) DCH
Director and Chief Dermatologist
Rita Skin Foundation
Kolkata, West Bengal, India

Surit Malakar MBBS MD(Dermatology)
Medical Director and Consultant Dermatologist
Rita Skin foundation
Kolkata, West Bengal, India

Preface to the Second Edition

Dermoscopy has carved its niche in the routine consultations of a dermatology clinic. It is a pleasure to present the Second Edition of our book *"Trichoscopy: A Text and Atlas"*, which has been updated to help the clinician be up to date with the basics, advances, and the varieties encountered in clinical practice. The meticulously compiled array of photographs encompassing various disorders and crisp texts to look for the pointers toward dermoscopic findings in particular disorders makes it an easy day-to-day guide for the students, academicians, and practitioners. The authors' personal experience and inputs in the trichoscopy world are especially useful to the clinicians. The user-friendly nature of the atlas with a uniform format, lucid language for easy understanding, and excellent quality images is expected to enthrall the readers. As our knowledge in the field of trichoscopy advances in leaps and bounds, we hope to see the dawn when it can safely avoid the need for biopsies in the future to come!

The authors/editors sincerely hope that this book will be a handy guide for students and physicians not only in the Indian subcontinent but also across the world. The well-illustrated dermoscopic images of hair disorders are expected to leave a lasting impression in the minds of the reader. We thank all the contributors for their mammoth efforts in compilation of this comprehensive text.

Subrata Malakar
Surit Malakar

Preface to the First Edition

Trichoscopy is fast gaining hold in daily clinical practice of dermatologists across India and the world. This book is written by the trichoscopy enthusiasts with a vision to help and enhance structured and step-by-step practice of trichoscopy by the students and practitioners. The idea of this book was conceived when the authors saw that there was a dearth of work and data related to trichoscopy in the skin of color and the absence of proper teaching modules related to the same. This book was envisioned as a ready-reckoner and a basic step-by-step module that helped to arrive at a trichoscopic diagnosis of a particular condition.

The authors are trichoscopy enthusiasts, who use trichoscopy in the same way that a physician would use his stethoscope. They concur with the words of Antonella Tosti and Lidia Rudnicka that the practice of trichology without trichoscopy is a professional practice gap.

Having said this, the author would like to extend his heartfelt thanks to the two doyens in the world of trichology at large and trichoscopy as well, Antonella Tosti and Lidia Rudnicka. Their relentless efforts in this field culminated in producing two of the best books for trichoscopy that are being relied upon from across the world. Since its inception way back in 1993, when Steven Kossard and Sam Zagarella described dermoscopy with dots in cicatricial alopecia to 2006, where the term 'trichoscopy' was first introduced and used, the knowledge in this field is growing by leaps and bounds worldwide.

As we compile the trichoscopic data in this book and guide our readers towards making a trichoscopic diagnosis, we are certain that every reader will make their new observations as they go along and we solemnly support and request them to share their work and knowledge to add to the existing knowledge in trichoscopy.

We hope this book delivers what you are looking forth to learn in the field of trichoscopy and, thereby, helps in your clinical practice to achieve maximum output for yourself and your patients.

Subrata Malakar

Acknowledgments

I would like to acknowledge my patients who have inspired me a lot to work on this project.

I would like to thank Dr Samipa S Mukherjee, Shri Jitendar P Vij (Group Chairman), Mr Ankit Vij (Managing Director), Ms Somoshri Banerji (Development Editor), Mr Sabyasachi Hazra (Associate Director—Publishing & Digital Sales) and the entire team of Jaypee Brothers Medical Publishers, New Delhi, India for their tireless efforts in producing the book in its final form.

Contents

SECTION 6: NONSCARRING ALOPECIAS

SECTION 7: SCARRING ALOPECIAS

SECTION 8: HAIR WEATHERING

SECTION 9: INFECTION AND INFESTATION

1

SECTION

Introduction

CHAPTER

1 Introduction

Samipa S Mukherjee

Hair loss is one of the most common dermatological problems encountered on a day-to-day basis, the diagnosis and treatment of which may be challenging owing to the numerable number of causes of the same. Although clinical tests such as card test, hair pull test, tug test, and light microscopy of the scalp hair may provide a clue to the diagnosis at times, histopathology still remains the most definitive way of diagnosing the disorder. In recent times, dermatoscopy/epiluminescence microscopy has been found to be a valuable tool in the diagnosis and differentiation of hair disorders. Being noninvasive in nature, prompt and quick, easy demonstration of the problem to the patient leading to increased acceptability and compliance in the patients has led to an increased interest in this field. Lidia Rudnicka and Malgorzata Olszewska coined the term "Trichoscopy" for dermoscopy of hair and the scalp.[1] For scalp examination, a manual dermoscope (×10 magnification) or a videodermoscope with lenses ranging from ×20 to ×1,000 magnification can be used.[2,3]

The trichoscopic diagnosis of a disorder is based on the four fundamental findings-follicular, vascular, pigmentary, and interfollicular patterns. It is the alteration, permutation, and combinations in four cardinal findings that lead to the diagnosing of particular disorders.

INDICATIONS FOR TRICHOSCOPY

- Diagnosis of hair disorders
- Monitoring response
- Explaining prognosis of hair disorders
- Choosing an optimum site for biopsy
- In forensic medicine
- For demonstration of nature of complaints to the patient

ADEQUATE TRICHOSCOPIC EXAMINATION CRITERIA

- *Diffuse hair loss:* In diffuse hair loss, the frontal and occipital areas must be evaluated.
- *Patchy hair loss:* The center of the patch and the margins need to be evaluated. It is advisable to look into the normal areas of the scalp as well to acquaint oneself with the pigmentary, vascular, and follicular patterns in that individual.

ADVANTAGES OF TRICHOSCOPY

- In vivo procedure
- Immediate results—no lag time for processing
- Magnification of up to 200× can be possible
- Three-dimensional viewing of the specimen
- Entire specimen can be viewed at the same time.
- Noninvasive

- Simple to use
- Hair washing/hair coloring does not alter the yield of results in dermatoscopy

LIMITATIONS

Adequate training in trichoscopy may be needed before a dermatologist can start appreciating changes on the scalp under a dermatoscope.

The devices available for trichoscopy range from manual handheld basic devices such as the eyepiece of a microscope at 10× magnification to the more advanced machine such as Fotofinder, which does not just give an insight to the basic structural details of the scalp but also the other details like follicular unit count and strength, anagen/telogen ratio, etc.

Low Magnification versus Higher Magnification

Lower magnification allows viewing a larger area whereas the higher magnification is warranted for viewing the finer structural details.

Contact Dermatoscopy versus Noncontact Dermatoscopy

Contact dermatoscopy refers to the lens of the dermoscope coming in direct contact with the scalp/lesion/linkage fluid. In this method, the most commonly utilized technique is the roll-on technique, where one edge of the dermatoscope makes contact with the surface at an angle of 45° and the rest of the lens is rolled on over the lesion/skin surface.

Nonpolarized versus Polarized Mode

Since majority of the publications in trichoscopy are done on nonpolarized light dermatoscopes, it is easier to use this mode for learning. However, keratotic structures are better seen in nonpolarized mode and vascular structures are seen best with polarized mode and pigment boost to enhance the contrast.

Dry Trichoscopy versus Use of Immersion Fluid

Dry trichoscopy in the nonpolarized mode allows better visualization of scales whereas a contact fluid may be needed to visualize the blood vessels under low pressure.

Choice of Dermatoscopy/Contact Fluids

The various immersion fluids used include alcoholic solutions, aqueous gels, and immersion oils. In a study conducted in 2003, the authors found that dermoscopic structures were clearly visible through alcoholic solutions and liquid paraffin and slightly burred with water and aqueous gel.[4] The same study also demonstrated that alcoholic fluids resulted in the least amount of air bubbles whereas liquid paraffin resulted in the most. The authors also opined that they prefer to use 70% ethanol in most circumstances because it has the advantage of being odorless, unlike its counterpart. Additionally, ethanol will not stain clothing, does not crystallize on the dermatoscope, and disinfects and evaporates immediately (does not need to be wiped off). For certain local considerations, such as dermoscopy on mucosa or the nail, it was reported that the same authors preferred to use ultrasound gel because it will not flow owing to its viscosity.

Tips for improving dermoscopic imaging:

- Clean the dermatoscope and camera lenses.
- Ensure that both dermatoscope and camera are fully charged.
- Ensure the dermatoscope is in contact with the skin
- Use interface medium to reduce surface light scatter and apply carefully to reduce air bubbles.

- Use ultrasound gel for imaging nails.
- For larger lesions, use a dermatoscope with a large field of view.
- Adjust horizontal and lateral pressure.
- Take multiple images and save the best!

Care of the dermatoscope:
- Keep the dermatoscope on its side and not resting on the lens.
- It should be disinfected in case of contact dermatoscopy.
- Keep the instrument detached from its attachment for storage.
- Clean the lens with a soft tissue or muller cloth.
- Do not over charge the instrument.

SCOPE OF THE BOOK

This book is aimed as a practical teaching guide to aid the practicing dermatologists as well as the students undergoing postgraduate training in dermatology. The chapters and the extent of the book have been designed in a way to help learn the basics and thus, form a strong foundation for going onto advanced learning. Focusing more on the "why" than the "what" has been maintained in all sections of the book. At a glance, images with descriptive legends provide an one-glance information to the reader regarding a topic. The self-assessment queries incorporated at the end of each section will help the reader to assess his recognition power of the trichoscopic structures, thus making him more and more adept to practicing trichoscopy in day-to-day clinical practice. The repetitions regarding certain terminologies in this book are intentional for better comprehensive understanding of the reader.

REFERENCES

1. Rudnicka L, Olszewska M, Rakowska A, Kowalska-Oledzka E, Slowinska M. Trichoscopy: a new method for diagnosing hair loss. J Drugs Dermatol. 2008;7:651-4.
2. Tosti A. Hair shaft disorders. In: Tosti A (Ed). Dermoscopy of Hair and Scalp: Pathological and Clinical Correlation, illustrated edition. USA: CRC Press; 2007. pp. 51-3.
3. Tosti A, Duque-Estrada B. Dermoscopy in hair disorders. J Egypt Womens Dermatol Soc. 2010;7:1-4.
4. Gewirtzman AJ, Saurat JH, Braun RP. An evaluation of dermoscopy fluids and application techniques. Br J Dermatol. 2003;149(1):59-63.

2

SECTION

Devices and Tools

CHAPTER

2

Devices and Tools

Subrata Malakar, Surit Malakar

INTRODUCTION

Trichoscopy is a method of evaluation of scalp and hair disorders using a dermatoscope. The term "trichoscopy" was first coined in 2006 by Lidia Rudnicka and Malgorzata Olszewska.[1] Dermatologists are trained to make diagnosis based on naked eye appearance of skin lesions. However, the shape, size, color, and distribution of a lesion may not always be sufficient to come to a diagnostic conclusion, wherein we are left with the option of biopsy. Dermoscopy is a noninvasive office procedure, which bridges the gap between clinical examination and biopsy.

The dermoscopic findings equate to histopathological correlation; hence, patients can be saved from the cost and trauma of undergoing invasive diagnostic procedures such as biopsy. Therefore, this simple diagnostic tool is rapidly gaining popularity among dermatologists.

WORKING PRINCIPLE OF DERMOSCOPY

Dermatoscope consists of a strong magnifying lens powered with a bright illumination source; this source can be either a halogen lamp or a light-emitting diode (LED). When light falls on the stratum corneum, it is reflected and refracted reducing the visibility of underlying structures. This scattering of light is overcome by polarized light in polarized dermatoscope, and contact fluid in nonpolarized dermatoscope allowing the visualization of subsurface skin structures in the epidermis, dermoepidermal junction, and upper dermis.

There are three types of dermatoscopes:

1. Nonpolarized
2. Polarized
3. Hybrid

Nonpolarized Devices

These devices require a contact medium/fluid (ideally with refractive index equal to that of skin), which optically links the skin surface with a glass plate mounted on the dermoscope. Contact fluids decrease the reflection and refraction of light on the skin surface, thus enabling visualization of the skin surface and subsurface structures. The liquids that can be used as a contact medium are alcohol solutions (70% ethanol), which have an added advantage of disinfection, hence preventing cross-infection. Aqueous solutions such as distilled water and normal saline can also be used. Gels are useful for convex surfaces.[2] The commonly used nonpolarized devices are Heine Delta 20 and DermLite II fluid.

Polarized Devices

Polarized devices have two filters in a process called cross-polarization; one filter is placed between the light source and skin, and the second is placed between the skin and light detector. This cross-polarization absorbs all the scattered light allowing only light in a single plane to pass through it, hence providing a very good visibility. The advantage of polarized devices over nonpolarized devices is the ability to visualize multiple lesions without the use of contact medium. The devices available in this category are DL100 and DermLite II PRO HR.

Hybrid Devices

These devices come incorporated with both polarized and nonpolarized lighting modes. Why the need for a hybrid device? There are certain structures which are better appreciated in polarized light, and while some are better visualized with a contact fluid. Nonpolarized light allows for better visualization more superficial structures such as milia-like cyst, comedo-like structures, and regression areas.[3] Vascular pattern, pigment distribution, and scar-like structures (in tumors with dermal component) are best appreciated in polarized light. The first device to have this combined facility was DermLite II Hybrid m. The latest in the series are DL3, DL4, and DL5, they have a very good image quality and is now preferred by many dermatologists. The images taken in this book are from DermLite DL3, DermLite DL4 and DermLite DL5.

Dermoscopy instruments are available as handheld dermatoscope or digital dermatoscope/video dermatoscope. Handheld devices are light weight and battery-powered devices, most of them providing a magnification of 10 fold. These devices can be attached to cameras; the newer ones can be attached to smartphones (e.g., DL3, DL4, and DL5) for taking video and still photographs. We can obtain an excellent image quality by zooming with smartphones. The above-mentioned devices are all handheld devices.

Digital dermatoscopes provide a magnification of 20–120-fold, allowing for better assessment of finer details and a good-quality image. The images obtained can be archived for follow-up assessment. They have software for expert diagnosis and reporting (mole mapping). An objective diagnosis of conditions such as telogen effluvium and androgenetic alopecia/female pattern hair loss can be achieved with the help of trichogram (anagen: telogen, terminal: vellus hair ratio is calculated). However, digital dermatoscopes are large and require installment space, and are quite expensive. The FotoFinder (FotoFinder Systems GmbH, Bad Birnbach) is once such videodermatoscope.

Dermoscopy is widely used in developed countries for diagnoses of melanoma. However, with time its diagnostic potentials in various pigmentary, inflammatory and infectious dermatoses as well as scalp/hair disorders have been recognized. Hence, despite its costs this novel diagnostic technique is gradually gaining its foothold in developing countries as well.

REFERENCES

1. Rudnicka L, Olszewska M, Magdalena M, Czuwara J. Presence and future of dermoscopy. Expert Rev Dermatol. 2006;1(6):769.
2. Rudnicka L, Rusek M, Borkowska B. Introduction. In: Rudnicka L, Olszewska M, Rakowska A, editors: Atlas of Trichoscopy: Springer; 2012. pp. 3-8.
3. Cristiane BA, Stephen WD, Agero ALC. Dermoscopy for the evaluation of skin lesions. Arch Dermatol. 2007;143(3):329-38.

3

SECTION

Trichoscopic Terminologies

CHAPTER 3

Trichoscopic Terminologies

Subrata Malakar

INTRODUCTION

This chapter is composed of terminologies which are new in the medical field to understand precisely an account of them are given accordingly in alphabetic order.

BLACK DOTS

- Hair follicle openings when viewed through dermoscopic lens appear as DOTS. This is how the term DOTS originated. These follicular openings may have other features like hair shaft residues, perifollicular fibrosis, follicular hyperkeratotic plugs, etc. Thereby the different terminologies such as black dots, yellow dots, white dots have been created.[1]
- *Black dots (cadaverized hairs)*: When pigmented hair is broken at scalp level, black dot is created.
- Black dots are not present in healthy individual and are present in nonscarring alopecias such as alopecia areata (AA), trichotillomania (TTM), tinea capitis, and chemotherapy-induced alopecia.
- A few isolated black dots are common in scarring alopecias, e.g., lichen planopilaris (LPP) and frontal fibrosing alopecia (FFA).

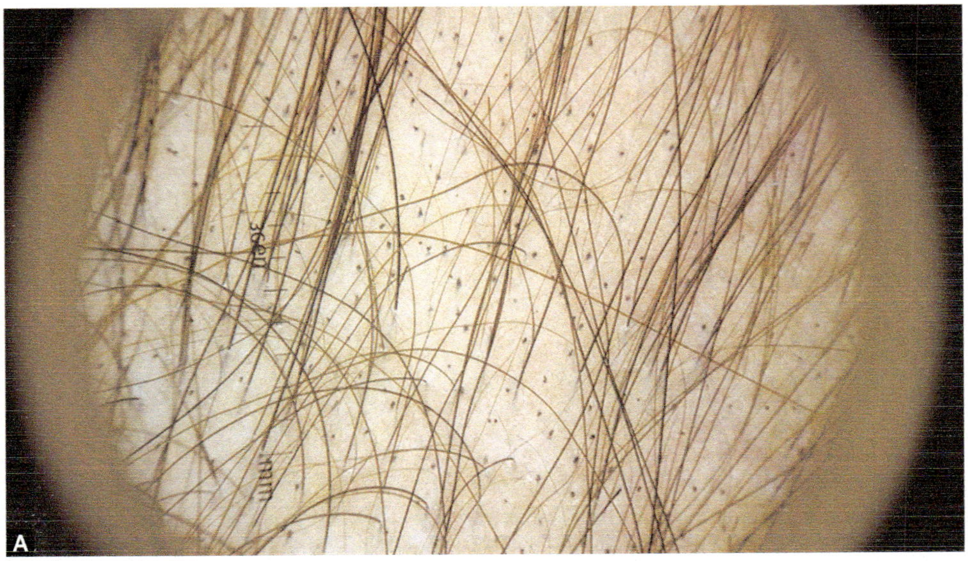

A

Continued

Continued

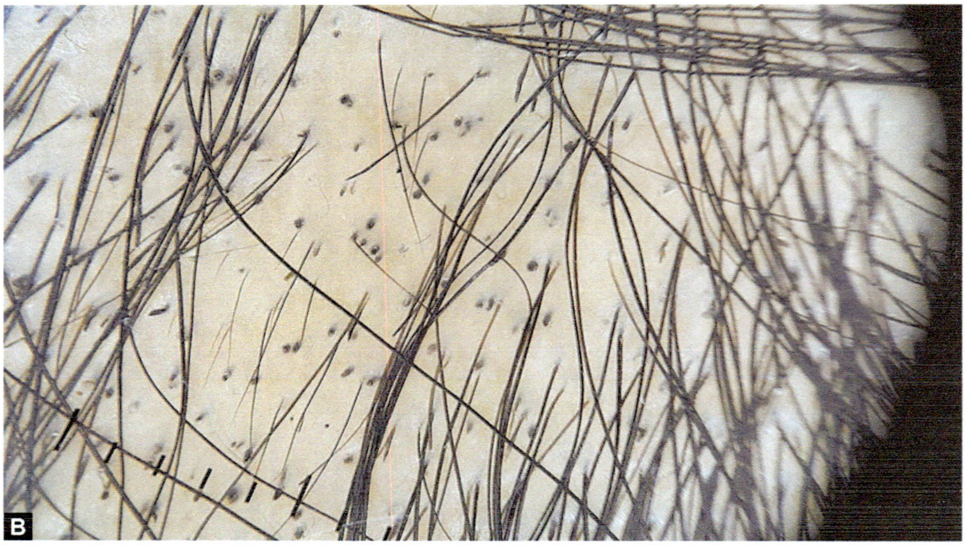

Figs. 1A and B: Black dots in alopecia areata (AA).

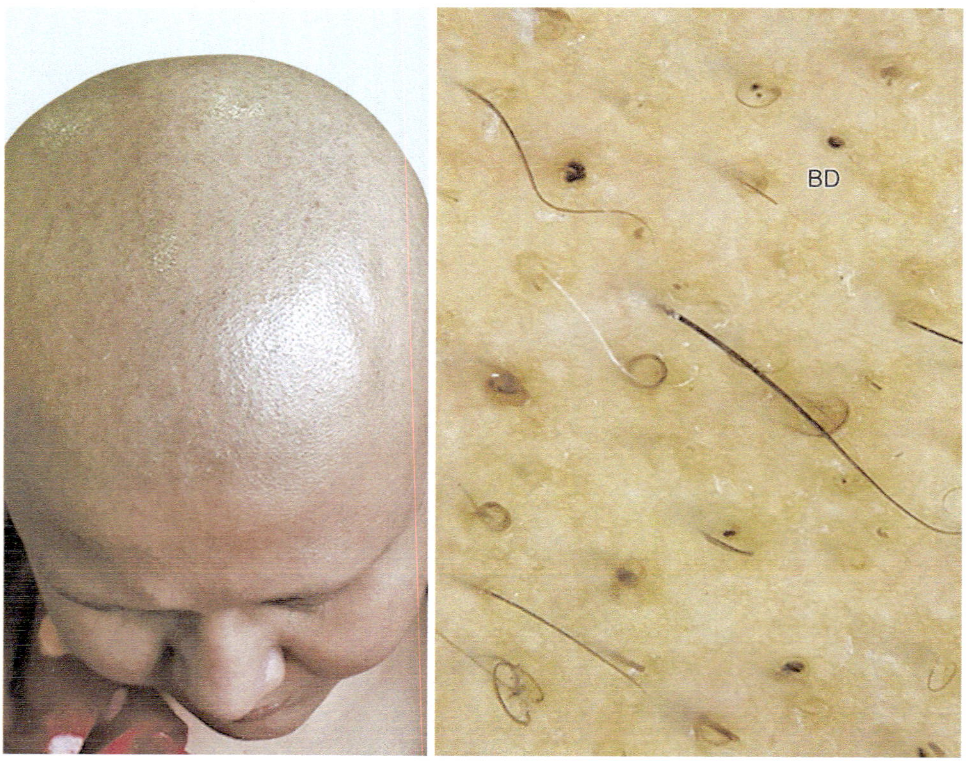

Fig. 2: Black dots (BD) in chemotherapy-induced alopecia.

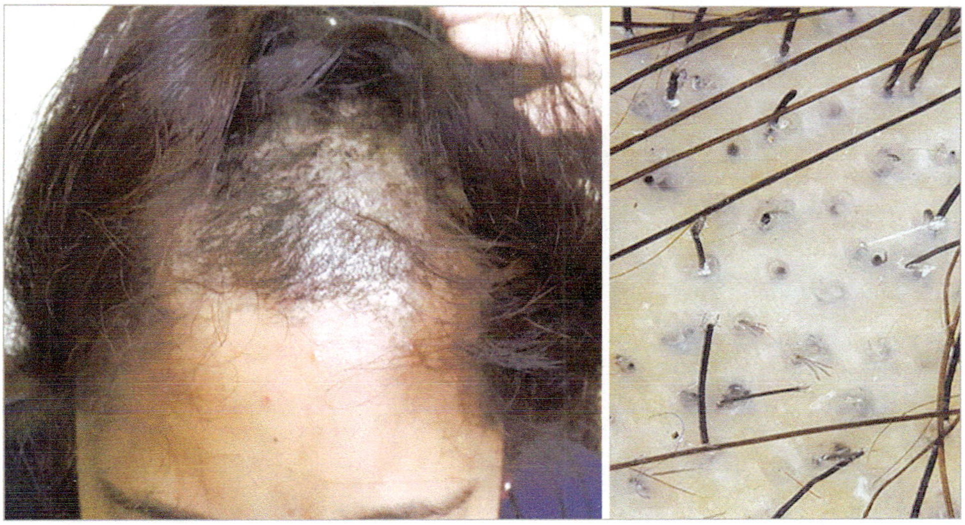

Fig. 3: Black dots in trichotillomania (TTM).

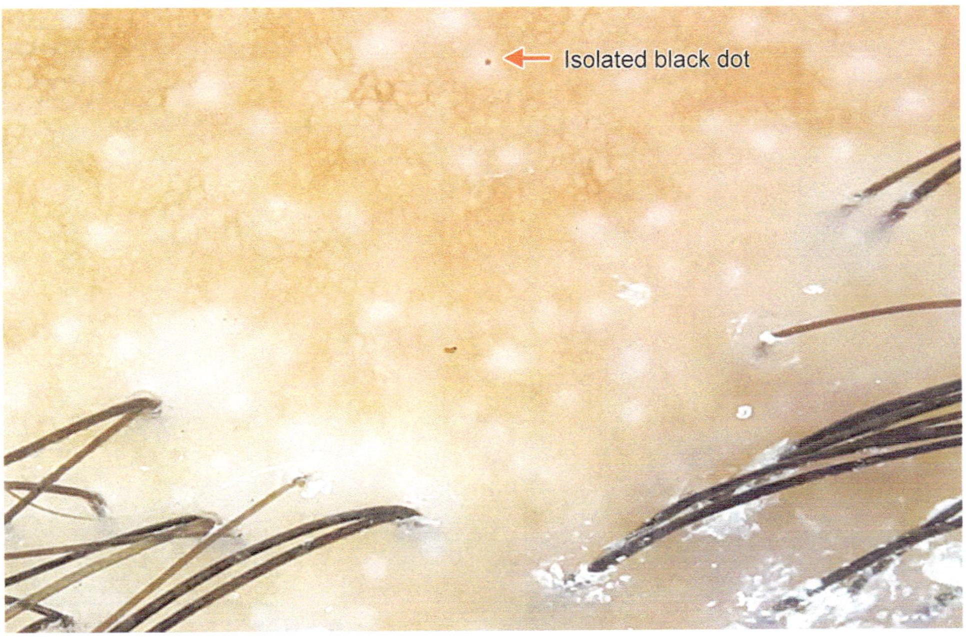

Fig. 4: Isolated black dot may be present in scarring alopecia.

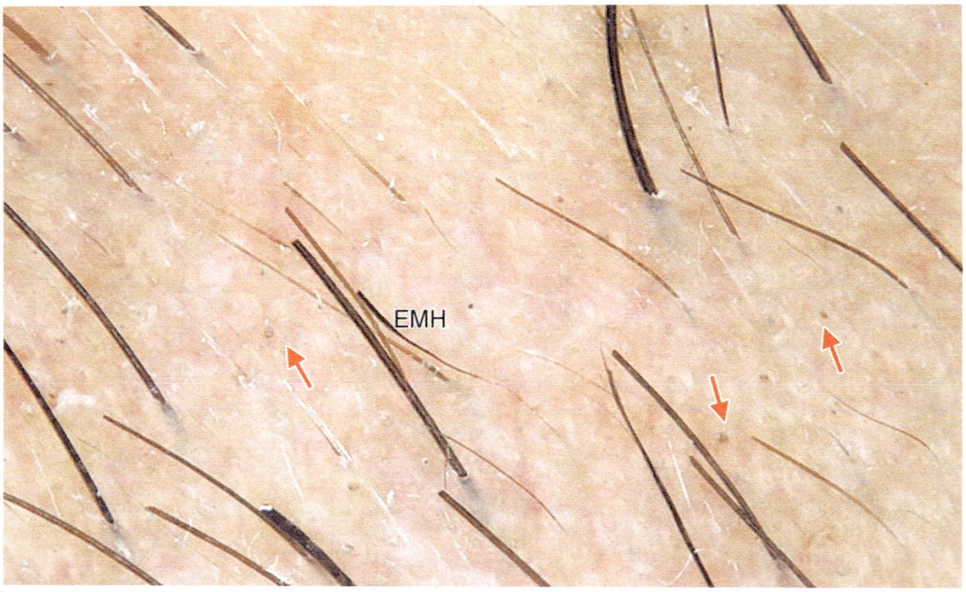

Fig. 5: Black dots in alopecia areata. Note exclamation mark hair (EMH) which is a marker of alopecia areata.

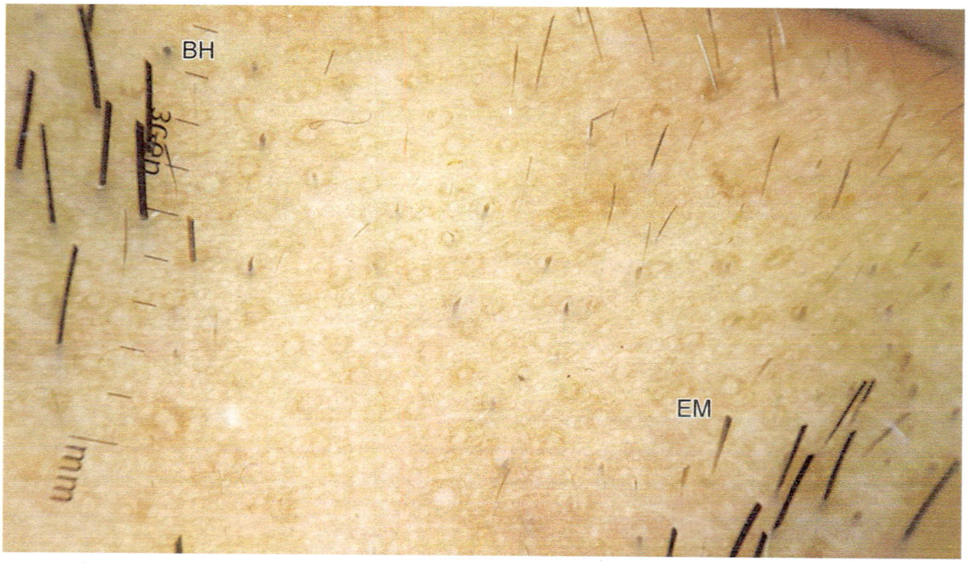

Fig. 6: Block hairs.[2] These are very short hairs with horizontal distal ends. Block hairs (BH) are found in many acquired conditions including tinea capitis. This is a case of alopecia areata where exclamation mark (EM) hairs are found at the periphery of the patch.

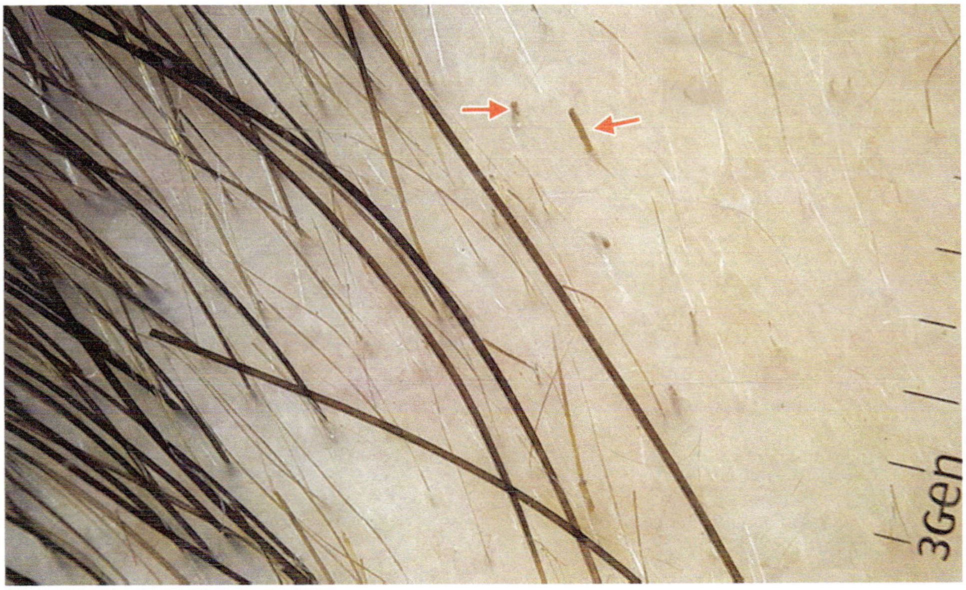

Fig. 7: Block hair.

BLUE-GRAY DOTS

- They correspond histopathologically to melanophages in the papillary dermis and are a sign of pigmentary incontinence.
- Blue-gray dots arranged in a target pattern are characteristic of LPP. This target pattern helps in differentiating LPP from other scarring alopecias.
- Blue-gray dots can also be seen in discoid lupus erythematosus (DLE) where they are present both perifollicularly as well as in speckled pattern.

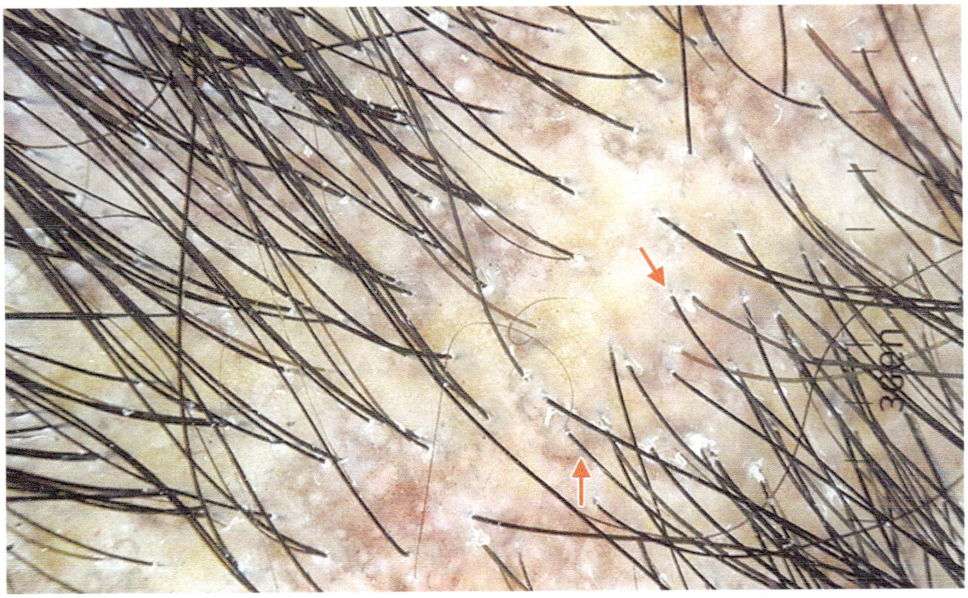

Fig. 8: Blue-gray dots. Round perifollicular blue-gray dots; the target pattern represents histopathologic melanophages around hair follicles.[3]

BROKEN HAIRS

- Hair shafts are broken at different levels from the scalp.
- They may be found in nonscarring and scarring alopecias.
- Broken hairs are mostly found in TTM, tinea capitis, alopecia areata, and after hair styling procedures.

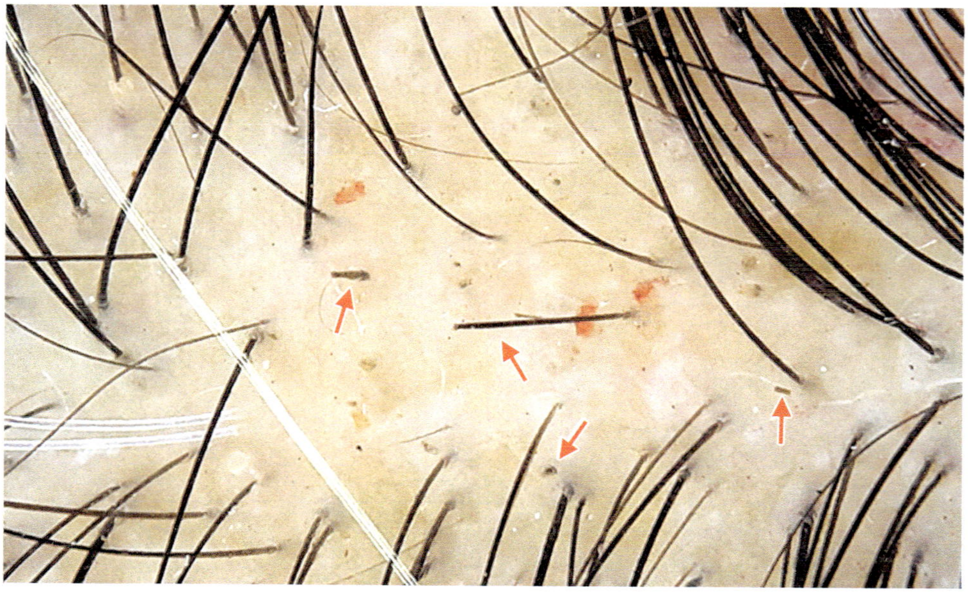

Fig. 9: Broken hair. Hairs may be broken at different levels from the scalp.[4,5]

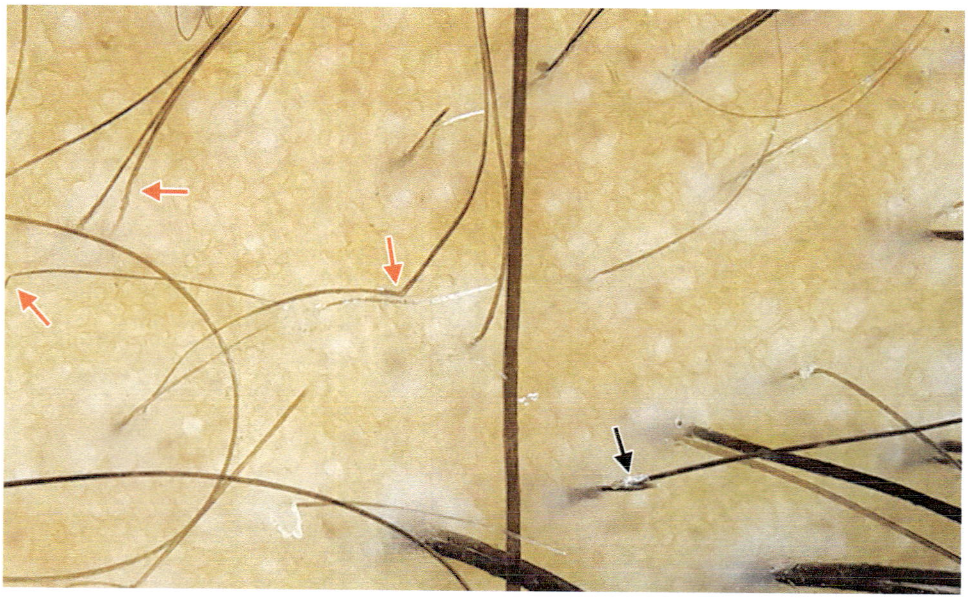

Fig. 10: Broken hairs in alopecia areata (AA), may develop in one of the two ways. Transverse fracture of the terminal hair shafts which are weakened by the inflammatory process. Here hair fracture is preceded by Pohl-Pinkus constrictions (red arrows) or by trichorrhexis nodosa (black arrow). Rapid regrowth of the incompletely destroyed hair shaft in the form of black dot is the other possibility.[4,5]

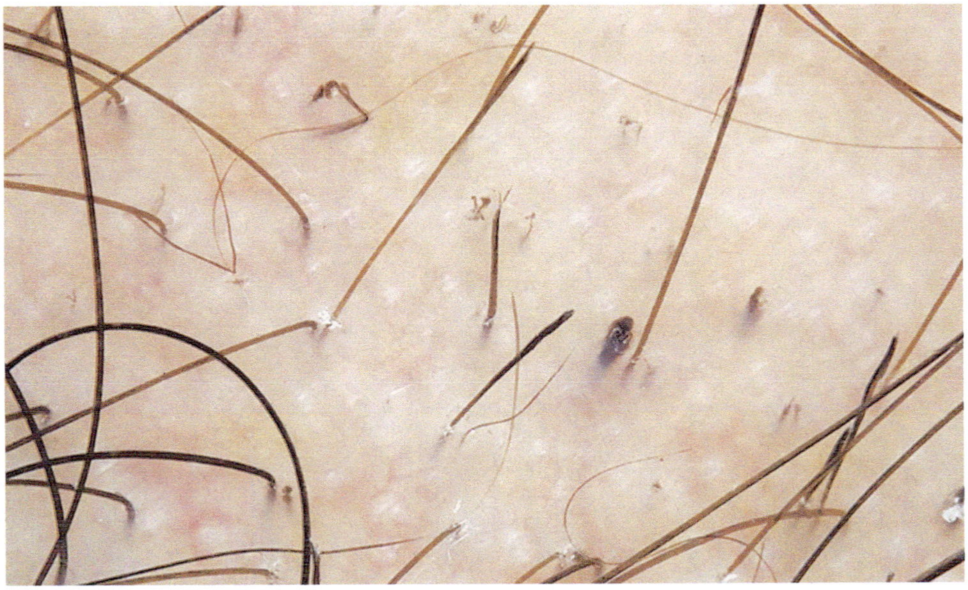

Fig. 11: Presence of hairs broken at different lengths is highly suggestive of trichotillomania (TTM). These hairs also have variable morphology.

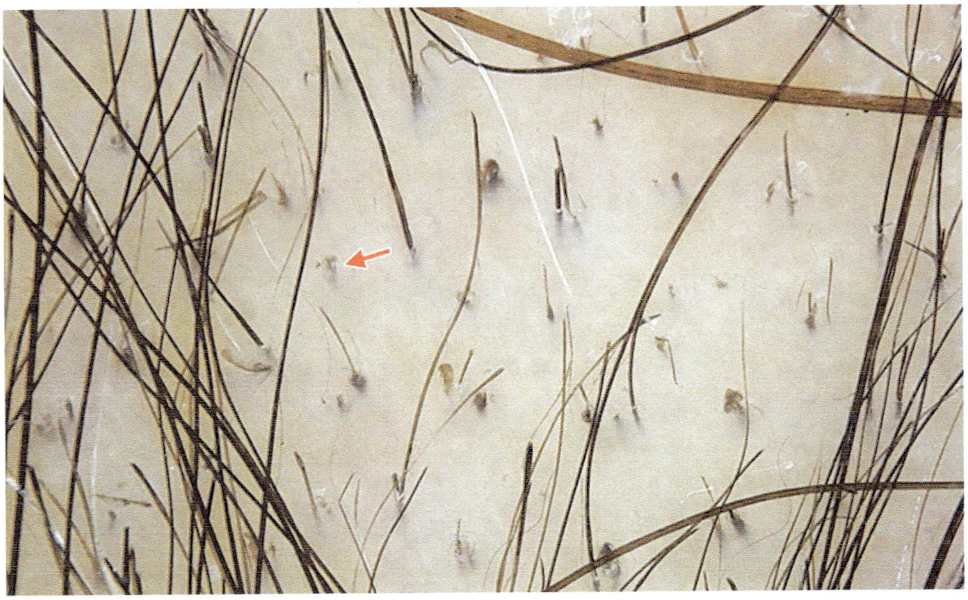

Fig. 12: In trichotillomania (TTM), broken hairs are formed by mechanical force of pulling the hairs. Hair may be broken at different lengths above the scalp surface. Sometimes, hairs are broken below the skin surface which is visible through the epidermis (red arrow).

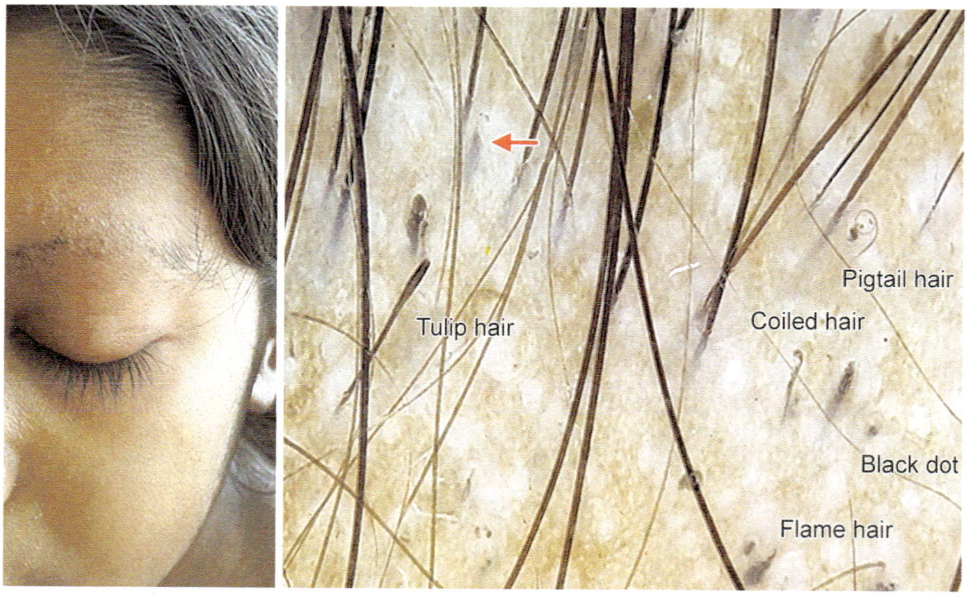

Fig. 13: Multiple hairs broken at different lengths showing extreme variability in morphology. Hair broken below the skin surface (red arrow) is seen through the epidermis; it is formed by mechanical force of pulling the hair. Pigtail hairs are new regrowing hairs which are regularly twisted and have tapered distal ends differentiating them from coiled hair.[4,5]

BROOM HAIR

- Broom hairs were originally described as two or more hair shafts emerging from a single follicular unit in a patient who otherwise has long hair.[6]
- On trichoscopic observations, broom hairs are redefined as multiple thin hairs emerging from a single follicular unit.[7,8]
- They reflect different pathologic mechanisms and histopathologies.[9]
- These may be seen in both cicatricial and noncicatricial alopecias, but has not been described in AA.

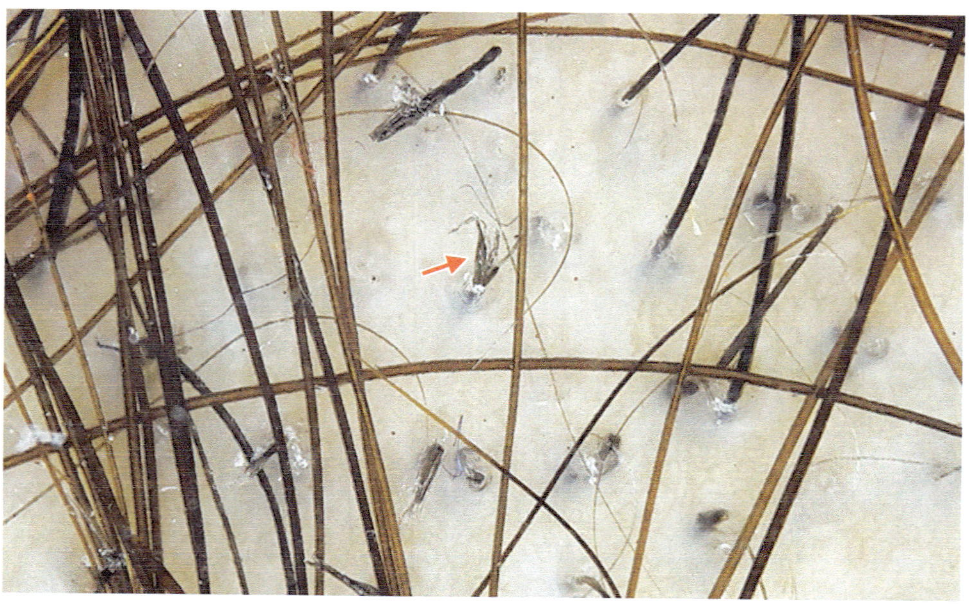

Fig. 14: Broom hairs in trichotillomania (TTM). Multiple thin hairs emerging from one follicular unit.

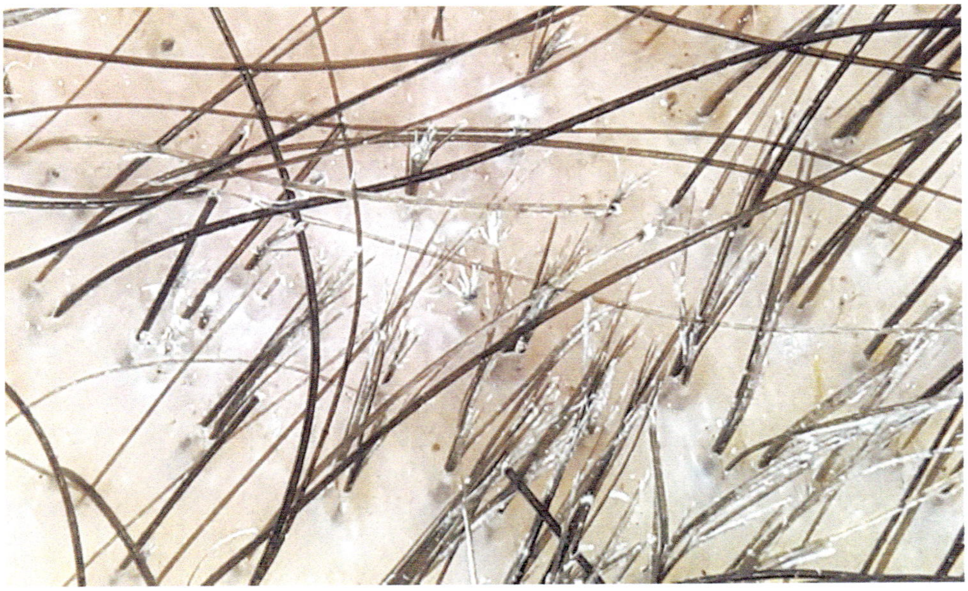

Fig. 15: Extensive broom hairs in trichotillomania (TTM).

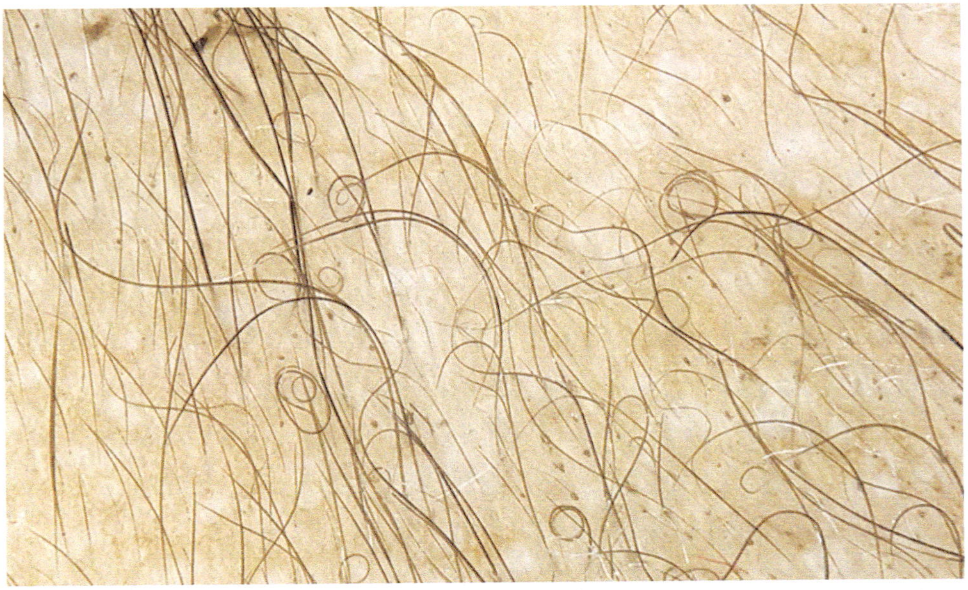

Fig. 16: Circle hair. Circle hairs appear as thin coiled hairs. They are also known as pigtail hairs. Presence of greater number of circle hairs strongly suggest alopecia areata (AA).[10] These hairs signify the active phase of the disease.

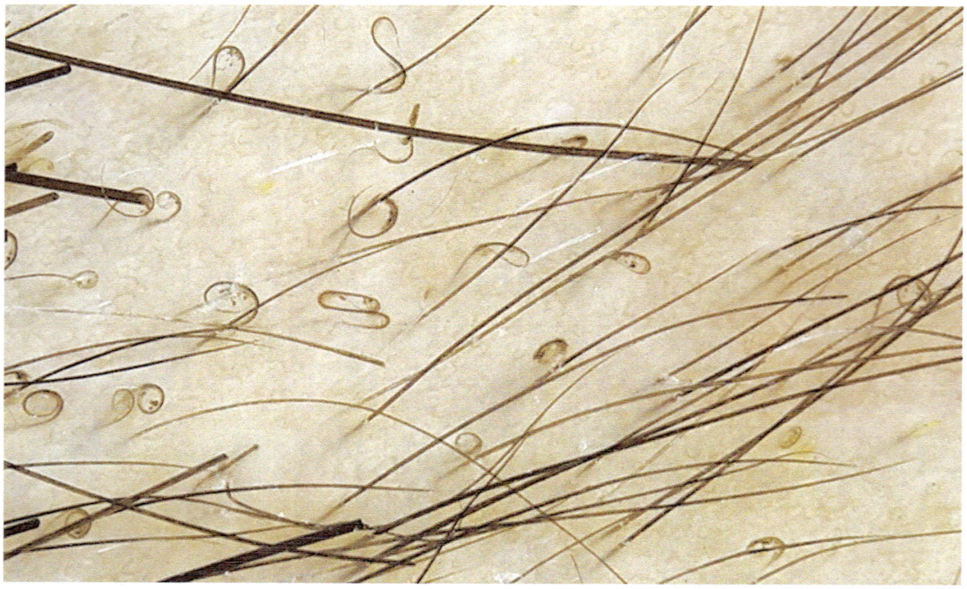

Fig. 17: Circle hairs (short vellus hairs) may be the solitary feature of alopecia areata (AA). It may also be found in androgenetic alopecia (AGA).[10]

COILED HAIRS

- Coiled hairs are broken hairs that curl back.
- Coiled hairs are most typical of TTM.
- But it may be present in small numbers in patients with traction alopecia.
- It may occur in healthy individual as a result of hair pulling during hair spa (style) procedures.

MECHANISM OF DEVELOPMENT OF COILED HAIRS

- It may occur in healthy individual as a result of hair pulling during hairspa (style) procedures.
- Hair shaft fractures in response to a pulling force → remaining hair shaft that is fixed to the scalp, may contract and coil coiled hairs.
- Partial coiling of the remaining hair shaft results in a hook-like appearance. This is called hook hairs or question mark hairs.

COILED HAIRS MUST BE DIFFERENTIATED FROM PIGTAIL HAIRS

Pigtail hairs are new regrowing hairs and are uniform in thickness and color and regular in shape.[11]

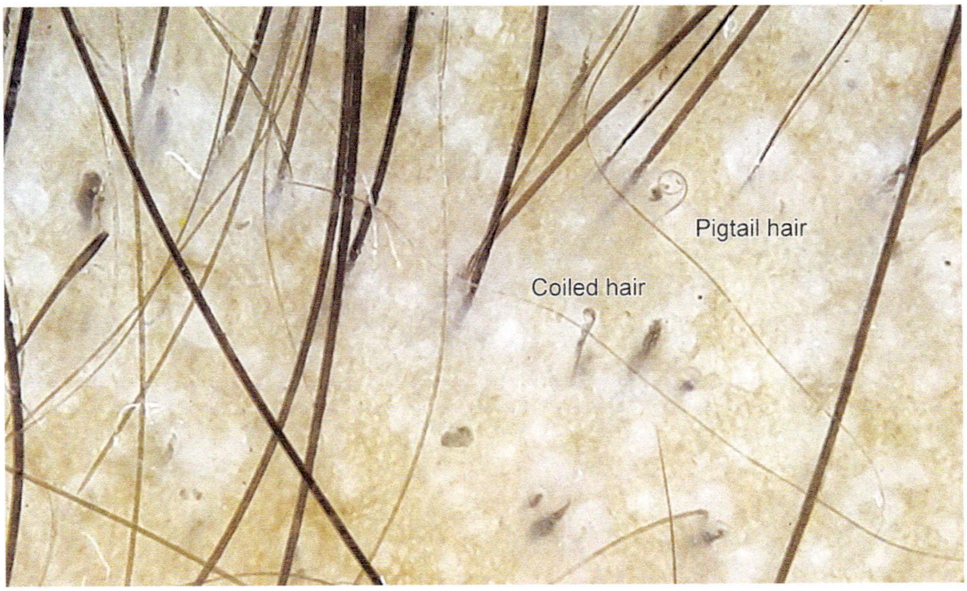

Fig. 18: Note the differentiation between coiled hair and pigtail hair. Coiled hairs have a hook-like appearance whereas pigtail hairs are circular with tapered ends. Pigtail hairs resemble a pig's tail.

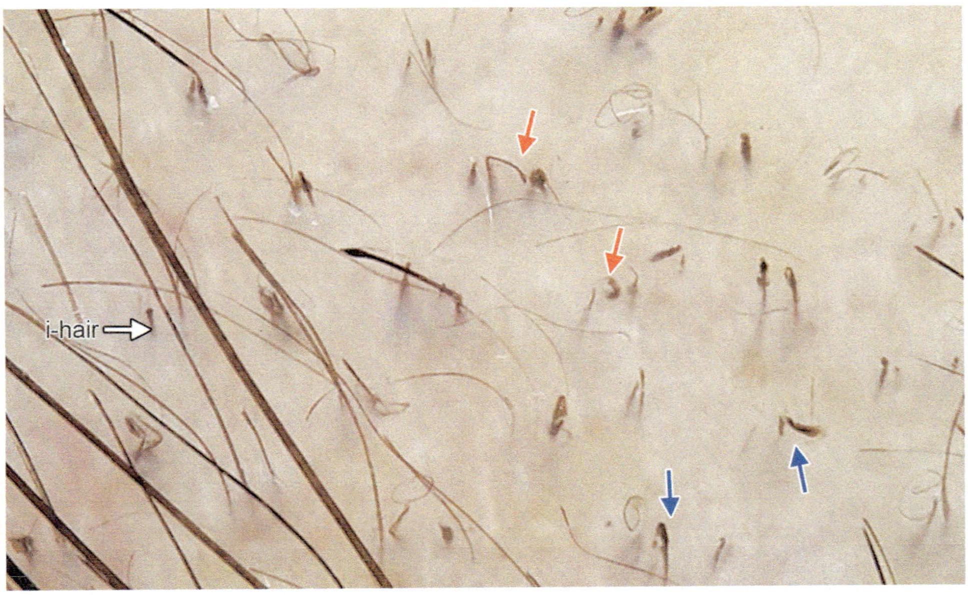

Fig. 19: Red arrows—coiled hairs, blue arrows—partially coiled hairs or question mark hairs, white arrow—i-hair.[10]

COMMA HAIR

- Focal alopecia with multiple comma hairs is pathognomonic for tinea capitis.
- Single hairs that curl into a comma-like appearance may be observed in healthy individuals with very short hair or remitting phase of AA.
- They are broken single hair shafts that curl into a comma-like structure due to hair ectothrix parasitation.[11,12]

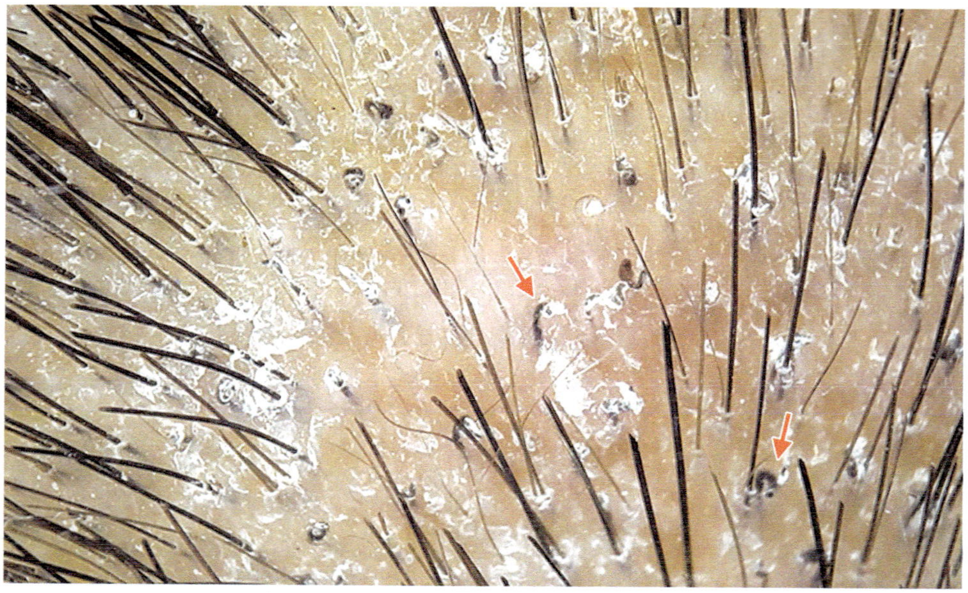

Fig. 20: Comma hairs (red arrows). Slightly curved short broken hairs. Comma hairs are dermoscopic markers of tinea capitis with microsporum canis.[11,12]

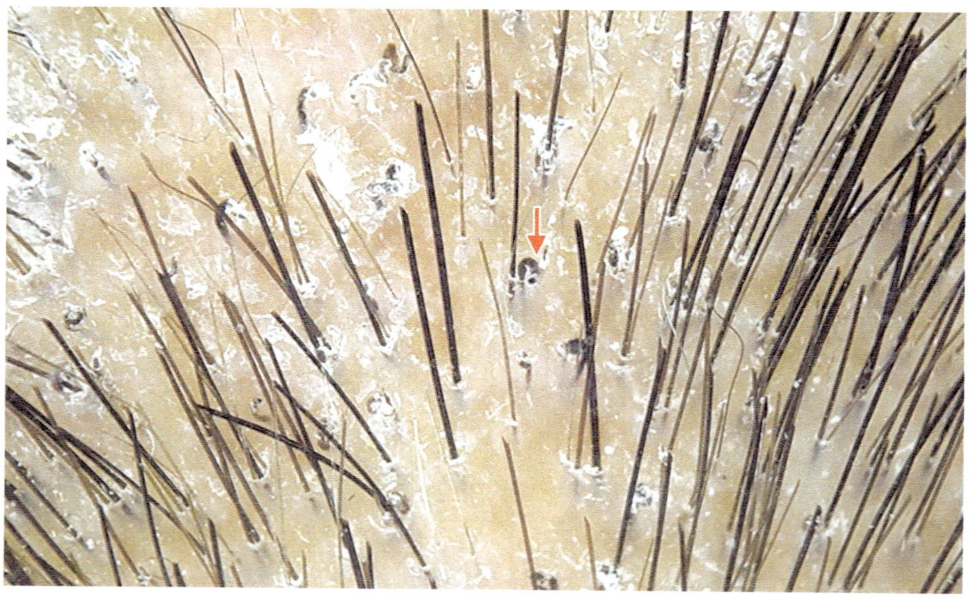

Fig. 21: Comma hairs (red arrow) are short broken hairs with hair ectothrix parasitation.

CORKSCREW HAIR

- Hairs curl into corkscrew structures
- These hairs are hallmark of tinea capitis in all phototypes[13]
- Comma hairs often coexist with corkscrew hairs
- Corkscrew hairs of tinea capitis differ from comma hairs by the presence of multiple twists and an intensely coiled shape, occurring from the same pathology as comma hairs.

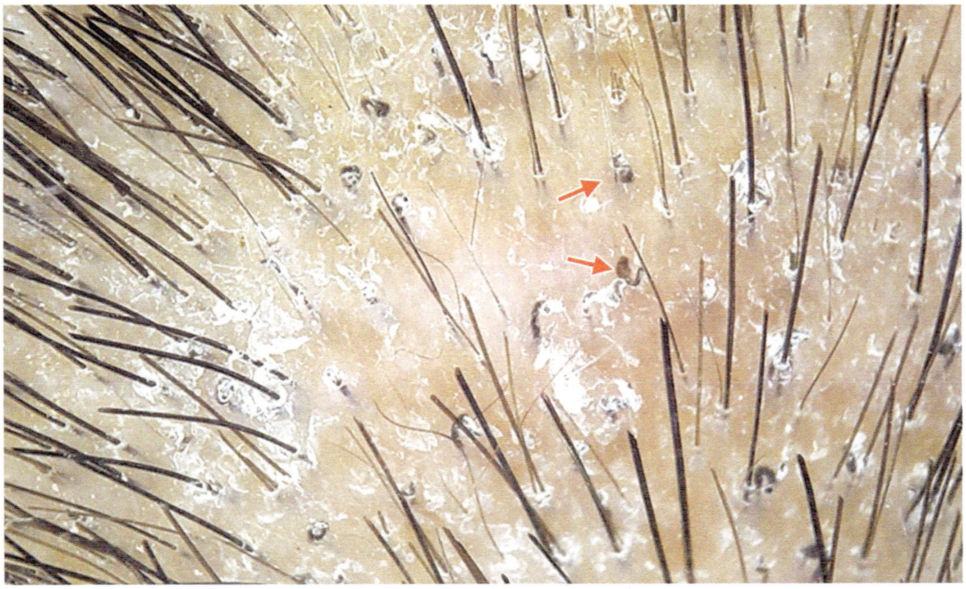

Fig. 22: Corkscrew hairs (red arrows): A child with tinea capitis and hairs curled into corkscrew shape was described by Huges et al.[14]

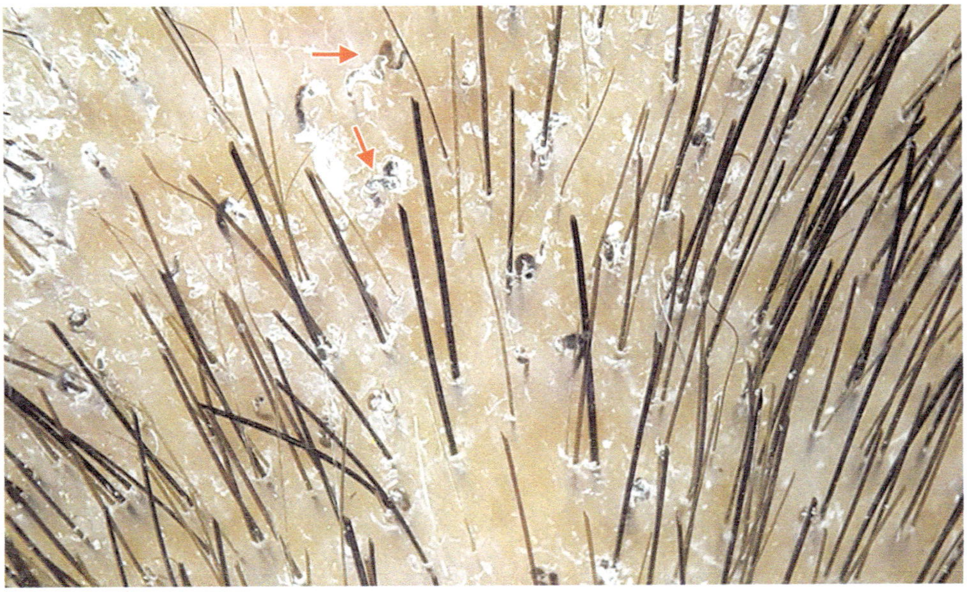

Fig. 23: Corkscrew hairs (red arrows) are short broken hairs with spiral shape.

COUDABILITY HAIR

- Coudability hairs are long hair with proximal hair shaft tapering.[15]
- Coudability hairs are trichoscopic marker of disease activity.[15]
- When coudability hair is pushed inwards toward the scalp, the proximal hair shaft tends to bend—this is called "coudability sign."[16]
- *Mechanism of formation of coudability hair*: (a) Rapid transition from anagen to catagen—it results in hair shaft narrowing. (b) These hairs may be the result of less severe injury to the hair follicle which then continue into an anagen, but a dystrophic anagen follicle and produce hair shaft narrowing.[16]

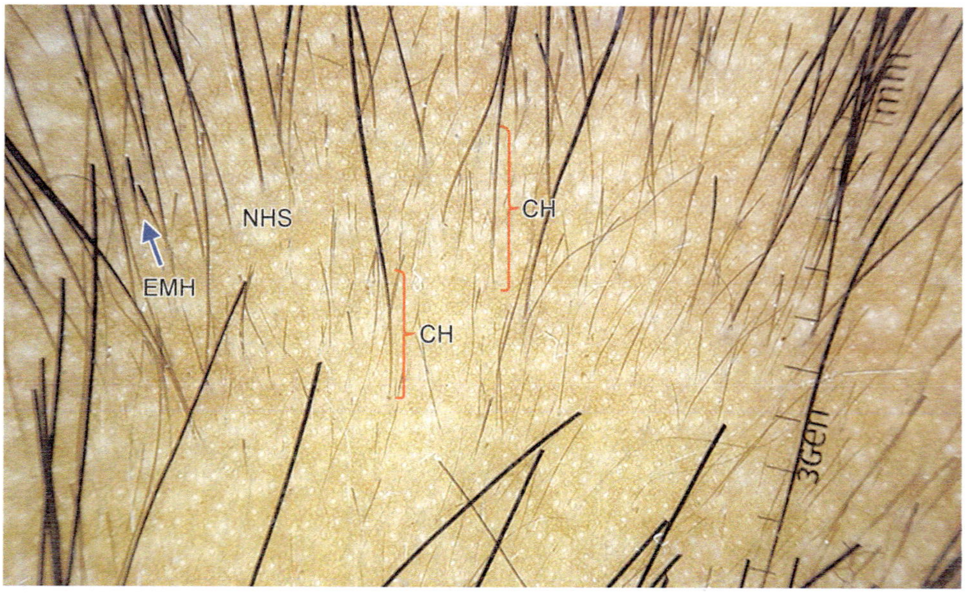

Fig. 24: Coudability hair (CH). Note the narrowing of the proximal hair shaft (red bracket) of long hairs. Try to appreciate and compare CH with the normal hair shaft (NHS) which is uniform in color and thickness all throughout its length. Numerous exclamation mark hairs can also be observed in this field.

DARK LINES[17]

- The follicular end of the hair is difficult to determine. Sometimes, the distinction between proximal and distal ends is impossible.
- These hairs are regrowing hairs and are thin, short and pigmented.

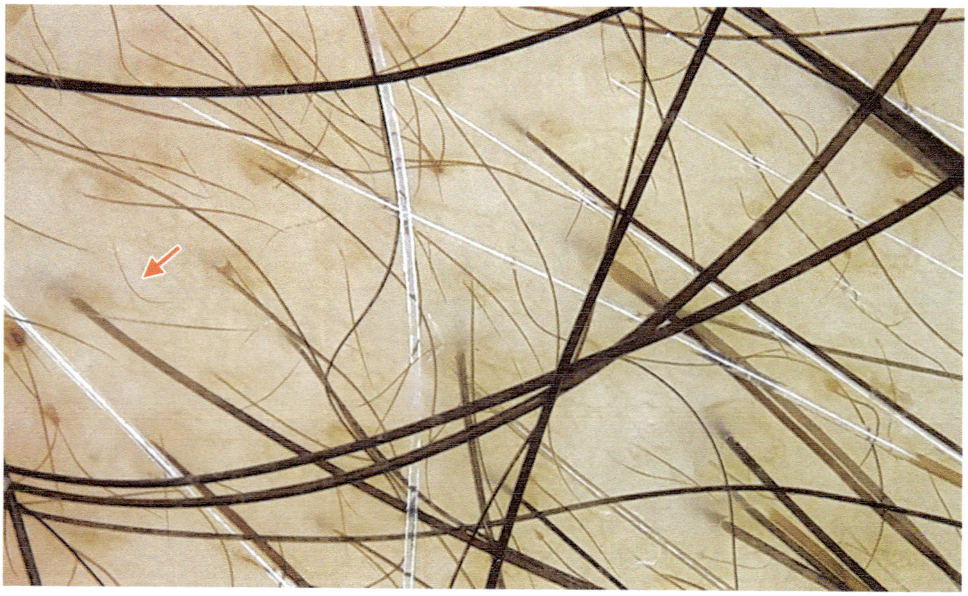

Fig. 25: Dark line (red arrow) in alopecia areata (AA) incognito.

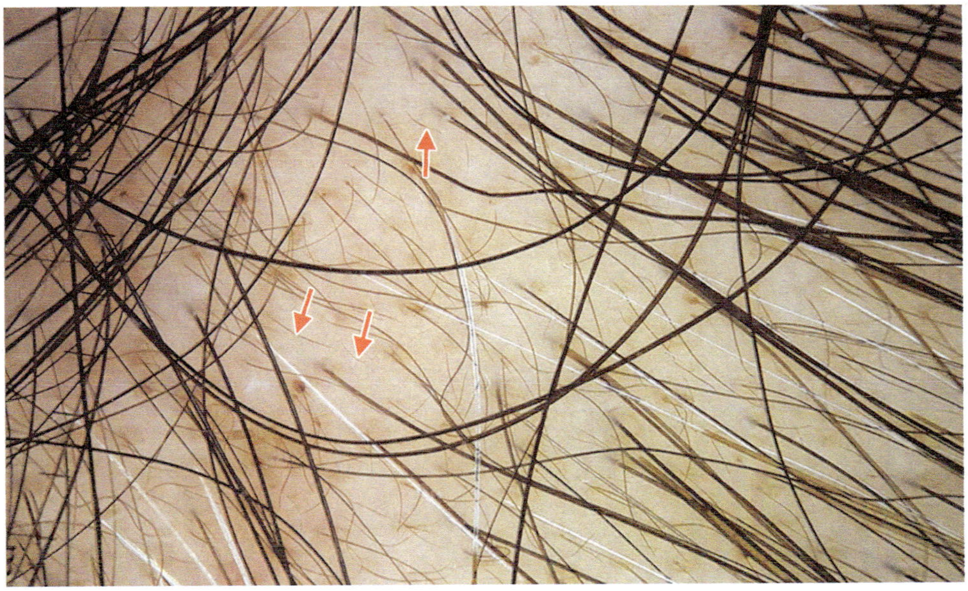

Fig. 26: Dark lines (red arrows) in alopecia areata incognito.

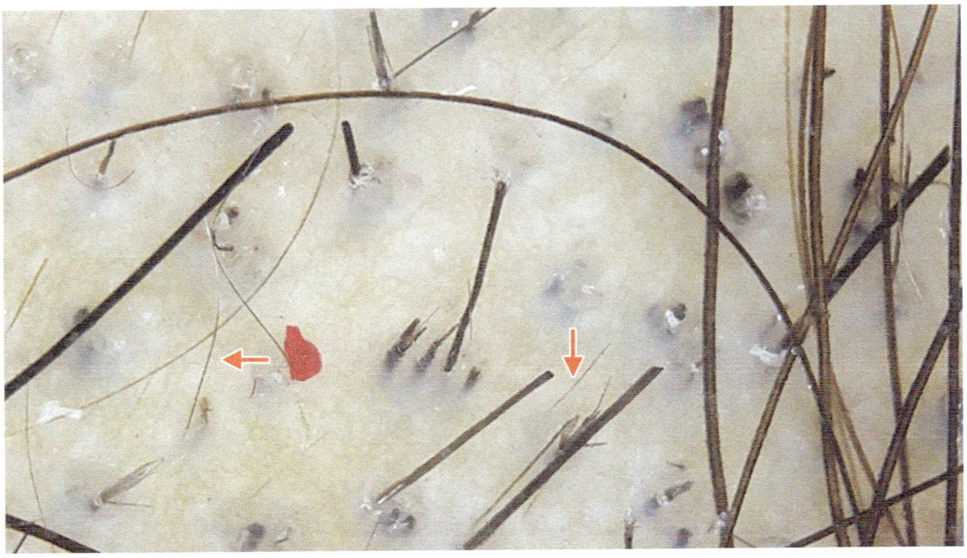

Fig. 27: Dark line (red arrows) in trichotillomania (TTM).

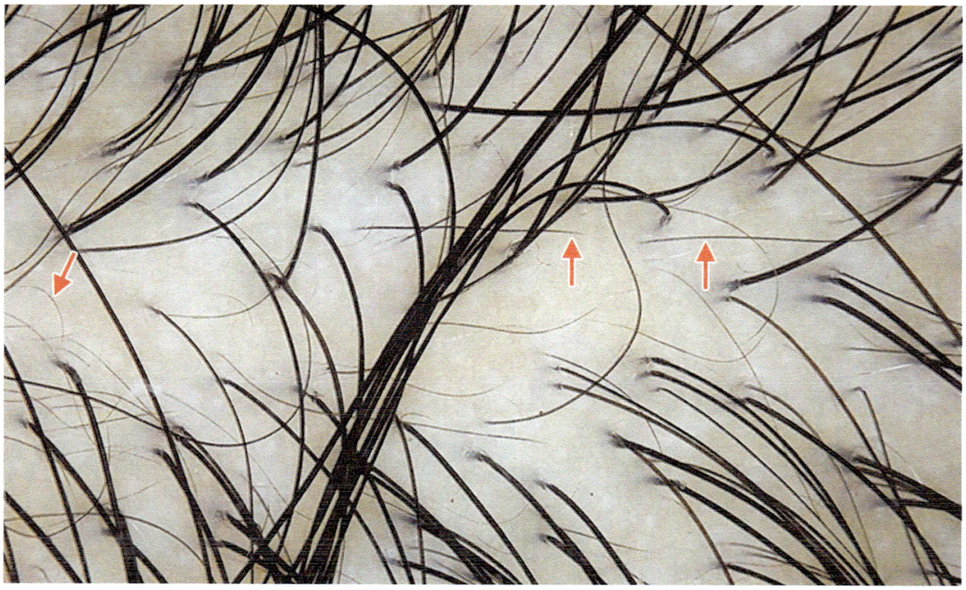

Fig. 28: Dark lines (red arrows) in acute telogen effluvium (TE).

DIRTY DOTS

Appear as brown or black tiny dots irregularly distributed on the scalp. Usually observed in the children, these particles are derived from the environment. Dirty dots are commonly found in children after playing outdoor games.[18] It can also be seen in manual laborers.

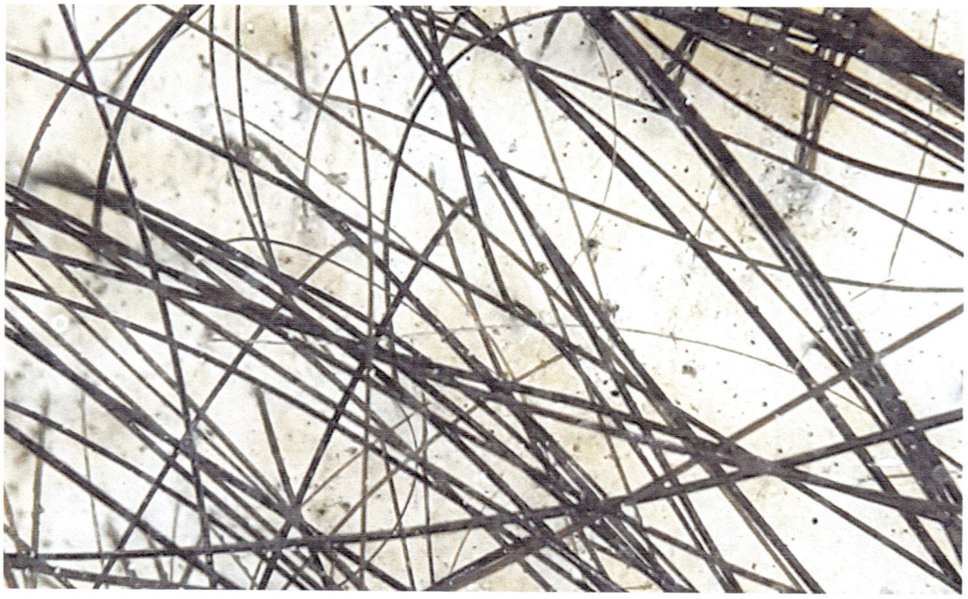

Fig. 29: Dirty dots.

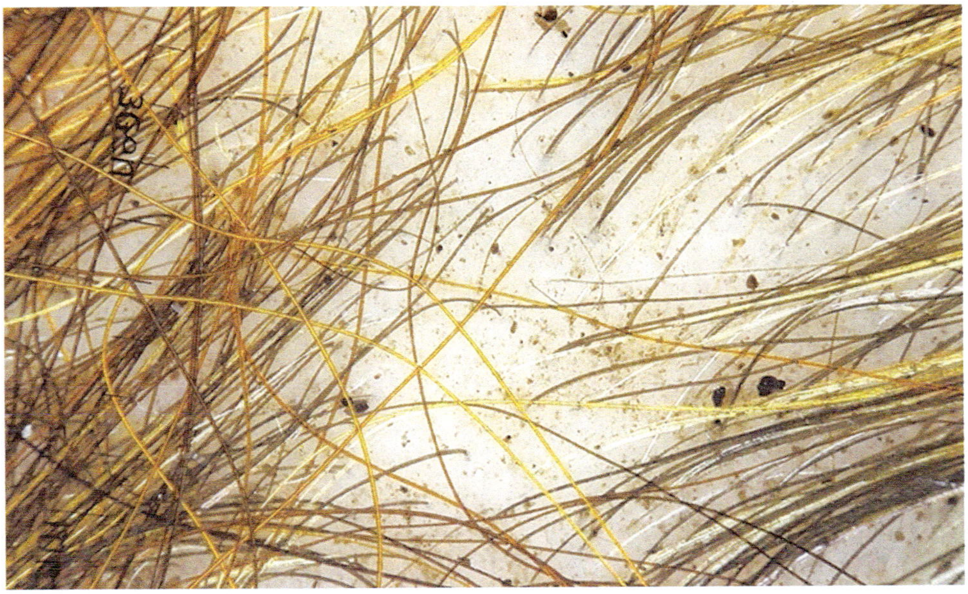

Fig. 30: Dirty dots appear as black or brown particles on the scalp are distributed in an irregular fashion.

EMPTY FOLLICLES

- They are seen as hair follicles without hairs.
- These blank follicles are found in androgenetic alopecia (AGA) and telogen effluvium and sometimes on healthy scalp.

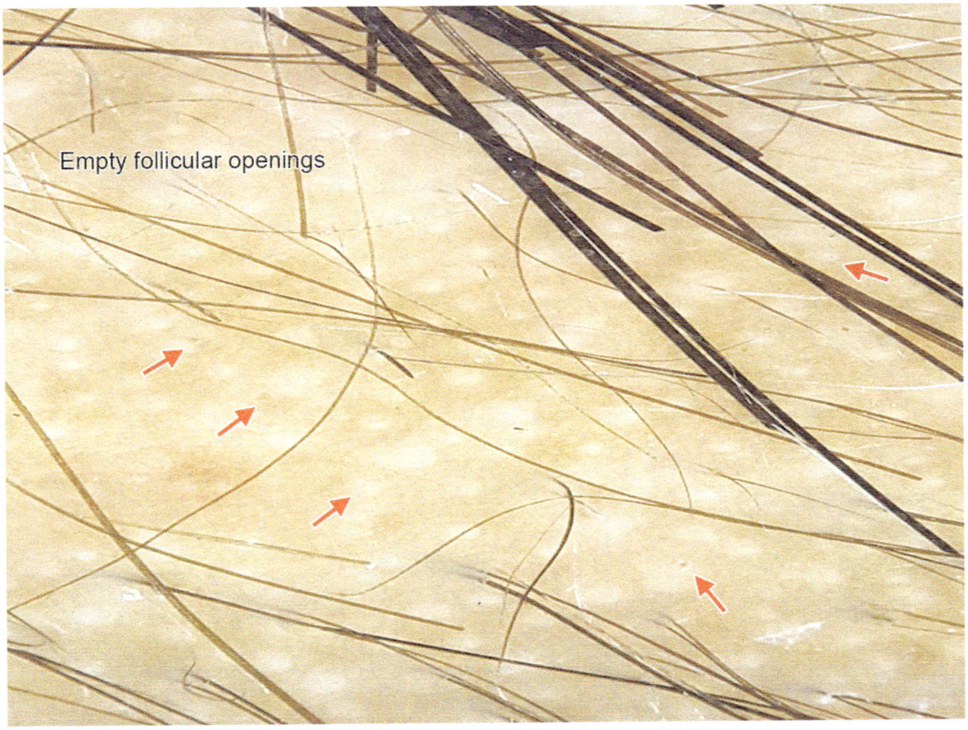

Fig. 31: Empty hair follicles (red arrows) are usually filled with keratosebaceous material.

EXCLAMATION MARK HAIRS

- Exclamation mark hairs present a frayed thicker tip. These are exclusively seen in AA, mainly along the edges.[19]
- It is mainly manifested due to the rapid transition from anagen to catagen, which results in hair shaft narrowing.[20]

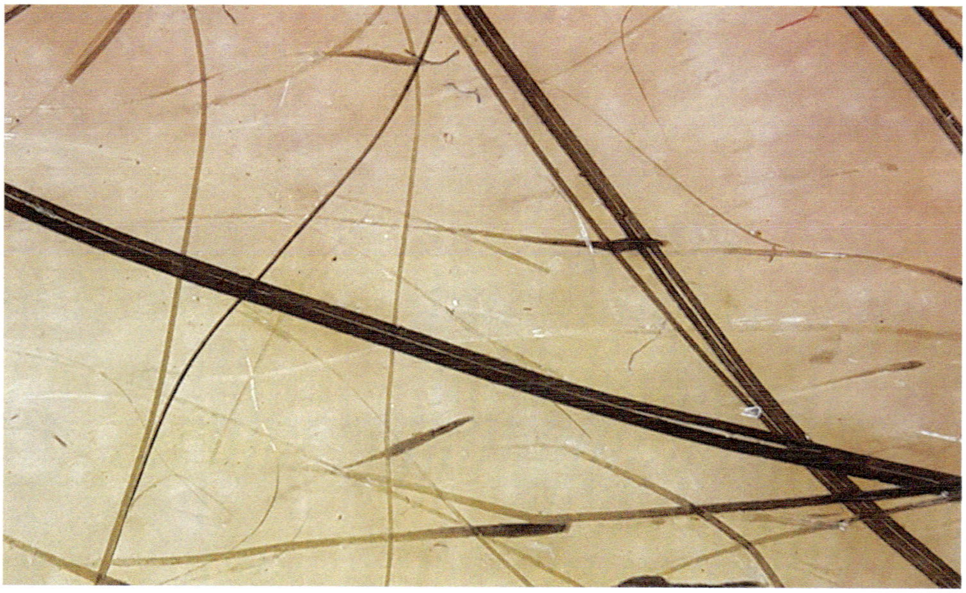

Fig. 32: Exclamation mark hairs: Tapered hairs with dark ends. Exclusively seen in alopecia areata (AA), mostly along the border of the patches.

FLAME HAIRS

- These are described as cone shaped, semitransparent, and wavy.
- This results from severe mechanical trauma due to hair pulling and because of their characteristic shape, these hairs are called flame hairs.
- Flame hairs are highly suggestive of TTM.
- There may be some variations of flame hairs such as they may appear thicker, more intensely pigmented, the flame may have two tongues or may be longer in size.[21]

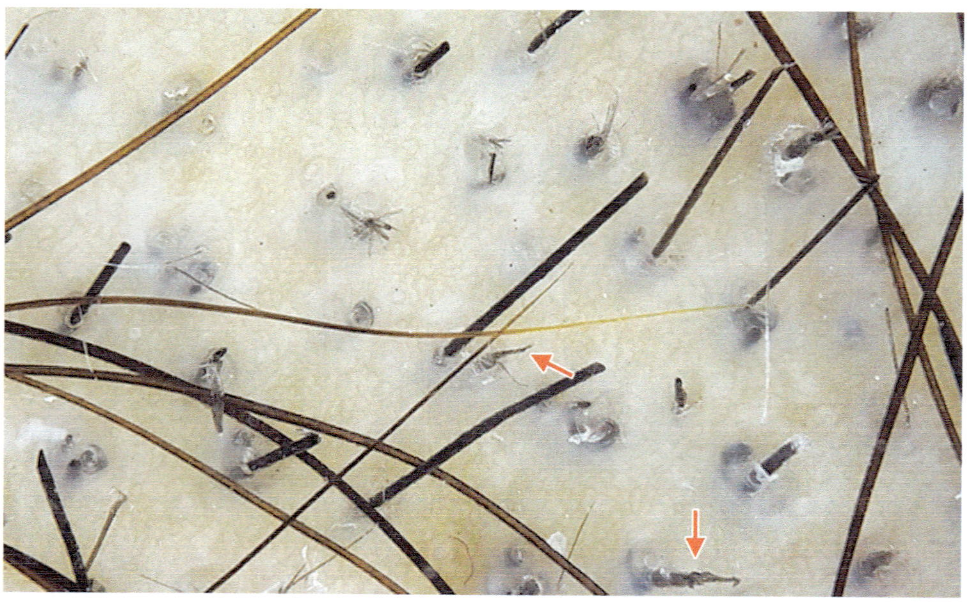

Fig. 33: Flame hairs (red arrows).

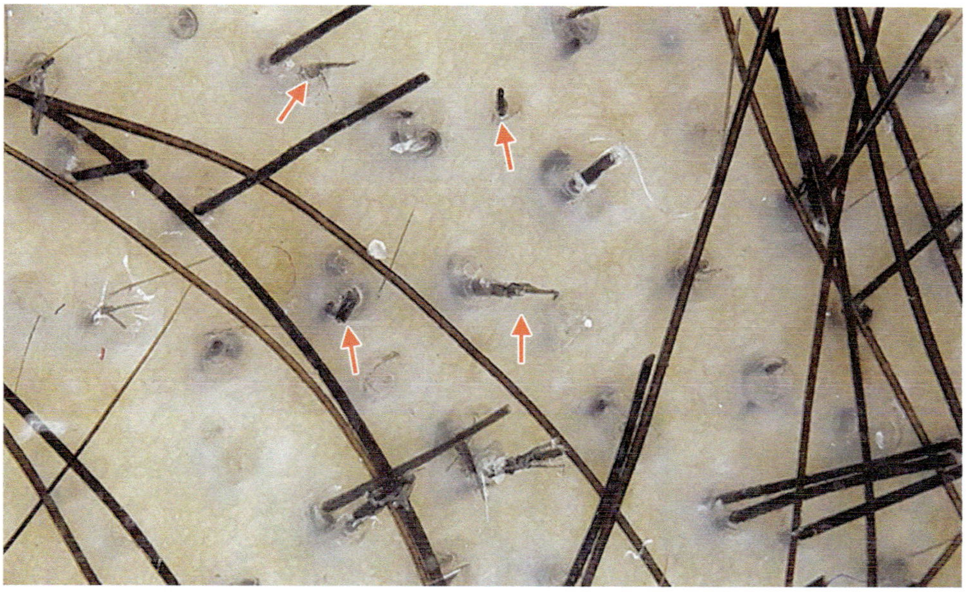

Fig. 34: Flame hair variations (red arrows).

HAIR TUFTS

- It is a group of several hairs (>5) emerging from one dilated follicular opening
- It may be seen in tufted folliculitis, folliculitis decalvans, LLP, DLE, central centrifugal cicatricial alopecia (CCCA), and acne keloidalis nuchae.[22]

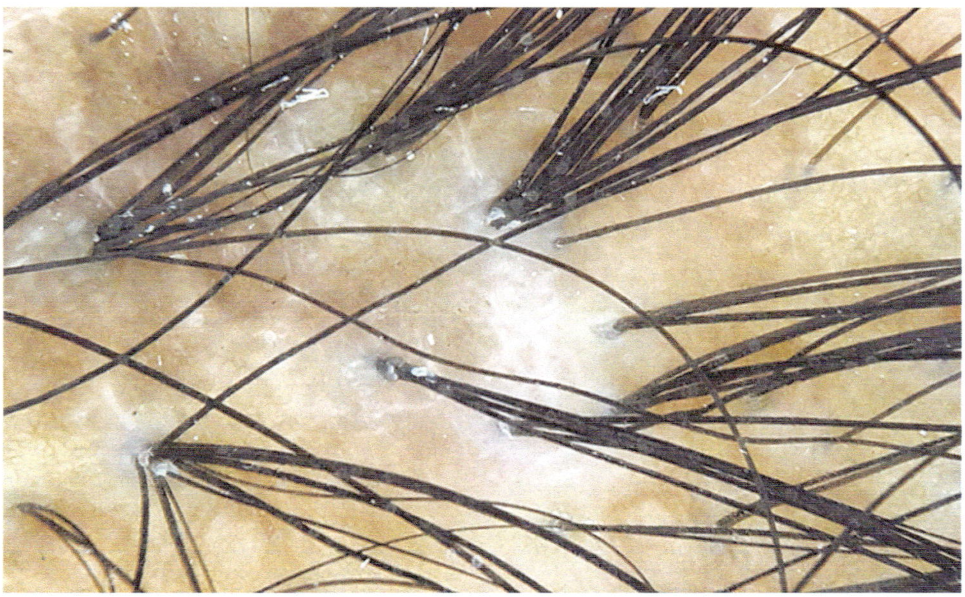

Fig. 35: Tufts may be small and is seen in lichen planopilaris (LPP) and tinea capitis, where it consists of five to seven hairs. When the tufts consist of more than eight to nine hairs, they are called large tufts and is observed in folliculitis decalvans.

HONEYCOMB PIGMENT

- Honeycomb pigmented network consists of homogeneous mosaic of contiguous brownish rings. It resembles pigmented network of melanocytes over skin on dermoscopy.
- The hyperchromic areas of this network correspond to rete ridge melanocytes whereas hypochromic areas correlate with suprapapillary epidermal melanocytes.
- This pattern is found in normal scalp, nonscarring alopecia, and scarring alopecia, except DLE.[23]

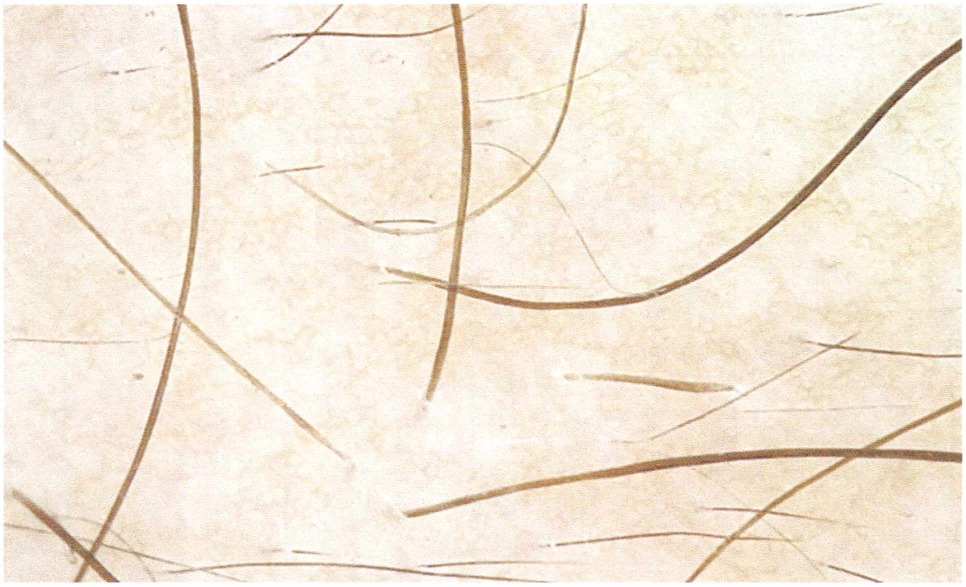

Fig. 36: Honeycomb pigment pattern.

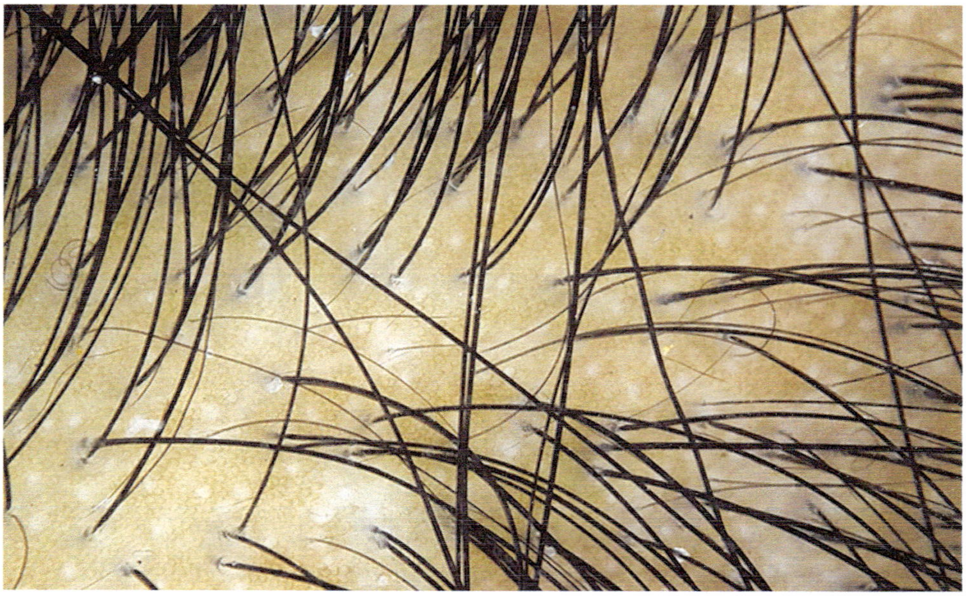

Fig. 37: Honeycomb pigmentation.

i-HAIR[24]

- i-hairs are described as short broken hairs with accentuated distal end forming the letter "i".
- If there is no distal accentuation, the same hair may be referred to as block hair.
- It may be seen in conditions with broken hair like trichotillomania and tinea capitis.

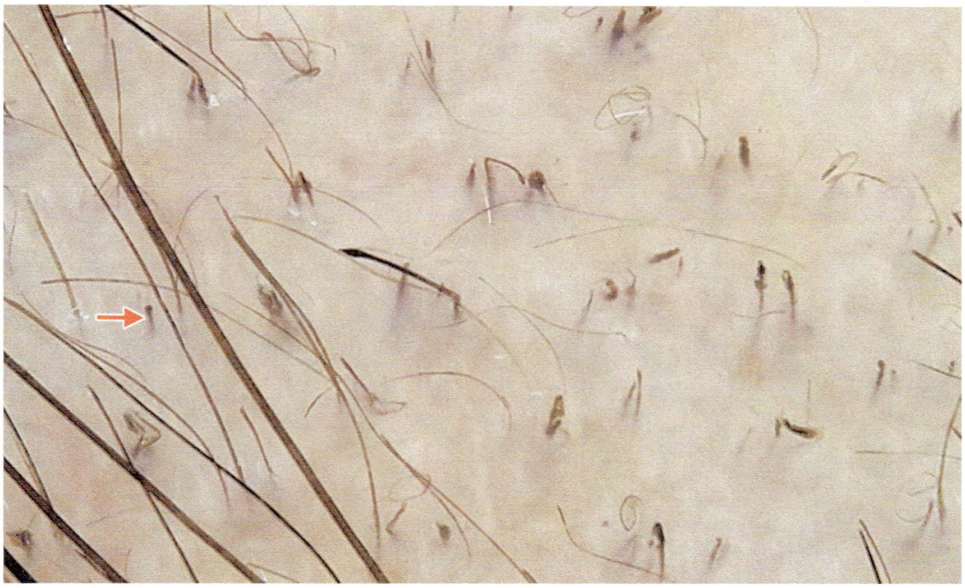

Fig. 38: i-hair (red arrow).

KERATOTIC PLUGS[25]

- Classically, they are found in DLE.
- Trichoscopically, they are seen as keratotic masses plugging follicular ostia. It varies in color and size and protrude from the scalp.
- Histologically, keratotic plugs correspond to keratin material occluding the dilated infundibular ostia.
- Isolated keratotic plug is observed in dissecting cellulitis.[26]

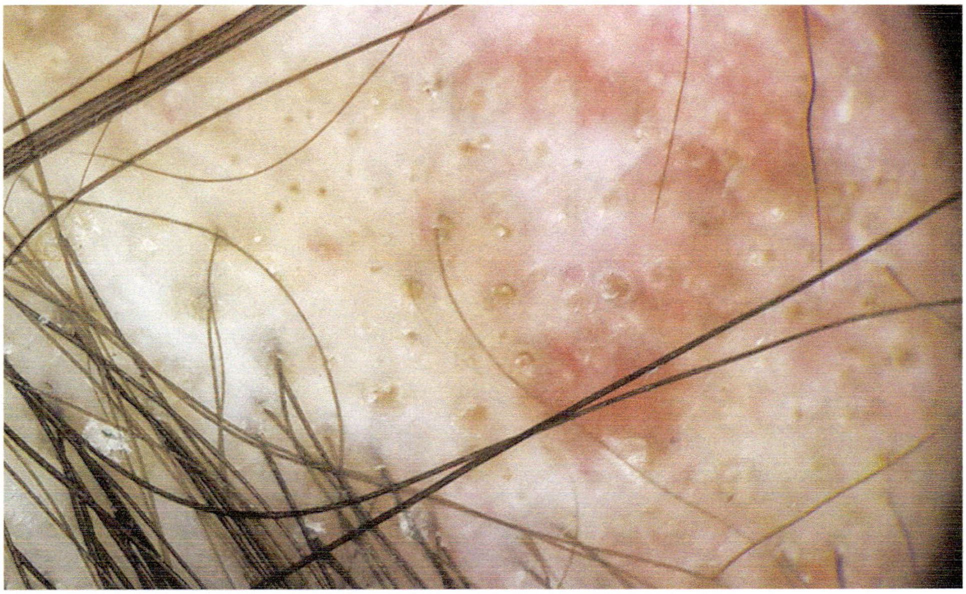

Fig. 39: Keratotic plugs in a case of discoid lupus erythematosus (DLE).

MONILETHRIX-LIKE PHENOMENON

- Monilethrix-like phenomenon occurs due to hair shaft thinning due to active stage of the disease followed by thickening during remission.
- This occurs in hair disorders with variable course such as AA, LPP, or in patients undergoing chemotherapy. This condition may be created artificially after using hair styling gels.[27]
- This differs from monilethrix in that monilethrix-like hairs have uneven length of the nodes which are arranged irregularly; whereas monilethrix hairs show regular nodes arranged in a regular fashion.[28]

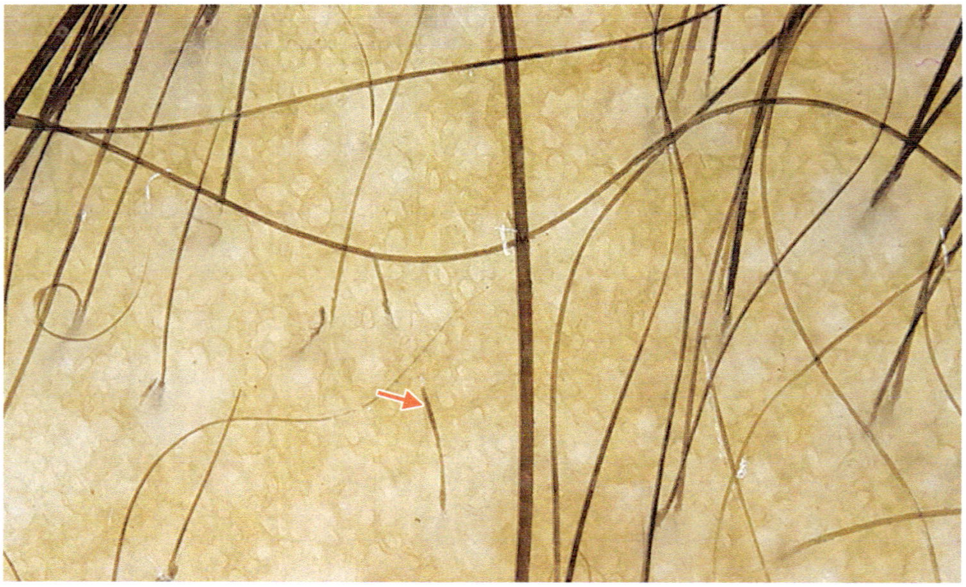

Fig. 40: Monilethrix-like hairs (red arrow).

MORSE-CODE HAIR (FOR THE TRICHOSCOPIC PICTURE REF. TO CH 25)

- These can also be called as interrupted hair. It is seen in tinea capitis.[29]
- On dry trichoscopy, they are observed as transparent transverse bands or gaps present at regular intervals along the hair shaft.
- It should be differentiated from trichorrhexis nodosa, which have white transverse bands.[29]

PERIPILAR SIGN[30]

- It is seen as a brown depressed halo of approximately 1 mm diameter at the follicular emergence. It correlates with perifollicular inflammation.
- Inui et al. hypothesized peripilar sign in Asians as a result of postinflammatory peripilar pigmentation.
- This sign is observed in 20–66% of patients.
- This is commonly found in patients with early androgenetic alopecia.
- Keradog et al. indicated that peripilar sign is specific for AGA. Less than 5% of hair follicle openings with brown peripilar discoloration are observed in healthy scalp.
- Extensive peripilar sign is a poor prognostic factor for AGA.

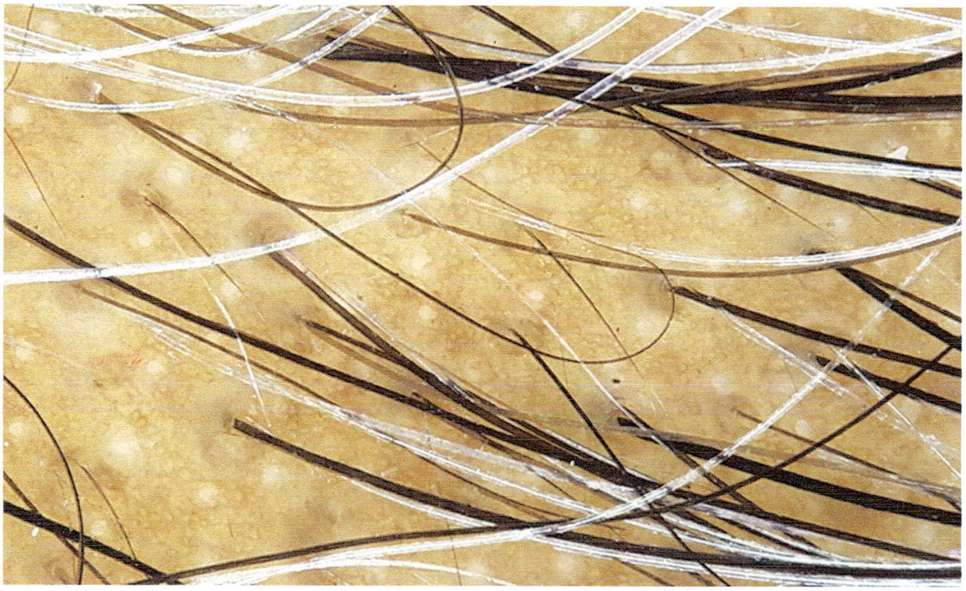

Fig. 41: Peripilar sign.

PIGTAIL HAIRS

- They are regrowing hairs and are seen trichoscopically as short hairs with tapered and coiled ends resembling pigtail.
- Short regrowing hairs and pigtail hairs are basically same, except their appearance. The end of short regrowing hairs are straight and do not resemble pigtail.
- Pigtail hairs should be differentiated from coiled hairs. Pigtail hairs are also coiled but they are uniform in thickness and color and regular in shape.[11]

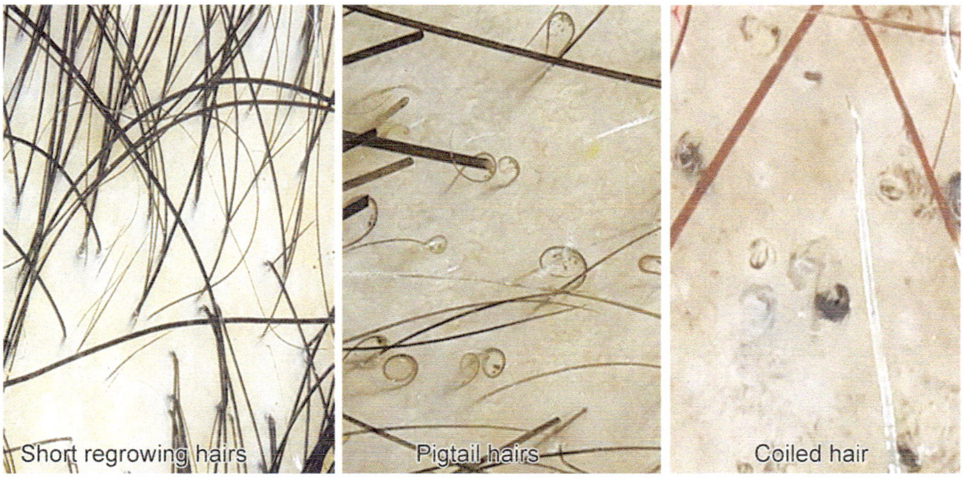

Fig. 42: Difference among pigtail, short regrowing, and coiled hairs.

PINPOINT WHITE DOTS

- There are two types of white dots.
- The pinpoint white dots are visible on pigmented skin and present as small regular white dots, sometimes with a rim of hyperpigmentation which corresponds to the acrosyringial portion of the eccrine sweat glands or empty hair follicles.[31,32]
- The other type is the fibrotic white dots which represent fibrosis as a result of selective follicular destruction as seen in LPP and other cicatricial alopecias with primary follicular involvement.[7,33]

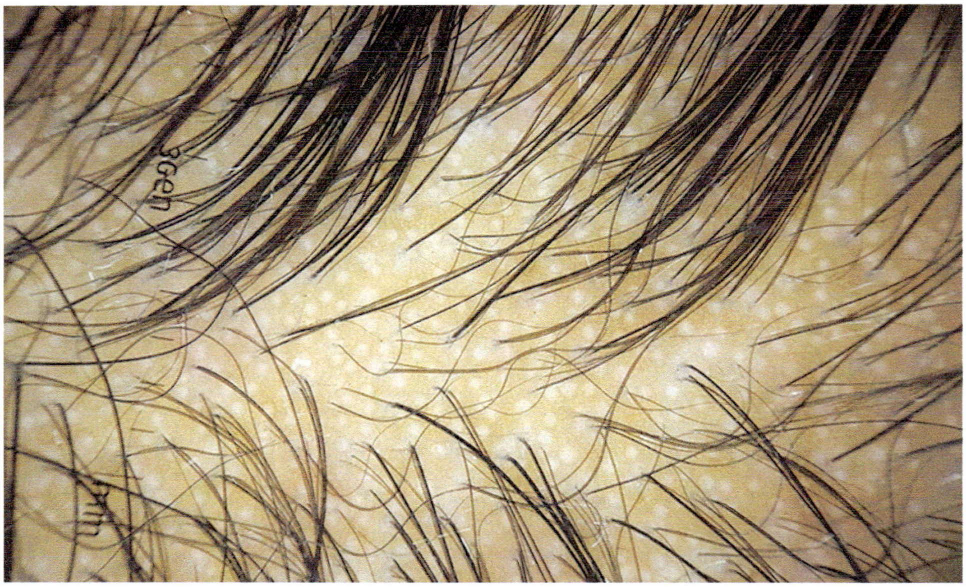

Fig. 43: Pinpoint white dots.

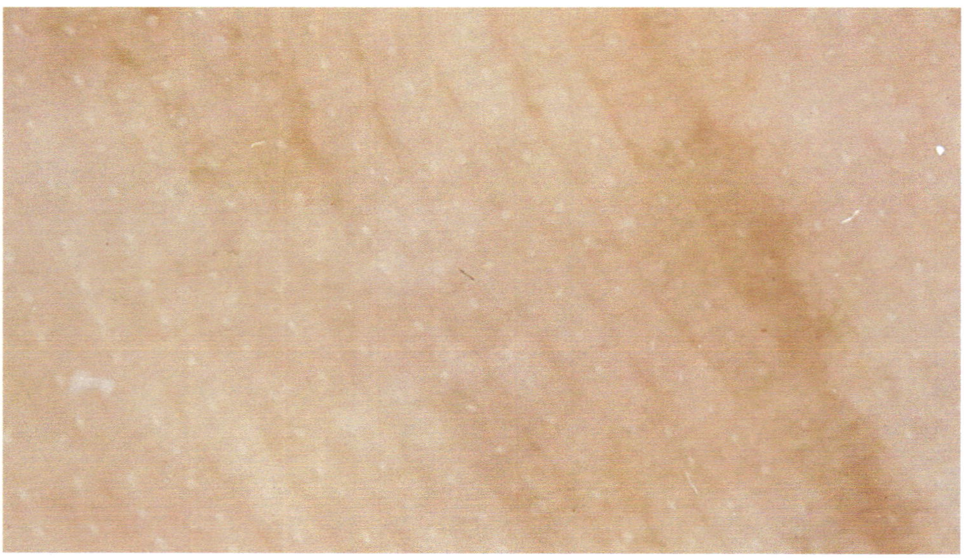

Fig. 44: Pinpoint white dots over palm due to acrosyringeal opening of eccrine glands.

POHL–PINKUS CONSTRICTIONS

- Pohl–Pinkus constrictions are irregularly placed constrictions on a hair shaft.
- These hairs with constrictions may follow one of the two fates.
- The hair shaft may regain its original stature with due course of time with only a residual constriction, which continues to be the weakest point of the shaft.
- If the ongoing pathology of the hair continues, the hair shaft becomes increasingly thinner and weaker leading to breakage, and thereby forming the black dots or broken hairs.[4,34]

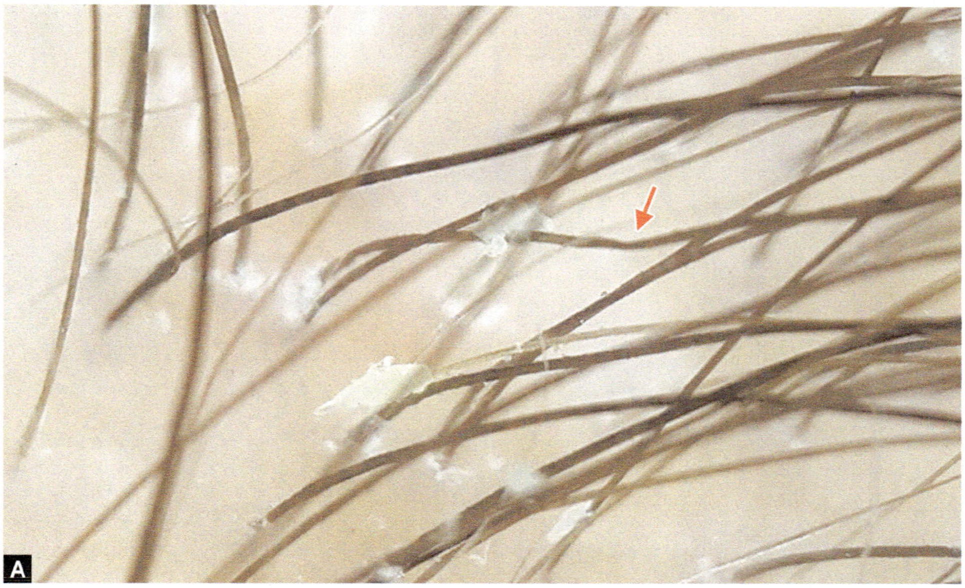

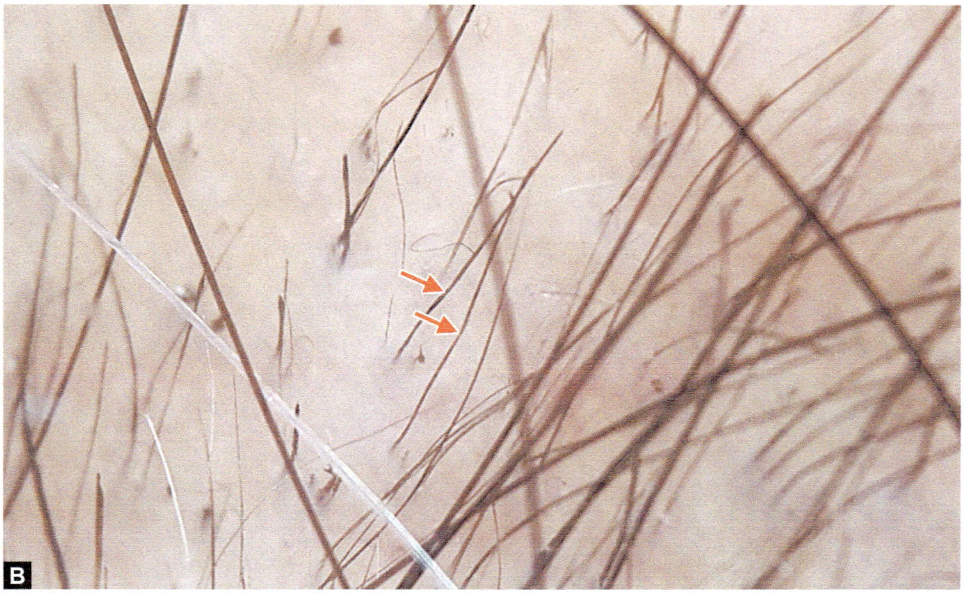

Continued

Continued

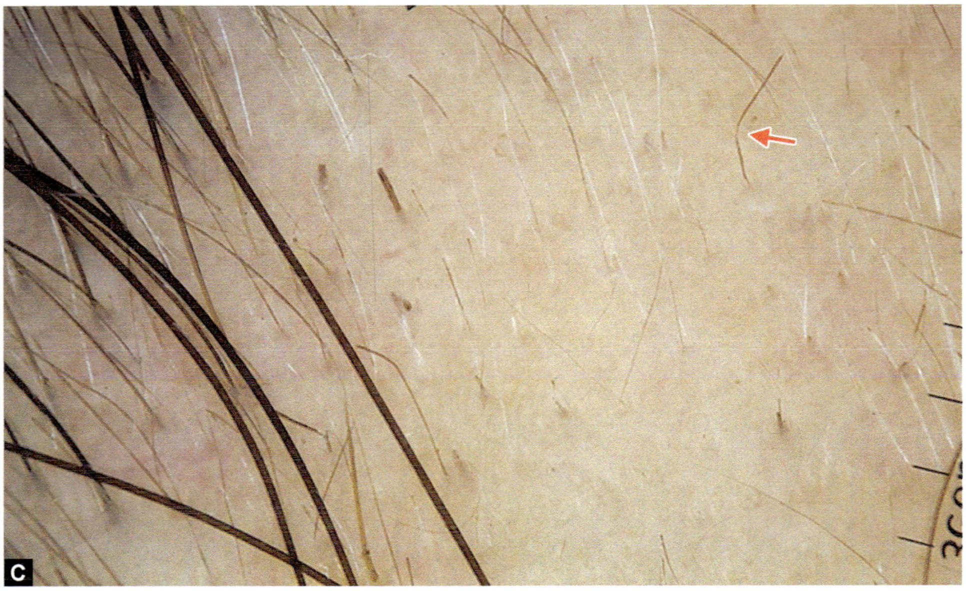

Figs. 45A to C: Pohl–Pinkus constriction (red arrows).

QUESTION MARK HAIR

- Partial coiling of the distal part of fractured hairs results in a hook-like appearance. They are also called question mark hair or hook hairs.[35]
- This appearance is highly characteristic of TTM.

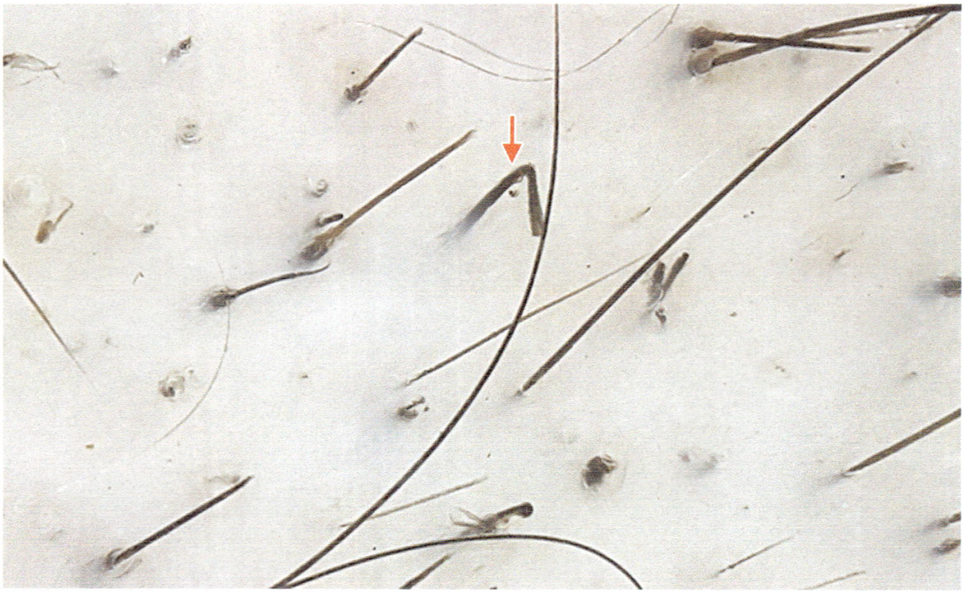

Fig. 46: Question mark hair (red arrow).

RED DOTS

- Red dots are one of the specific features of DLE. The other two specific features of DLE are keratotic plugs and enlarged branching vessels.[36]
- They correspond to dilated follicular openings surrounded by dilated vessels.
- These dots are typically seen in DLE in black, where the hypopigmented scalp is present.
- Red dots indicate early disease and so if treated promptly hair regrowth is a possibility.
- They may be seen in the glabella of patients with FFA because of involvement of eyebrows.
- These red dots are different from those in psoriasis. In DLE, it is related to follicular openings whereas in psoriasis it is due to dilated papillary capillaries in the interfollicular scalp.

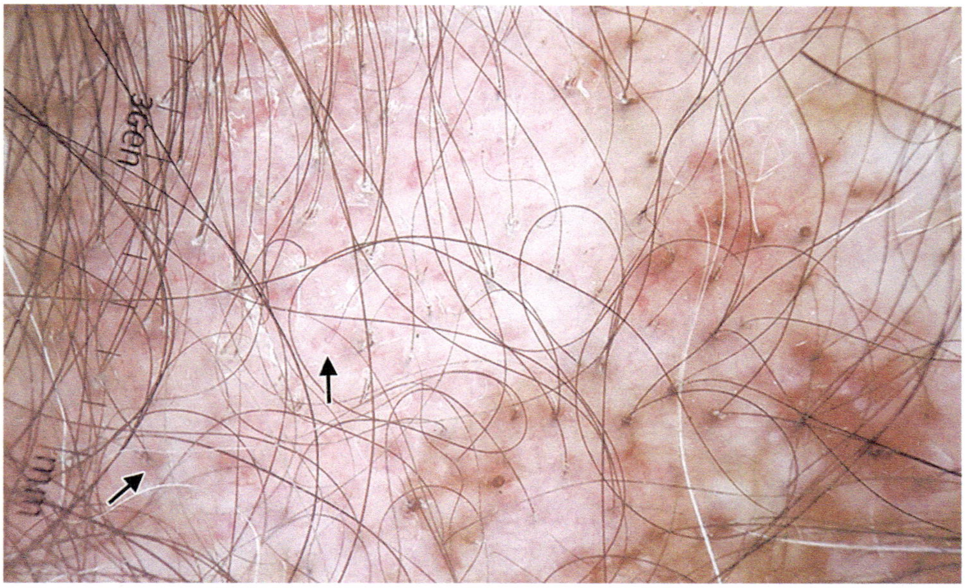

Fig. 47: Red dots (arrows).

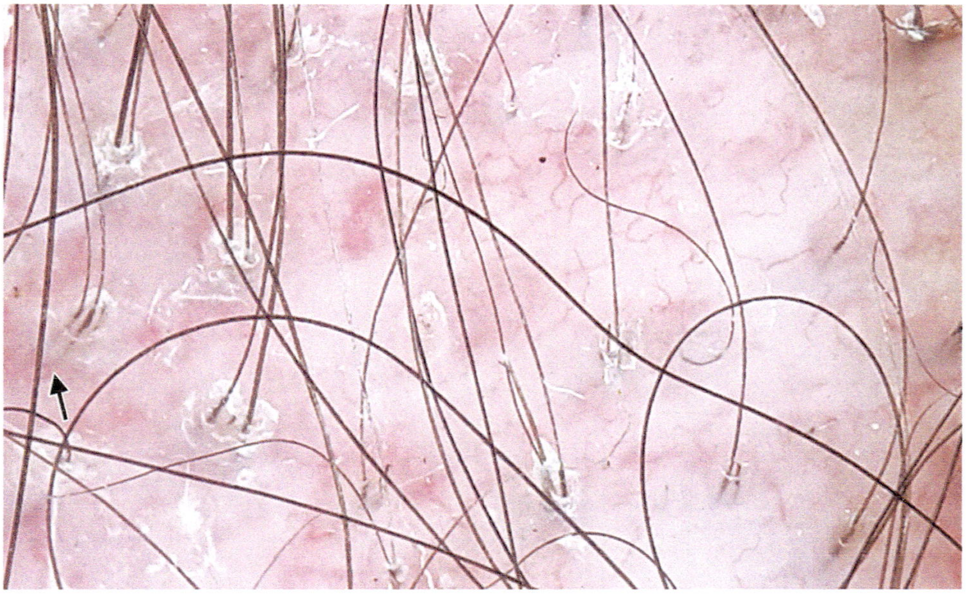

Fig. 48: Red dots (arrow) after zooming.

ROLLED HAIRS

- Rolled hairs are present as keratotic inflammatory follicular papules with twisted hairs.
- Rolled hairs are probably caused by trauma due to vigorous rubbing.[37]
- These are more common than circle hairs.
- Its association has been reported with treatment with cyclosporin and corticosteroid, keratosis pilaris, xerosis, ichthyosis, etc.[37]
- They are present over extensor of extremities, back, buttocks, and shoulder.
- It is postulated that rolled hair is the result of inability of the hair follicle to emerge through the infundibulum.
- They correspond to follicular hyperkeratosis on histology.
- On trichoscopy, rolled hairs will be seen as irregularly twisted hair in a hyperkeratotic papule.

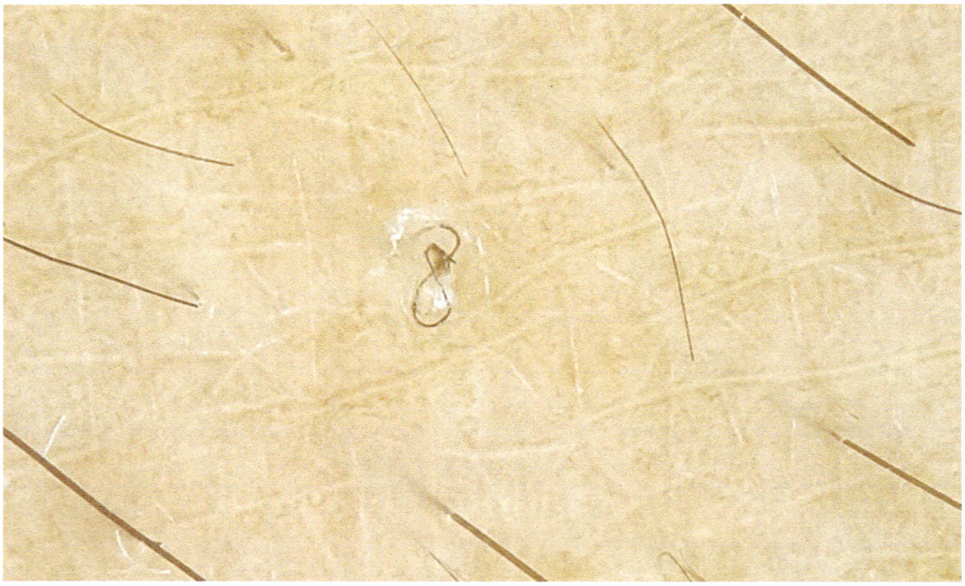

Fig. 49: Rolled hairs. Irregularly twisted subcorneal hairs on dermoscopy.[38]

SHORT REGROWING HAIRS

- They are also called upright regrowing hairs.
- They are found in the normal scalp, in the remitting phase of AA and TE.
- Thin URH are found in AGA and persisting AA.
- These regrowing hairs may have a normal thickness (>0.03 mm) or less than that.
- Upright regrowing hairs (URH: The presence of multiple URH is typical of TE and can also be found in other noncicatricial alopecias. They have tapered end and their thickness are increased continuously toward the root. They have a normal thickness of >0.03 mm or less than that.)

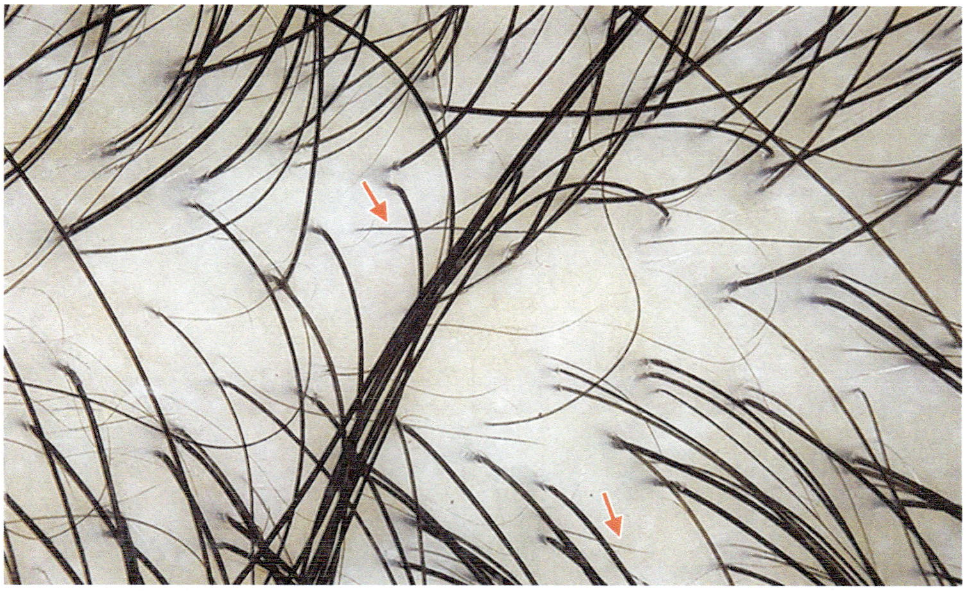

Fig. 50: Short regrowing hairs (red arrows).

STARRY SKY PATTERN

- Pinpoint white dots inside the honeycomb pigment pattern give rise to starry sky appearance.
- It is classically seen in lichen planopilaris.[39]

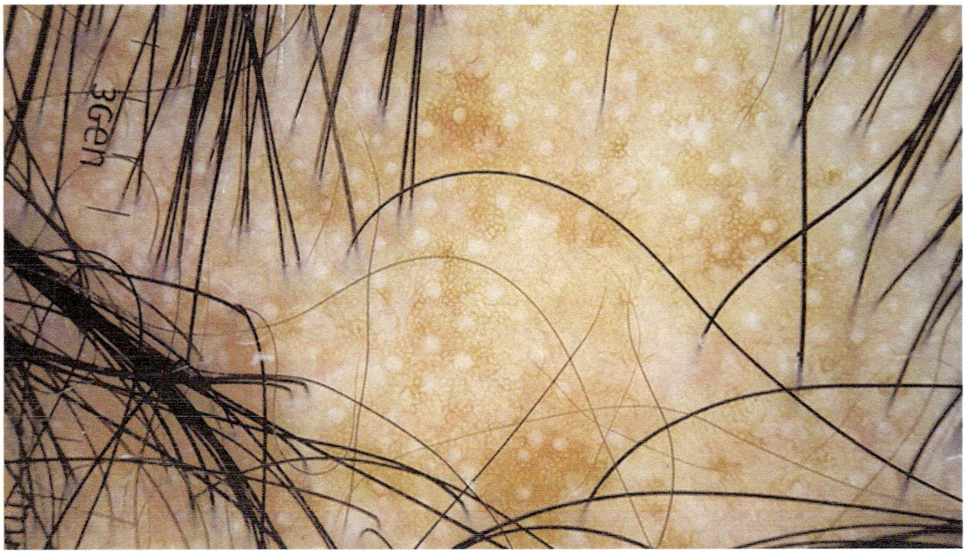

Fig. 51: Starry sky pattern in lichen planopilaris (LPP).

TADPOLE HAIR

- Tadpole hairs are defined as new regrowing hair with a bulge at the emerging point of the hair.
- It is found in alopecia areata incognito (AAI).[40]

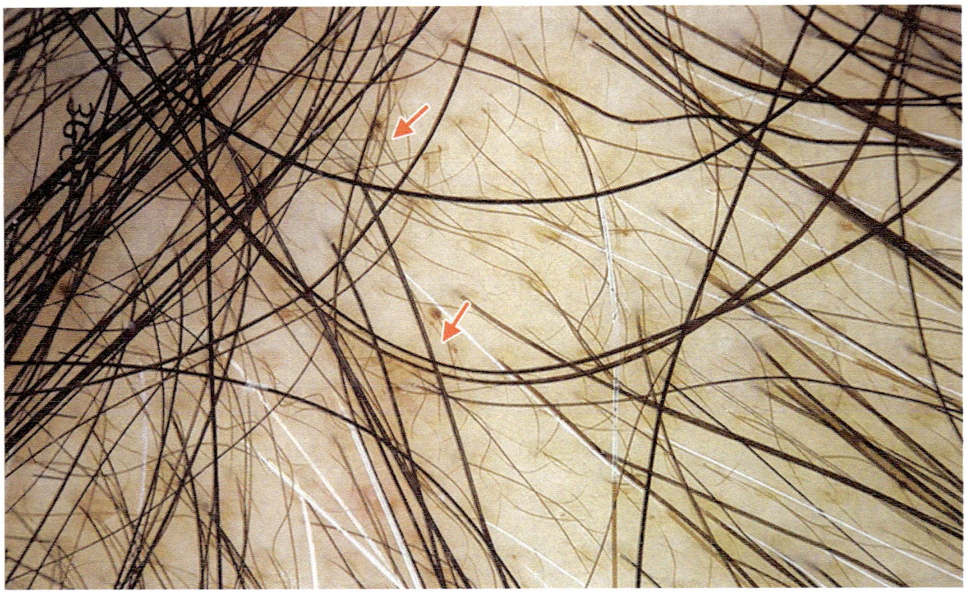

Fig. 52: Tadpole hair (red arrows).

TARGET PATTERN

- In patients with dark phototype, blue-gray dots arranged in a target pattern are characteristic of LPP.[41]
- They correspond histopathologically to melanophages in the papillary dermis and are a sign of pigmentary incontinence confined to the hair follicles.
- Blue gray dots can also be seen in DLE where they are present both perifollicularly as well as in speckled pattern.

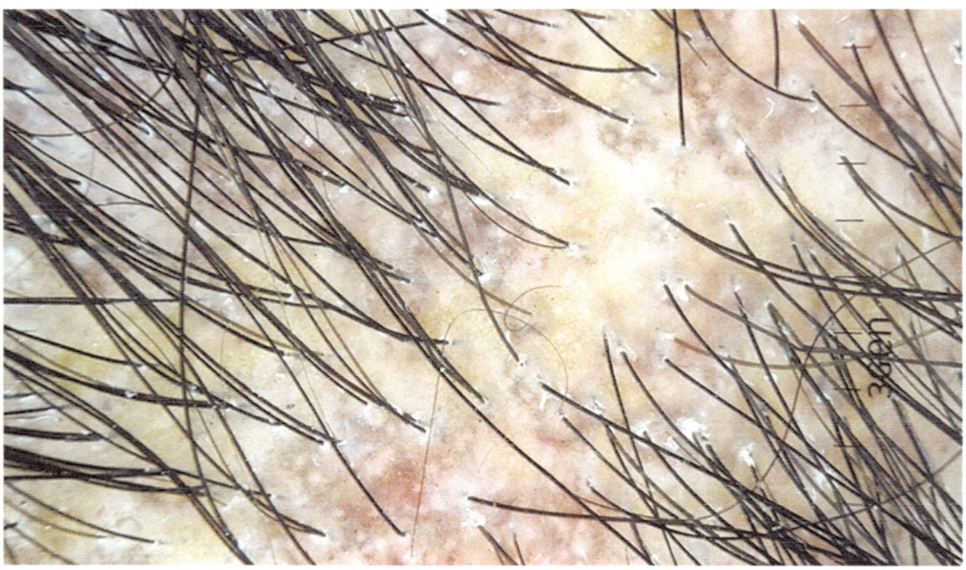

Fig. 53: Target pattern.

TRICHOCLASIS

- It is defined as a transverse fracture in the hair shaft.[42]
- Many a times, the two parts may remain attached at one point.
- It may be seen due to external trauma to the hair in the form of perming, traction combing, etc.

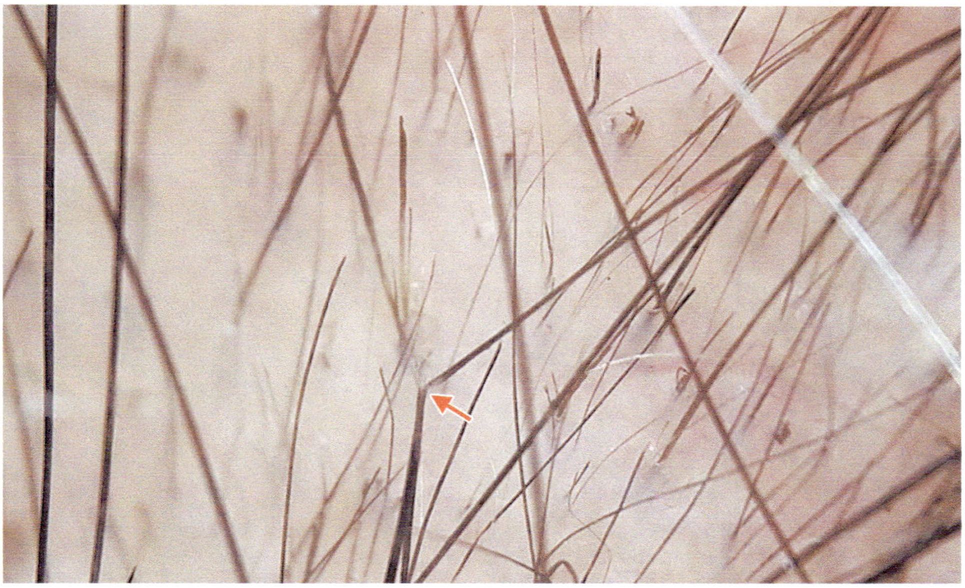

Fig. 54: Trichoclasis (red arrow).

TRICHONODOSIS

- It is defined as knotting of hair shaft in a single or double knot.
- It may occur spontaneously or due to scratching.[43]
- It is seen more commonly in dry, frizzy, and curly hair.
- It may be an incidental finding.

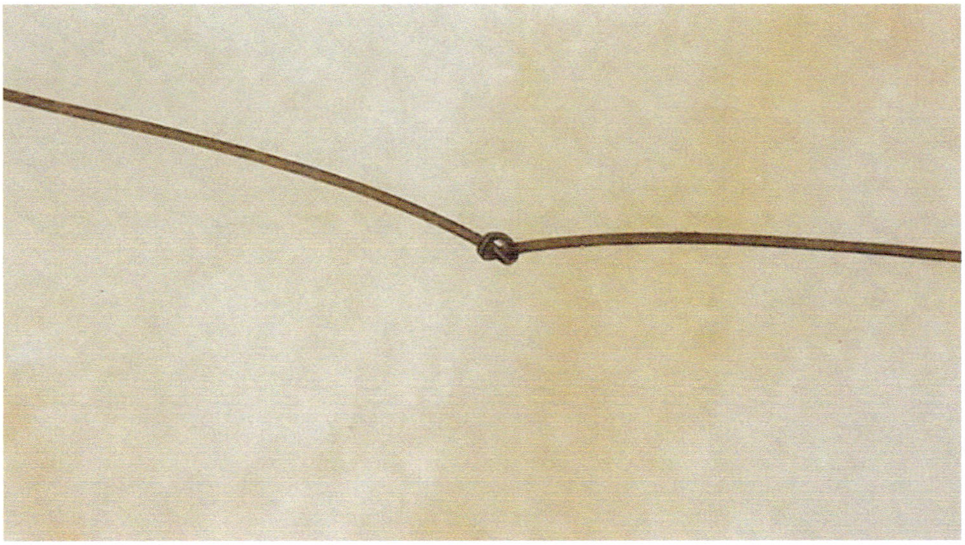

Fig. 55: Trichonodosis.

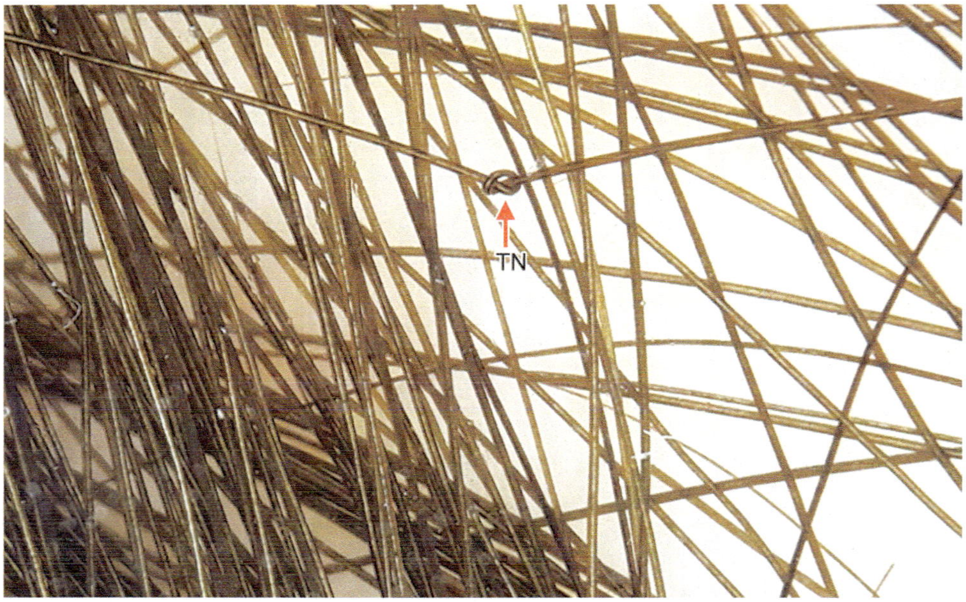

Fig. 56: Trichonodosis.

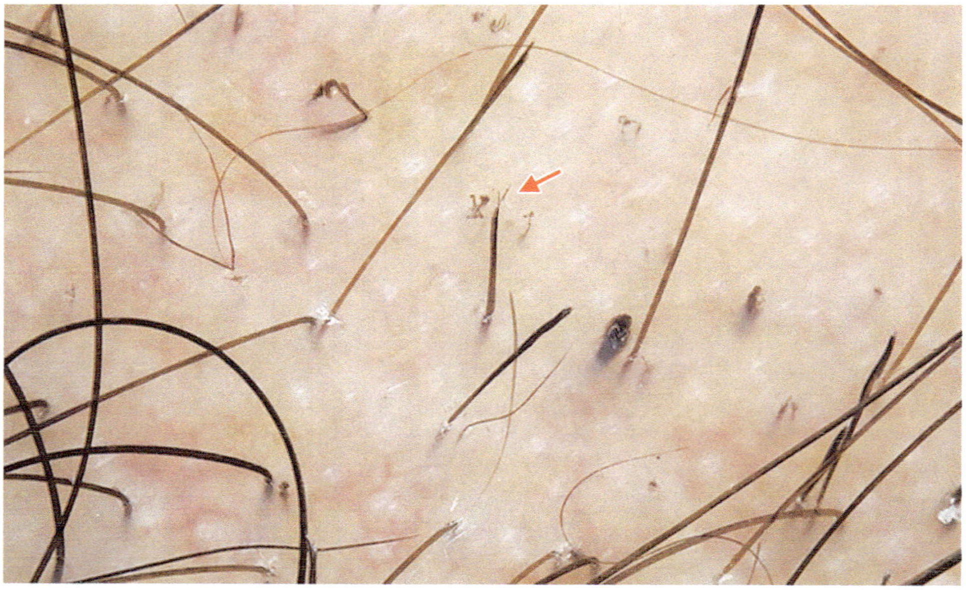

Fig. 57: Trichoptilosis (red arrow). It refers to the longitudinal splitting of the distal end of hair shaft. It is a symptom of hair shaft damage and may be seen after hair styling procedures. Not pathognomonic for any type of hair disorders and may be seen in healthy individuals.[44]

TRICHORRHEXIS NODOSA[45]

- It is a condition where hair shafts split longitudinally in numerous small fibers in localized zones.
- On zooming trichoscopically, the split hair shaft appears as two paint brushes aligned in opposition.
- Trichoscopy shows nodular thickenings along the hair shaft in low magnification.
- It is found in several inherited and acquired conditions such as ectodermal dysplasias, physical and chemical trauma, nutritional deficiencies, and as a part of syndromes.
- As an isolated finding, without any associations it may be seen in 5.6% of children.

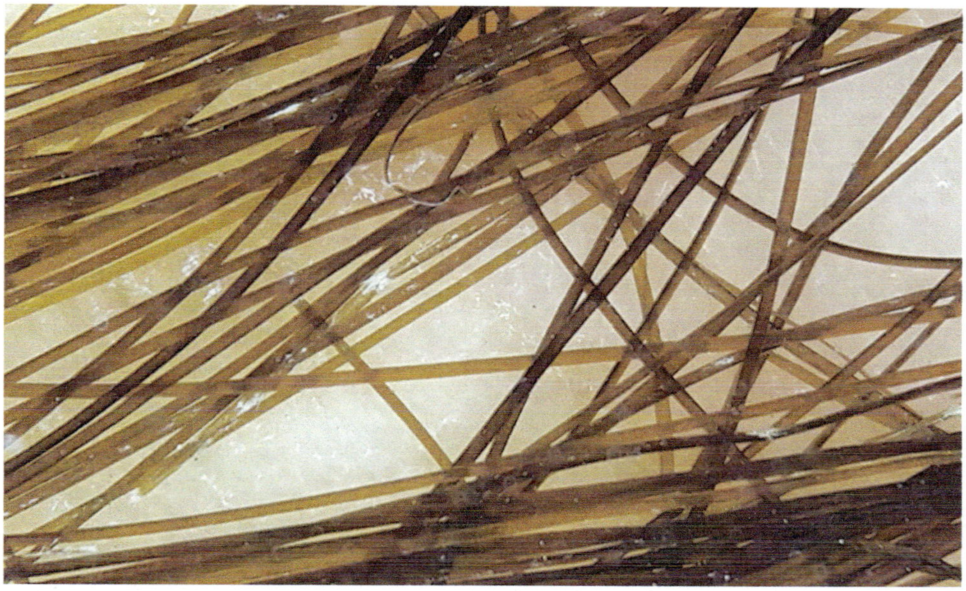

Fig. 58: Trichorrhexis nodosa.

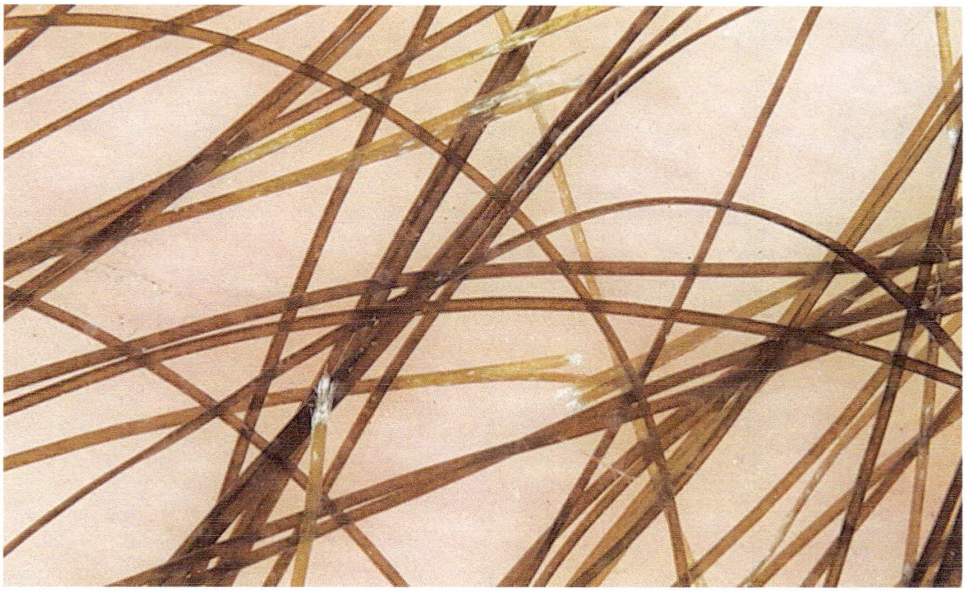

Fig. 59: Trichorrhexis nodosa (split hair shaft appears as two paint brushes aligned in opposition).

TULIP HAIRS[24]

- Tulip hairs look like tulips and appear as light-colored hair shafts with dark distal ends.
- They are regarded as broken hairs.
- These hairs are highly suggestive of TTM.
- They are also found in AA and traction alopecia.

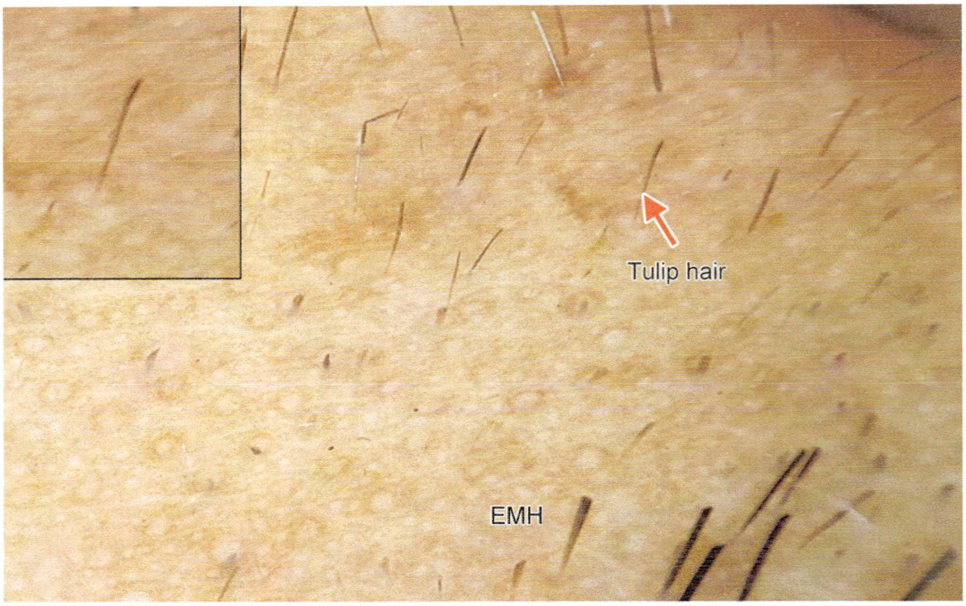

Fig. 60: Tulip hair in a case of alopecia areata. Zoomed tulip hair is shown in the inset. Note the exclamation mark hair (EMH).

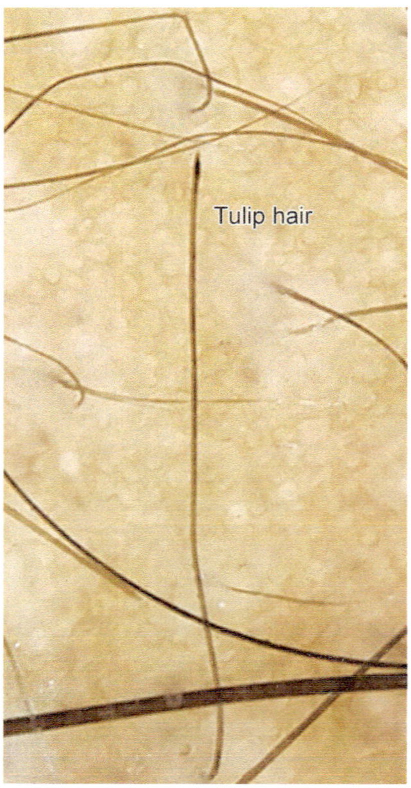

Fig. 61: Tulip hair.

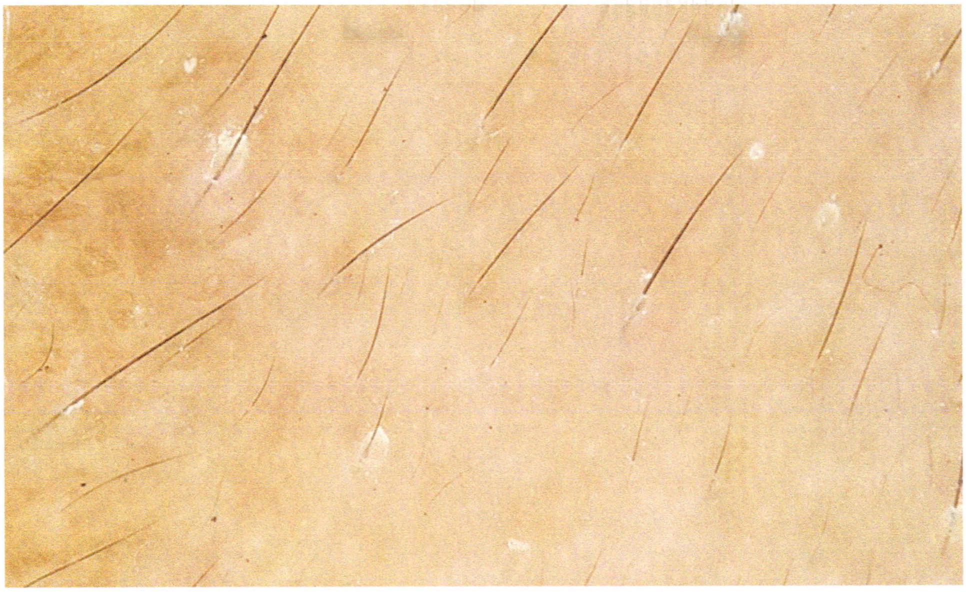

Fig. 62: Upright regrowing hairs (also called as short regrowing hair and have been discussed before).

VELLUS HAIR

- It is defined as hypopigmented, nonmedullated hairs <30 mm thick and <2–3 mm long; upto about 10% of normal scalp hair are vellus hairs.[46,47]
- During the process of hair follicle miniaturization, vellus hairs replace terminal ones. Vellus hairs are increased in male and female androgenetic alopecia.[48,49]
- Vellus hairs should be differentiated from regrowing hairs. Regrowing hairs are short and thin, not hypopigmented, they are firm and have pointed ends, whereas vellus hairs are hypopigmented and thin.

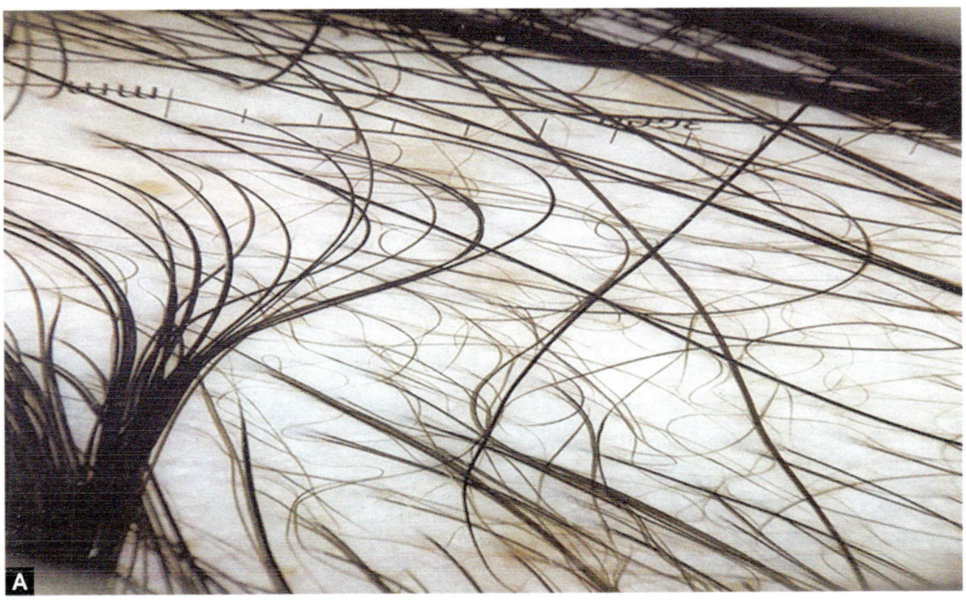

Continued

Continued

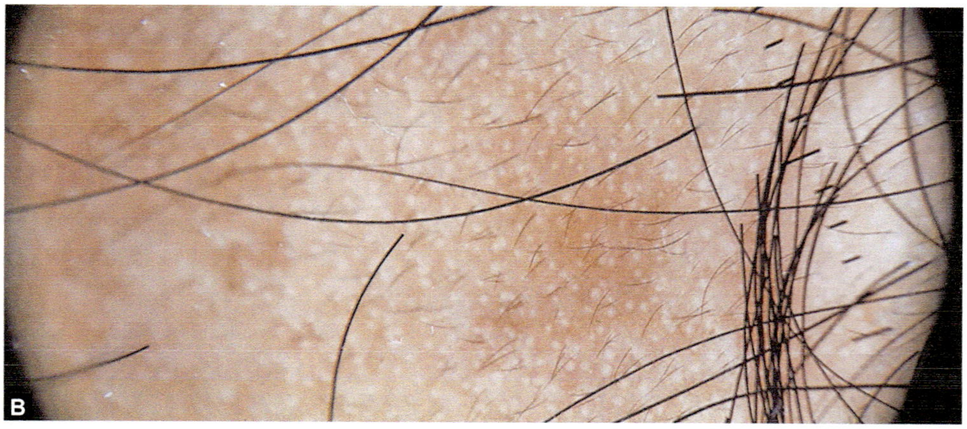

Fig. 63: Vellus hairs.

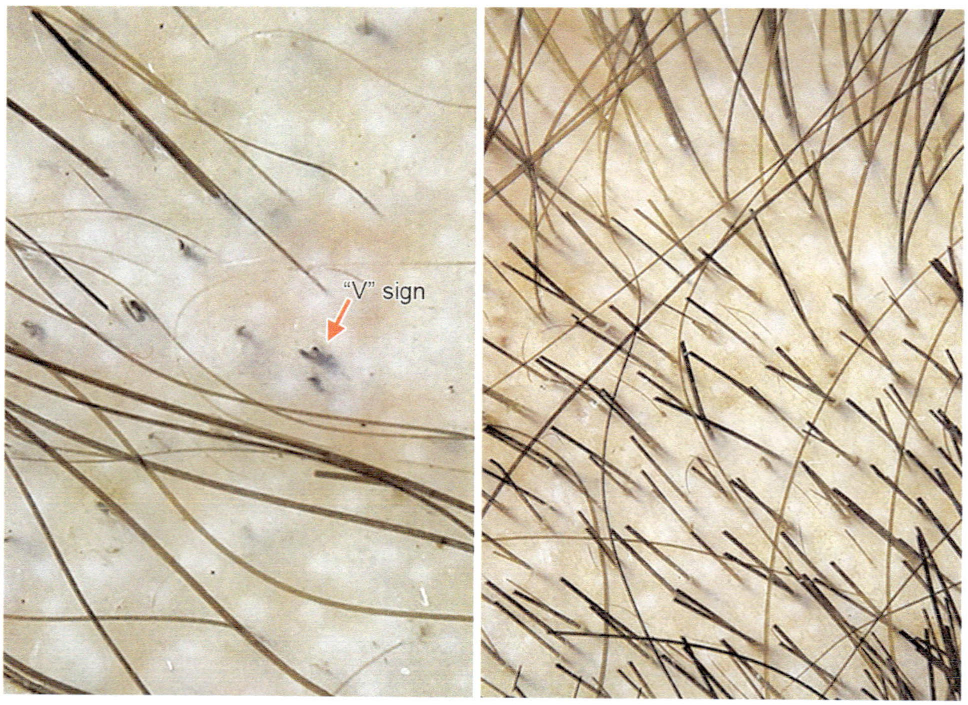

Fig. 64: "V" sign in trichotillomania (TTM). When two hairs of a follicular unit are broken at the same time it is seen as the letter ""V." It should be differentiated from "V" sign seen after regrowth of shaving hairs. In TTM, surrounding hairs are of normal length whereas "V" sign is present in all the shaving hairs.

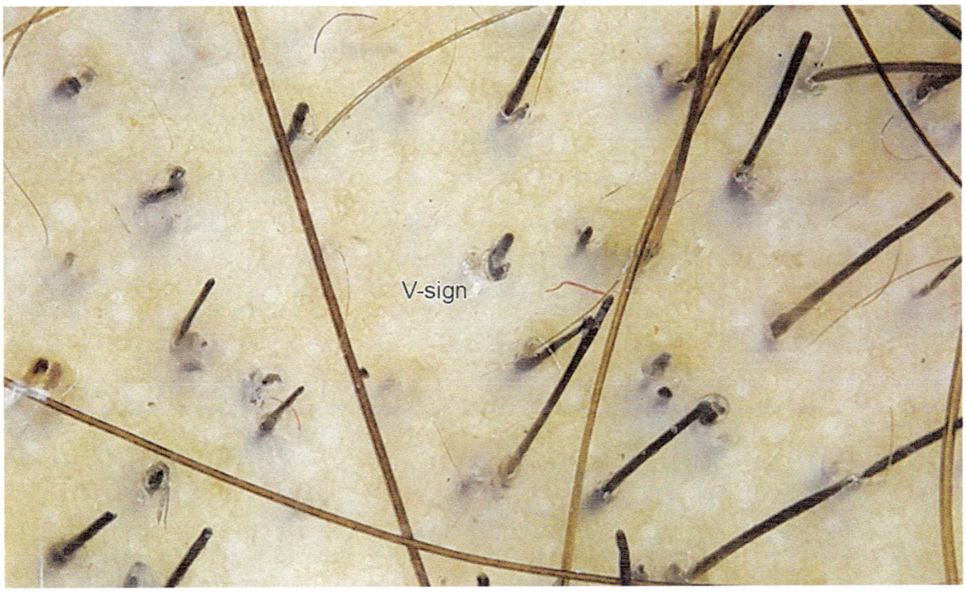

Fig. 65: V-sign. When two hairs emerge from one follicular unit and are broken at the same level above the scalp, V-sign is formed. It can be seen in trichotillomania (TTM) and traction alopecia.

WHITE-GRAY PERIPILAR HALO

- Peripilar white-gray halo around the emergence of hairs are observed in 94% of patients and is highly specific and sensitive for in all clinical stages.
- It appears as a white-grayish circle of 0.3–0.5 mm in diameter surrounding a single hair or more commonly, a group of 2–3 hairs emerging from same follicular unit.
- It was also noted surrounding the emergence of vellus or miniaturized hairs and around both pigmented and white hairs.
- It corresponds histologically to lamellar fibrosis around hair follicle.[50]

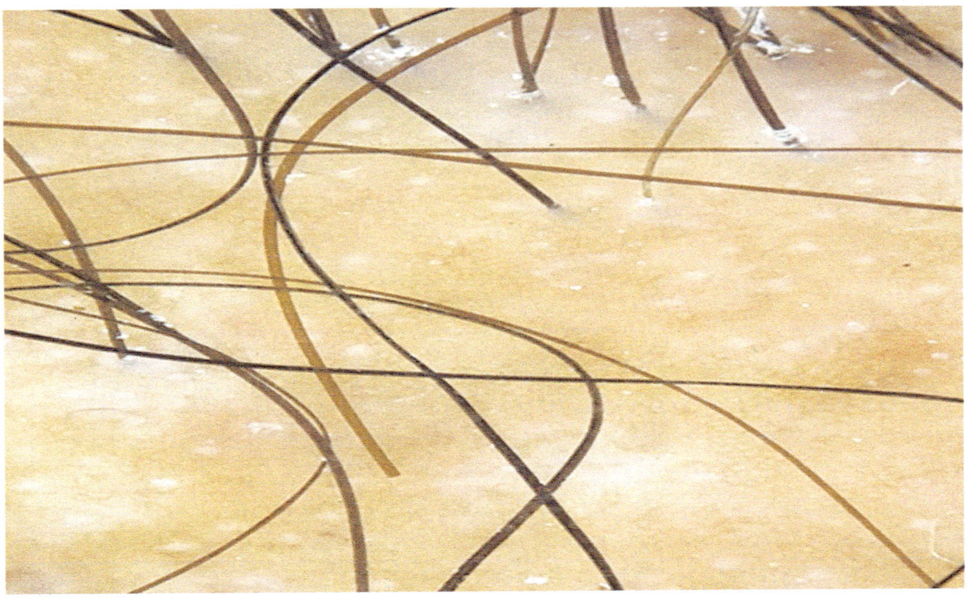

Fig. 66: White-gray peripilar halo.

WHITE PATCHES

- White dots have two variants: (a) pinpoint white dots and (b) fibrotic white dots.
- Pinpoint white dots correspond to empty hair follicles or acrosyringeal openings of eccrine ducts.
- Fibrotic white dots are observed in primary, folliculocentric cicatricial alopecia, most commonly lichen planopilaris. This is the trichoscopic finding of the longitudinal wedge-shaped tracts of fibrosis, which results from inflammatory destruction of hair follicles and perifollicular area.
- Fibrotic white dots become confluent to form white patches or white areas.

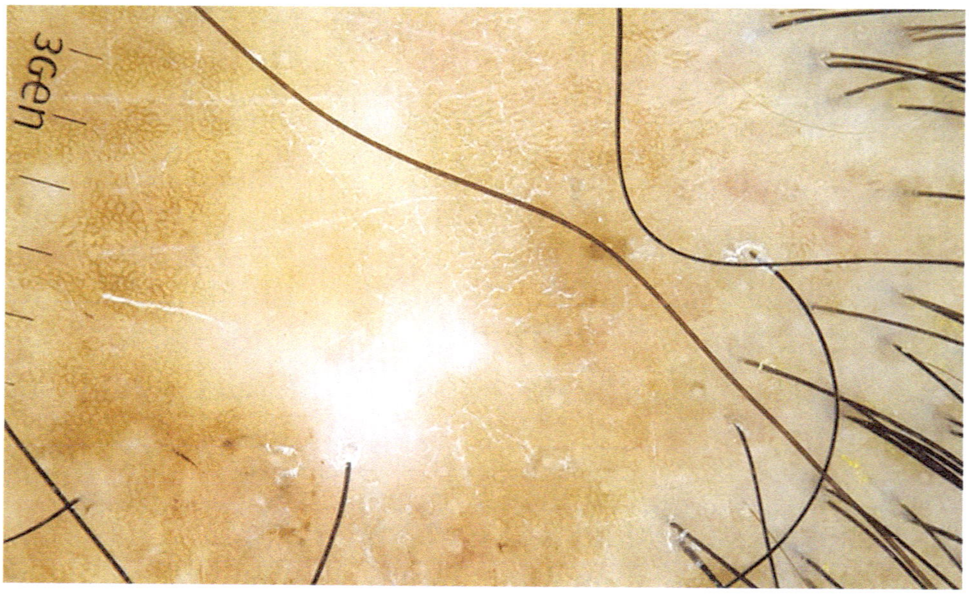

Fig. 67: White patches.

YELLOW DOTS

- Yellow dots are round yellowish dots over the scalp observed in all the magnifications.
- They can be empty, or may contain vellus hairs, or broken hairs.
- They correspond histopathologically to dilated infundibulum filled with keratosebaceous material.[7,51,52]
- They may not be visible in dark phenotypes but are easily recognized in Caucasians.
- Yellow dots are typical of AA, where they are regularly distributed and are marker of disease activity.[53]
- Large brownish-yellow dots are found in DLE which correspond to wide infundibula filled with keratotic material.[7]
- In AGA, yellow dots consist mainly of sebum and the amount of keratotic material is usually minimum.[54]
- In FPHL, yellow dots are present mainly over the frontal scalp in comparison to occipital area.[54]
- Yellow dots may also be present in AAI, TTM, and chemotherapy alopecia.

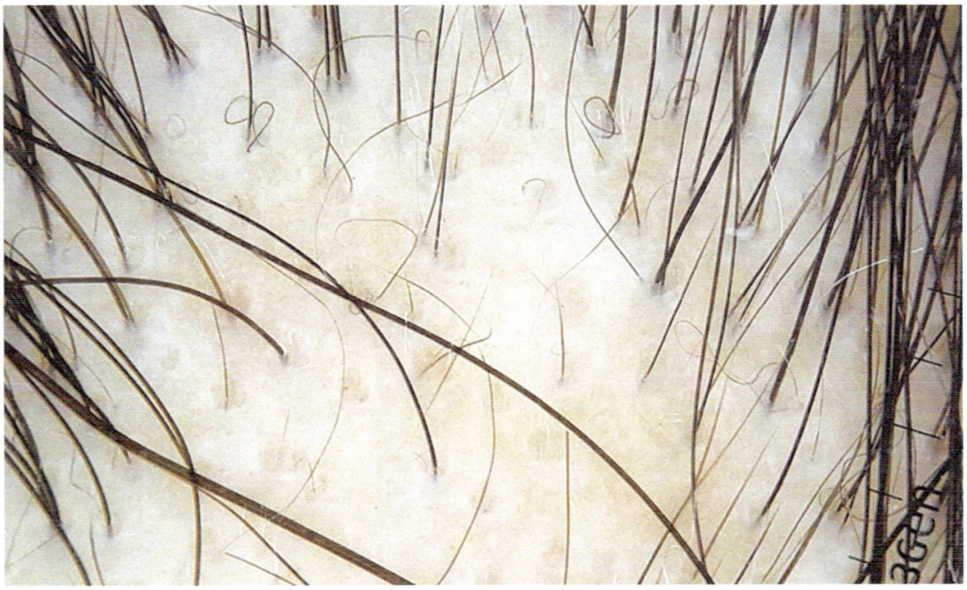

Fig. 68: Yellow dots in alopecia areata (AA).

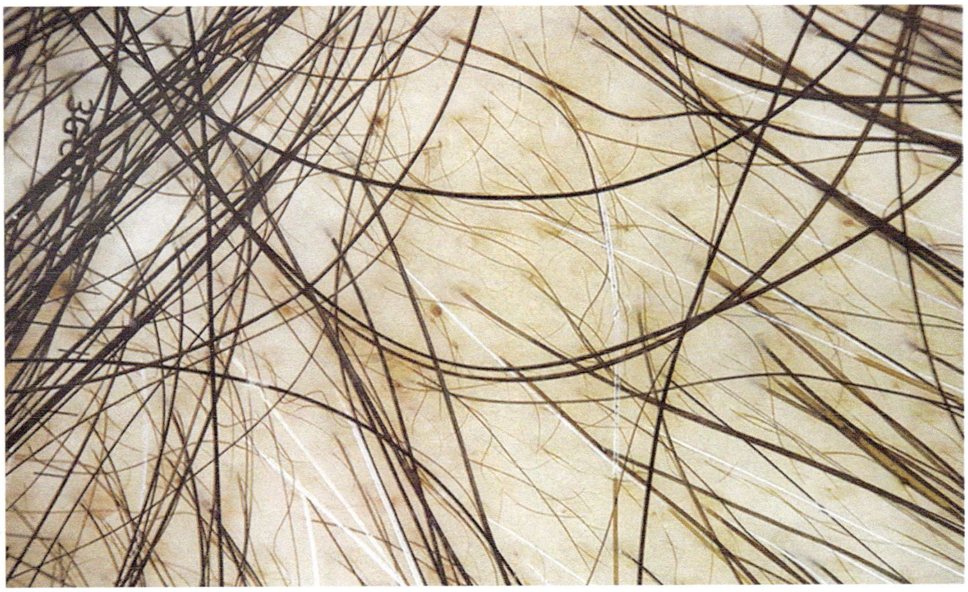

Fig. 69: Yellow dots in alopecia areata incognito.

ZIG-ZAG HAIRS

- Zig-zag hairs are sharply bent hairs at multiple points due to focal weakening of the hair shaft giving rise to zig-zag patterns or "z" shape.
- They are not specific but can be found in tinea capitis, trichorrhexis nodosa, AA, and monilethrix.
- The mechanism of formation is not known.

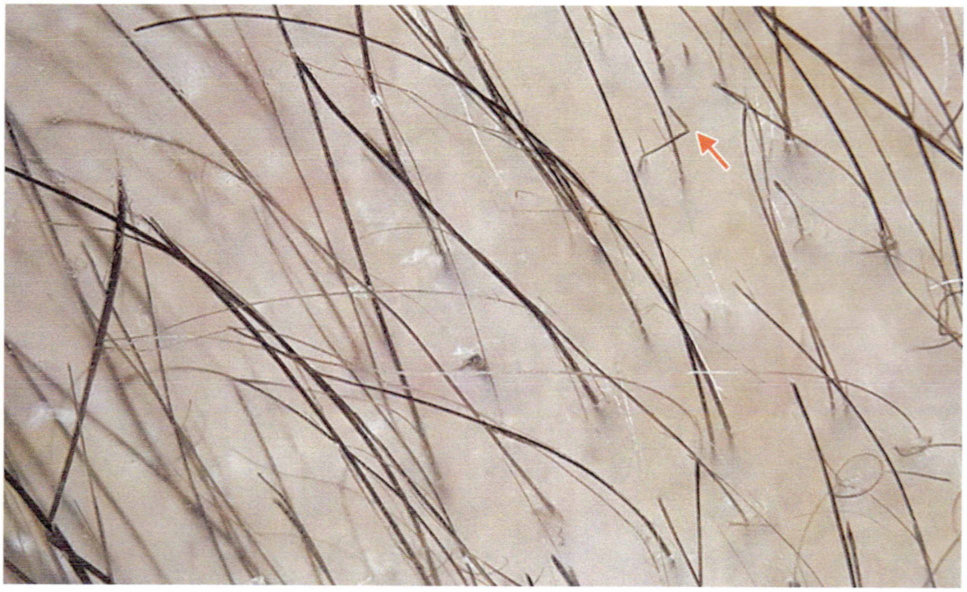

Fig. 70: Zig-zag hair (red arrow).

REFERENCES

1. Rudnicka L, Olszewska M, Rakowska A, Kowalska-Oledzka E, Slowinska M. Trichoscopy: a new method for diagnosing hair loss. J Drugs Dermatol. 2008;7(7):651-4.
2. Rudnicka L, Olszewska M, Rakowska A. Hair shaft. In: Rudnicka L, Olszewska M, Rakowska A, (eds). Atlas in Trichoscopy, 1st edition. Berlin, Germany: Springer; 2012. p. 38.
3. Duque-Estrada B, Tamler C, Sodre CT, Barcaui CB, Pereira FBC . Dermoscopic pattern of cicatricial alopecia resulting from discoid lupus erythematosus and lichen planopilaris. An Bras Dermatol. 2010;85:179-83.
4. Rudnicka L, Olszewska M, Rakowska A. Alopecia Areata. In: Rudnicka L, Olszewska M, Rakowska A, (eds). Atlas in Trichoscopy, 1st edition. Berlin, Germany: Springer; 2012. pp. 211-2.
5. Rudnicka L, Olszewska M, Rakowska A. Trichotillomania and Tractional Alopecia; In: Rudnicka L, Olszewska M, Rakowska A, (eds). Atlas in Trichoscopy, 1st edition. Berlin, Germany: Springer; 2012. pp. 260-2.
6. Pinkus H. Multiple hairs: report of two cases of pili multigemini and discussion of some other anomalies of the primary complex. J Inves Dermatol. 1951;17(5):291-301.
7. Rudnicka L, Olszewska M, Rakowska A, Slowinska M. Trichoscopy update 2011. J Dermatol Case Rep. 2011;5(4):82-8.
8. Rudnicka L, Olszewska M, Rakowska A. Trichotillomania and Tractional Alopecia; In: Rudnicka L, Olszewska M, Rakowska A, (eds). Atlas in Trichoscopy, 1st edition. Berlin, Germany: Springer; 2012. p. 268.
9. Rudnicka L, Olszewska M, Rakowska A. Hair shaft; In: Rudnicka L, Olszewska M, Rakowska A, (eds). Atlas in Trichoscopy, 1st edition. Berlin, Germany: Springer; 2012. p. 40.
10. Lacarruba F, Misciali C, Gibilisco R, Micali G. Circle Hair: Clinical, trichoscopic and histological finding. Int J of Trichol. 2013;5(4):211-3.
11. Slowinska M, Rudnicka L, Schwartz RA, Kowalska-Oledzka E, Rakowska A, Sicinska J, et al. Comma hairs: a dermoscopic marker for tinea capitis: a rapid diagnostic method. J Am Acad Dermatol. 2008;59(5 suppl):s77-9.
12. Rudnicka L, Olszewska M, Rakowska A. Hair shaft; In: Rudnicka L, Olszewska M, Rakowska A, (eds). Atlas in Trichoscopy, 1st edition. Berlin, Germany: Springer; 2012. p. 46.
13. Rudnicka L, Olszewska M, Rakowska A. Hair shaft; In: Rudnicka L, Olszewska M, Rakowska A, (eds). Atlas in Trichoscopy, 1st edition. Berlin, Germany: Springer; 2012. p. 30.
14. Huges R, Chiaverini C, Bahadoran P, Lacour JP. Corkscrew hair: a new dermoscopic sign for diagnosis of tinea capitis in black children. Arch Dermatol. 2011;147(3):335-6.
15. Inui S, Nakajima T, Itami S: Coudability hairs: a revisited sign of alopecia areat assessed by trichoscopy. Clic Exp Dermatol. 2010;35:361-5.
16. Shuster S. 'Coudability': a new physical sign of alopecia areata. Br J Dermatol. 1984;111;629.
17. Rudnicka L, Olszewska M, Rakowska A. Hair shaft; In: Rudnicka L, Olszewska M, Rakowska A, (eds). Atlas in Trichoscopy, 1st edition. Berlin, Germany: Springer; 2012. p. 37.

18. Tosti A, Torres F. Dermoscopy in the diagnosis of hair and scalp disorders. Actas Dermosifiliogr. 2009;100:(Supl):1:114-9.
19. Inui S, Nakajima T, Itami S. Scalp dermatoscopy of androgenetic alopecia in Asian people. J Dermatol 2009;36:82-5.
20. Inui S, Nakajima T, Itami S: Coudability hairs: a revisited sign of alopecia areata assessed by trichoscopy. Clin Exp Dermatol. 2010;35:361-5.
21. Miteva M, Tosti A: Skin appendage disorder. 2015;1(2):105-9.
22. Otberg N, Kang H, Alzolibani AA, Shapiro J. Folliculitis decalvans. Dermatol Ther. 2008;21:238-44.
23. Tosti A. Normal scalp; In: Tosti A: Dermoscopy of the hair and nails: CRC Press;2016. p. 22.
24. Rudnicka L, Olszewska M, Rakowska A. Hair shaft; In: Rudnicka L, Olszewska M, Rakowska A, (eds). Atlas in Trichoscopy, 1st edition. Berlin, Germany: Springer; 2012. p. 38.
25. Lanuti E, Miteva M, Romanelli P, Tosti A. Trichoscopy and histopathology of follicular keratotic plugs in scalp discoid lupus erythematosus. Int J Trichology. 2012;4:36-8.
26. Tosti A. Trichoscopy pattern. In: Tosti A, (ed). Dermoscopy of the hair and nails. 2nd edition. Florida, United States: CRC Press; 2016. p. 5.
27. Rakowska A, Slowinska M, Czuwara J, Olszewska M, Rudnicka L. Dermoscopy as a tool for rapid diagnosis of monilethrix. J Drugs Dermatol. 2007;6(2):222-4.
28. Rakowska A, Rudnicka L. Monilethrix, Pseudomonas, and Monilethrix-like hairs; In: Rudnicka L, Olszewska M, Rakowska A, (eds). Atlas in Trichoscopy, 1st edition. Berlin, Germany: Springer; 2012. p. 145.
29. Rudnicka L, Szepietowski JC, Slowinska M. Pinherio. Tinea capitis; In: Rudnicka L, Olszewska M, Rakowska A, (eds). Atlas in Trichoscopy, 1st edition. Berlin, Germany: Springer; 2012. pp. 365-66.
30. Deloche C, de Lacharriere O, Piraccini BM, Piraccini BM, Vincenzi C, Bastien P, et al. Histological features of peripilar signs associated with androgenetic alopecia. Arch Dermatol Res. 2004;295:422-8.
31. de Moura LH, Duque-Estrada B, Abraham LS, Barcaui CP, Sodre CT. Dermoscopy findings of alopecia areata in an African-American patient. J Dermatol Case Rep. 2008;2(4):52-4.
32. Abraham LS, Pineiro-Maceira J, Duque-Estrada, Barcaui CP, Sodre CT . Pinpoint white dots in the scalp: dermoscopic and histopathological correlation. J Am Acad Dermatol. 2010;63(4):721-2.
33. Ross EK, Vincenzi C, Tosti A. Videodermoscopy in the evaluation of hair and scalp disorders. J Am Acad Dermatol. 2006;55(5):799-806.
34. Mane M, Nath AK, Thappa DM. Utility of dermoscopy in alopecia areata. Indian J Dermatol. 2011;56(4):407-11.
35. Rudnicka L, Olszewska M, Rakowska A. Trichotillomania and Tractional Alopecia; In: Rudnicka L, Olszewska M, Rakowska A, (eds). Atlas in Trichoscopy, 1st edition. Berlin, Germany: Springer; 2012. p. 267.
36. Rudnicka L, Olszewska M, Rokowska A. Discoid Lupus Erythematosus. In: Rudnicka L, Olszewska M, Rakowska A, (eds). Atlas in Trichoscopy, 1st edition. Berlin, Germany: Springer; 2012. p. 313.
37. Panchaprateep R, Tanus A, Tosti A. Clinical dermoscopic and histological features of body hair disorders. Am Acad Dermatol. 2015;72(5):893.
38. R Psnchaprateep, Tanus A, Tosti A. Clinical, dermoscopic, and histopathologic features of body hair disorders. J Am Acad Dermatol.2015;72:890-900.
39. Olszewska M, Rokowska A, Slowinska M, et al. Classical Lichen Planopilaris and Graham Little Syndrome; In: Rudnicka L, Olszewska M, Rakowska A, (eds). Atlas in Trichoscopy, 1st edition. Berlin, Germany: Springer; 2012. p. 279.
40. Rebora A. Alopecia areata incognito: a hypothesis. Dermatologica. 1987;174:214-8.
41. Duque-Estrada B, Tamler C, Sodre CT, Barcaui CB, Pereira FBC. Dermatoscopy pattern of cicatricial alopecia resulting from discoid lupus erythemotosus and lichen planopilaris. An Bras Dermatol. 2010;85:179-83.
42. Rokowska A, Olszewska M. Trichothiodystrophy; In: Rudnicka L, Olszewska M, Rakowska A, (eds). Atlas in Trichoscopy, 1st edition. Berlin, Germany: Springer; 2012. p. 186.
43. Rudnicka L, Olszewska M, Rakowska A. Hair shaft; In: Rudnicka L. Olszewska M, Rakowska A, (eds). Atlas in Trichoscopy, 1st edition. Berlin, Germany: Springer; 2012. p. 26.
44. Rudnicka L, Olszewska M, Rakowska A. Hair shaft; In: Rudnicka L. Olszewska M, Rakowska A, (eds). Atlas in Trichoscopy, 1st edition. Berlin, Germany: Springer; 2012. p. 18.
45. Rudnicka L, Olszewska M, Rakowska A. Trichorrhexis Nodosa; In: Rudnicka L, Olszewska M, Rakowska A, (eds). Atlas in Trichoscopy, 1st edition. Berlin, Germany: Springer; 2012. p. 159.
46. Rakaowsky A. Trichoscopy in the healthy female. J Dermatol Case Rep. 2009;3(1):14-9.
47. Vogt A, MacElwee KJ, Blume-Peytavi U. (eds). Hair: From Basis Science to Clinical Application. Berlin: Springer; 2008. pp. 1-22.
48. Inui S, Nakajima T, Itami S. Scalp dermoscopy of androgenic alopecia in Asian people. J dermatol. 20009;36(2):82-5.
49. Van Neste D. Natural scalp hair regression in preclinical stage of male androgenetic alopecia and its reversal by finasteride. Skin Pharmacol Physiol. 2006;19(3):82-5.
50. Tosti A. Primary scarring alopecia; In: Tosti A (ed). Dermoscopy of the Hair and Nails, 2nd edition. Florida, United States: CRC Press; 2016. p. 66.

51. Ross EK, Vincenzi C, Tosti A. Videodermoscopy in the evaluation of hair and scalp disorders. J Am Acad Dermatol. 2006;55 (5):799-806.
52. Lacarrubba F, Dall'Oglio F, Rita Nasca M, Micali G. Videodermatoscopy enhances diagnostic capability in some forms of hair loss. Am J Clin Dermatol. 2004;5(3):205-8.
53. Inui S, Nakajima T, Itami S. Clinical significance of dermoscopy in alopecia areata: Analysis of 300 cases. Int J Dermatol. 2008;47(7):688-93.
54. Rakowska A, Slowinska M, Kowalska-Oledzka E, Olszewska M, Rudnicka L. Dermoscopy in female androgenic alopecia: method standardization and diagnostic criteria. Int J Trichol. 2009;1(2);123-30.

4

SECTION

Trichoscopic Language and Pattern Analysis

CHAPTER 4

Follicular and Perifollicular Patterns

Subrata Malakar, Purva Mehta Movdawalla

FOLLICULAR AND PERIFOLLICULAR PATTERNS

- Yellow dots
- White dots
- Black dots
- Red dots
- Blue-gray dots
- Gray-white halo
- Peripilar sign
- Keratotic plugs
- Empty follicles
- Loss of follicular openings
- Perifollicular scales

Black Dots

- They are hairs broken at scalp level.[1]
- They appear as black dots at the hair follicle opening.
- Black dots are not specific for any conditions and are commonly plenty in alopecia areata, trichotillomania, tinea capitis, etc.
- Only a few black dots may be seen in some scarring alopecias.

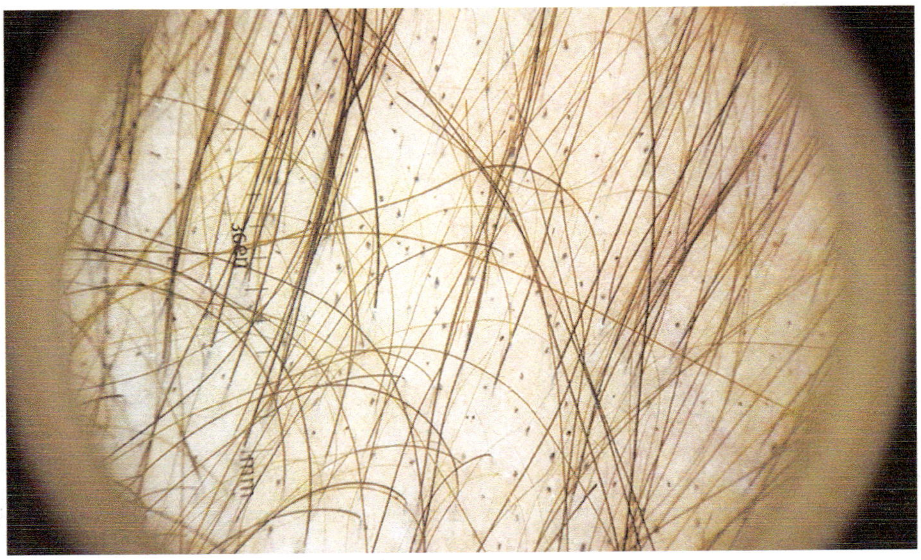

Fig. 1: Presence of plenty of black dots in alopecia areata. They are not diagnostic as numerous black dots are present in other nonscarring alopecia also.

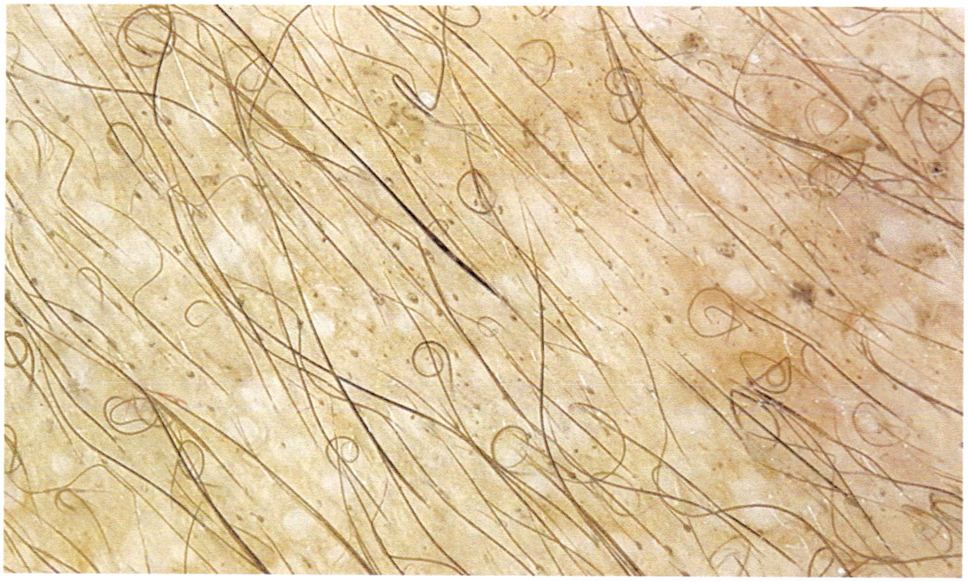

Fig. 2: Numerous black dots in trichotillomania of eyebrow. Note the circle hairs or pigtail hairs which are nothing but short vellus hairs.

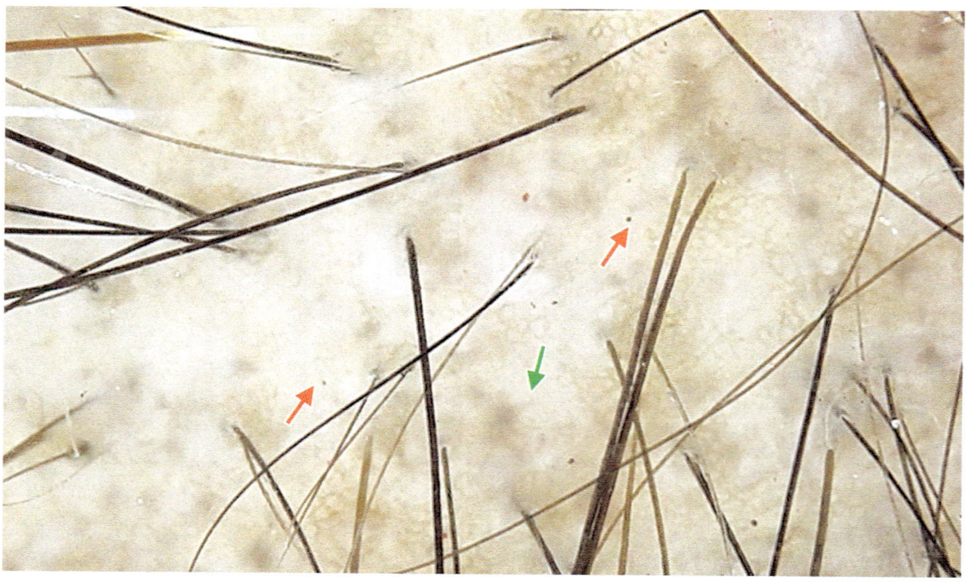

Fig. 3: Few black dots (red arrows) in lichen planopilaris (LPP). Note the blue–gray dots (green arrow) which is a feature of LPP due to pigment incontinence.

Pinpoint white dots:[2]

The characteristics of white dots are:

- They are regularly distributed in the normal scalp interspersed between the hair follicles.
- A diameter of 0.2–0.3 mm
- Present in normal scalp. It may be seen in scalp disorders with normal interfollicular scalp.
- Increased in number in all types of alopecia
- Scattered/absent in scalp discoid lupus erythematosus (DLE) and folliculitis decalvans

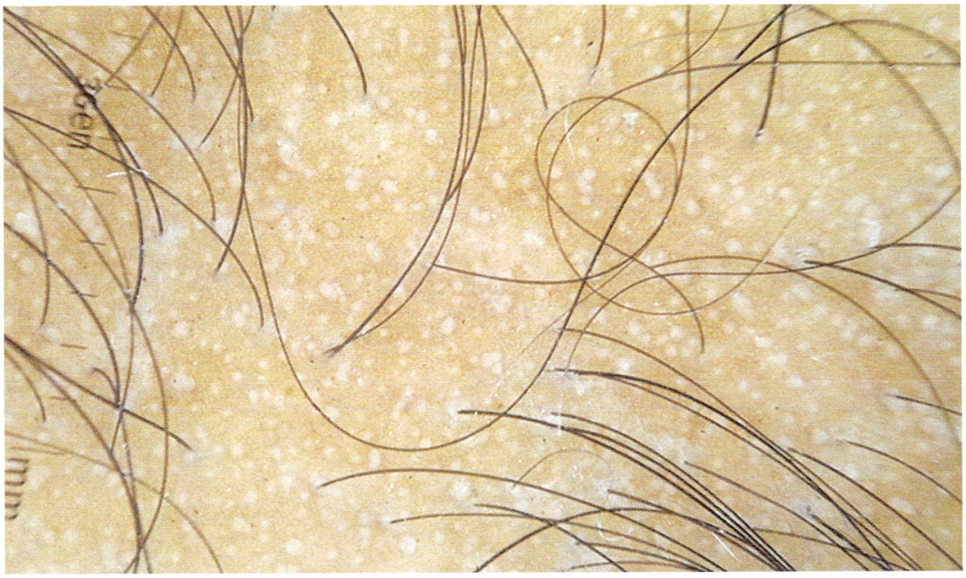

Fig. 4: Pinpoint white dots: 0.2–0.3 mm dots distributed regularly in the interfollicular scalp, dispersed among the mosaics of honeycomb pattern. They correspond to follicular and acrosyringium of eccrine sweat glands.

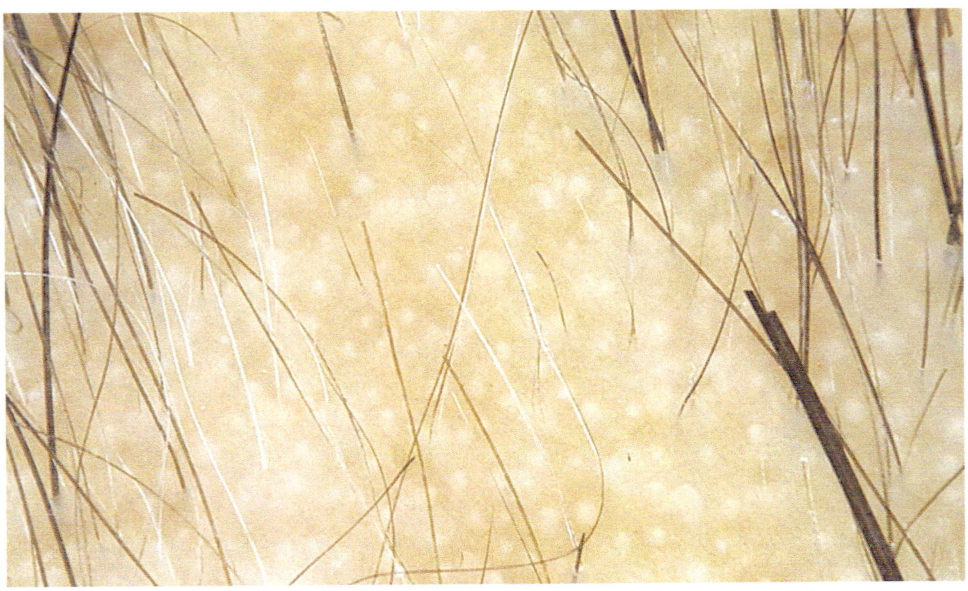

Fig. 5: Pinpoint white dots in alopecia areata.

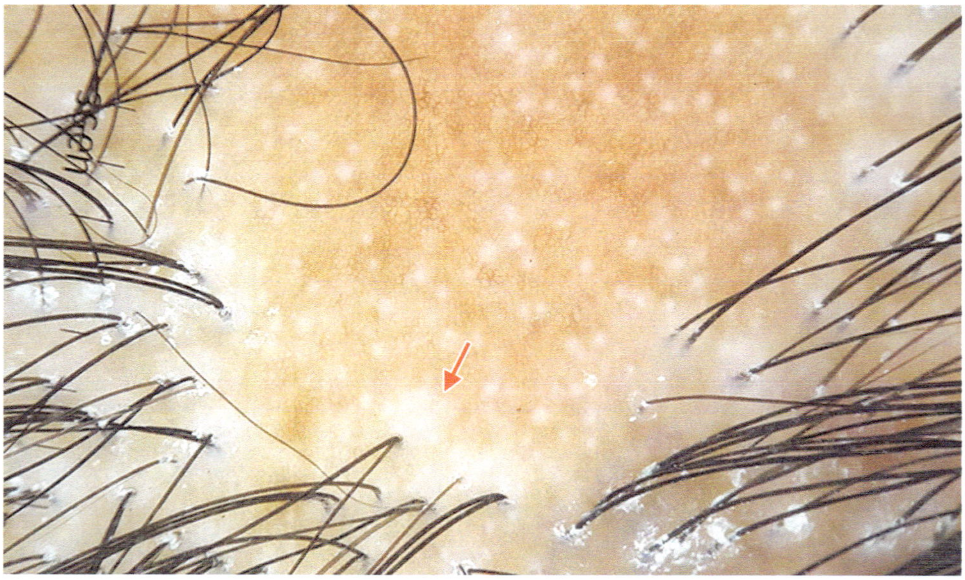

Fig. 6: Pinpoint white dots in scarring alopecia; their distribution is irregular. Note the perifollicular scaling and white patches (red arrow).

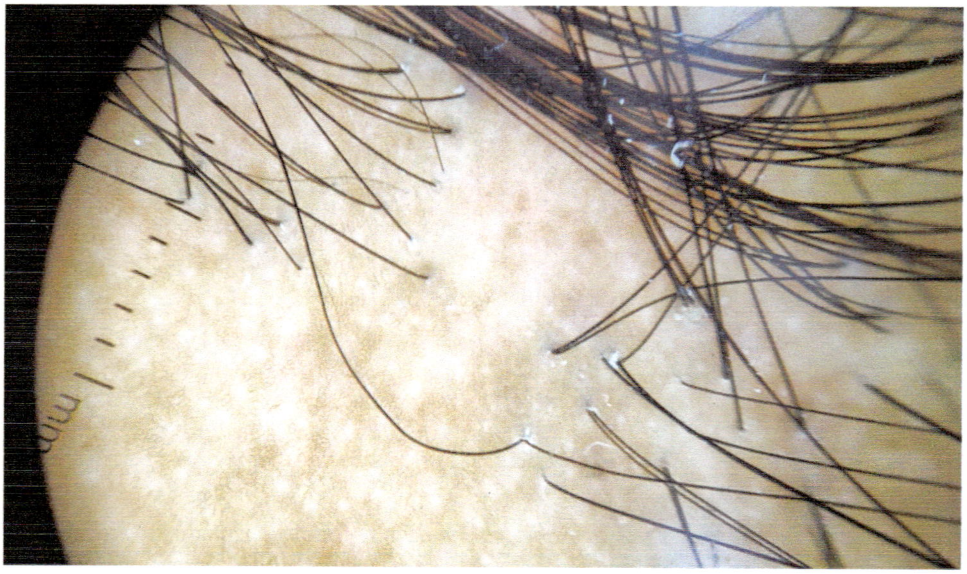

Fig. 7: Another picture showing pinpoint white dots in scarring alopecia; their distribution is irregular. Note the perifollicular scaling and white patches.

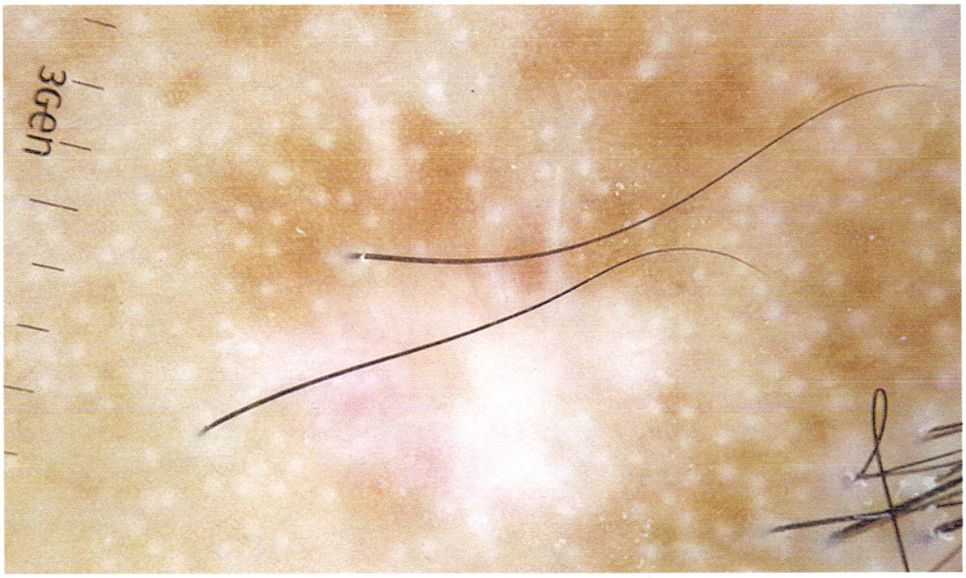

Fig. 8: In scarring alopecia, pinpoint white dots are irregularly distributed and interspersed with white patches.

Yellow Dots[1,3,4]

- They are round yellow dots, may be arranged singularly or in groups of 2–3 reflecting the number of hairs per follicular unit.
- A double margin may be observed in most dots.
- They are usually not visible in dark patients but an important diagnostic marker in Caucasians.
- Yellow dots correspond to dilated infundibular ostia filled with keratosebaceous material.
- It may contain vellus hair or broken hair shaft; often it is empty.
- Typically present in alopecia areata, yellow dots also can be revealed in androgenetic alopecia (AGA), trichotillomania (TTM), alopecia areata incognito, etc.

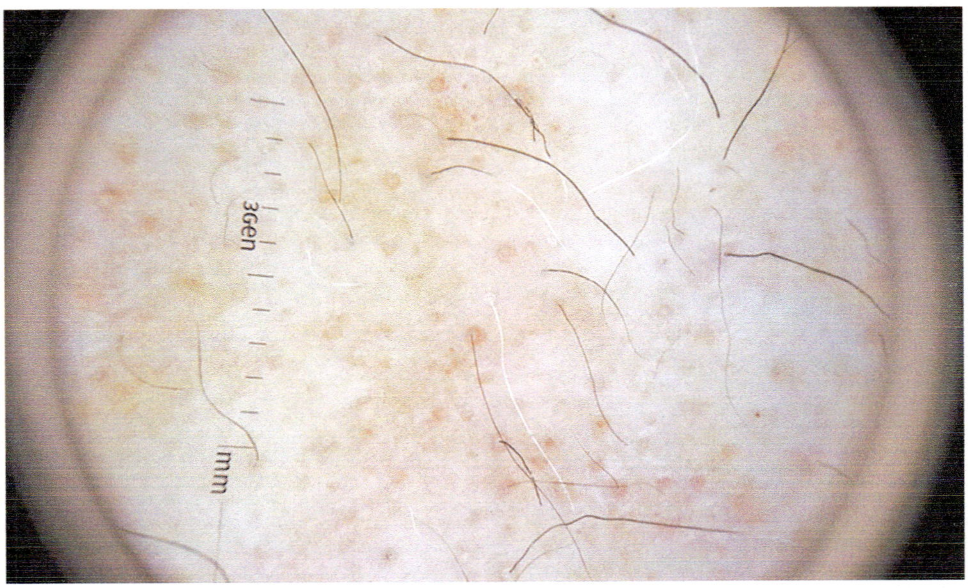

Fig. 9: Yellow dots can be appreciated better owing to the whitish background. Here the whitish background is due to widespread fibrosis in a case of lichen planopilaris (LPP). Note the lone hairs characteristic of LPP.

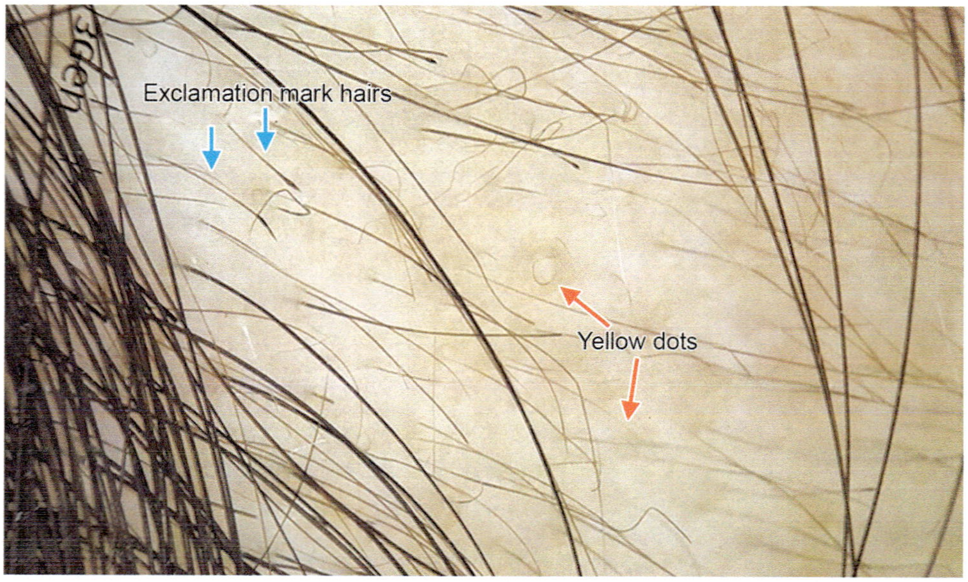

Fig. 10: Yellow dots in alopecia areata (red arrows). Upper yellow dot contains vellus hair. In pigmented skin, yellow dots appear more whitish. Several exclamation mark hairs as well as many vellus hairs are present in the field.

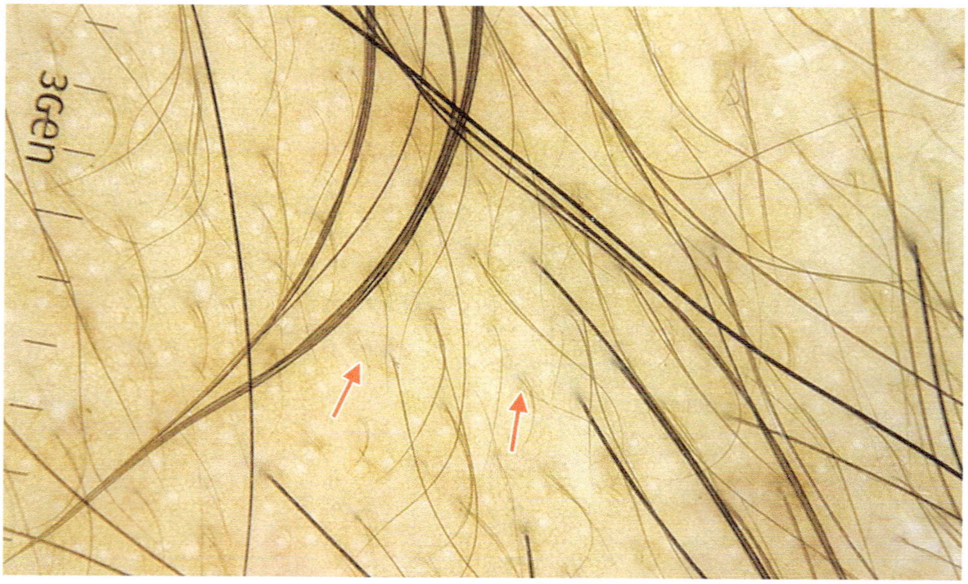

Fig. 11: Yellow dots in androgenetic alopecia (AGA) (red arrows). Miniaturized hairs are plenty and are present singularly or in groups of 2–3. Only few terminal hairs are present in this field.

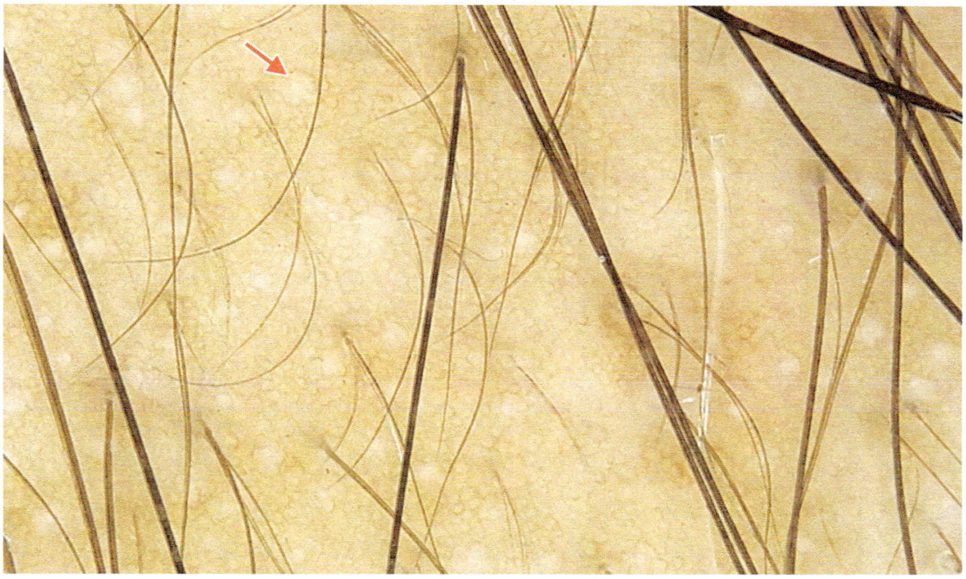

Fig. 12: More close-up view of yellow dots in androgenetic alopecia (AGA). Yellow dot marked by red arrow has two borders and contains no hair follicle. Most of the miniaturized hairs are present in groups of 2 per follicular unit.

Red Dots

- Red dots are one of the specific features of DLE. The other two specific features of DLE are keratotic plugs and enlarged branching vessels.
- They correspond to dilated follicular openings surrounded by dilated vessels.
- Typically seen in DLE in the black where the hypopigmented scalp is present.
- Red dots indicate early disease and so, if treated promptly, hair regrowth is a possibility.[5]
- They may be seen in the glabella of FFA patients because of involvement of eyebrows.
- These red dots are different from those in psoriasis. In DLE, it is related to follicular openings, whereas in psoriasis, it is due to dilated papillary capillaries in the interfollicular scalp.

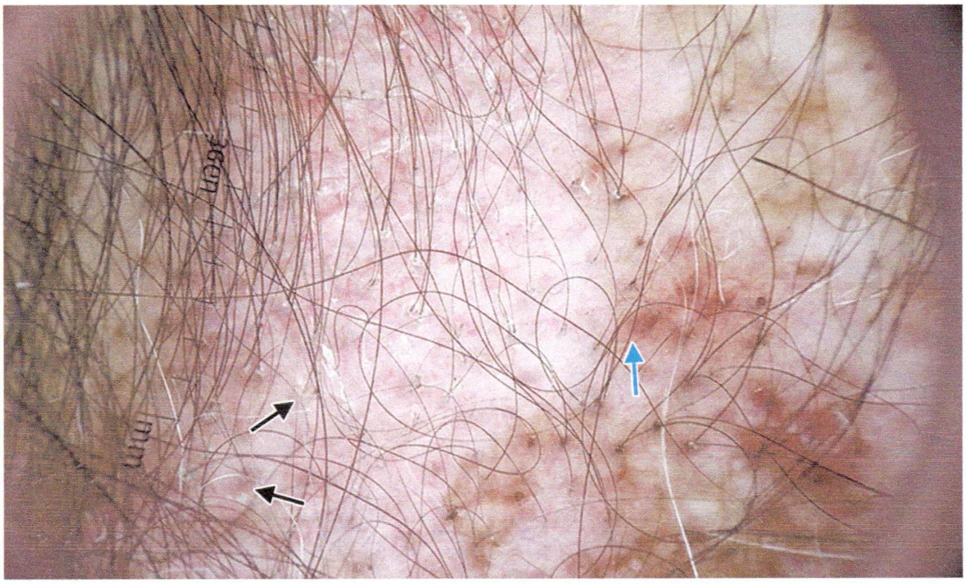

Fig. 13: Red dots (black arrows) in discoid lupus erythematosus (DLE. They are present around hair follicles. Note other features of DLE like keratotic plugging and brown–gray dots (blue arrow) are also present.

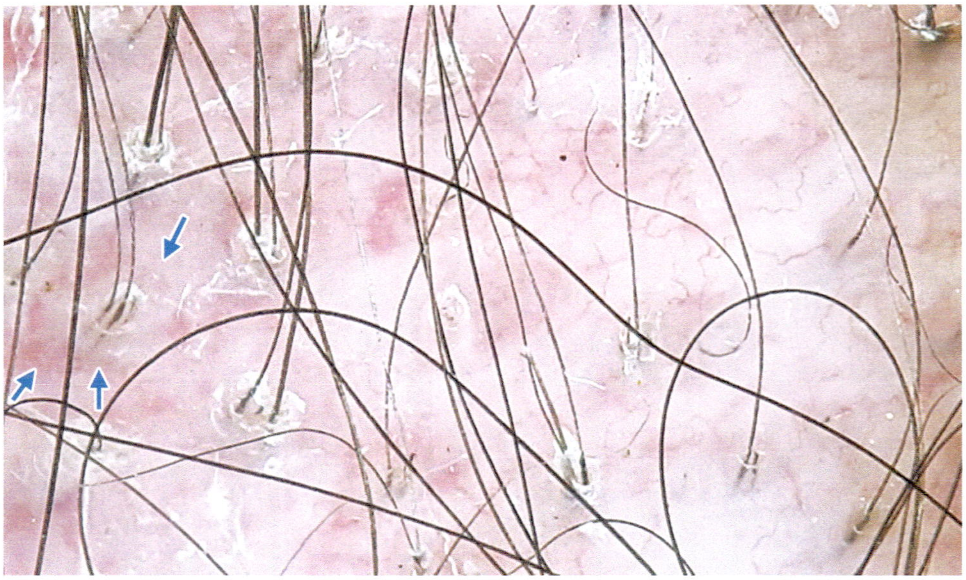

Fig. 14: Close-up view of red dots. Hair follicular unit with group of two hairs in this follicular unit is surrounded by dilated vessels marked by blue arrows. Enlarged branching vessels, another feature of discoid lupus erythematosus (DLE), are present in the right side of the field.

Blue–Gray Dots[6]

- In patients with dark phototype, blue-gray dots arranged in a target pattern are characteristic of LPP.
- They correspond histopathologically to melanophages in the papillary dermis and are a sign of pigmentary incontinence confined to the hair follicles.
- Blue-gray dots can also be seen in DLE where they are present both perifollicularly and in speckled pattern.

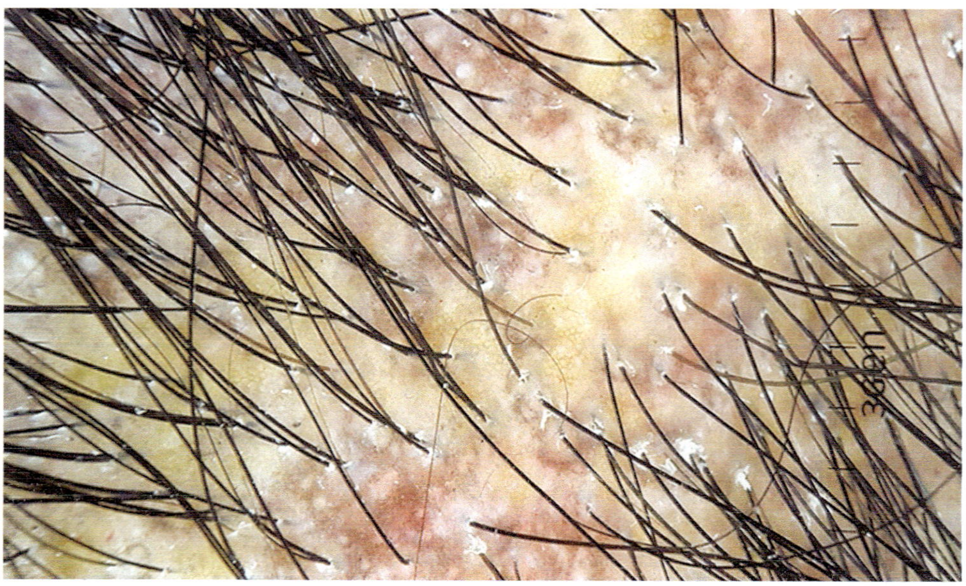

Fig. 15: Blue-gray dots in target pattern in a case of lichen planopilaris (LPP). Target pattern is due to melanin incontinence surrounding only the perifollicular area and sparing interfollicular region.

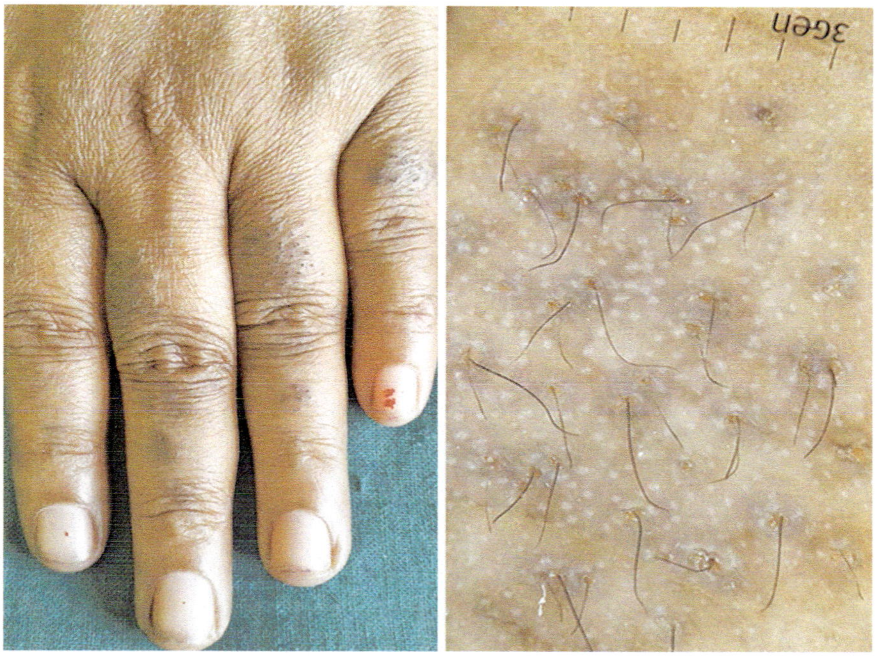

Fig. 16: Blue–gray dots in target pattern involving body hairs.

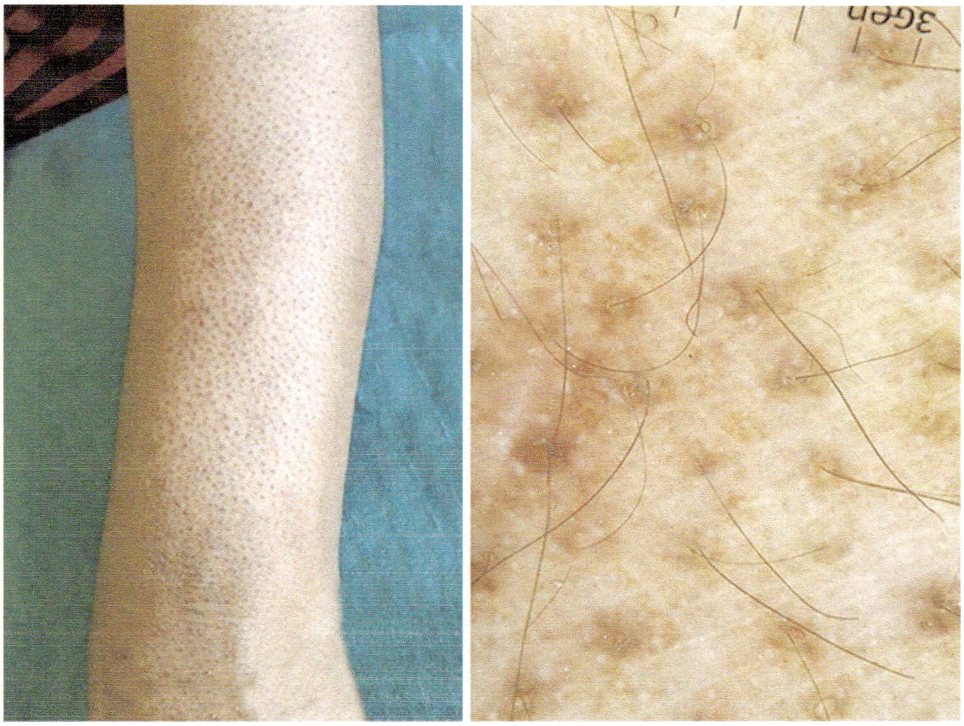

Fig. 17: Blue–gray target pattern over forearm hairs.

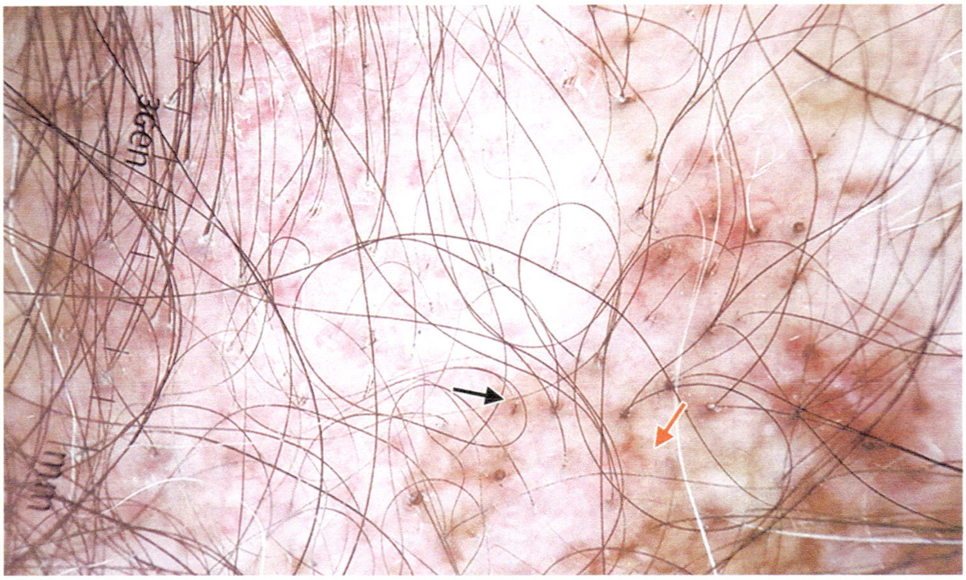

Fig. 18: In discoid lupus erythematosus (DLE), blue–gray dots are present peri- (black arrow) and inter-follicularly (red arrow).

Peripilar Sign[7]

- It is a brown halo of roughly 1 mm in diameter around the emergence of the hair shaft. It corresponds pathologically to perifollicular inflammation.
- Typically, it is seen in early AGA. It can also be found in late AGA and telogen effluvium.
- They appear as brown to brown-gray discoloration surrounding the follicular opening.

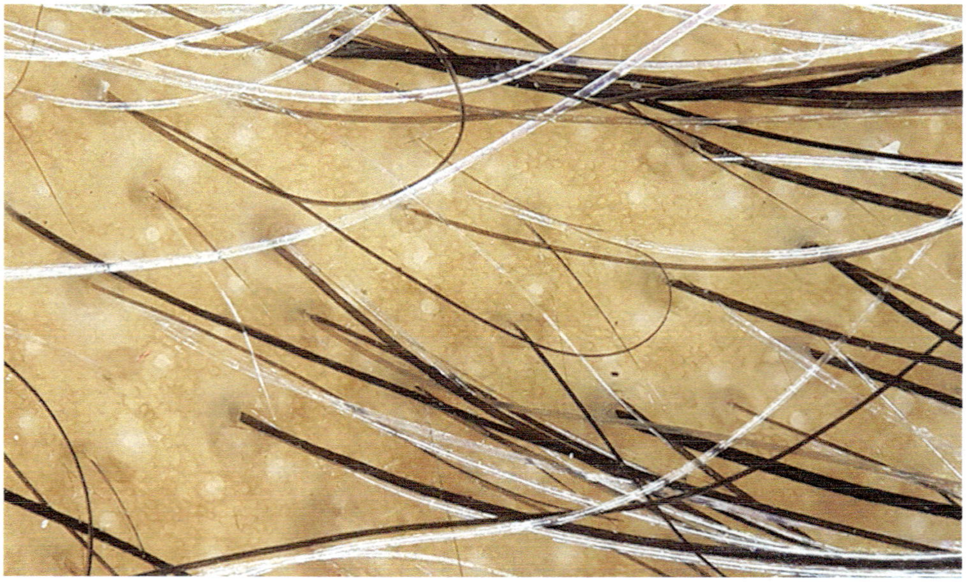

Fig. 19: Peripilar sign.

Loss of Follicular Opening

- It is a feature of all types of scarring alopecia.
- To differentiate different scarring alopecias, specific trichoscopic findings can help.

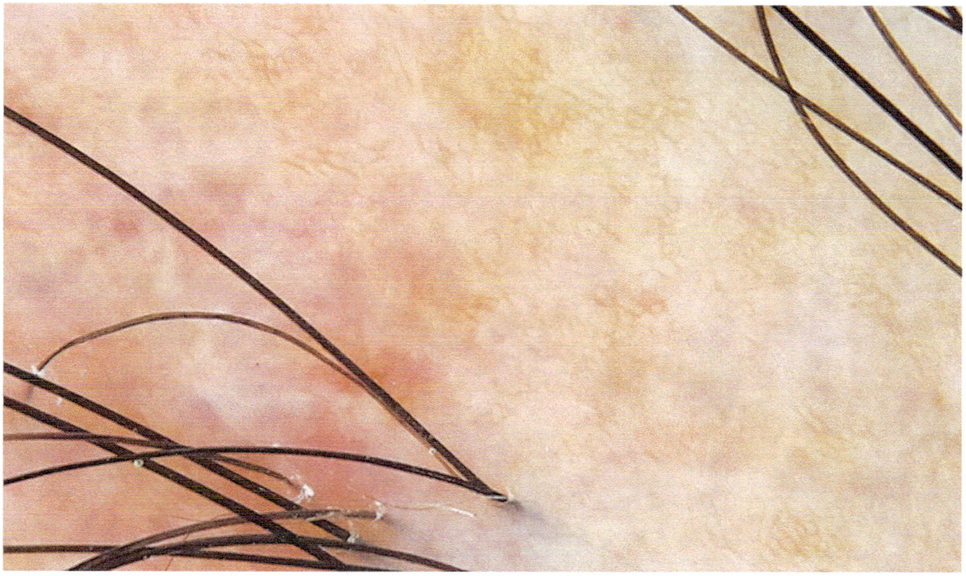

Fig. 20A: Loss of follicular openings.

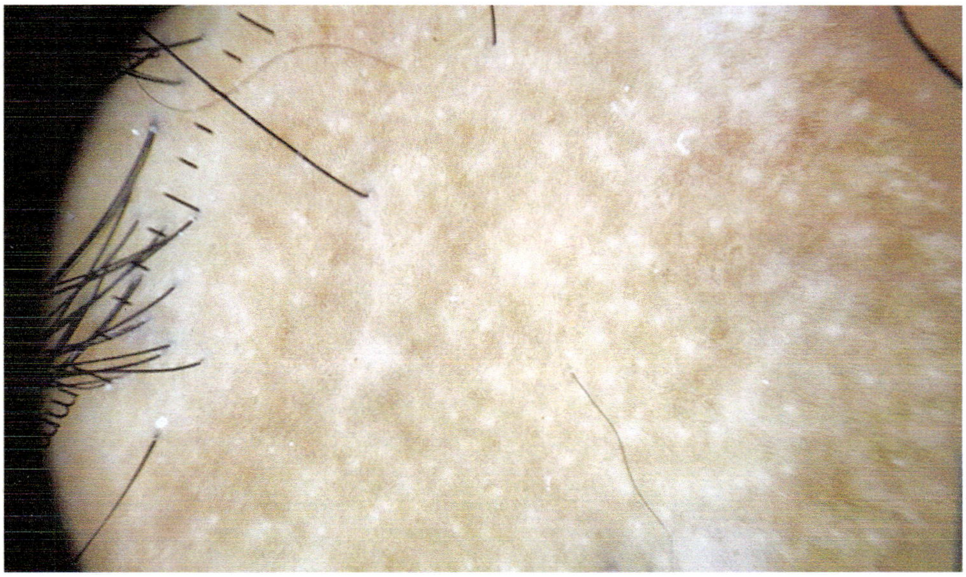

Fig. 20B: Another picture showing loss of follicular openings.

Empty Follicles

- They are seen as hair follicles without hairs.
- These blank follicles are found in AGA and telogen effluvium and also sometimes in healthy scalp.

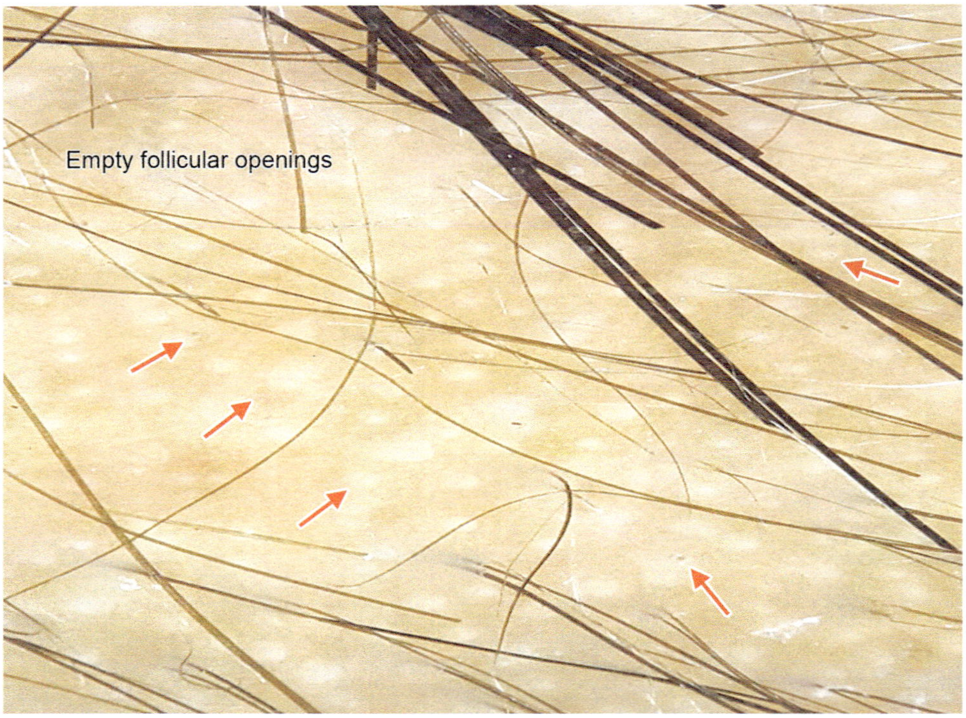

Fig. 21: Empty follicular openings.

REFERENCES

1. Ross EK, Vincenzi C, Tosti A. Videodermoscopy in the evaluation of hair and scalp disorders. J Am Acad Dermatol. 2006;55(5):799-806.
2. Abraham LS, Maceira JP, Estrada BD, Barcaui CB, Sodré CT. Pinpoint white dots in the scalp: dermoscopic and histopathological correlation. J Am Acad Dermat. 2009;63(4):721.
3. Rudnicka L, Olszewska M, Rakowska A, Slowinska M. Trichoscopy update 2011. J Dermatol Case Rep. 2011;5(4):82-8.
4. Lacarrubba F, Dall' Oglio F, Rita Nasca M, Micali G. Videodermatoscopy enhances diagnostic capability in some forms of hair loss. Am J Clin Dermatol. 2004;5(3):205-8.
5. Tosti A, Torres F, Misciali C, Vincenzi C, Starace M, Miteva M, et al. Follicular red dots: a novel dermoscopic pattern observed in scalp discoid lupus erythematosus. Arch Dermatol. 2009;145(12):1406-9.
6. Duque-Estrada B, Tamler C, Sodre CT, Barcaui CB, Pereira FB. Dermoscopic pattern of cicatricial alopecia resulting from discoid lupus erythematosus and lichen planopilaris. An Bras Dermatol. 2010;85:179-83.
7. Deloche C, de Lacharriere O, Miscali C, Piraccini BM, Vincenzi C, Bastien P, et al. Histological features of peripilar signs associated with androgenetic alopecia. Arch Dermatol Res. 2004;295(10):422-8.

CHAPTER 5

Interfollicular Pattern

Subrata Malakar, Surit Malakar

INTERFOLLICULAR PATTERNS

- Honeycomb pigment
- Interfollicular scales (see Chapter 7: Pattern of Scaly Scalp)
- White patches
- Vessels

Honeycomb Pigment

- *Honeycomb pigmented network* consists of homogenous mosaic of contiguous brownish rings. It resembles pigmented network of melanocytic lesions on dermoscopy.[1]
- The hyperchromic areas of this network correspond to rete ridge melanocytes, whereas hypochromic areas correlate with suprapapillary epidermal melanocytes.
- This pattern is found in normal scalp, nonscarring alopecia, and scarring alopecia except discoid lupus erythematosus (DLE).

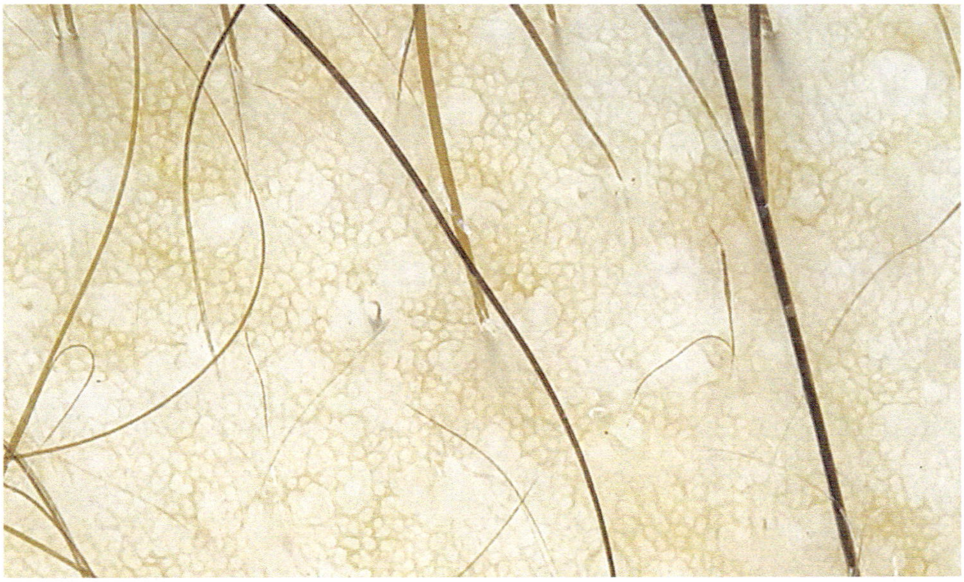

Fig. 1: Honeycomb pigment.

Vessels

- Normal scalp vessels include—(1) interfollicular red loops and (2) arborizing red lines.[2,3]
- Interfollicular red loops correspond to the capillaries in the dermal papillae and are seen as erythematous hairpin-shaped structures.
- Whereas arborizing red lines correlate with the subpapillary vascular plexus. They have larger caliber than the red loops.[4]
- Exaggerated arborizing vessels are seen in seborrheic dermatitis and contact dermatitis.
- In psoriasis, twisted capillary loops are found. These twisted loops appear as red dots in low magnification.[5]
- Giant enlarged capillaries are seen in dermatomyositis.

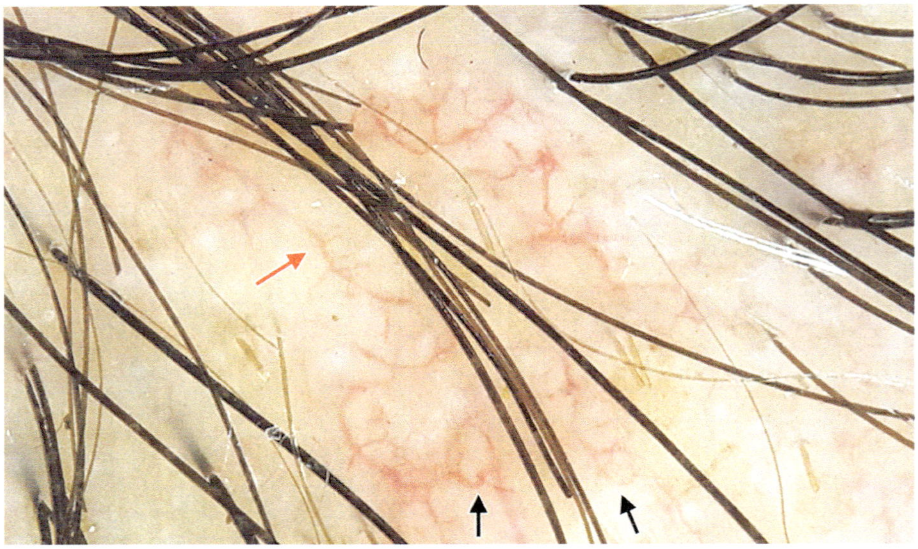

Fig. 2: Red loops (black arrows) and arborizing red lines (red arrow). These are exaggerated in seborrheic dermatitis and contact dermatitis.

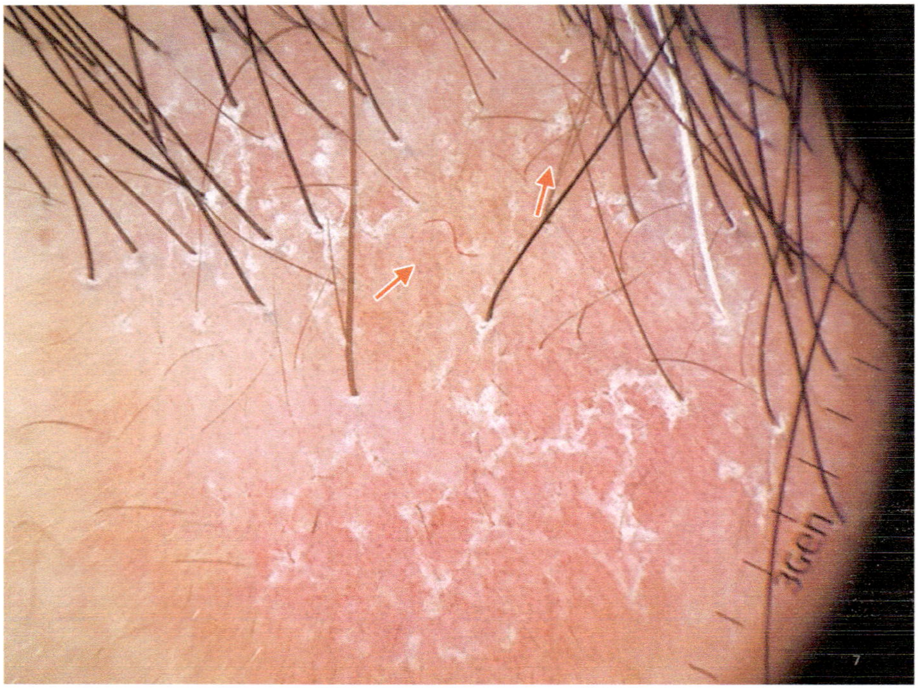

Fig. 3: Twisted capillary loops in psoriasis. Note silvery white scales.

White Patches

- White patches are described as white structureless areas present on the skin/scalp.
- They correspond histologically to the areas of fibrosis representing the process of scarring.
- Usually, it is seen in scarring alopecias, like LPP, DLE, etc.[6]

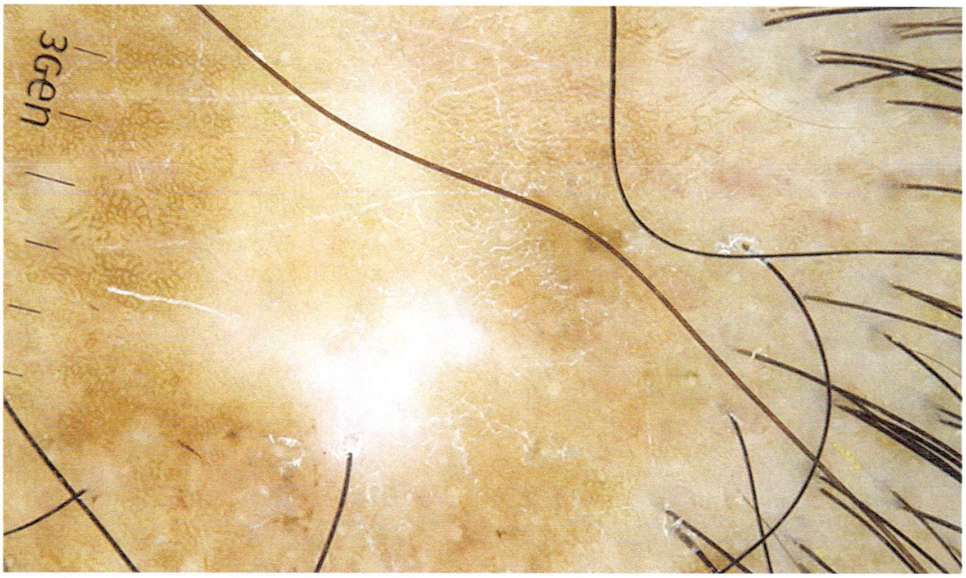

Fig. 4: White patches.

REFERENCES

1. Braun RP, Rabinovitz HS, Oliviero M, Kopf AW, Saurat JH. Dermoscopy of pigmented skin lesions. J Am Acad Dermatol. 2005;52:109-21.
2. Tosti A. Dermatoscopy of hair and scalp disorders. London: Informa Healthcare; 2007.
3. Ross EK, Vincenzi C, Tosti A. Videodermatoscopy in the evaluation of hair and scalp disorders. J Am Acad Dermatol. 2006;55:799-806.
4. Bull RH, Bates DO, Mortimer PS. Intravital video-capillaroscopy for the study of the microcirculation in psoriasis. Br J Dermatol. 1992;126:436-45.
5. Kim GW, Jung HJ, Ko HC, Kim MB, Lee WJ, Lee SJ, et al. Dermoscopy can be useful in differentiating scalp psoriasis from seborrheic dermatitis. Br J Dermatol. 2011;164:652-6.
6. Miteva M, Tosti A. Hair and scalp dermatoscopy. J Am Acad Dermatol. 2012;67:1040-8.

CHAPTER

6 Pattern of Hair Shafts

Subrata Malakar

PATTERNS OF HAIR SHAFTS

- Upright regrowing hairs (URH)
- Circle hairs
- Broken hairs
- Tapering hairs (exclamation mark hairs, coudability hairs)
- Comma hairs
- Corkscrew hairs
- Coiled hairs/question mark hairs
- Flame hairs
- Monilethrix-like hairs
- Hair diameter diversity
- Hair tufting

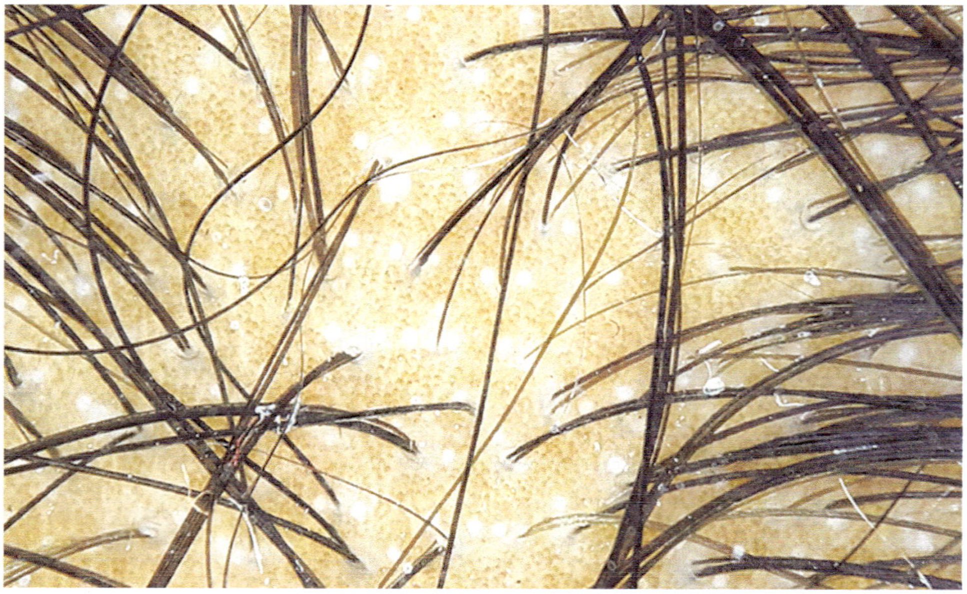

Fig. 1: Normal hair shafts are uniform in color and diameter. Normal hairs are >55 µm thick.[1] Various hair shaft abnormalities can be evaluated by trichoscopy.

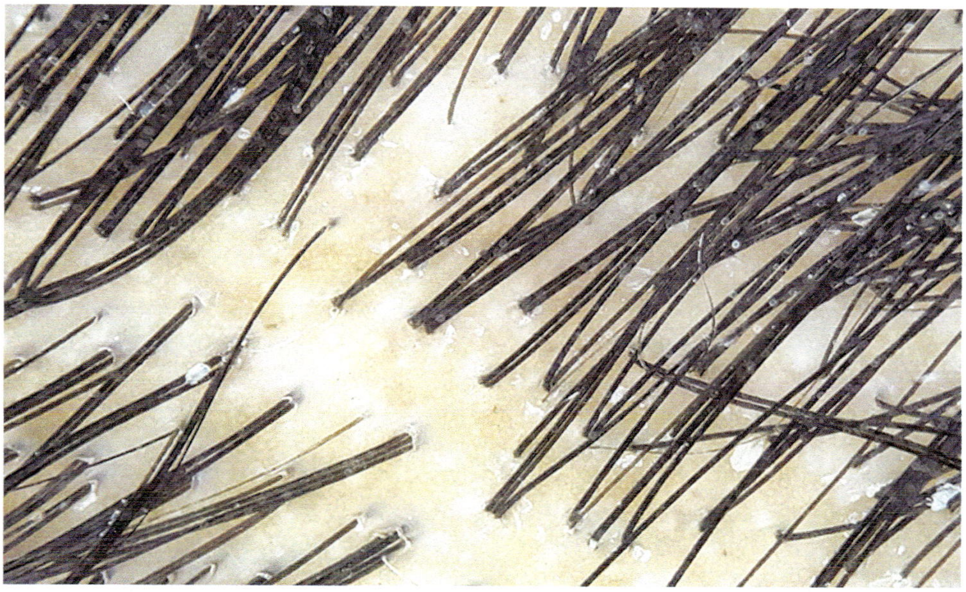

Fig. 2: Percentage of one follicular units with only one emerging hair shaft is usually <30% in healthy individual. Usually two to three follicular units and occasionally four follicular units may be found.[1,2]

Upright Regrowing Hairs

- They are also called short regrowing hairs.
- They are found in the normal scalp, in the remitting phase of alopecia areata (AA) and telogen effluvium (TE).
- Thin upright regrowing hairs (URH) are found in androgenetic alopecia (AGA) and persisting AA.
- These regrowing hairs may have a normal thickness (>0.03 mm) or less than that.[3]

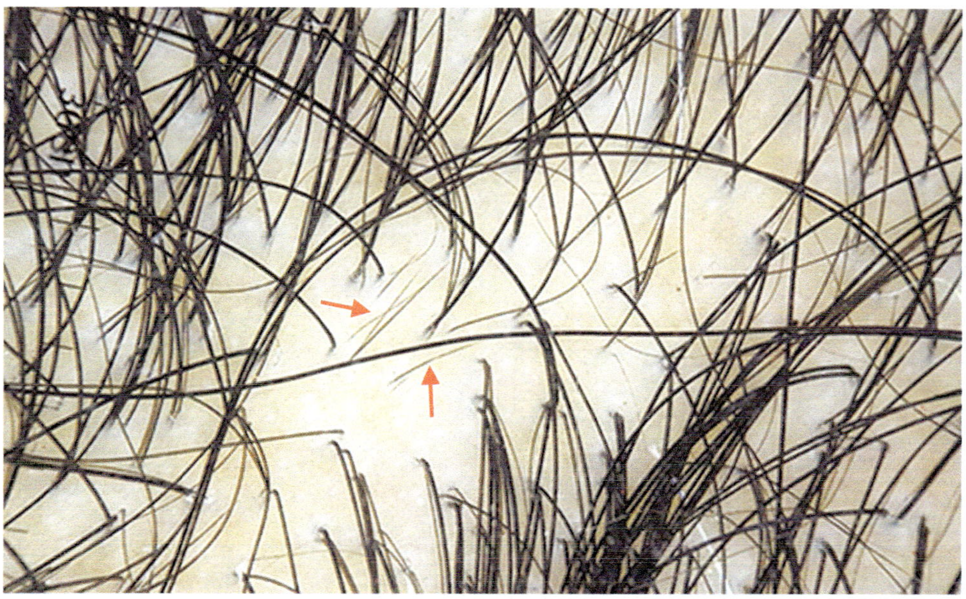

Fig. 3: Upright regrowing hairs (URH). The presence of multiple URH is typical of TE and can also be found in other noncicatricial alopecias. They have tapered end and their thickness is increased continuously toward the root. They have a normal thickness of >0.03 mm or less than that.[3]

Vellus Hair

- It is defined as hypopigmented, nonmedullated hairs <30 µm thick and <2–3 mm long; up to about 10% of normal scalp hair are vellus hairs.[4]
- During the process of hair follicle miniaturization, vellus hairs replace terminal ones.[5] Vellus hairs are increased in male and female AGA.[6,7]
- Vellus hairs should be differentiated from regrowing hairs. Regrowing hairs are short and thin, not hypopigmented, they are firm and have pointed ends. Whereas, vellus hairs are hypopigmented and thin hairs.[8]

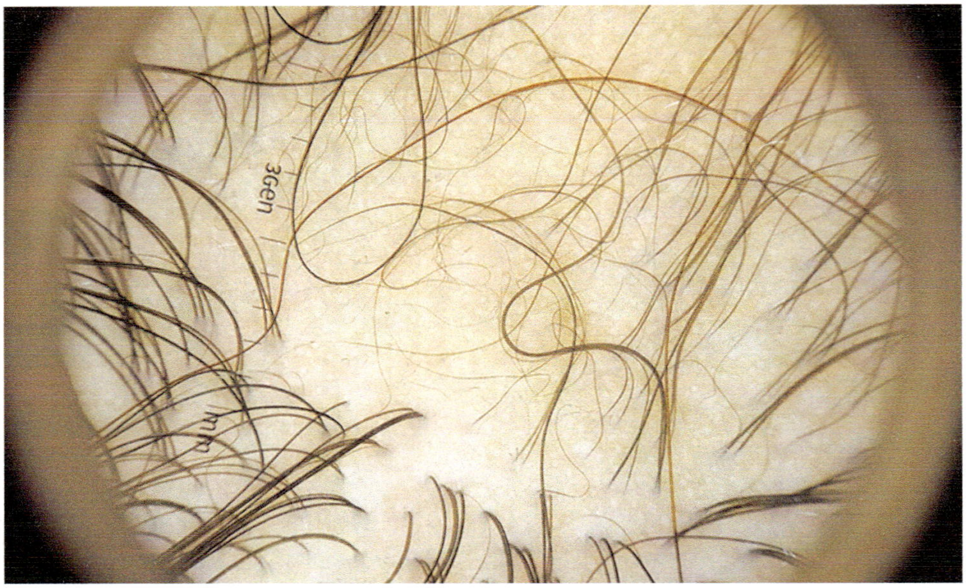

Fig. 4: Vellus hairs, clustered vellus hairs (>10 mm) are a common finding in alopecia areata (44.37%).[9]

Circle Hairs

- They are short vellus hairs and are also known as pigtail hairs.
- They appear as thin coiled hairs and can be found in AA and AGA.
- High number of coiled hairs in a field of trichoscopy are almost diagnostic of AA.[10]

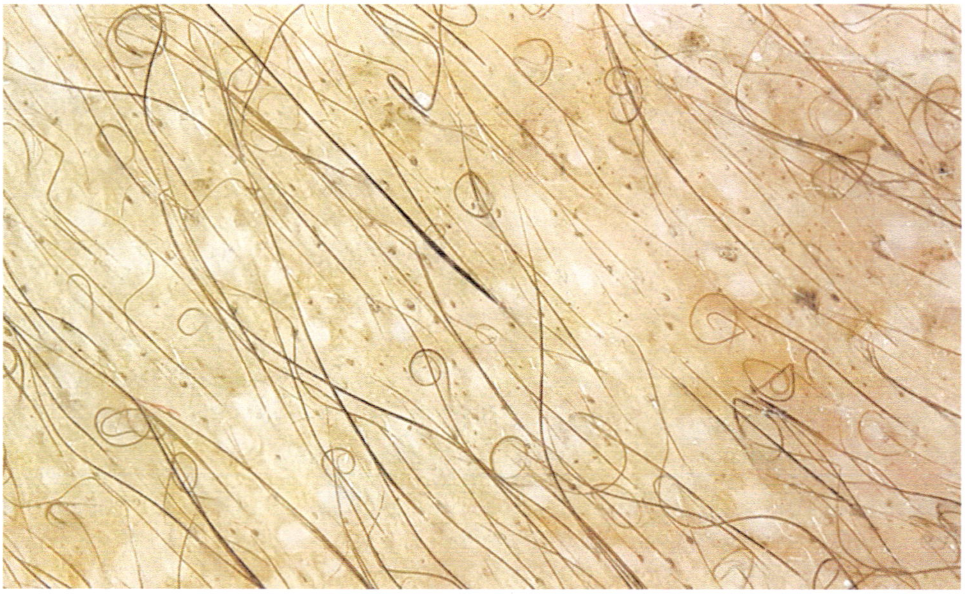

Fig. 5: Circle hairs in alopecia areata (AA) may be the predominant feature.[10]

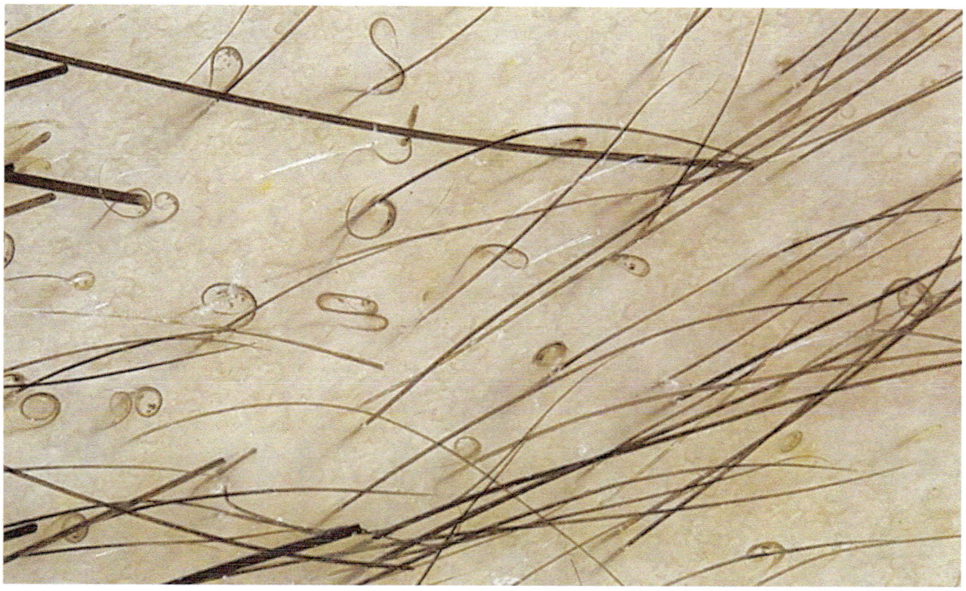

Fig. 6: Circle hairs (short vellus hairs) may be the solitary feature of alopecia areata (AA).

Broken Hairs

- Hair shafts are broken at different levels from the scalp.
- They may be found in nonscarring and scarring alopecias.
- Broken hairs are mostly found in trichotillomania (TTM), tinea capitis, alopecia areata, and after hair styling procedures.[11]

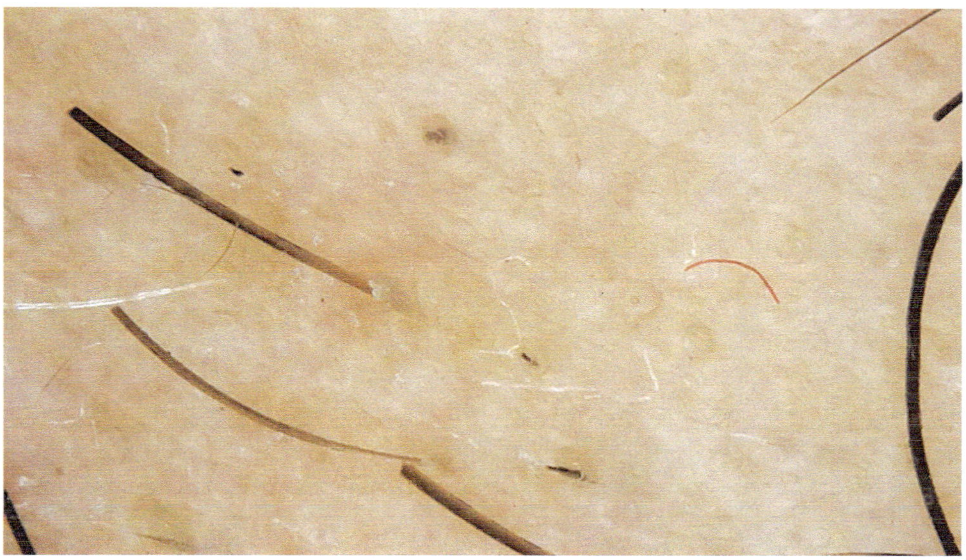

Fig. 7: Broken hairs in alopecia areata.[11]

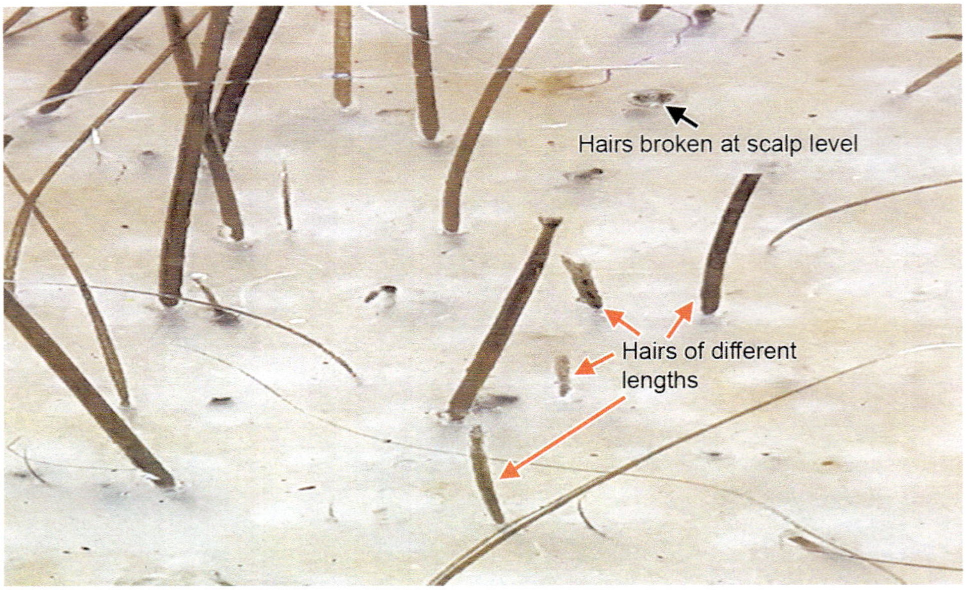

Fig. 8: Hairs of different heights are seen in the field. This feature is highly suggestive of trichotillomania (TTM).

Trichoptilosis

- These hairs have split ends and characteristically they are irregular and uneven.
- It is a frequent finding in healthy individual where it affects the distal ends of long hairs that have not been cut for a while.
- In trichotillomania, it affects the short hairs.[12]

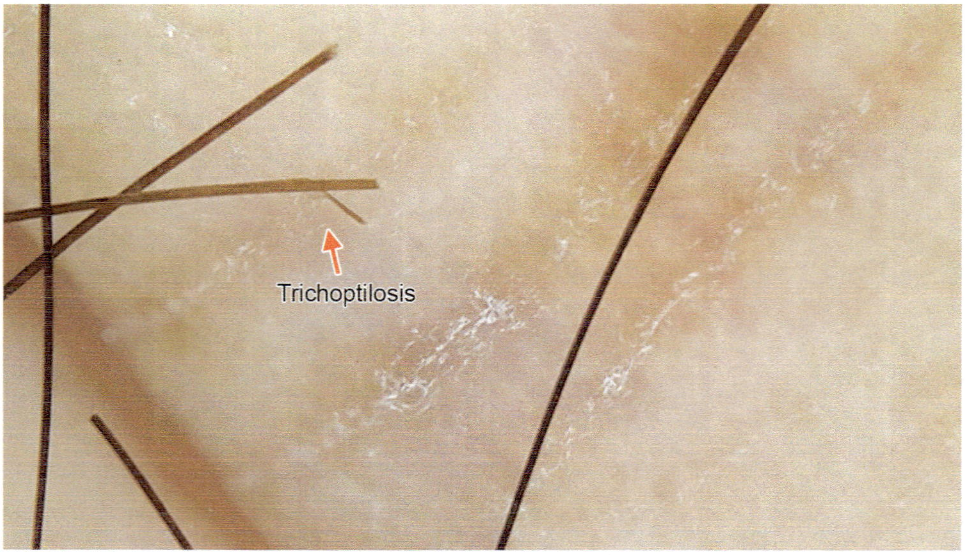

Fig. 9: Trichoptilosis is shown by red arrow. Short hairs[12] are affected in this field.

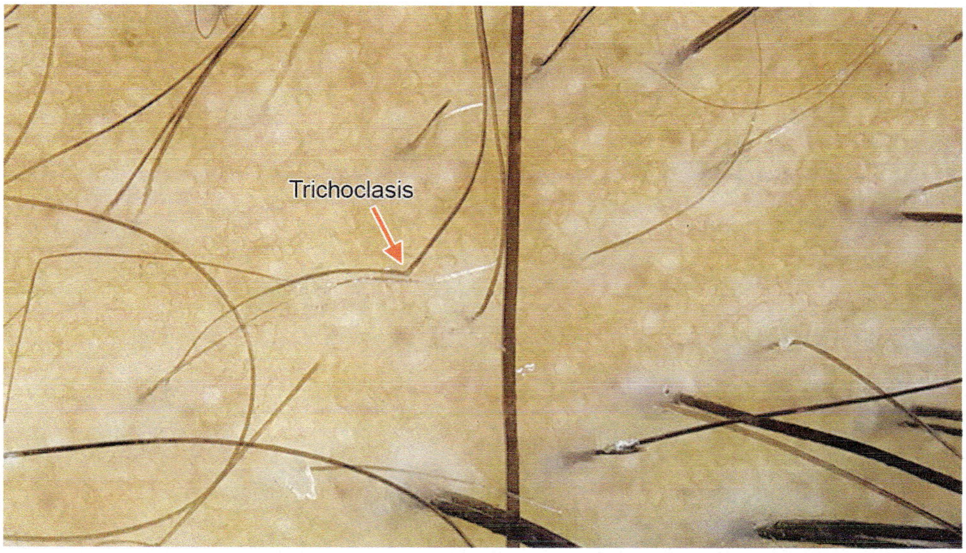

Fig. 10: Trichoclasis: a clean transverse fracture across hair shaft. Develops secondary to conditions that weaken the hair.[13]

Tapering Hairs

- Tapering hairs include exclamation mark hairs and coudability hairs.[9,14]
- Exclamation mark hair is a broken hair with a dark, frayed, thick tip; its proximal portion is thin and hypopigmented. They are typically seen in AA. Also can be found in chemotherapy-induced alopecia.[15]
- Coudability describes hairs of normal length with a narrowed proximal tip.[9,14] They are highly suggestive of AA where they are found at the periphery of the patches.

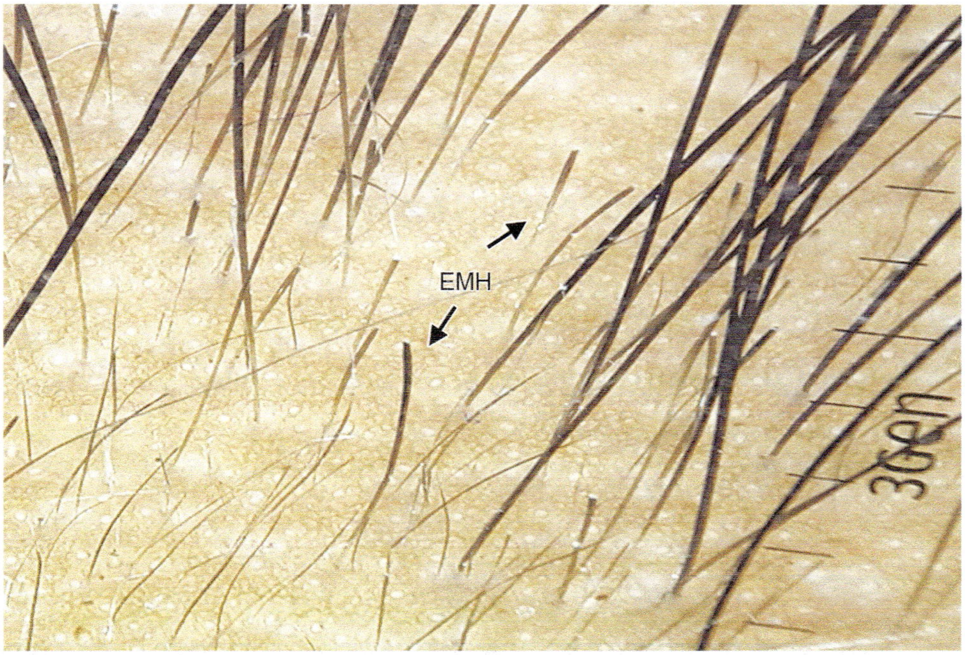

Fig. 11: Exclamation mark hairs (EMH): tapered hairs with dark ends. Highly suggestive of alopecia areata (AA), mostly along the border of the patches.[15]

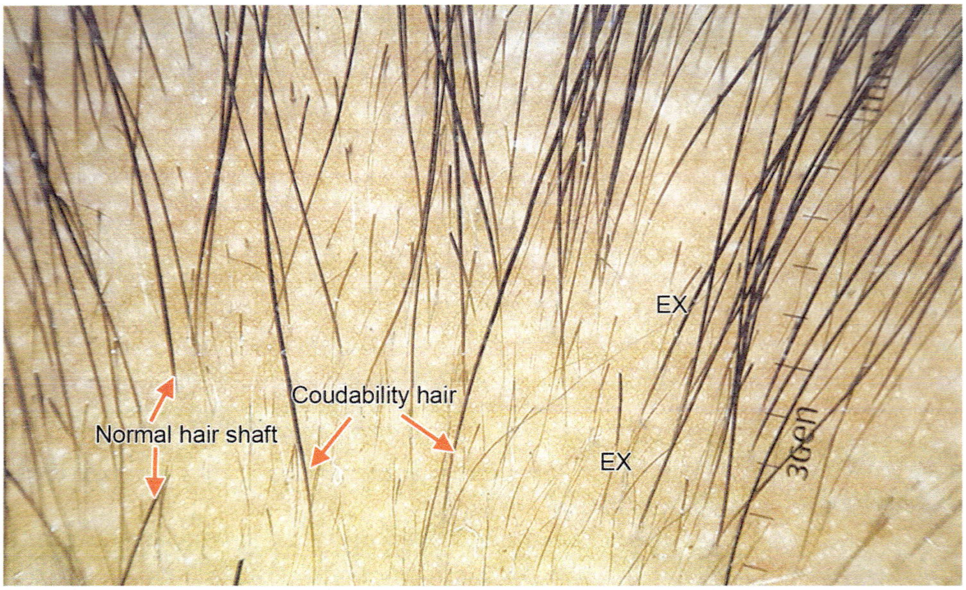

Fig. 12: Coudability hairs and exclamation mark hairs (EMH): coudability hairs are hairs of normal length with a narrowed proximal shaft. Mostly found in the scalp surrounding the patch. Compare it with normal hairs that have normal thickness throughout its whole length. The field is full of exclamation mark and coudability hairs that are marker of active disease.[9]

Flame Hairs

- Hairs become wavy and cone-shaped due to violent hair pulling. These hairs are called flame hairs because of their characteristic shape.
- They are highly diagnostic of TTM.
- They are found also in other nonscarring alopecias like AA, chemotherapy alopecia, etc.
- Flame hairs correlate to pigmented casts at histopathology.[16]
- They may sometimes have variations (described in trichotillomania chapter).

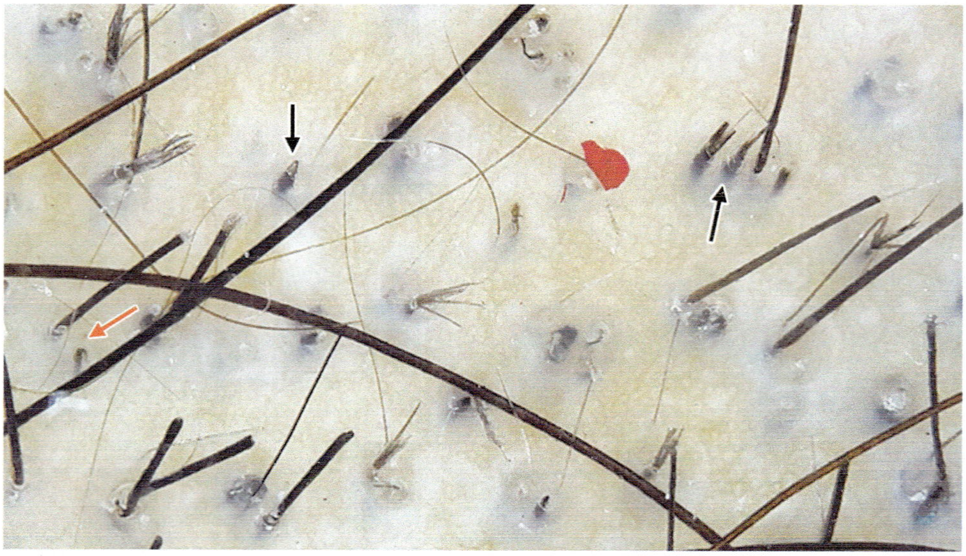

Fig. 13: Wavy and cone-shaped hairs (black arrows) are flame hairs. They are highly diagnostic of trichotillomania (TTM). Note the presence of coiled hair (red arrow) which is also a characteristic feature of TTM.[16]

Coiled Hairs

- Coiled hairs are broken hairs that curl back.
- Coiled hairs are most typical of TTM.
- But it may be present in small numbers in patients with traction alopecia.
- It may occur in healthy individual as a result of hair pulling during hairstyle procedures.[16]

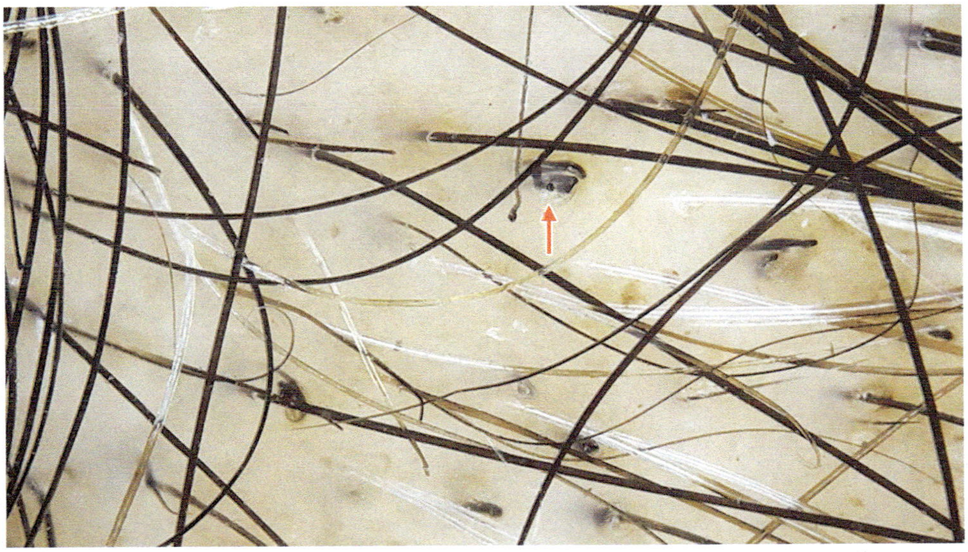

Fig. 14: Coiled hairs.

Mechanism of Development of Coiled Hairs

- Hair shaft fractures in response to a pulling force → remaining distal part that is fixed to the scalp, may contract and coil → coiled hairs.
- Partial coiling of the distal part results in a hook-like appearance. This is called hook hairs or question mark hairs.[16]

Coiled Hairs must be Differentiated from Pigtail Hairs

Pigtail hairs are new regrowing hairs. They are also coiled but they are uniform in thickness and color and regular in shape.[16]

Comma Hairs

- Comma hairs are a short c-shaped hair resembling comma.
- Highly diagnostic of tinea capitis
- Seen both in endo- and ectothrix parasitation.[17]

Corkscrew Hairs

- Short hairs, spiral in shape resembling corkscrew
- Found in tinea capitis
- Seen both in endo- and ectothrix parasitation.[18]

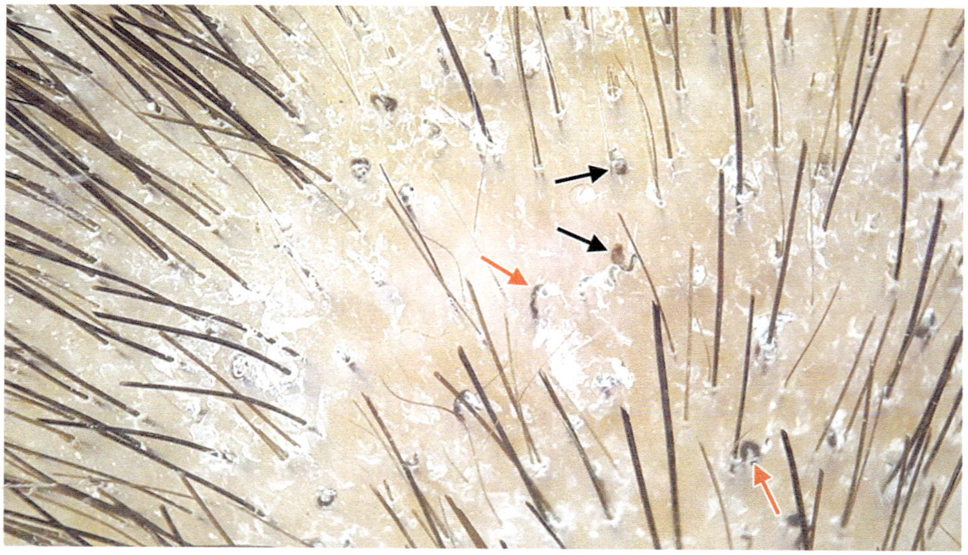

Fig. 15: Comma hairs (red arrows) and corkscrew hairs (black arrows) in tinea capitis.

Tufted Hairs

- When a bunch of hairs are present in a hair follicle, it is called tufted hairs.
- Tufting is found in scarring alopecias such as folliculitis decalvans, LPP, acne keloidalis nuchae, etc.
- It may be surrounded by peripilar cast.[19]

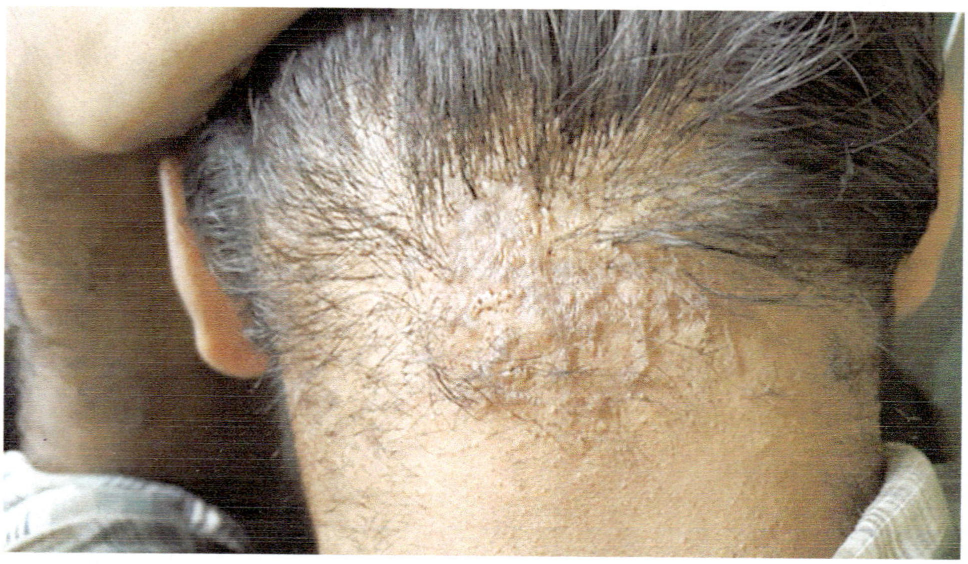

Fig. 16: A case of acne keloidalis nuchae (AKN).

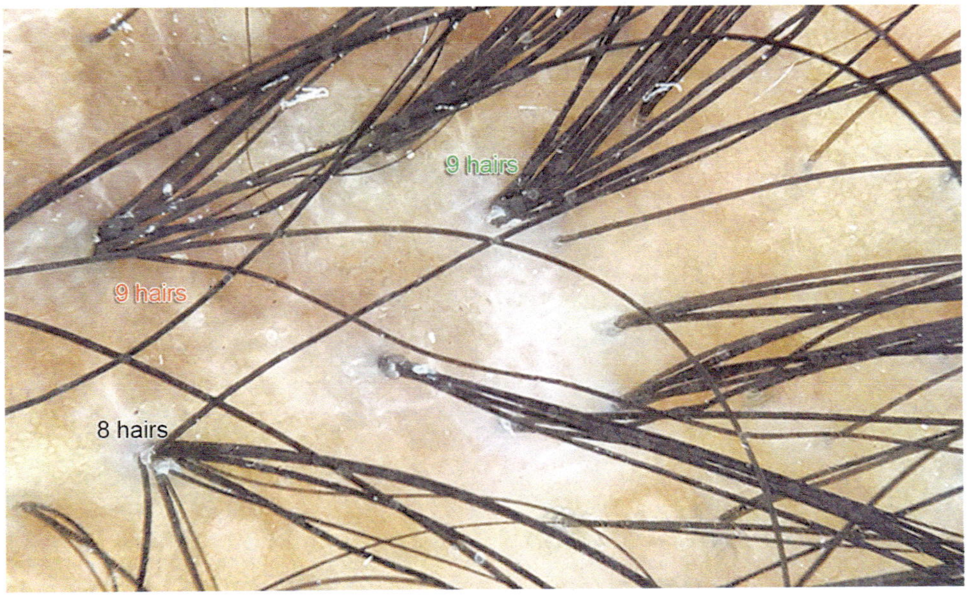

Fig. 17: Tufted hairs. The field is full of tufts. Shown are tufts of various sizes. The number indicates the number of hairs per hair follicle.[19]

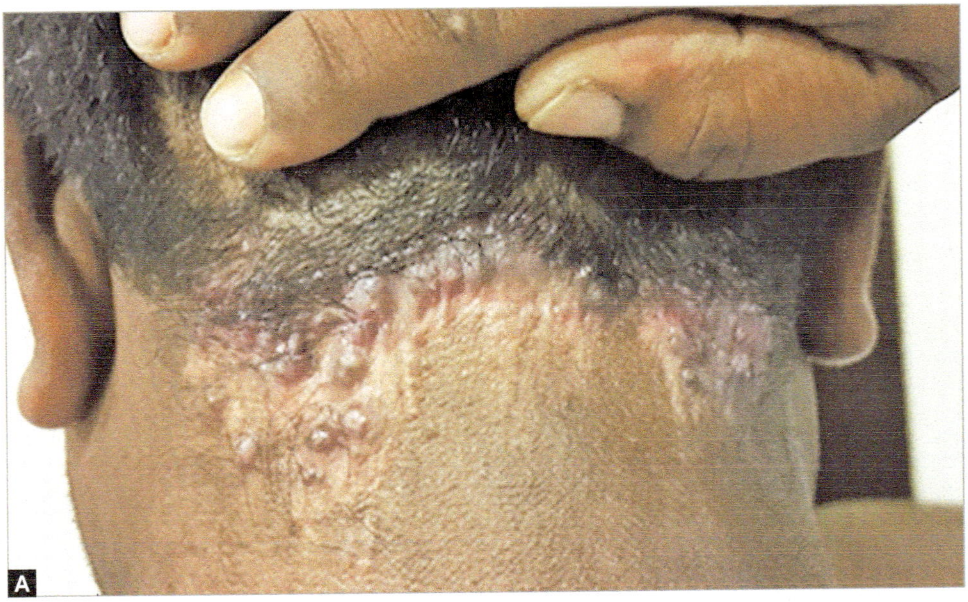

Continued

Continued

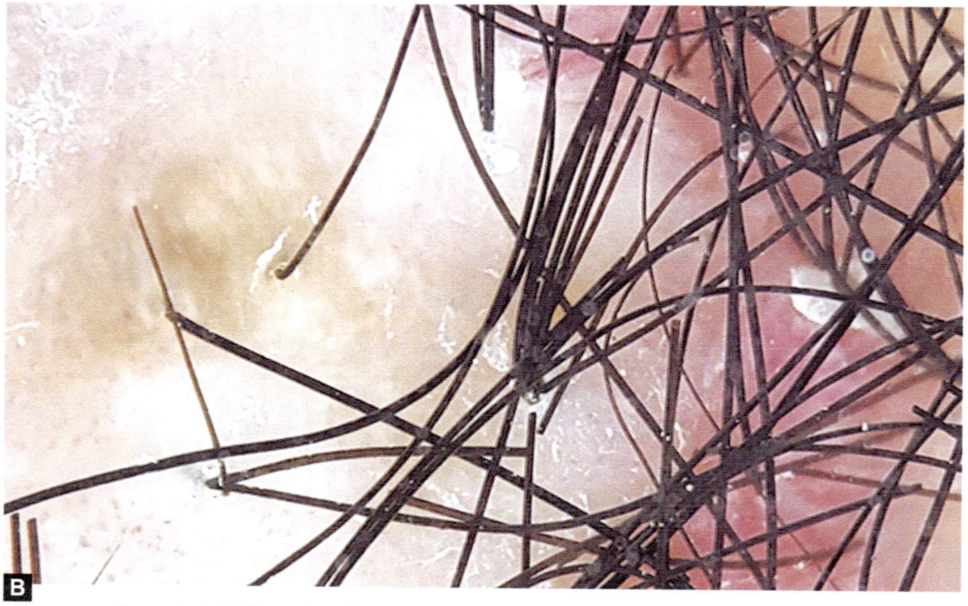

Figs. 18A and B: Another case of acne keloidalis nuchae (AKN) with tufted hairs.[20] The left part of the image shows an area of scarring alopecia characterized by lack of follicular openings.

Hair Diameter Diversity

- Hallmark of AGA.
- It means simultaneous presence of thin, intermediate, and thick hairs. This finding corresponds to hair follicle miniaturization. The miniaturization affects different follicles to different degrees. When a follicle is fully miniaturized, it produces thin vellus hairs.[6,21]
- Hair diameter diversity >20% is diagnostic of AGA.
- This feature can also be found in AA. However in AA, it shows uniform miniaturization instead of hair shafts with different degrees of thinning which is characteristic of AGA.

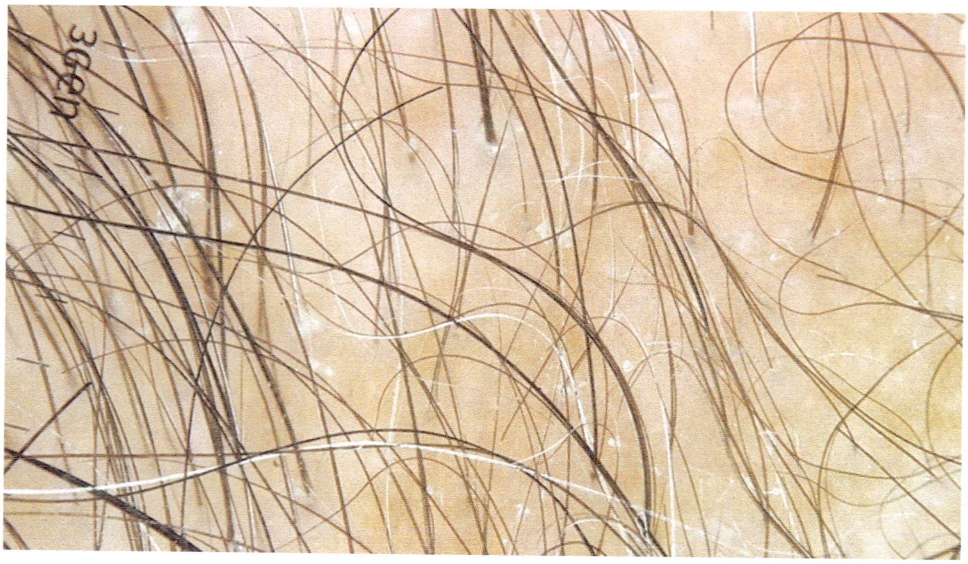

Fig. 19: Hair diameter diversity in androgenetic alopecia (AGA). Miniaturization affects different follicles to different degrees. Note the presence of thin, intermediate, and thick hairs.

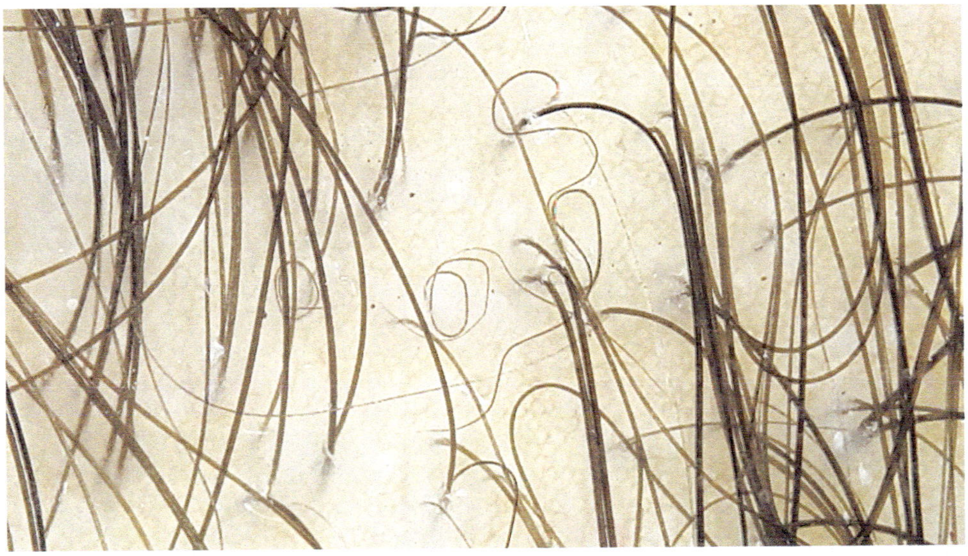

Fig. 20: This trichoscopic picture highlighted the thin wavy hairs which are intermediate in thickness between vellus and terminal hairs. Apart from androgenetic alopecia (AGA), it is also seen in alopecia areata (AA) incognito.

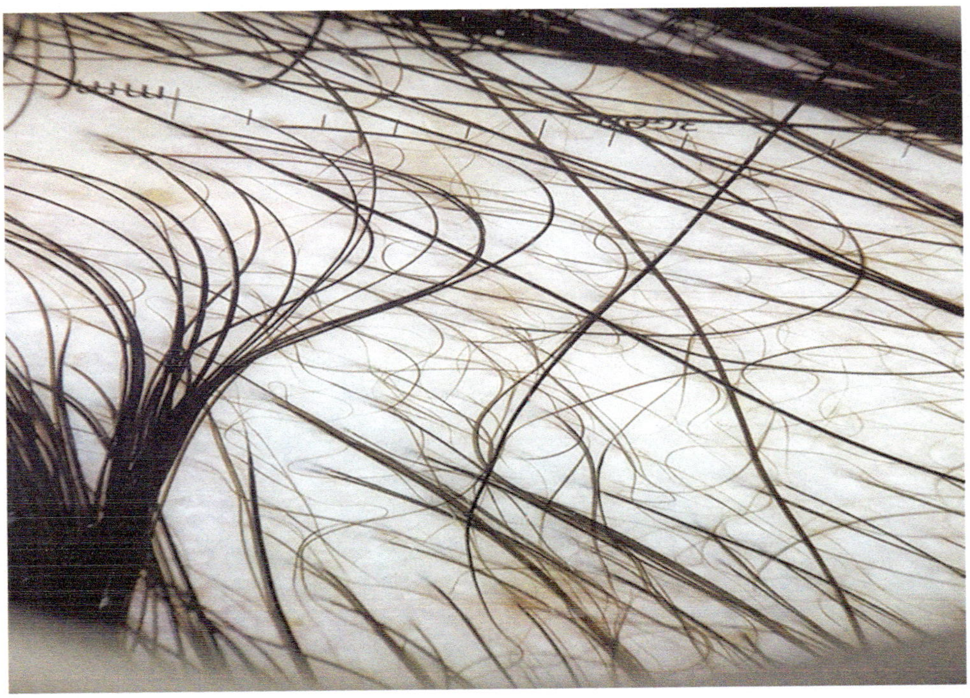

Fig. 21: Hair diameter diversity is seen in both androgenetic alopecia (AGA) and alopecia areata (AA). However in AA, there is uniform miniaturization.

DARK LINES[22]

- The follicular end of the hair is difficult to determine. Sometimes, the distinction between proximal and distal ends is impossible.
- These hairs are regrowing hairs and are thin, short, and pigmented.

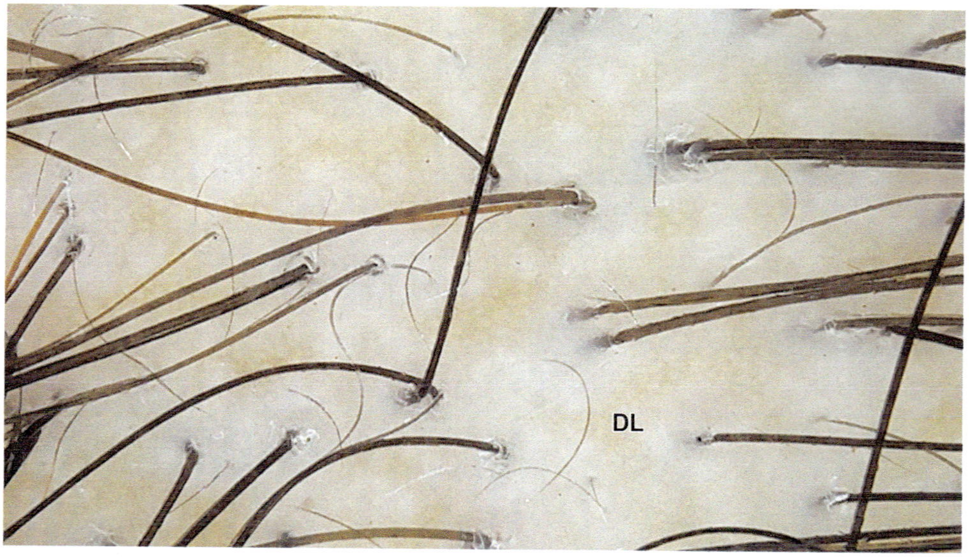

Fig. 22: Dark lines (DL).

ZIGZAG HAIRS/Z HAIRS[23]

- Zigzag hairs are sharply bent hairs at multiple points due to focal weakening of the hair shaft giving rise to zigzag patterns or "z" shape.
- They are not specific but can be found in tinea capitis, trichorrhexis nodosa, alopecia areata, and monilethrix.
- The mechanism of formation is not known.

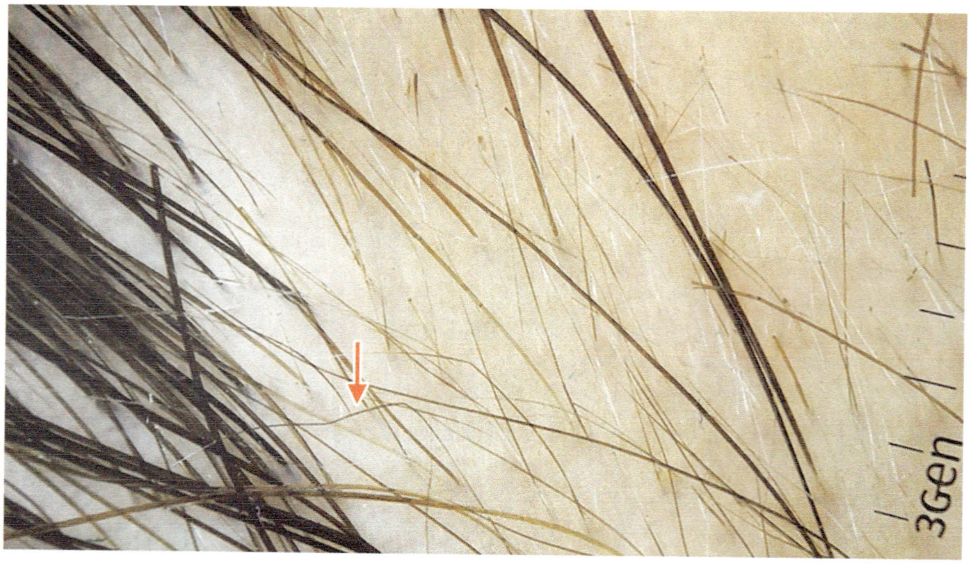

Fig. 23: Z hair in alopecia areata (AA).[24,25]

MEDULLA[26]

- Trichoscopy helps visualization of medulla that in normal individuals may be continuous, interrupted, or absent and these variations have no influence on their shaft properties.[26]

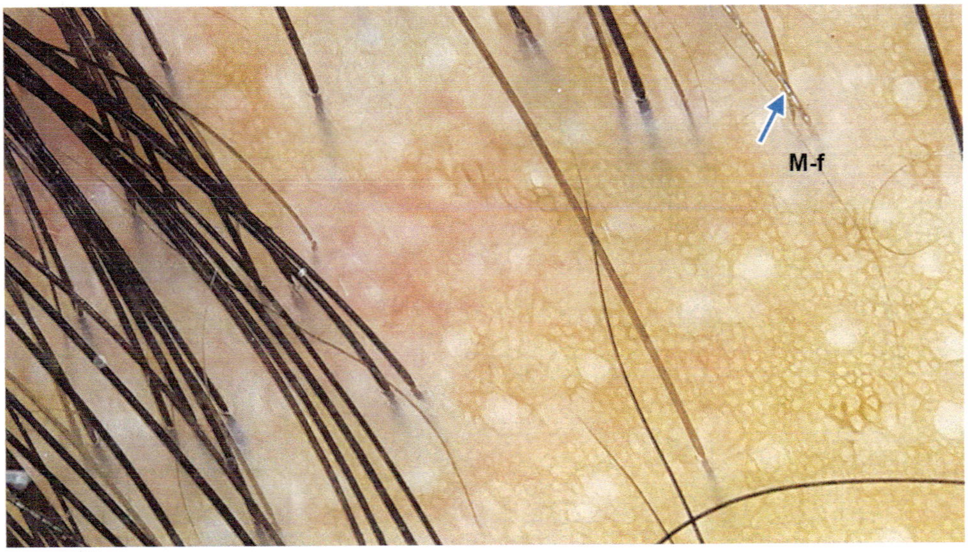

Fig. 24: Medulla—fragmented (M-f).

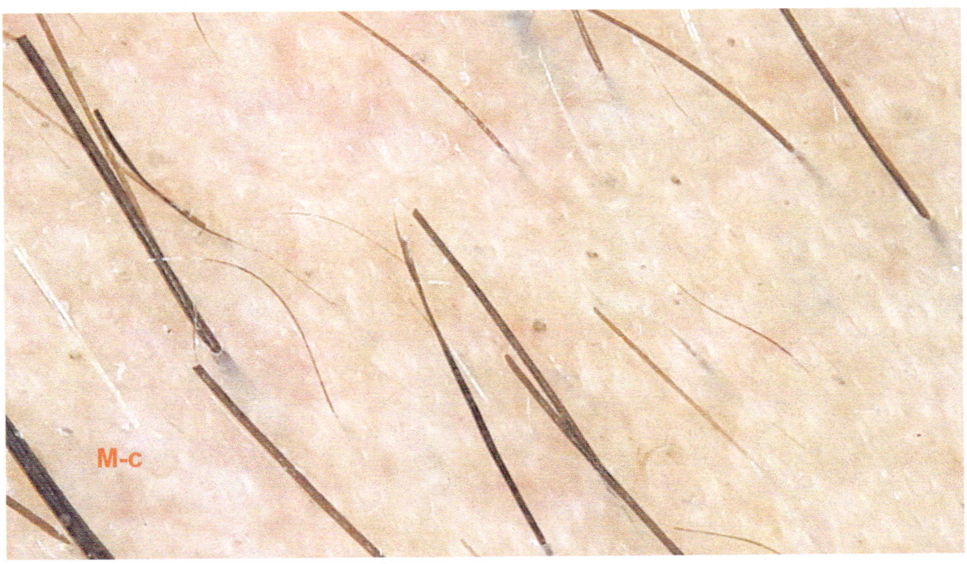

Fig. 25: Medulla—continuous (M-c).

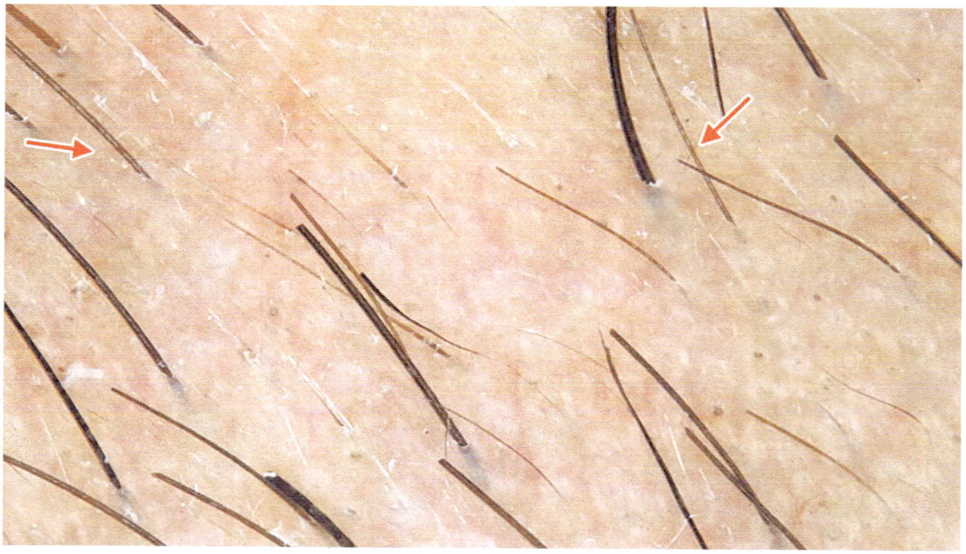

Fig. 26: Medulla—continuous and broken.

POHL-PINKUS CONSTRICTION

- Pohl-Pinkus constrictions are irregularly placed constrictions on a hair shaft.
- These hairs with constrictions may follow one of the two fates.
- The hair shaft may regain its original stature with due course of time with only a residual constriction which continues to be the weakest point of the shaft.
- If the ongoing pathology of the hair continues, the hair shaft becomes increasingly thinner and weaker leading to breakage, thereby forming the black dots or broken hairs.[27,28]

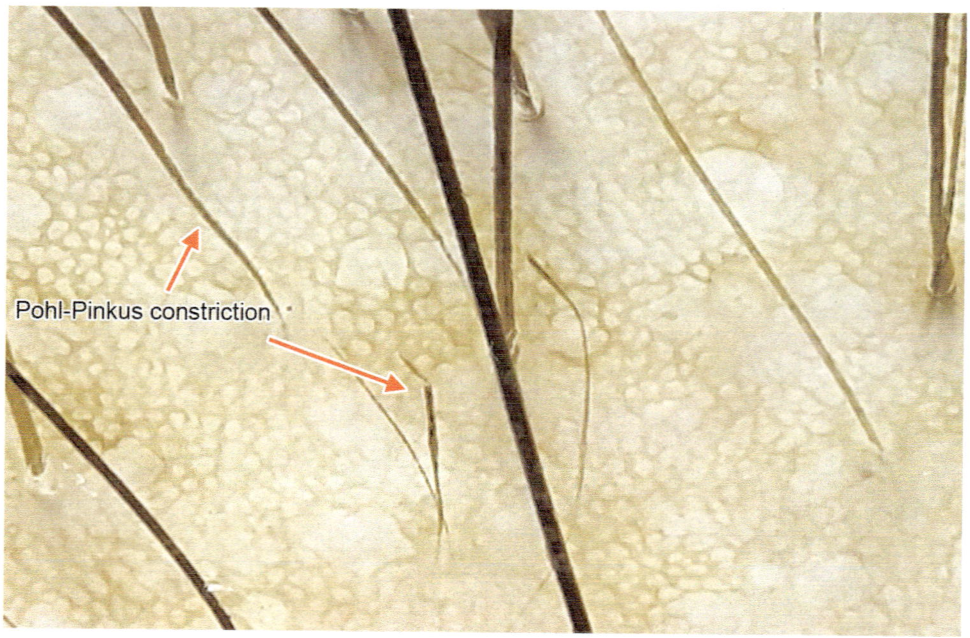

Fig. 27: Pohl-Pinkus.

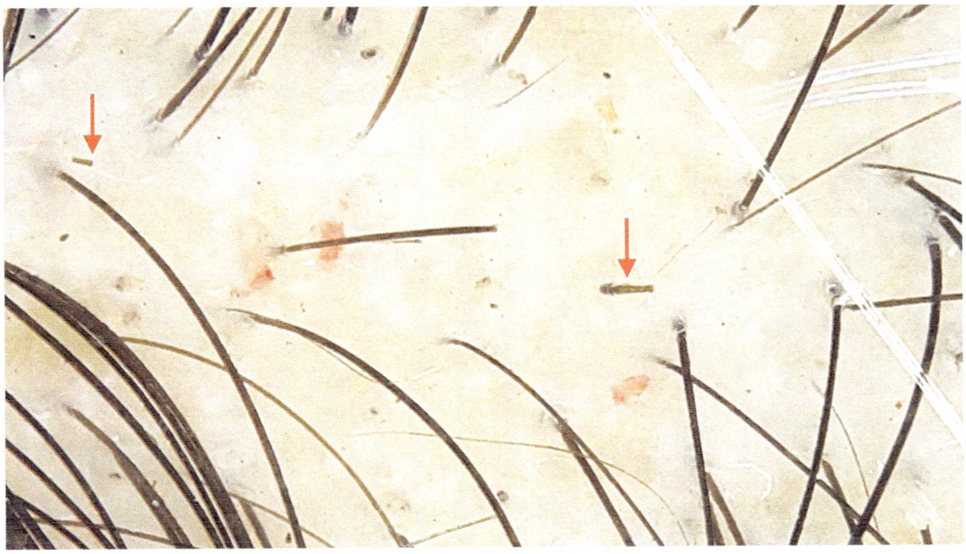

Fig. 28: Block hairs. They are very short hairs with horizontal distal ends. Block hairs are found in many acquired conditions including tinea capitis.[29]

i-hAIRS[29]

- i-hairs are described as short broken hairs with accentuated distal end forming the letter "i".
- If there is no distal accentuation, the same hair may be referred to as block hair.
- It may be seen in conditions with broken hair like trichotillomania and tinea capitis.

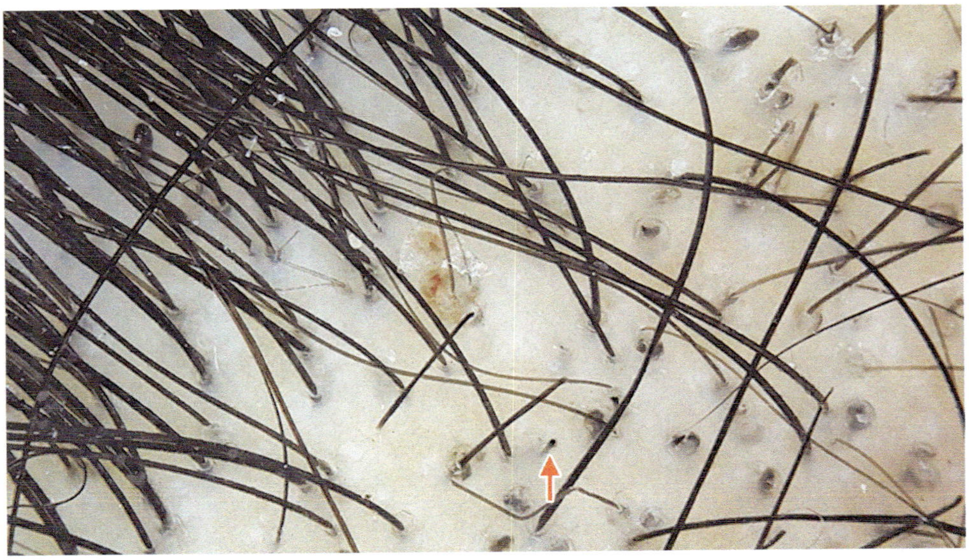

Fig. 29: i-hair (resembles the letter "i"). Otherwise chaotic picture seen commonly in trichotillomania (TTM).

REFERENCES

1. Rakowsky A. Trichoscopy in the healthy female. Method standardization and norms for measurable parameters. J Dermatol Case Rep. 2009;3(1):14-9.
2. Yazdabadi A, Magee J, Harrison S, Sinclair R. The Ludwig pattern of androgenetic alopecia is due to a hierarchy of androgen sensitivity within follicular units that leads to selective miniaturization and a reduction in the number of terminal hairs per follicular unit. Br J Dermatol. 2008;159(6):1300-2.

3. Rakowsa A, Olszewska M, Rudnica L. Telogen effluvium. In: Rudnica L, Olszewska M, Rakowsa A (Eds). Atlas of Trichoscopy. London: Springer; 2012. pp. 241-44.
4. Rakaowsky A. trichoscopy in the healthy female. J Dermatol Case Rep. 2009;3(1):14-9.
5. Vogt A, MacElwee KJ, Blume-Peytavi U. Hair: From basic science to clinical application. Berlin: Springer; 2008. pp. 1-22.
6. Inui S, NakajimaT, Itami S. Scalp dermoscopy of androgenic alopecia in Asian people. J Dermatol. 2009;36(2):82-5.
7. Van Neste D. Natural scalp hair regression in preclinical stage of male androgenetic alopecia and its reversal by finasteride. Skin Pharmacol Physiol. 2006;19(3):82-5.
8. Rakowsa A, Olszewska M, Rudnica L, Slowinska M, Czuwara J, Rusek M, et al. Hair shafts. In: Rudnica L, Olszewska M, Rakowsa A (Eds). Atlas of Trichoscopy. London: Springer; 2012. p. 11.
9. Inui S, Nakajima T, Itami S. Coudability hairs: a revisited sign of alopecia areata assessed by trichoscopy. Clin Exp Dermatol. 2010;35:361-5.
10. Rakowsa A, Olszewska M, Rudnica L, Slowinska M, Czuwara J, Rusek M, et al. Hair shafts. In: Rudnica L, Olszewska M, Rakowsa A (Eds). Atlas of Trichoscopy. London: Springer; 2012. p. 28.
11. Rudnica L, Olszewska M, Rakowsa A, Czuwara J. Alopecia areata. In: Rudnica L, Olszewska M, Rakowsa A (Eds). Atlas of Trichoscopy. London: Springer; 2012. p. 211.
12. Rudnica L, Olszewska M, Rakowsa A. Trichotillomania and traction alopecia. In: Rudnica L, Olszewska M, Rakowsa A (Eds). Atlas of Trichoscopy: London: Springer; 2012. p. 263.
13. Rakowsa A, Olszewska M, Rudnica L, Slowinska M, Czuwara J, Rusek M, et al. Hair shafts. In: Rudnica L, Olszewska M, Rakowsa A (Eds). Atlas of Trichoscopy. London: Springer; 2012. p. 19.
14. Shuster S. 'Coudability': a new physical sign of alopecia areata. Br J Dermatol. 1984;111:629.
15. Rakowsa A, Olszewska M, Rudnica L, Slowinska M, Czuwara J, Rusek M, et al. Hair shafts. In: Rudnica L, Olszewska M, Rakowsa A (Eds). Atlas of Trichoscopy. London: Springer; 2012. p. 25.
16. Rudnica L, Olszewska M, Rakowsa A. Trichotillomania and traction alopecia. In: Rudnica L, Olszewska M, Rakowsa A (Eds). Atlas of Trichoscopy. London: Springer; 2012. pp. 264-7.
17. Slowniska M, Rudnicka L, Schwartz RA, Kowalska-Oledzka E, Rakowska A, Sicinska J, et al. Comma hairs: a dermatoscopic marker for tinea capitis: a rapid diagnostic method. J Am Acad Dermatol. 2008;59(5 Suppl):S77-9.
18. Hughes R, Chiaverini C, Bahadoran P, Lacour JP. Corkscrew hair: a new dermoscopic sign for diagnosis of tinea capitis in black children. Arch Dermatol. 2011;147(3):355-6.
19. Otberg N, Kang H, Alzolibani AA, Shapiro J. Folliculitis decalvans. Dermatol Ther. 2008;21:238-44.
20. Rudnicka L, Olszewska M, Rakowska A, Slowinska M, Czuwara J, Rusek M, et al. Hair shaft. In: Rudnicka L, Olszewska M, Rakowska A (Eds). Atlas in Trichoscopy. London: Springer; 2012. p. 45.
21. De Lacharriere O, Deloche C, Misciali C, Piraccini BM, Vincenzi C, Bastien P, et al. Hair diameter diversity: a clinical sign reflecting the follicle miniaturization. Arch Dermatol. 2001;137(5):641-6.
22. Rudnicka L, Olszewska M, Rakowska A, Slowinska M, Czuwara J, Rusek M, et al. Hair shaft. In: Rudnicka L, Olszewska M, Rakowska A (Eds). Atlas in Trichoscopy. London: Springer; 2012. p. 37.
23. Rudnicka L, Olszewska M, Rakowska A, Slowinska M, Czuwara J, Rusek M, et al. Hair shaft. In: Rudnicka L, Olszewska M, Rakowska A (Eds). Atlas in Trichoscopy. London: Springer; 2012. p. 41.
24. Rudnicka L, Olszewska M, Rakowska A, Slowinska M, Czuwara J, Rusek M, et al. Hair shaft. In: Rudnicka L, Olszewska M, Rakowska A (Eds). Atlas in Trichoscopy. London: Springer; 2012. p. 31.
25. Rudnicka L, Olszewska M, Rakowska A, Czuwara J. Alopecia Areata. In: Rudnicka L, Olszewska M, Rakowska A (Eds). Atlas of Trichoscopy. London: Springer; 2012. p. 216.
26. Wagner R, Joekes I. Hair medulla morphology and mechanical properties. J Cosmet Sci. 2007;58(4):359-68.
27. Mane M, Nath AK, Thappa DM. Utility of dermoscopy in alopecia areata. Indian J Dermatol. 2011;56(4):407-11.
28. Rudnicka L, Olszewska M, Rakowska A, Czuwara J. Alopecia Areata. In: Rudnicka L, Olszewska M, Rakowska A (Eds). Atlas of Trichoscopy. London: Springer; 2012. pp. 211-2.
29. Rudnicka L, Olszewska M, Rakowska A, Slowinska M, Czuwara J, Rusek M, et al. Hair shaft. In: Rudnicka L, Olszewska M, Rakowska A (Eds). Atlas in Trichoscopy. London: Springer; 2012. p. 38.

CHAPTER 7

Pattern of Scaly Scalp

Subrata Malakar

KEY TRICHOSCOPIC FEATURES

- Scales can be seen around the follicles, around the hair shafts and in the interfollicular space. Scales could be a useful clue to reach a diagnosis.
- *Perifollicular scales* may be found in lichen planopilaris (LPP), frontal fibrosing alopecia (FFA), discoid lupus erythematosus (DLE), ichthyosis vulgaris, folliculitis decalvans, etc.[1]
- *Scales surrounding the hair shaft* (hair casts) can be present in psoriasis, tinea capitis, seborrheic dermatitis, folliculitis decalvans, etc.
- *Interfollicular scales* are seen in psoriasis, seborrheic dermatitis, ichthyosis vulgaris, tinea capitis, DLE, etc.[2]
- In seborrheic capitis, a mixed pattern of peri- and interfollicular scales are seen.
- Caution should be exercised while differentiating between hair casts and nits.
- Hair casts can be appreciated by its cylindrical shape which surround the hair shafts.[3]
- Nits have an oval shape and do not surround the hair shaft.
- *Tips*: Dry dermoscopy is preferred to identify scales.

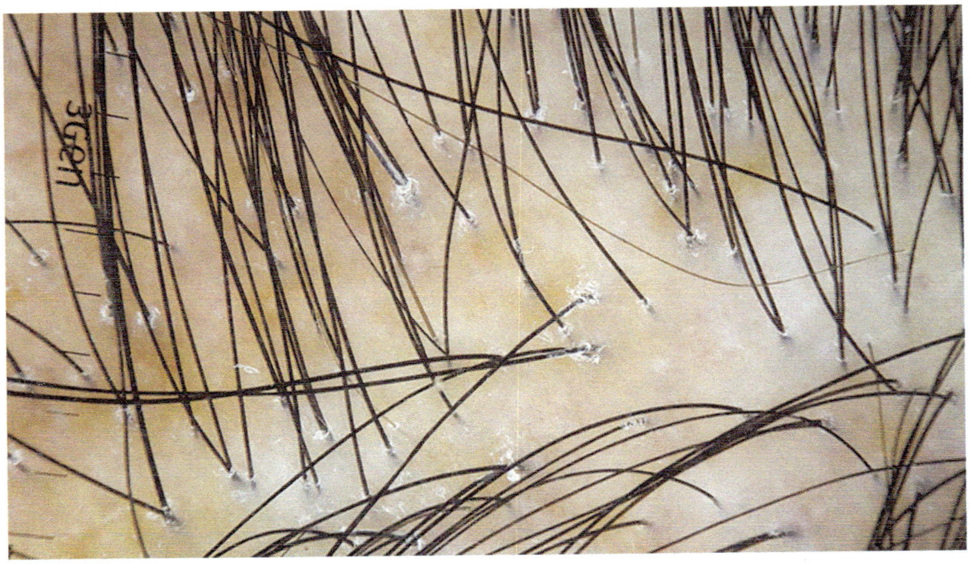

Fig. 1A: Perifollicular scales.

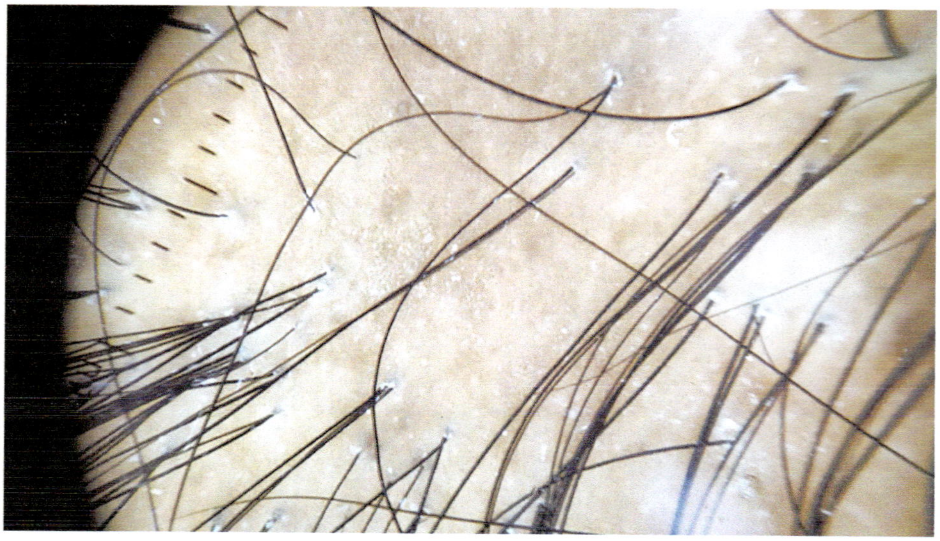

Fig. 1B: Another picture showing perifollicular scales.

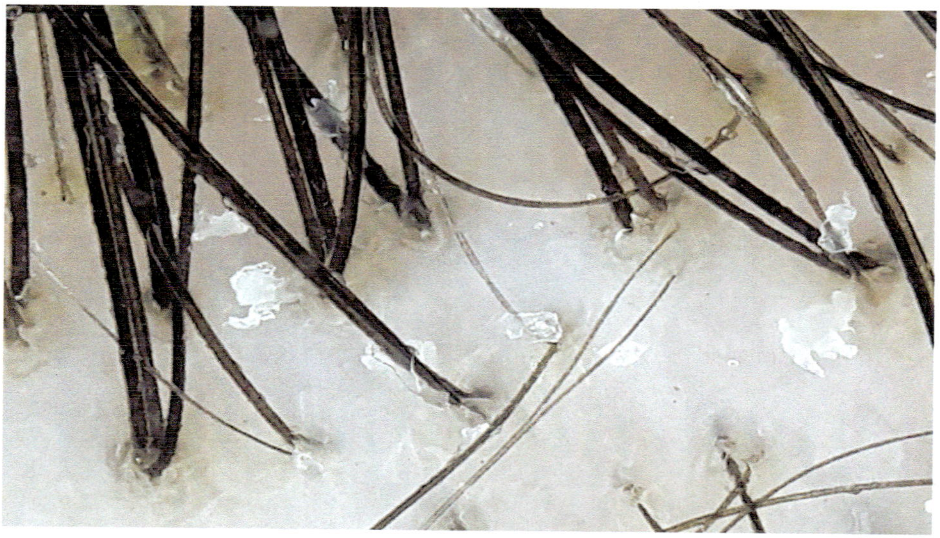

Fig. 2: Interfollicular scales.

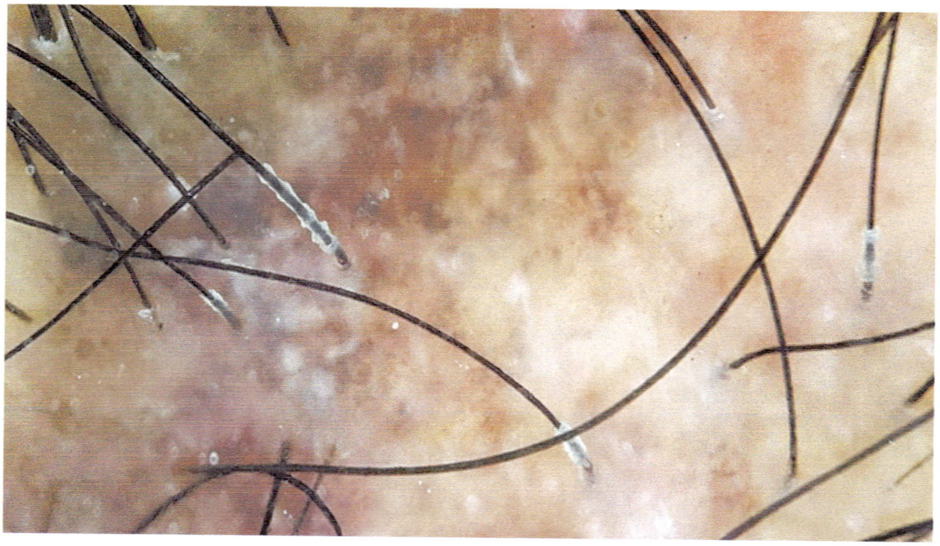

Fig. 3: Peripilar casts (hair casts).

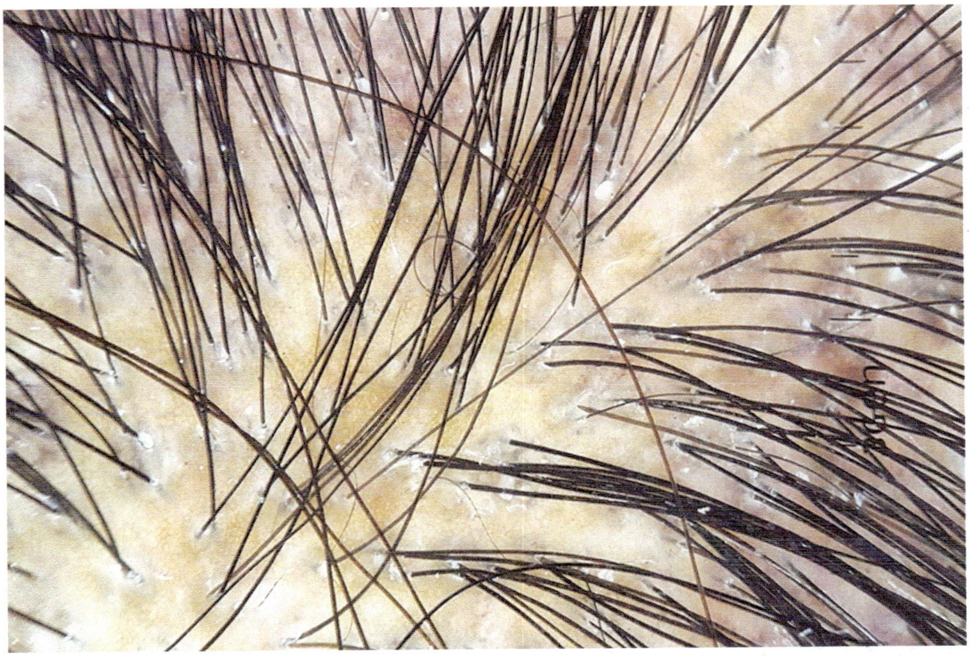

Fig. 4: Perifollicular scales in lichen planopilaris (LPP). Note the presence of blue–gray dots in target pattern which is highly suggestive of LPP.

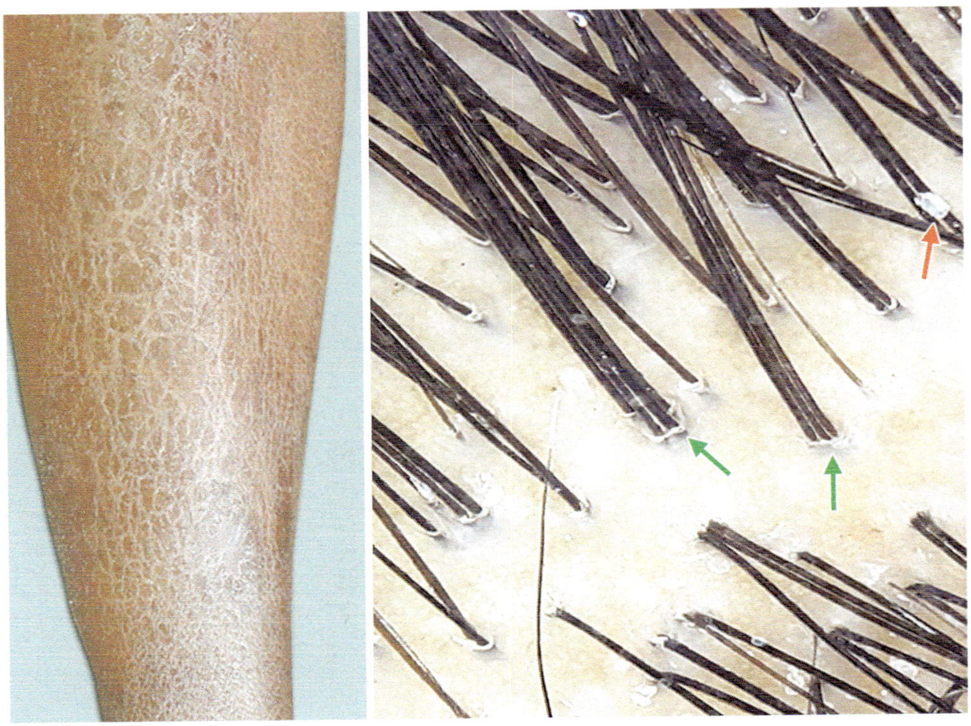

Fig. 5: Peripilar scales (green arrows) and hair casts (red arrow) in ichthyosis vulgaris.

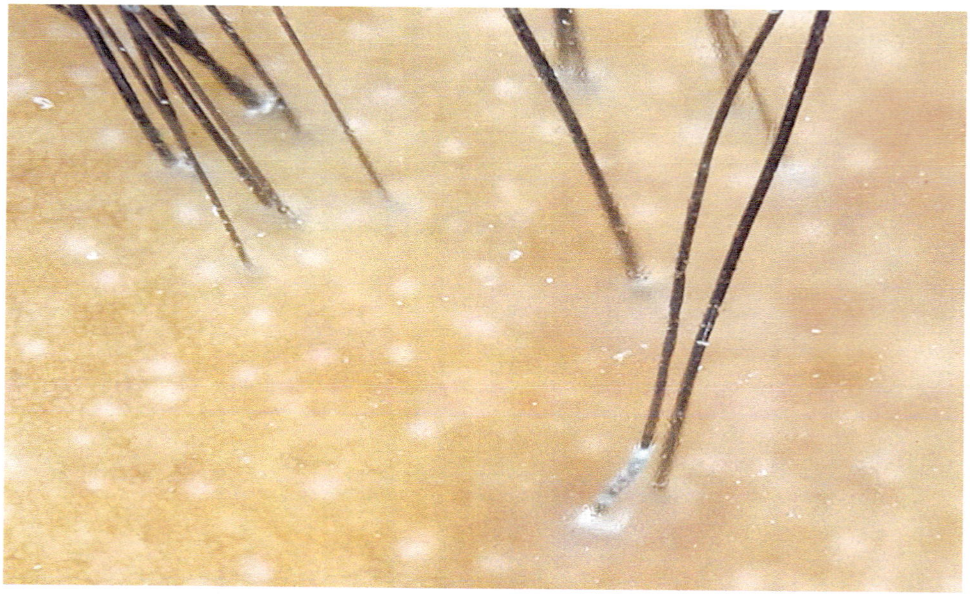

Fig. 6: Hair cast forms a silvery white tubular structure around the emerging hair shaft and is seen reaching a little distance above scalp surface. This is called perifollicular collar scaling which is a hallmark of lichen planopilaris (LPP).[2]

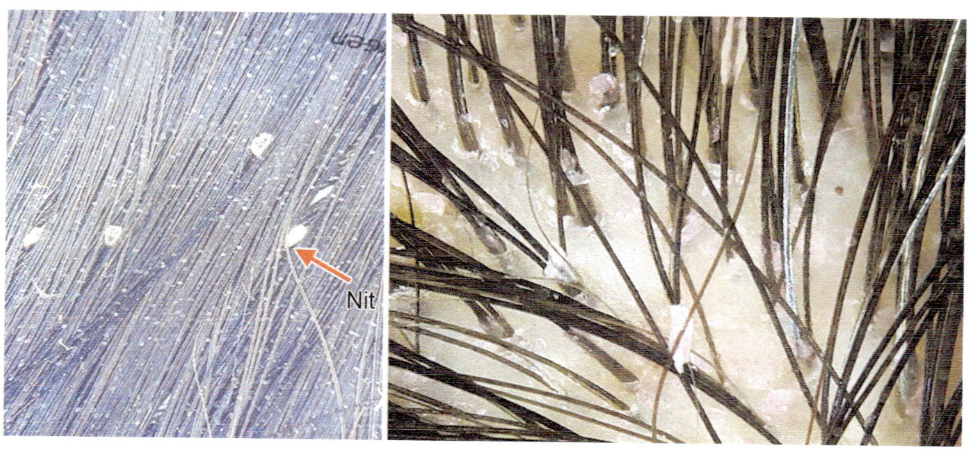

Fig. 7: Appreciate the difference between hair cast and nit. Nits have an oval shape and do not surround the shaft whereas hair casts surround the shaft.

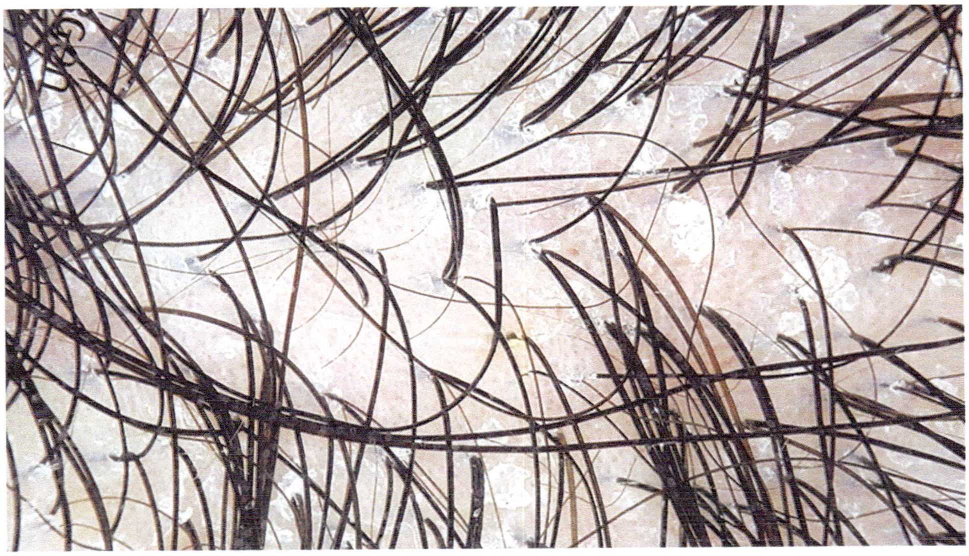

Fig. 8: Extensive interfollicular scales in psoriasis. Scales are silvery white. Red dots and twisted capillaries characteristic of psoriasis are arranged regularly.

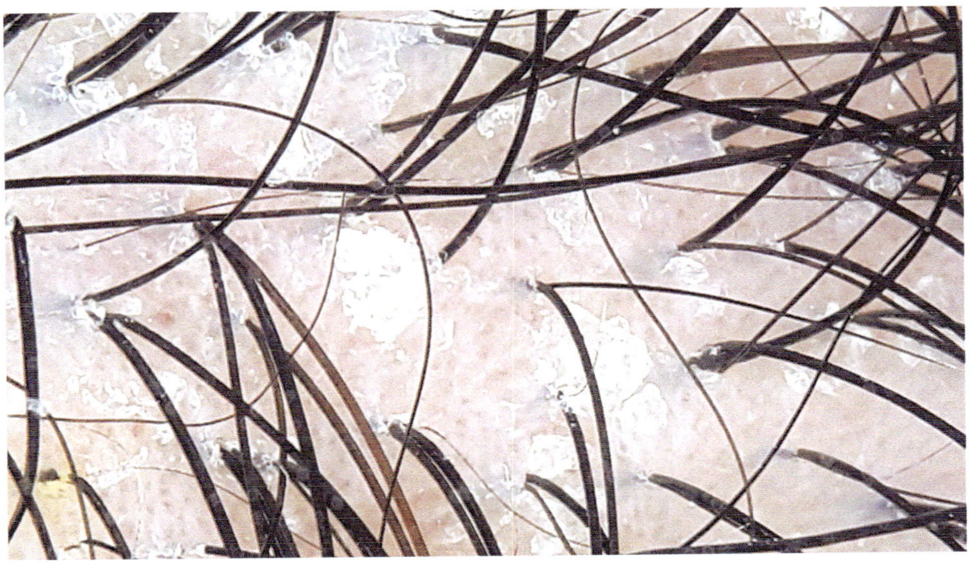

Fig. 9: Close-up view of interfollicular scales in a case of psoriasis.

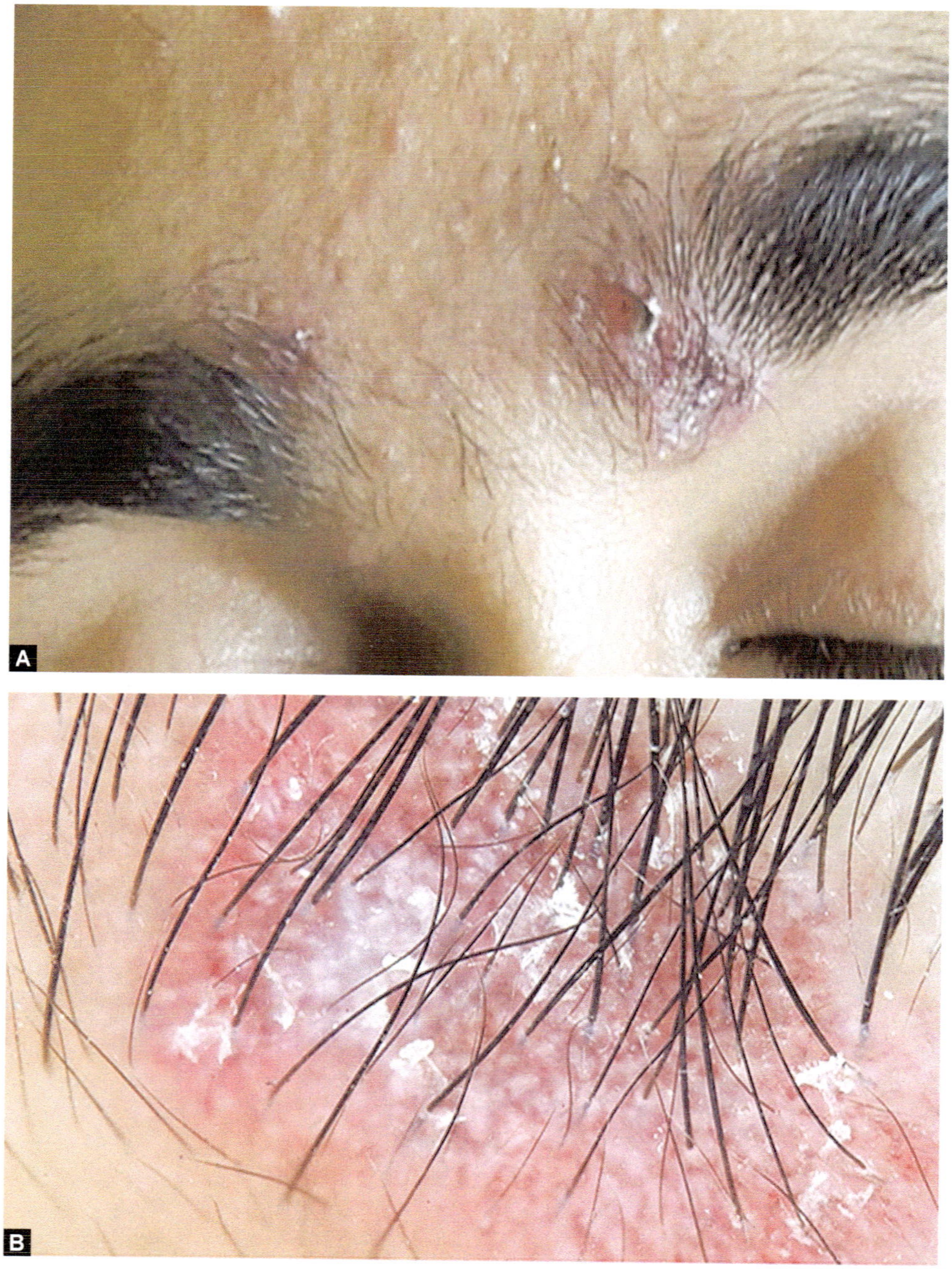

Figs. 10A and B: Seborrheic dermatitis of eyelid is commonly associated with seborrheic capitis. Note perifollicular and interfollicular scales.

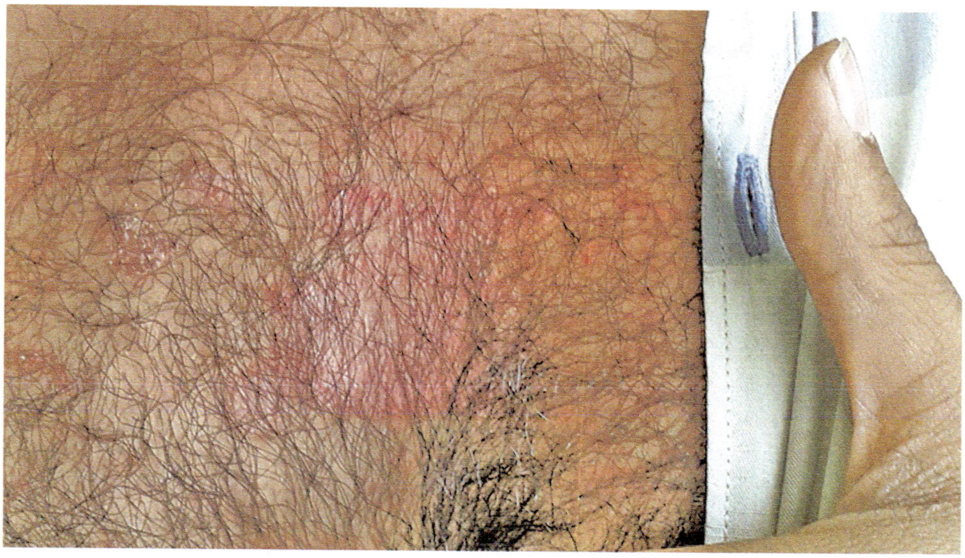

Fig. 11: Seborrheic dermatitis of chest and back is usually associated with seborrheic capitis.

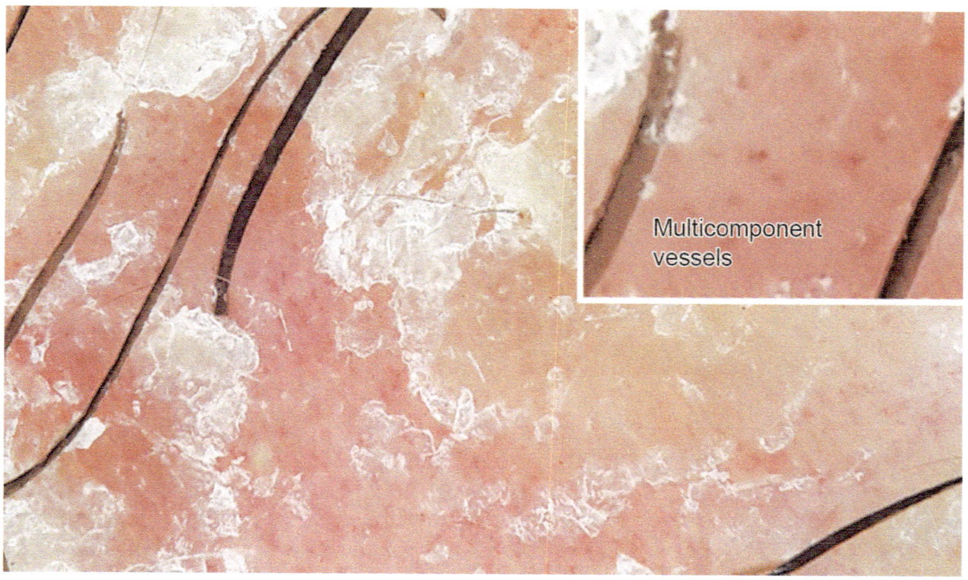

Fig. 12: Trichoscopy of the previous patient. Interfollicular scales seen in this image are yellowish in color. Note the background erythema with multicomponent vessels (refer to Chapter 27).

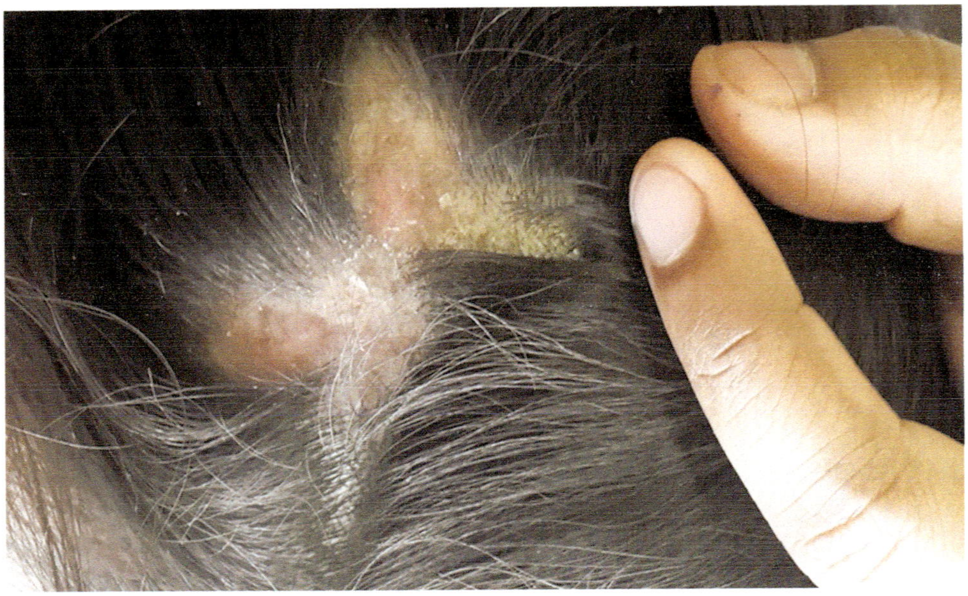

Fig. 13: Scarring alopecia in a longstanding case of discoid lupus erythematosus (DLE).

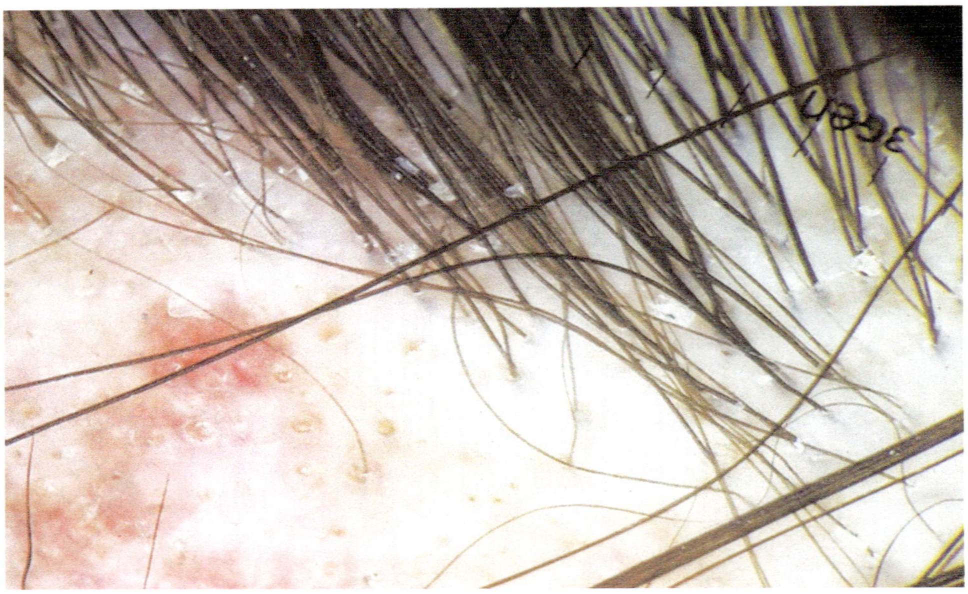

Fig. 14: Trichoscopy of the previous patient. Appreciate peripilar scaling, hair casts, and mild interfollicular scaling.

REFERENCES

1. Rakowska A, Slowinska M, Kowalska-Oledzka E, Warszawik O, Czuwara J, Olszewska M, et al. Trichoscopy of cicatricial alopecia. J Drugs Dermatol. 2012;11:753-8.
2. Rudnicka L, Olszewka M, Rakowska A, Slowinska M. Trichoscopy update 2011. J Dermatol Case Rep. 2011;5:82-8.
3. Rudnicka L, Rakowska A, Olszewka M. Trichoscopy: how it may help the clinician. Dermatol Clin. 2013:31:29-41.

ASSESSMENT IMAGE-BASED QUESTIONS

1. What is the location of the scales? What are the conditions where these type of trichoscopic scales are found?

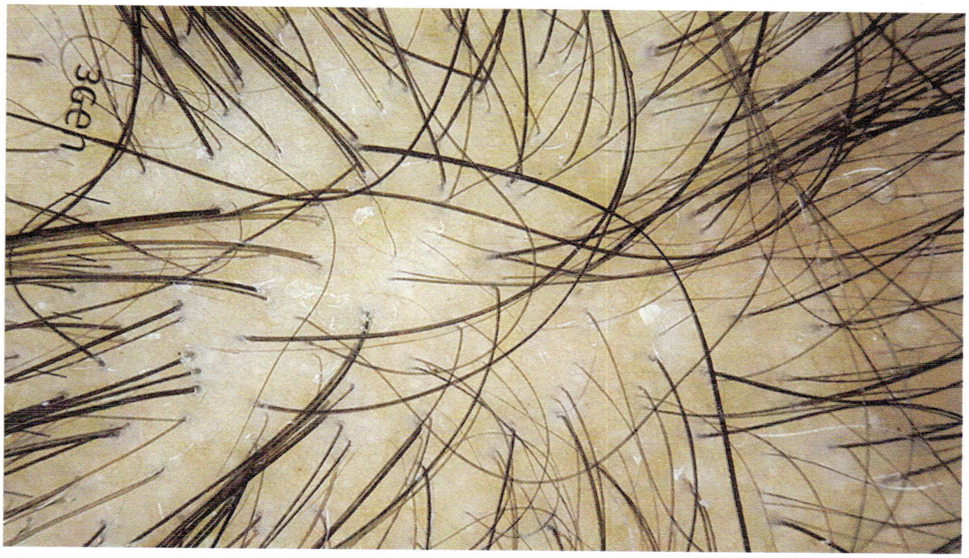

2. Image of the inset shows scarring alopecia with itching. This is the trichoscopic image of the same patient. What type of scales are seen? Can you diagnose the condition?

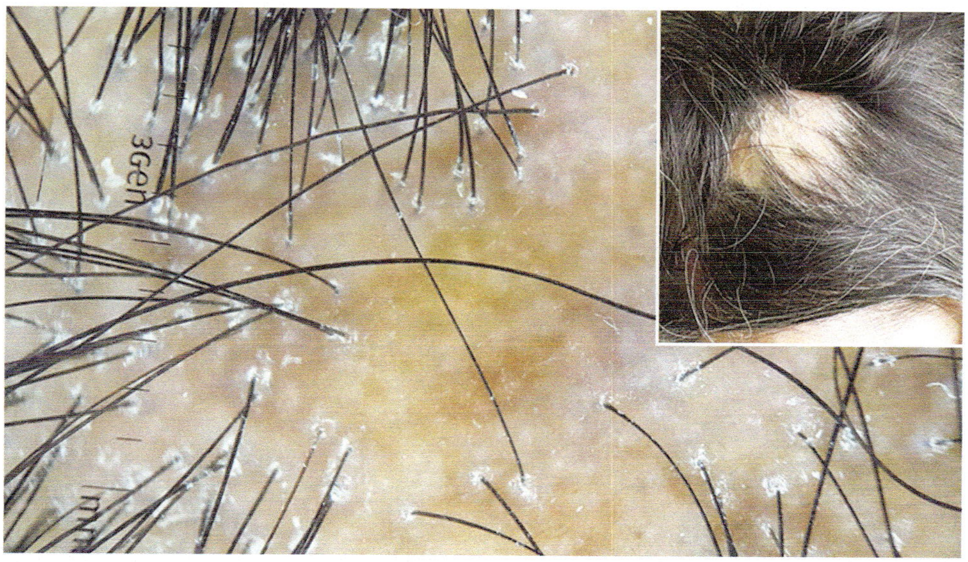

3. Mention the type of scale seen in this trichoscopic image.

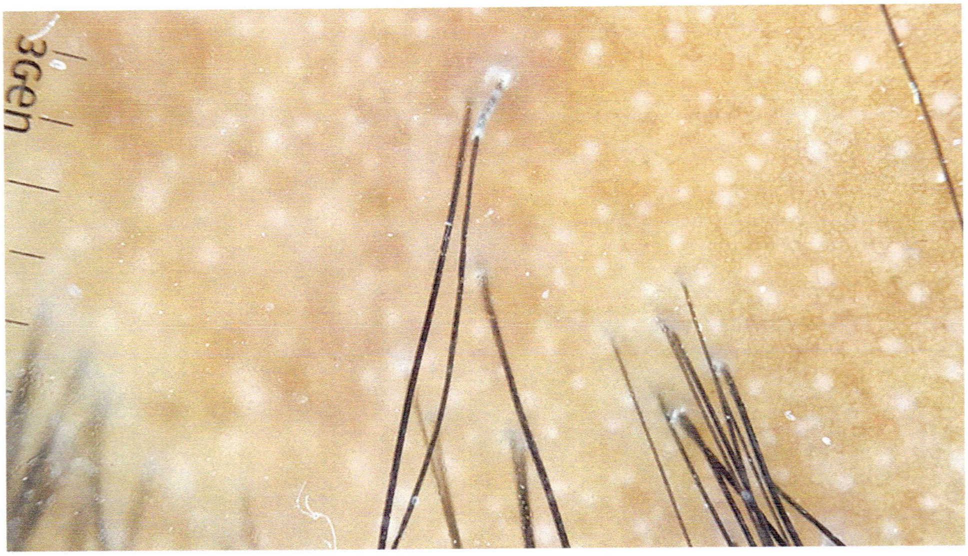

ANSWERS

1. Location of the scale is interfollicular. Interfollicular scales are found in psoriasis, seborrheic dermatitis, ichthyosis vulgaris, tinea capitis, DLE, etc.
2. Perifollicular scales are seen in this image. The diagnosis is lichen planopilaris because perifollicular scales are seen mostly around single hair and double hair containing follicles, blue-gray pigmentation in target pattern, less hair density and absence of hair follicles in the hairless area.
3. Perifollicular scale.

5

SECTION

Normal Scalp

CHAPTER

8

Normal Scalp

Subrata Malakar

KEY TRICHOSCOPIC FEATURES

- Honeycomb pigmented network
- Interfollicular white dots
- Hairs from follicular units emerge commonly in groups of twos. Single hair and groups of three hairs are also seen.
- Dirty dots
- Residues of products
- Interfollicular red loops and arborizing vessels

THREE STEPS OF TRICHOSCOPIC EXAMINATION OF NORMAL SCALP

1. Hair follicle openings
2. Hair shafts
3. Perifollicular and interfollicular scalp

Hair Follicle Openings

- The term "dots" were used to describe hair follicular openings by a dermoscopy device and the terms black dots, white dots, and yellow dots were applied for hair shaft residues, perifollicular fibrosis, and keratosebaceous material in the infundibulum respectively.[1]
- Black dots are residues of pigmented hairs broken at scalp level.[1] They are not present in healthy individuals.[2]
- White dots are of two types. Fibrotic white dots represent follicular fibrosis. In advanced cases of scarring alopecias, white dots merge with each other and form white areas lacking follicular openings. The other type of white dots are pinpoint white dots observed in skin of color.[3,4] They correspond to empty hair follicles or to the openings of acrosyringium of eccrine sweat glands.

Yellow Dots

- Yellow dots are round yellowish dots over the scalp observed in all the magnifications.
- They can be empty, or may contain vellus hairs or broken hairs.
- They correspond histopathologically to dilated infundibulum filled with keratosebaceous material.[1,5,6]
- They may not be visible in dark phenotypes but are easily recognized in Caucasians. Yellow dot, however, looks more whitish than yellow on a pigmented scalp and more precisely it is centrally white with a yellowish halo (author's observation).
- Yellow dots are typical of alopecia areata (AA) where they are regularly distributed and are a marker of disease activity.[7]
- Large brownish-yellow dots are found in discoid lupus erythematosus (DLE) which correspond to wide infundibula mainly filled with keratotic material.[5]

- In AGA, yellow dots consist mainly of sebum and the amount of keratotic material is usually minimum.[8]
- In female pattern hair loss (FPHL), yellow dots are present mainly over the frontal scalp in comparison to the occipital area.[8]
- Yellow dots may also be present in alopecia areata incognito (AAI), trichotillomania (TTM) and chemotherapy alopecia.

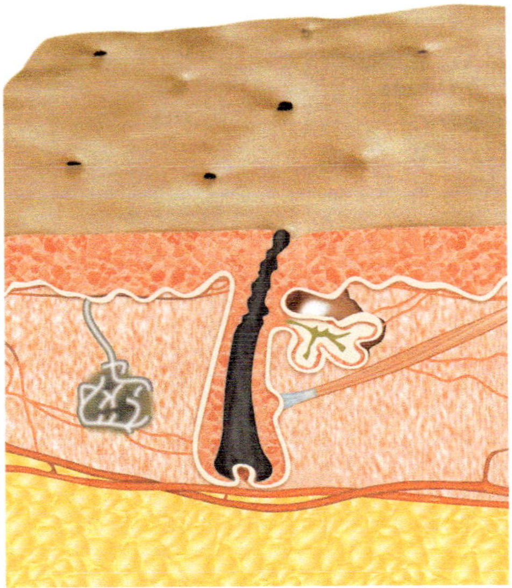

Fig. 1: "Dots". Hair follicle openings seen from the perspective of a dermoscopic lens. These hair follicle openings may have different features depending on the presence of hair follicle residues, e.g., "black dots" (as depicted in the image).

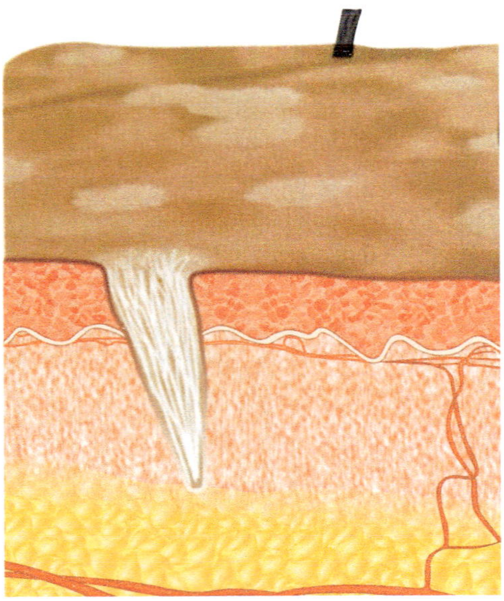

Fig. 2: "White dots" (fibrotic). Observed in scarring alopecias mainly lichen planopilaris. Trichoscopic fibrotic white dots correspond to histopathologic wedge-shaped fibrosis of scarring alopecia.

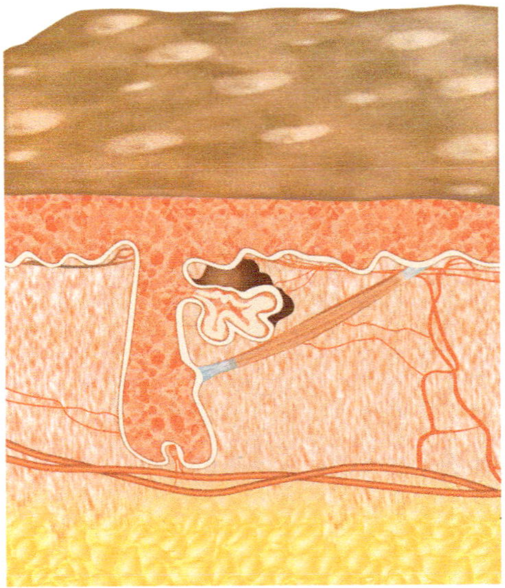

Fig. 3: "Pinpoint white dots". Correspond to the empty follicle openings and to the acrosyringium of eccrine sweat glands. Observed in most forms of non-cicatricial alopecia and in healthy individuals.

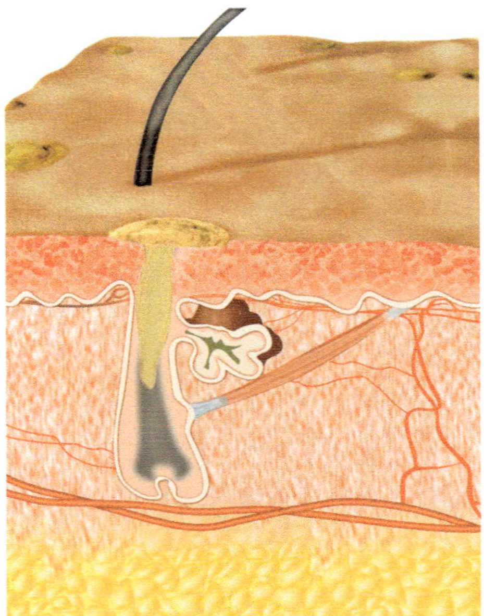

Fig. 4: "Yellow dots". They contain keratotic material and sebum. Sebum is responsible for the yellowness of the dots.

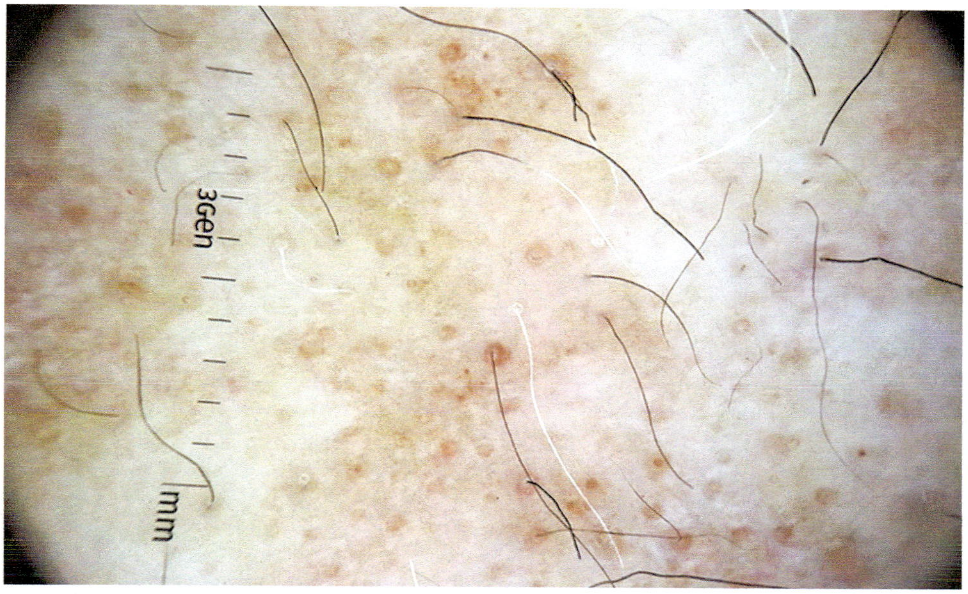

Fig. 5: Yellow dots in a case of extensive lichen planopilaris (LPP). Note the whitish color of the scalp is due to diffuse fibrosis. The color of the dots looks yellow as described in Caucasian scalp whereas in darker skin type, the yellow dots look more whitish. Note the lone hair shafts characteristic of LPP.

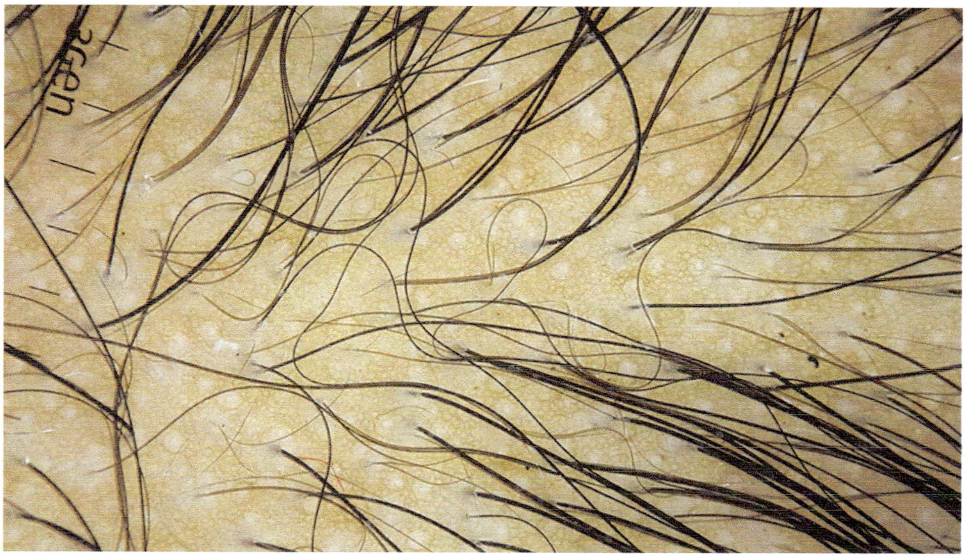

Fig. 6: Yellow dots in a case of androgenetic alopecia (AGA) which are more whitish than yellow in dark skin type. Note the hair diameter diversity.

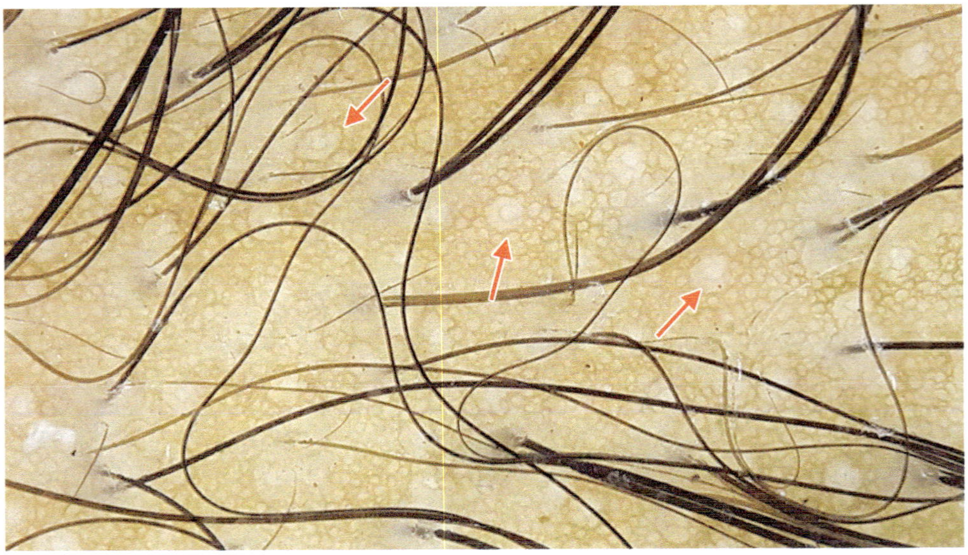

Fig. 7: Zooming of the previous image showing yellow dots (arrows) more clearly in a case of androgenetic alopecia (AGA). The dots are centrally white with a yellowish halo (author's observation) which correlates well with the description of double margin of the yellow dots. Note vellus and thin wavy hairs along with terminal hairs which is consistent with AGA.

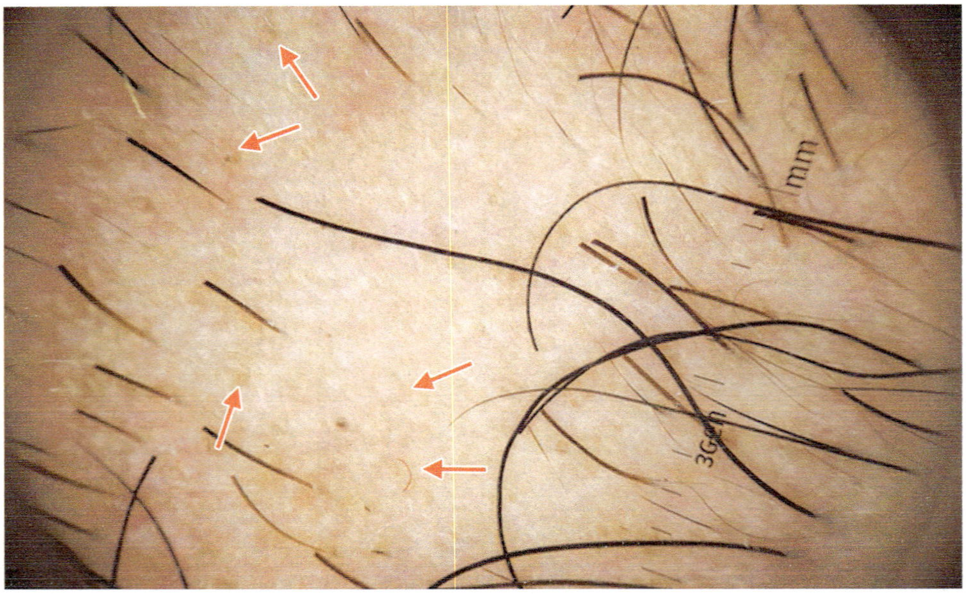

Fig. 8: Yellow dots are a marker of disease activity in alopecia areata. In darker skin type, they are observed with difficulty (red arrows). Note the exclamation mark hairs at the periphery of the alopecic patch.

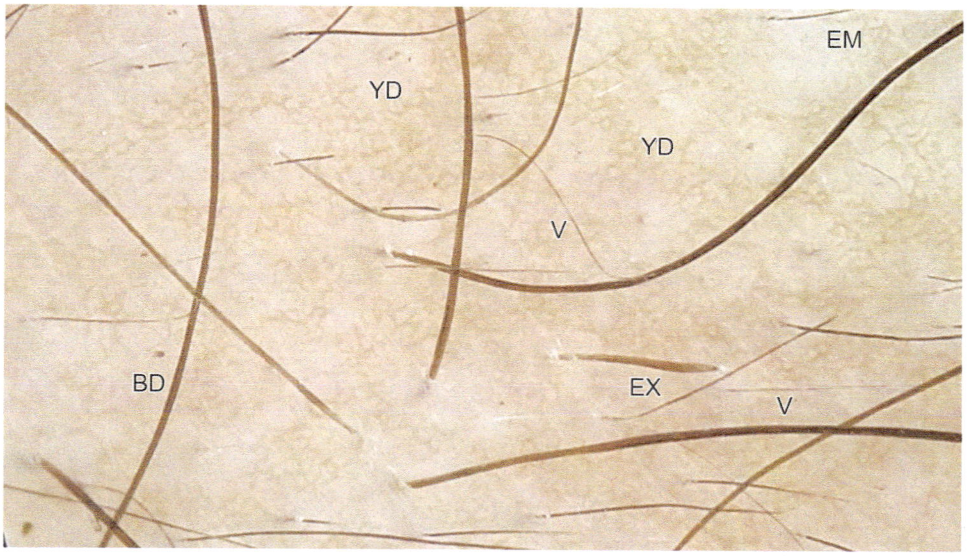

Fig. 9: Yellow dots (YD) seen in Caucasians look whitish in dark skin type (author's observation). Note that this is a case of active alopecia areata with exclamation mark (EX) and vellus hairs (V). Most of the yellow dots in this image are empty (EM), few have vellus hairs (V), and follicles with black dots (BD) are also present.

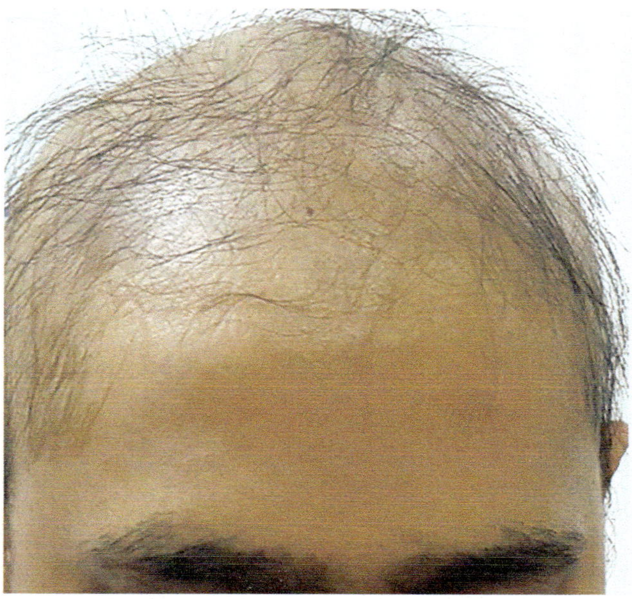

Fig. 10: Chemotherapy alopecia.

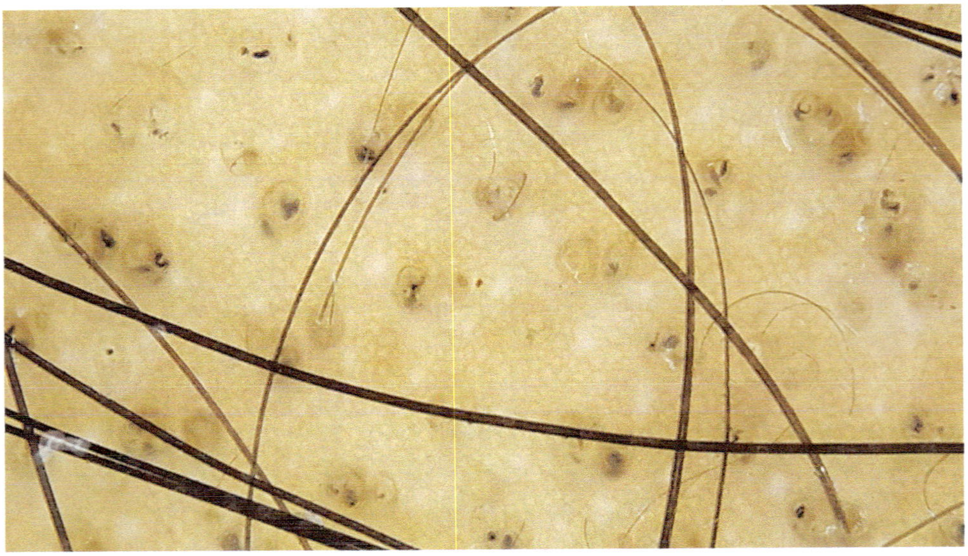

Fig. 11: Yellow dots in chemotherapy alopecia.

Hair Shafts

- Normal hairs are uniform in thickness and color when viewed through a dermoscope and they are >55 μm in diameter.[1,7] Hair shaft may be classified trichoscopically as thin, thick, and normal. Accurate measurement of shaft thickness is not essential for diagnosis in hair and scalp disorder; however, gross hair diameter diversity >20% points toward patterned hair loss.
- Trichoscopy helps visualization of medulla that, in normal individuals, may be continuous, interrupted, or absent and this variation has no influence on hair shaft properties.[9]
- Up to 10% of scalp hairs are vellus hairs. They are defined as hypopigmented, nonmedullated hairs <30 μm thick, and <3 mm long.[1,7]
- Vellus hairs should be differentiated from short regrowing hairs which have black color, pointed ends, and are upright.
- Number of hairs per follicular unit can be evaluated by trichoscopy. One to three hairs have been observed most commonly to emerge per follicle.[1,10] In healthy individuals, single hair units are <30% in the occipital, 35% in the frontal, and 40% in the temporal areas.[1]

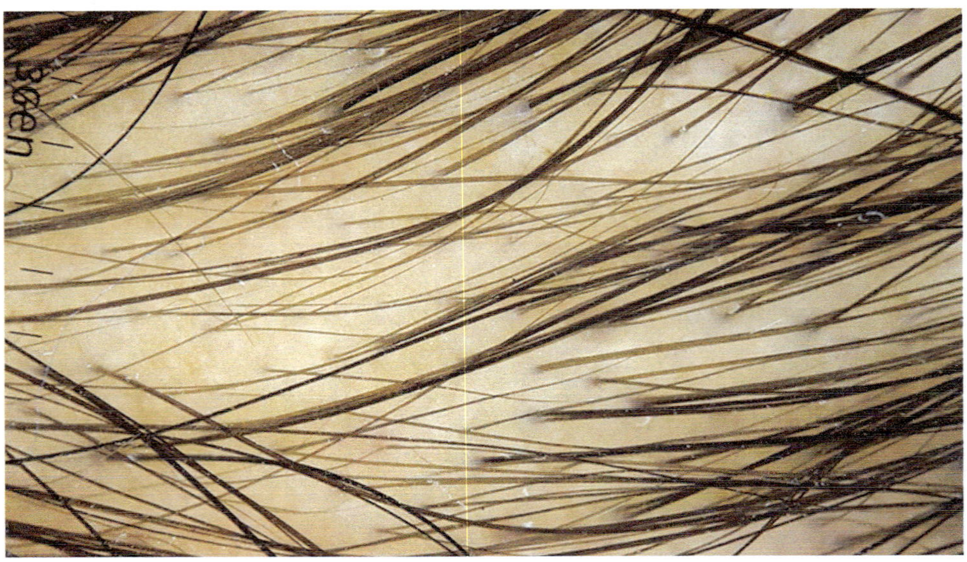

Fig. 12: Mostly single-hair units in temporal area of scalp (40%).

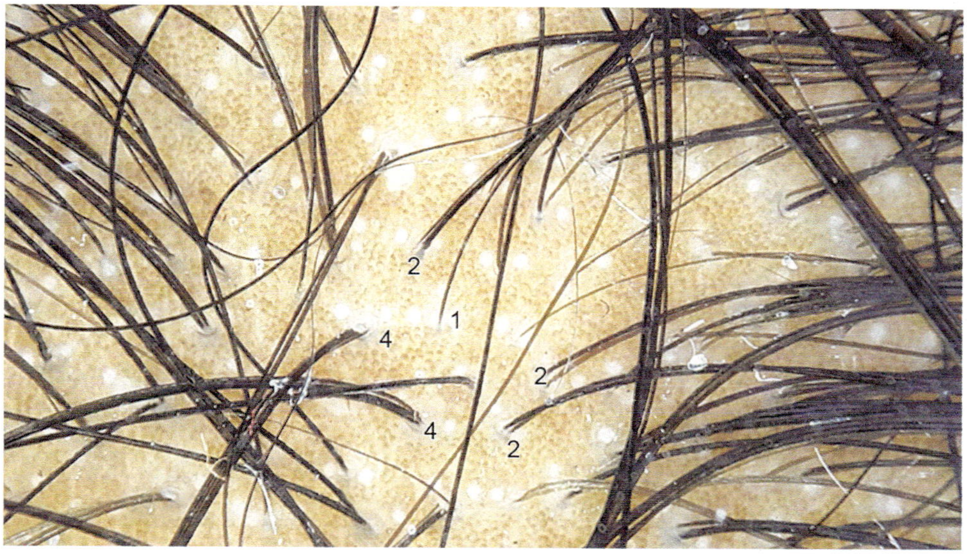

Fig. 13: Follicular units: Denoted by the digits. Note most follicular units have 2–4 hairs.

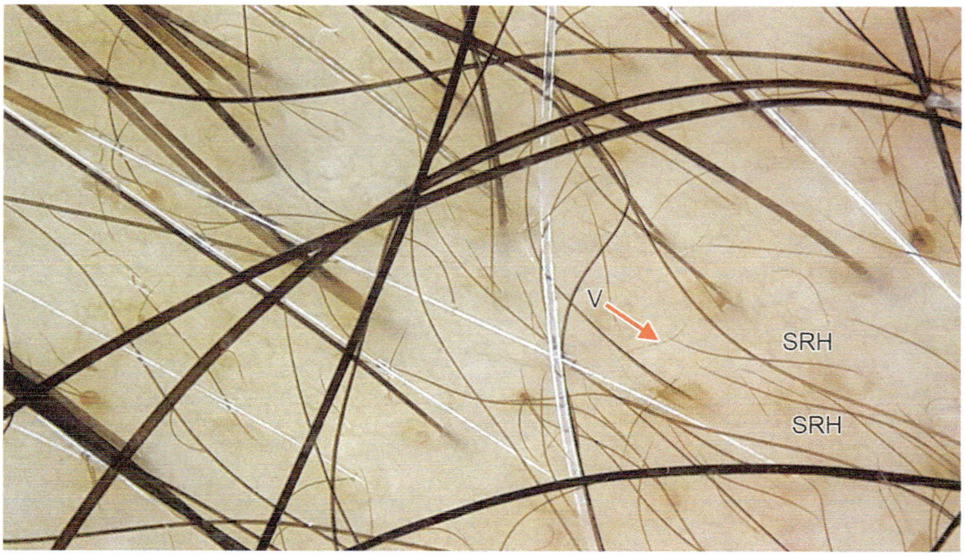

Fig. 14: Both vellus hairs (V) and short regrowing hairs (SRH) are observed in this image. Vellus hairs are hypopigmented and <3 mm in length whereas SRH are pigmented and have a pointed tip.

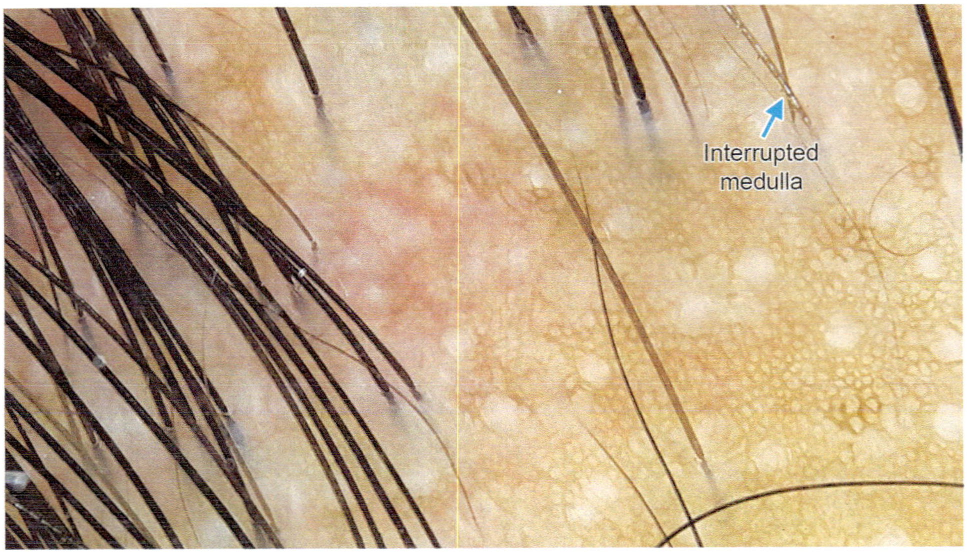

Fig. 15: While examining hair shafts, medulla may be visible as continuous, interrupted, fragmented or absent. Presence of medulla appears to have no clinical significance.

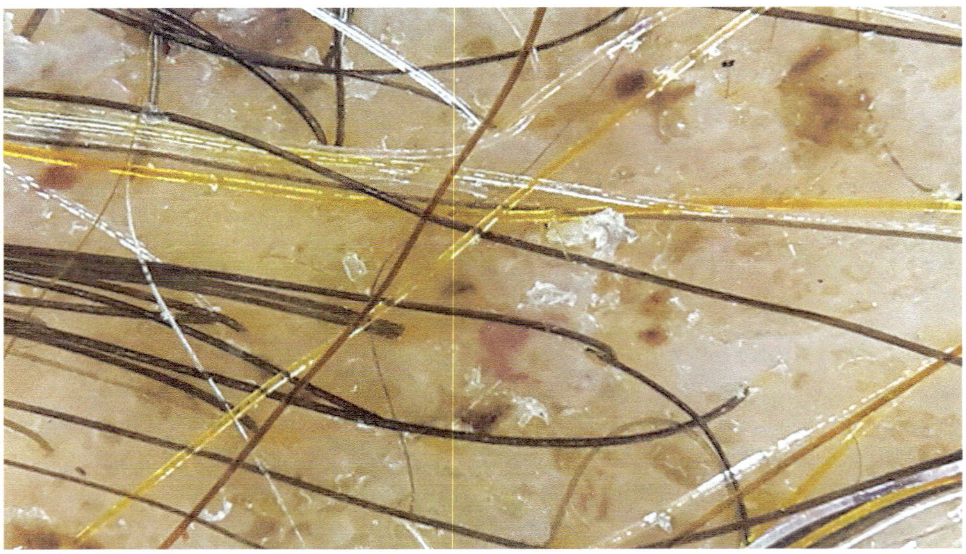

Fig. 16: Medulla: Continuous, absent, and interrupted. Note the black rhomboidal structures on the scalp due to hair dye.

Peri- and Interfollicular Area

- *Honeycomb pigmentation*: It is a steady finding in skin of color which consists of contiguous brownish rings. It can also be found in Caucasians with bald areas that are exposed to sun.[11]
- *Interfollicular scaling* is usually seen in various inflammatory disorders as well as in healthy individuals. Intensity, color, and localization of scaling may guide to a division between normal and diseased skin. Mild scaling is a common finding in healthy individuals with dry skin.[7]
- *White dots* (described in "hair follicle openings") appear as 0.2–0.3 mm in size and are distributed regularly in the interfollicular scalp and correspond to follicular openings or openings of eccrine sweat glands.[4,12]

- *Perifollicular scaling*: Mild perifollicular scaling is a nonspecific finding and may be found in healthy persons with dry skin.
- *Scalp vessels*: Interfollicular simple red loops and arborizing red lines are normally present in interfollicular scalp.[1,11] Red loops are fine hairpin-shaped structures and correspond to dermal papillae capillaries. Whereas arborizing red lines correspond to subpapillary vascular plexus; they are vessels of larger caliber.[13]
- *Dirty dots*: Appear as brown or black particles irregularly distributed on the scalp. They are environmental particles observed in children after playing outdoors and can easily be removed after shampooing.
- *Residues of dye*: They are multiple brown to black rhomboidal structures present in the interfollicular scalp.
- Residues of hair care products, e.g., cosmetic hair fibers—these fibers consist of keratin protein and/or synthetic ingredients. They are found trichoscopically as short lines in-between the follicular units. They are significantly thinner than the natural hair shafts.

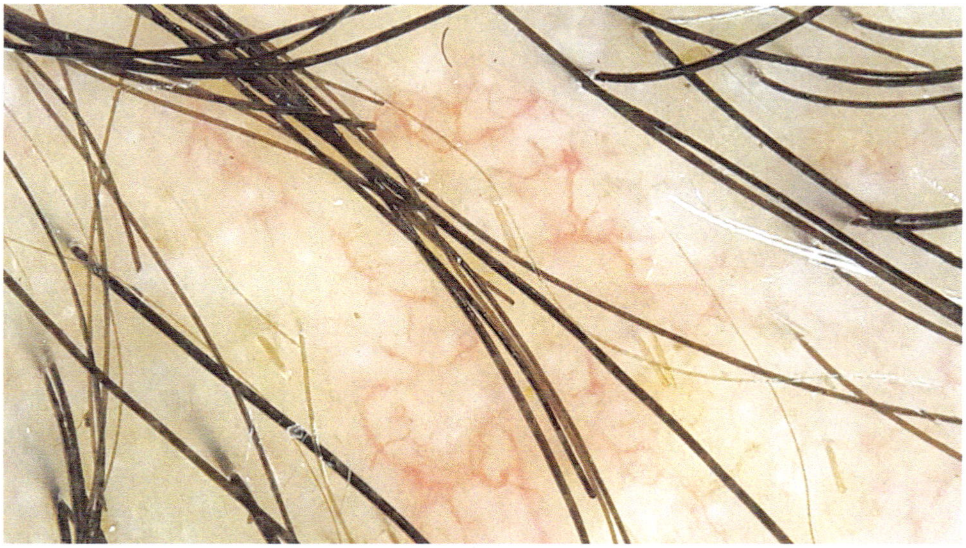

Fig. 17: Normal scalp vessels include red loops and arborizing red lines.

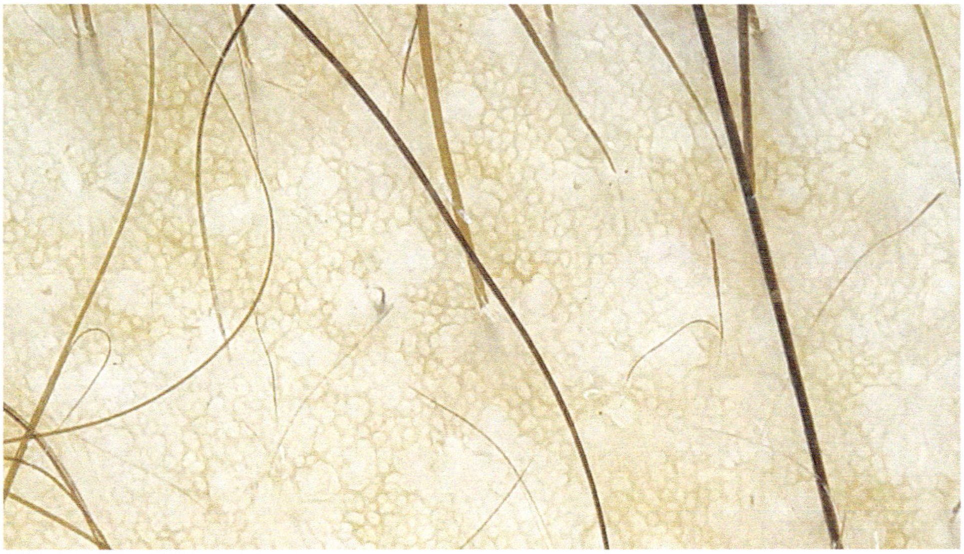

Fig. 18: *Honeycomb pigmented network*: It consists of homogeneous mosaic of contiguous brownish rings with interspersed white areas. These brownish rings are due to rete ridge melanocytes.

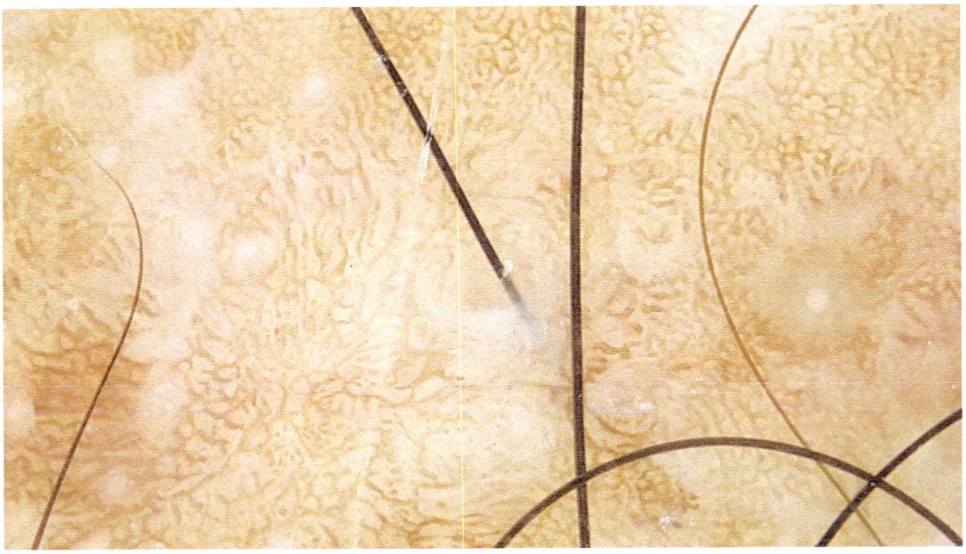

Fig. 19: Honeycomb pigmented network after zooming. It is a normal finding in darker skin individuals; also can be found in Caucasians with chronic sun exposure.

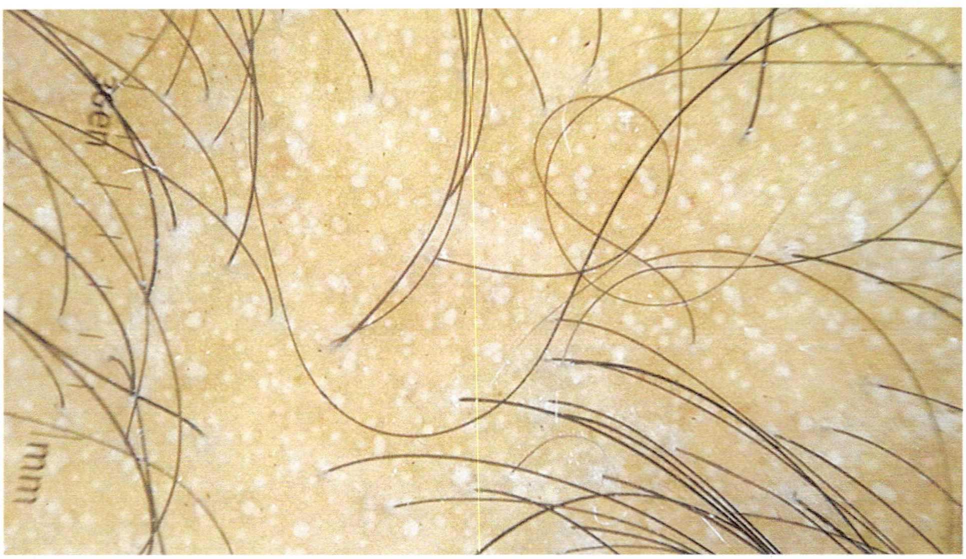

Fig. 20: Pinpoint white dots distributed regularly in the interfollicular scalp. The dots are scattered among the honeycomb pigmented network.

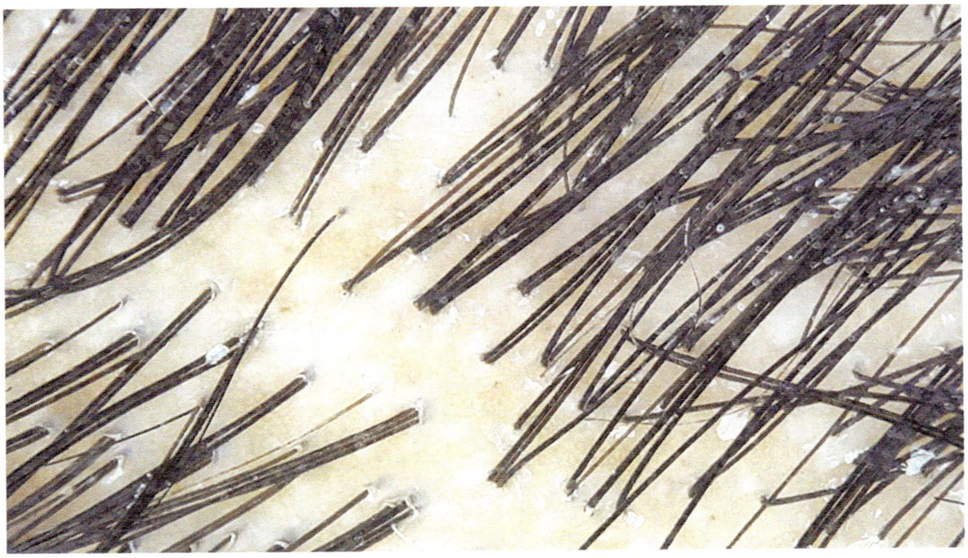

Fig. 21: Peri- and interfollicular scale in a healthy individual.

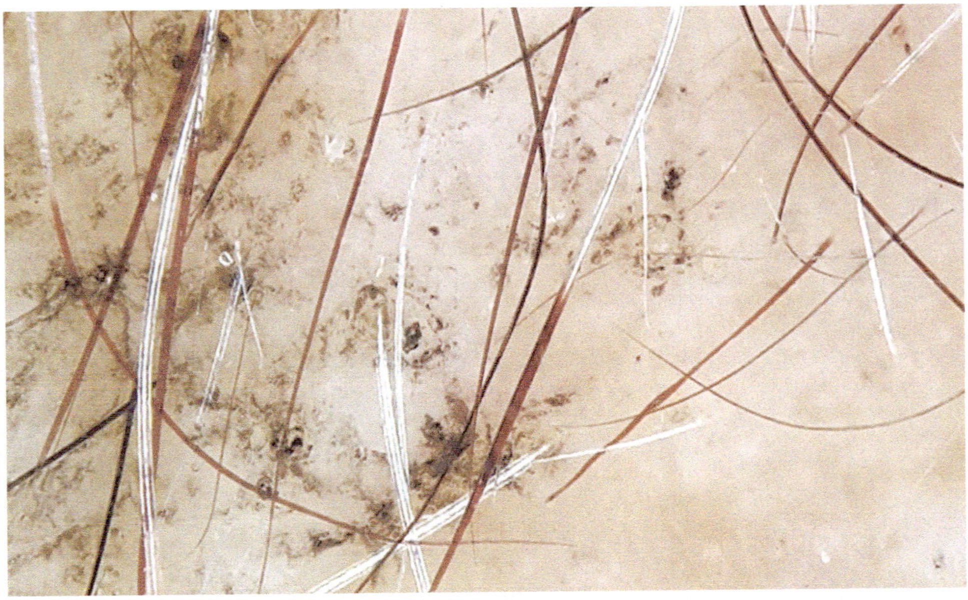

Fig. 22: Blackish rhomboidal structures and dots in interfollicular distribution. This is hair dye remnant. Closest differential diagnosis is postinflammatory hyperpigmentation. To remove the dye remnant, patient should be advised to wash the scalp 2–3 times after dyeing.

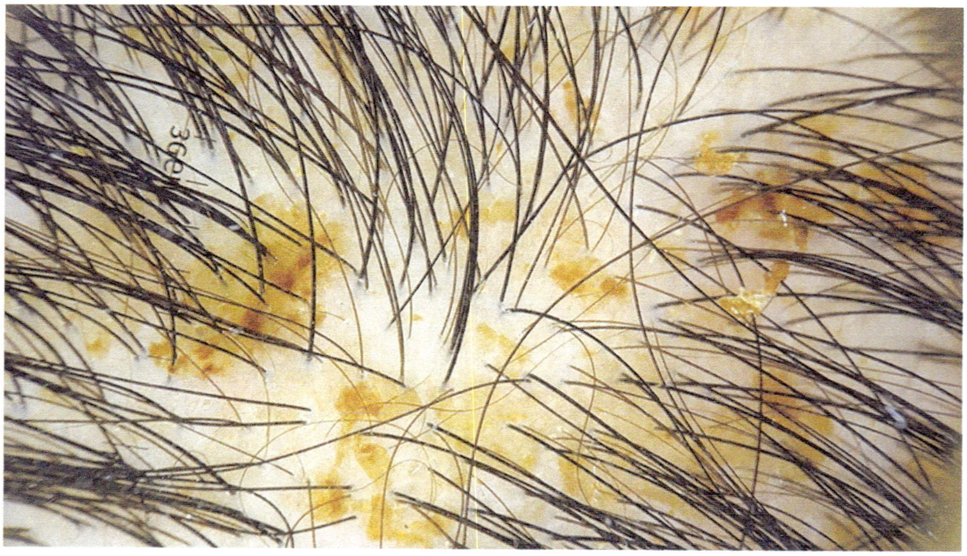

Fig. 23: Trichoscopically, *mehendi* residues on interfollicular scalp are seen as rhomboidal structures. *Mehendi* is used commonly for coloring of hair.

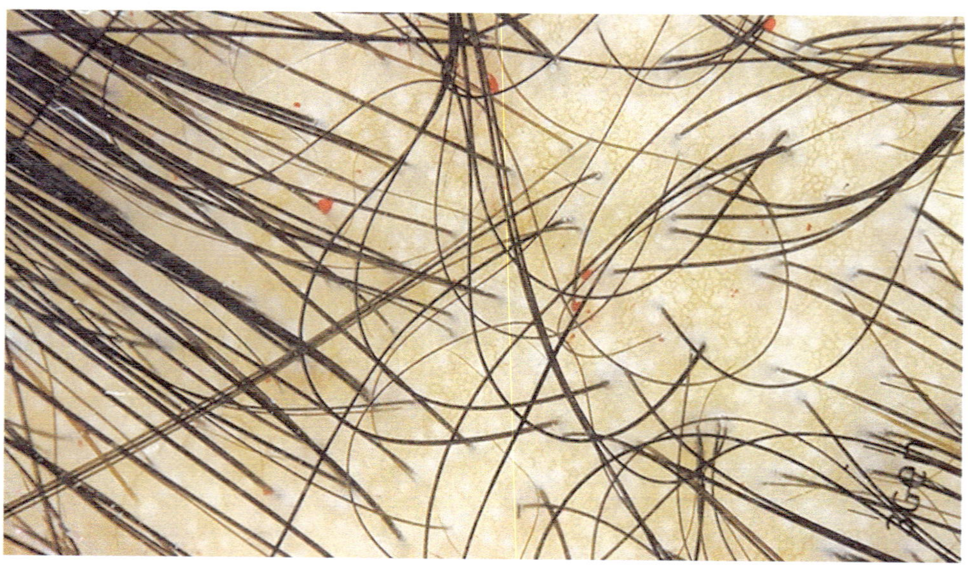

Fig. 24: Product residue: Vermillion. While examining normal scalp, these red dots should not be confused with vascular hemorrhages.

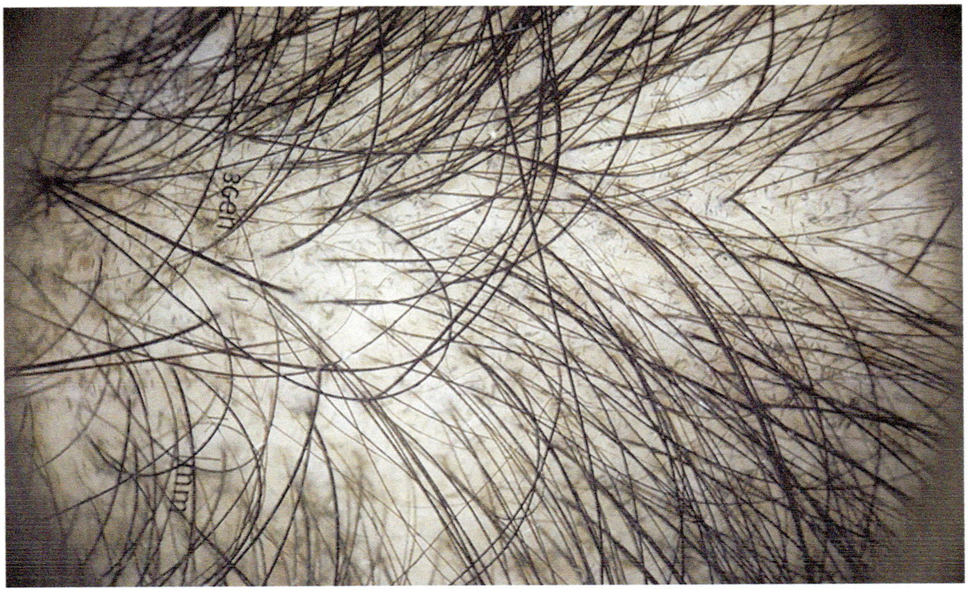

Fig. 25: The image shows black cosmetic hair fibers that match the color of hair. These synthetic hair fibers most commonly consist of keratin proteins and are used to camouflage thinning of hair.

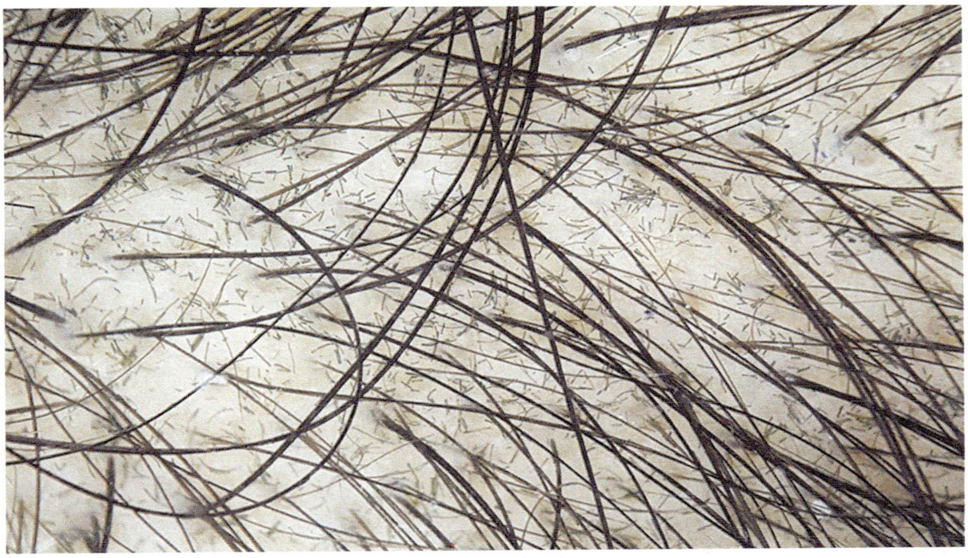

Fig. 26: High magnification reveals that the cosmetic hair fibers are markedly thinner than the normal hair shafts. If trichoscopy is done after a few hours of haircut, hair fragments similar to hair fibers may be visible; the differentiating point from cosmetic hair fibers is that the thickness of the cut hair fragments is the same as that of normal hair.

REFERENCES

1. Ross EK, Vincenzi C, Tosti A. Videodermoscopy in the evaluation of hair and scalp disorders. J Am Acad Dermatol. 2006;55(5):799-806.
2. Rakowska A. Trichoscopy (hair and scalp videodermoscopy) in the healthy female. Method standardization and norms for measurable parameters. J Dermatol Case Rep. 2009;3(1):14-9.
3. de Moura LH, Duque-Estrada B, Abraham LS, Barcaui CB, Sodre CT. Dermoscopy findings of alopecia areata in an African American patient. J Dermatol Case Rep. 2008;2(4):52-4.
4. Abraham LS, Pinerio-Maceira J, Duque-Estrada B, Barcaui CB, Sodré CT. Pinpoint white dot in the scalp: dermoscopic and histopathological correlation. J Am Acad Dermatol. 2010;63(4):721-2.

5. Rudnicka L, Olszewska M, Rakowska A, Slowinska M. Trichoscopy update 2011. J Dermatol Case Report. 2011;5(4):82-8.
6. Lacarrubba F, Dall'Oglio F, Rita Nasca M, Micali G. Videodermatoscopy enhances diagnostic capability in some forms of hair loss. Am J Clin Dermatol. 2004;5(3):205-8.
7. Inui S, Nakajima T, Nakagawa K, Itami S. Clinical significance of dermoscopy in alopecia areata: analysis of 300 cases. Int J Dermatol. 2008;47(7):688-93.
8. Rokowska A, Slowinska M, Kowalska-Oledzka E, Olszewska M, Rudnicka L. Dermoscopy in female androgenic alopecia: method standardization and diagnostic criteria. Int J Trichol. 2009;1(2):123-30.
9. Rudnicka L, Olszewska M, Rakowska A, Kowalska-Oledzka E, Slowinska M. Trichoscopy: a new method for diagnosing hair loss. J Drugs Dermatol. 2008;7(7):651-4.
10. Rokowska A, Slowinska M, Kowalska-Oledzka E, Warszawik O, Czuwara J, Olszewska M, et al. Trichoscopy in cicatricial alopecia. J Drugs Dermatol. 2012;11(6):753-8.
11. Tosti A. Dermatoscopy of hair and scalp disorders. London: Informa Healthcare; 2007.
12. Ardigo M, Tosti A, Cameli N, Vincenzi C, Misciali C, Berardesca E. Reflectance confocal microscopy of the yellow dot pattern in alopecia areata. Arch Dermatol. 2011;147:61-4.
13. Bull RH, Bates DO, Mortimer PS. Intravital video-capillaroscopy for the study of microcirculation in psoriasis. Br J Dermatol. 1992;126:436-45.

ASSESSMENT IMAGE-BASED QUESTIONS

1. What is responsible for the yellowness of the dots? Identify the yellow dots.

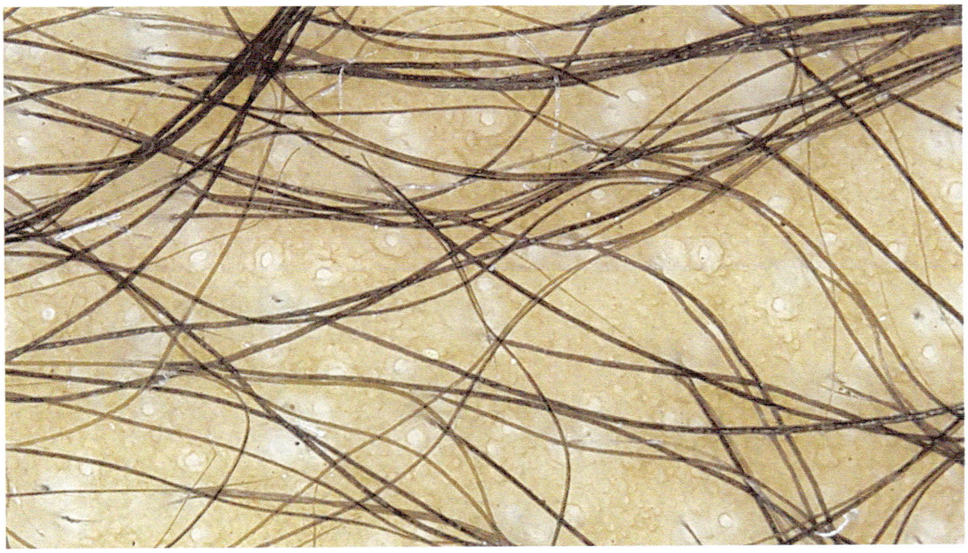

2. In normal hair shafts, medulla may be visualized by trichoscopy that appear as continuous, interrupted, or fragmented. Identify the hair with medulla.

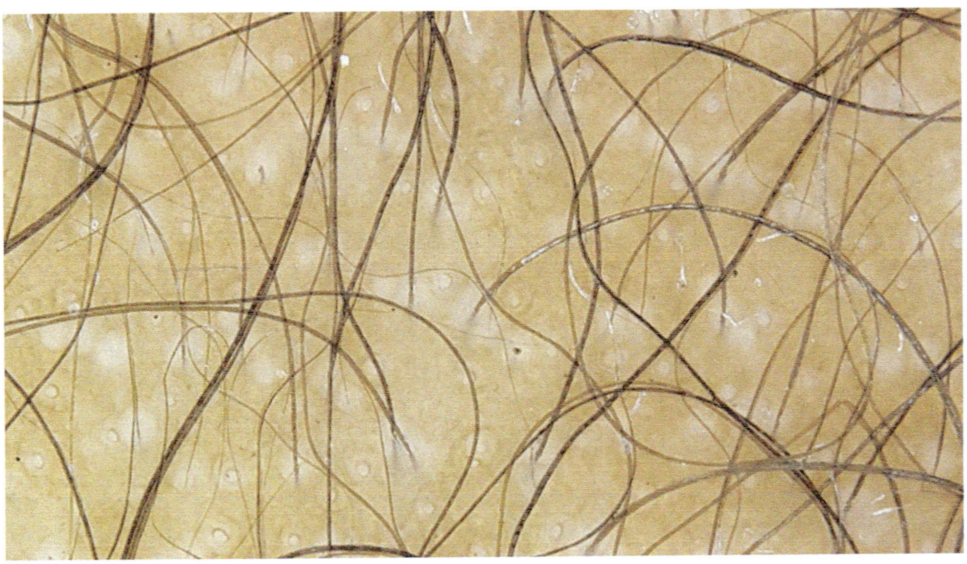

3. Homogeneous rings of contiguous brownish rings are seen in the interfollicular scalp. What is the name given to it? What is its histopathological correlation?

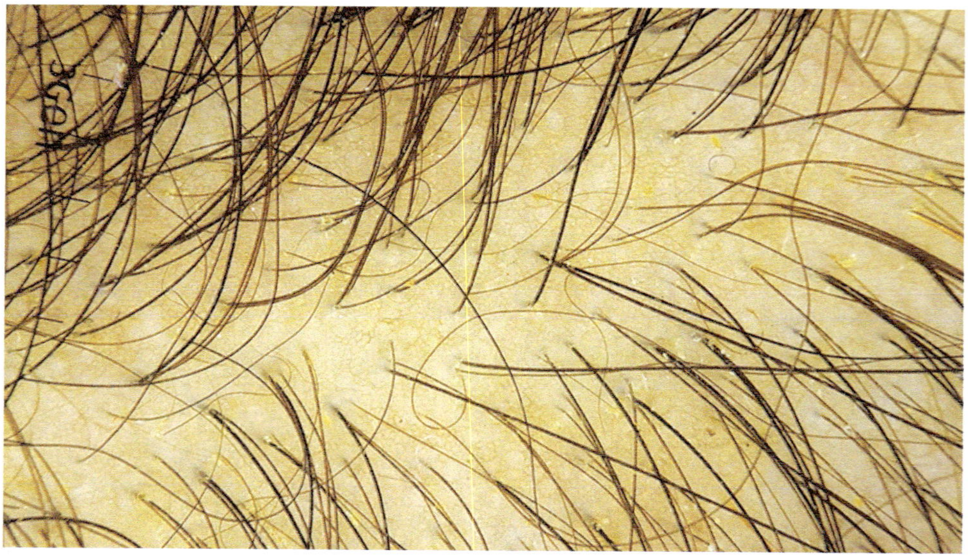

4. Pinpoint white dots are observed in this image. What are the types of white dots? What are their histological correlates?

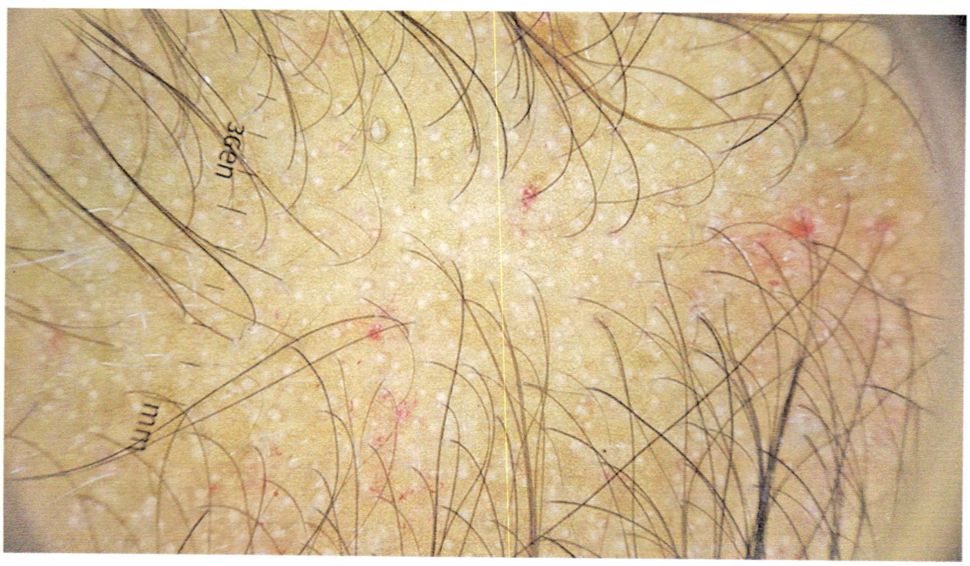

5. Usually 1–3 hairs emerge from a follicular unit. In healthy individual, the percentage of follicular units with single hairs is >30%. Most follicular units consist of two hairs. Mention the number of hairs emerging from follicular units that are denoted by alphabets in this image.

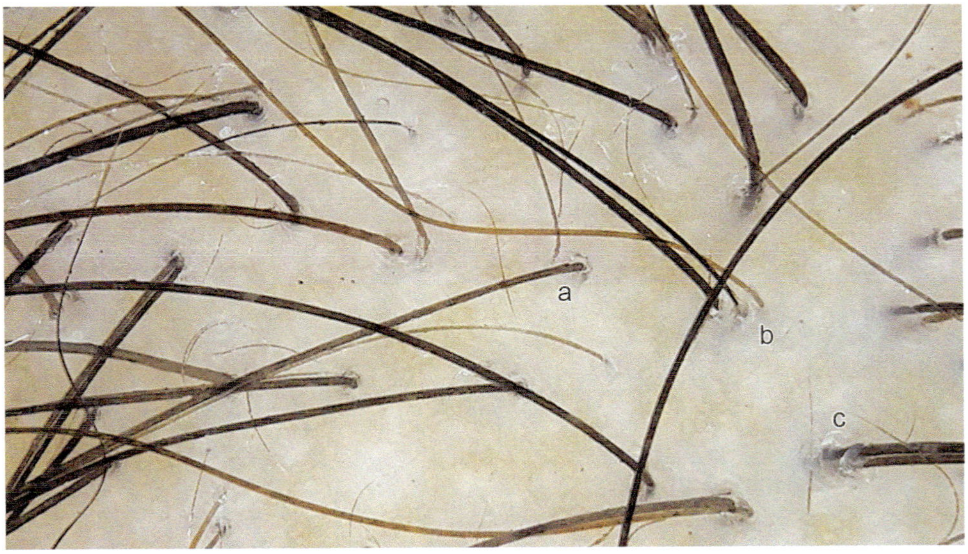

6. Which vascular pattern is seen in this image? What is the normal vascular pattern of scalp?

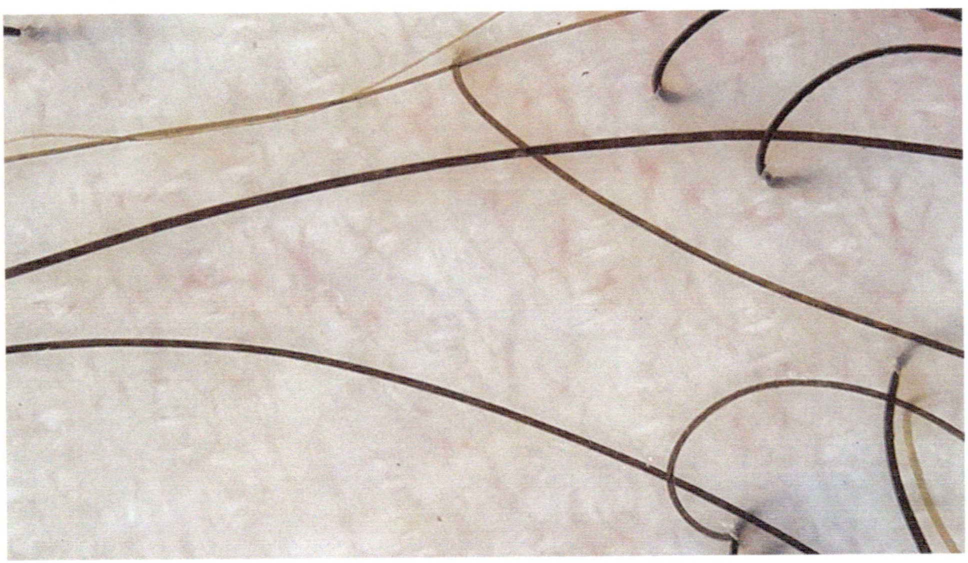

7. What do the black structures indicate? (a) dirty dots (b) remnant of dye (c) hair fibers.

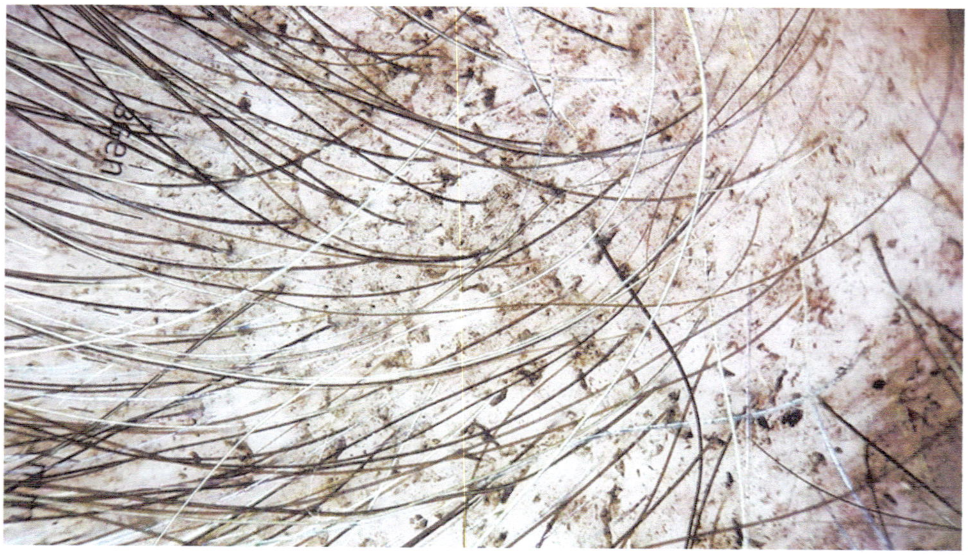

8. What is seen in the interfollicular scalp?

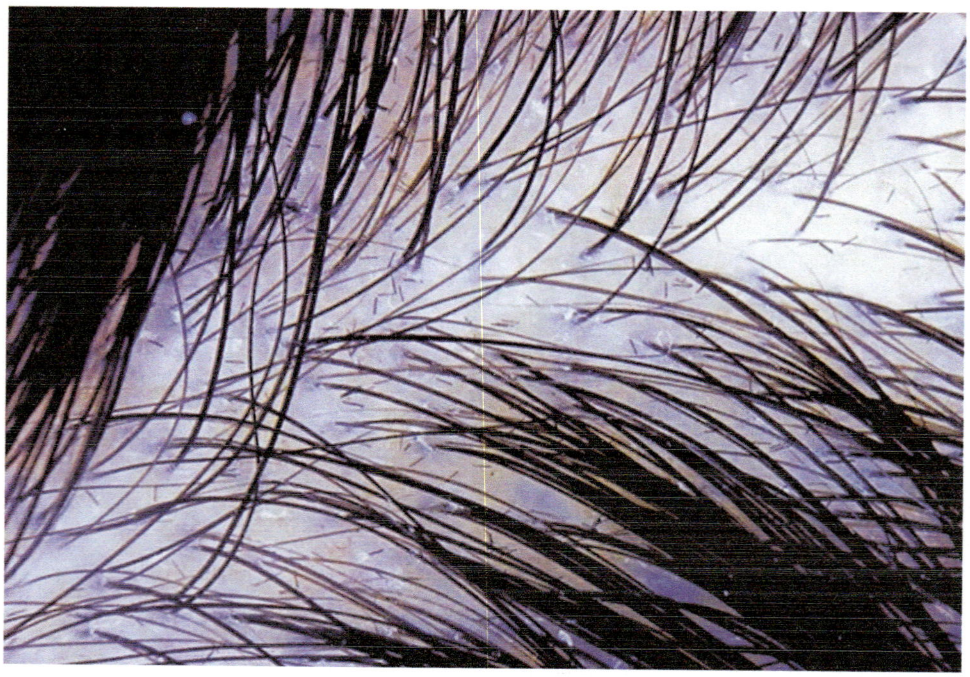

ANSWERS

1. Sebum
2. No influence
3. Honeycomb appearance. Rete ridge melanocytes
4. Two types of white dots—pinpoint and fibrotic. Pinpoint white dots correspond to openings of hair follicle or to the acrosyringium of eccrine ducts.
5. a. 1
   b. 3
   c. 2
6. Telangiectatic vessels are visible probably due to overapplication of topical steroid on scalp. Normal scalp vessels include simple red loops and arborizing red lines.
7. b.
8. Cosmetic hair fibers

CHAPTER

8A Scalp Dysesthesia

Surit Malakar, Subrata Malakar

INTRODUCTION

- Scalp dysesthesia is an abnormal sensation of the scalp in the absence of cutaneous disease.[1]
- It is characterized by a burning and/or itching sensation and can be related to a variety of neurogenic or psychogenic causes.

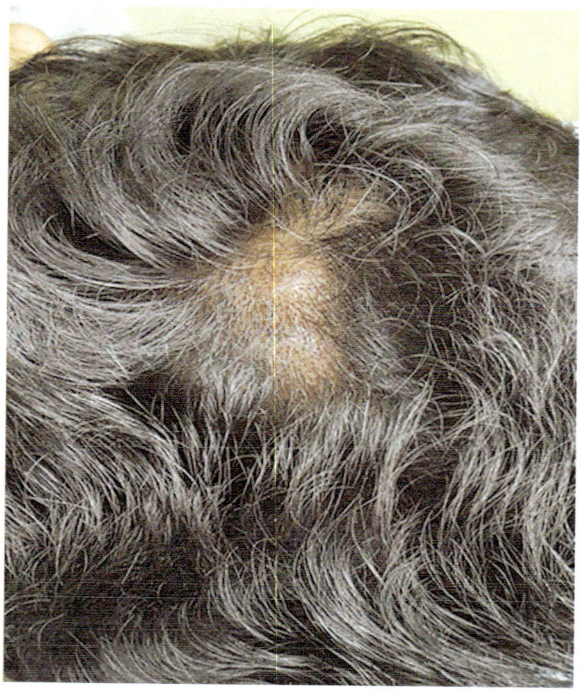

Fig. 1: Scalp dysesthesia.

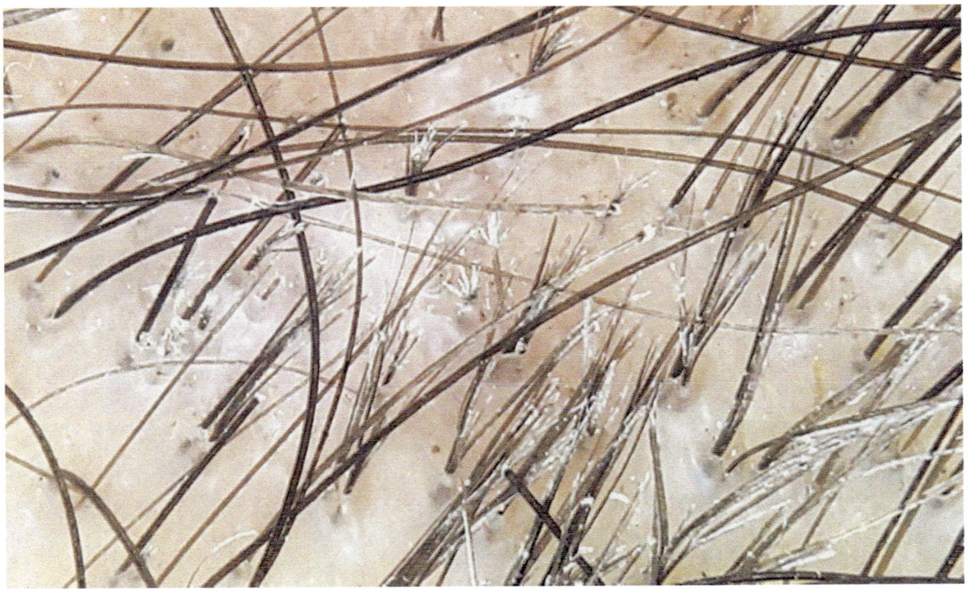

Fig. 2: Extensive broom hairs (multiple thin hairs emerge from single follicular unit), block hairs, and trichorrhexis nodosa.

KEY TRICHOSCOPIC FEATURES

- Broom hairs
- Block hairs
- Trichorrhexis nodosa

REFERENCE

1. Ju T, Vander Does A, Yosipovitch G. Scalp dysesthesia: a neuropathic phenomenon. J Eur Acad Dermatol Venereol. 2022;36(6):790-6.

CHAPTER 8B

Fox–Fordyce Disease

Surit Malakar, Subrata Malakar

INTRODUCTION

- Fox–Fordyce disease is a rare disease of apocrine sweat glands.[1]
- Diagnosis is based on clinical presentation of monomorphic skin-colored follicular papules in apocrine-rich sites like axilla.

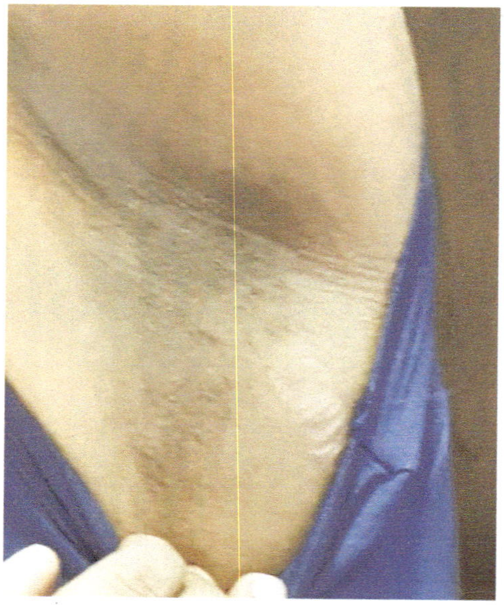

Fig. 1: Fox–Fordyce disease.

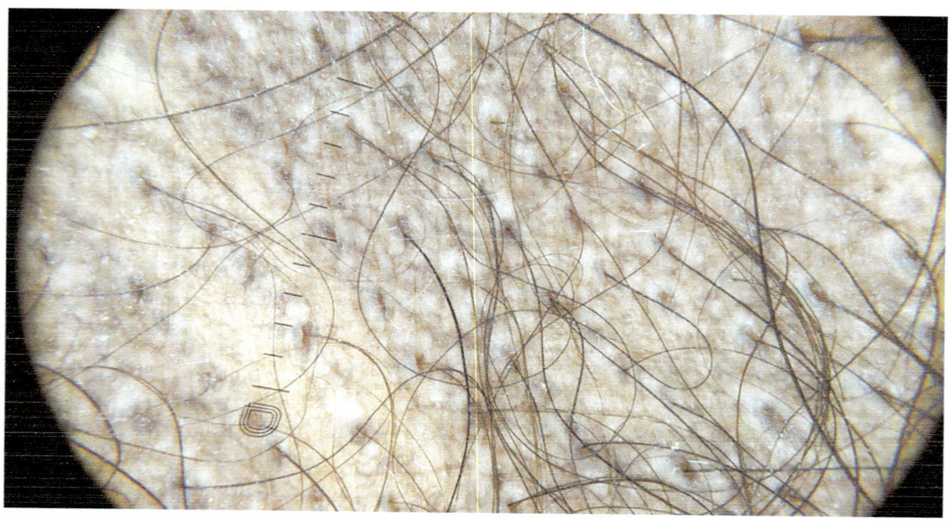

Fig. 2: Light brown to dark brown structureless areas (lacking any specific pigment network) and hyperkeratotic follicular plugging.

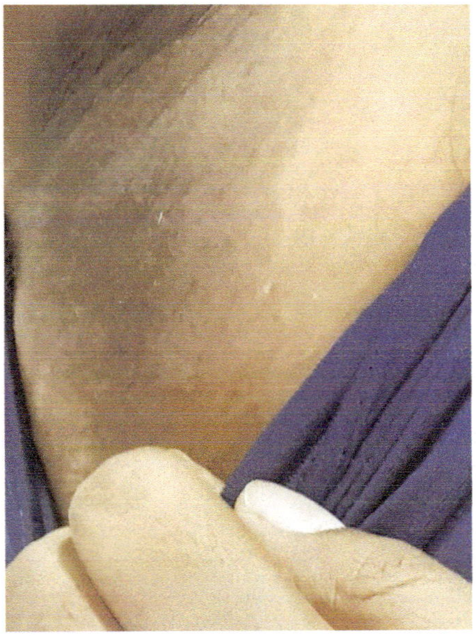

Fig. 3: Fox–Fordyce disease.

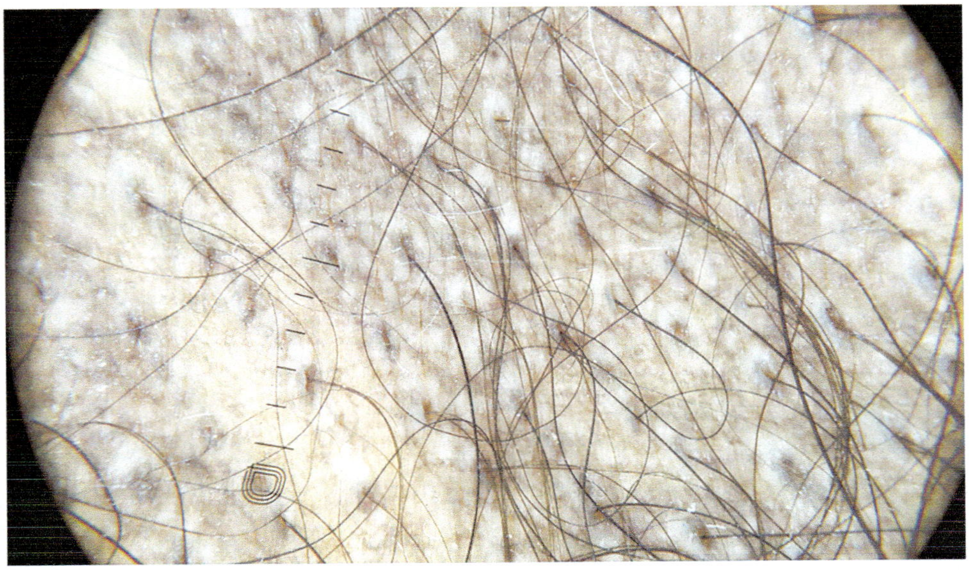

Fig. 4: Light brown to dark brown structureless areas (lacking any specific pigment network).

KEY TRICHOSCOPIC FEATURES

- Light brown to dark brown structureless areas (lacking any specific pigment network)
- Hyperkeratotic follicular plugging

REFERENCE

1. Singal A, Jakhar D, Kaur I, Sharma S. Fox-Fordyce Disease: Dermoscopic Perspective. Skin Appendage Disord. 2020;6(4):247-9.

6

SECTION

Nonscarring Alopecias

CHAPTER

9 Androgenetic Alopecia

Subrata Malakar, Purva Mehta Movdawalla, Surit Malakar

INTRODUCTION

- Both androgenetic alopecia (AGA) and female pattern hair loss (FPHL) are androgen-dependent conditions which develop in genetically predisposed persons.[1] AGA affects around 80% of males whereas FPHL affects around 50% of females.[1-4]
- They share the same histopathological criteria of hair follicle miniaturization.
- They also share the same pathway of pathogenesis. Dihydrotestosterone (DHT) binds to androgen receptor in susceptible hair follicles. This activates the genes responsible for the transformation of terminal follicles to miniaturized ones.[1-4]
- AGA affects the front-temporal areas and vertex which follows a pattern corresponding to Hamilton–Norwood scale.
- Whereas FPHL produces diffuse thinning of the crown where the frontal hairline is maintained (Ludwig pattern). It can easily be demonstrated by making a central parting.

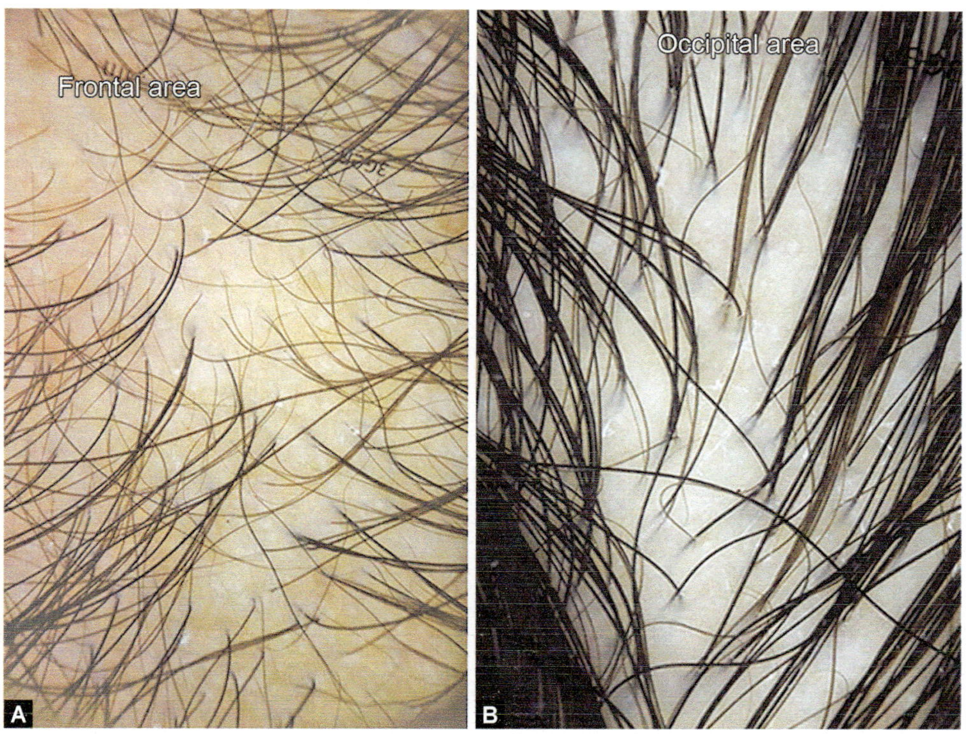

Figs. 1A and B: Androgenetic alopecia is more prominent in frontal than occipital area.

KEY FEATURES

- Hair diameter diversity of > 20%
- Peripilar sign
- Yellow dots
- Vellus hairs
- Reduced number of hairs per follicular unit
- AGA is more pronounced in the frontal rather than occipital area in trichoscopic examination.
- Coexistence of other causes of hair loss is not uncommon which can be excluded trichoscopically.

HAIR DIAMETER DIVERSITY

- A diversity of >20% per field of dermoscope in frontal area is diagnostic for AGA.
- However, an exception to this if found across scalp one has to suspect diffuse unpatterned alopecia (DUPA).
- It is characterized by simultaneous presence of hairs of different diameters such as thick, thin, intermediate, and vellus hairs. It reflects follicular miniaturization.[5,6]
- Trichoscopy is highly effective in differentiating FPHL from acute and chronic telogen effluvium.[7]

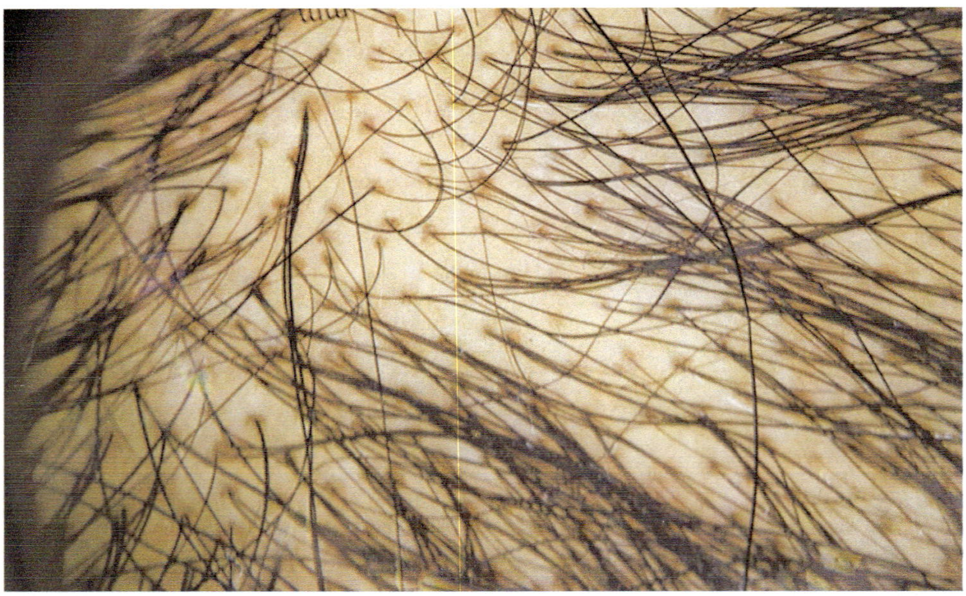

Fig. 2: Peripilar sign and hair diameter variability.

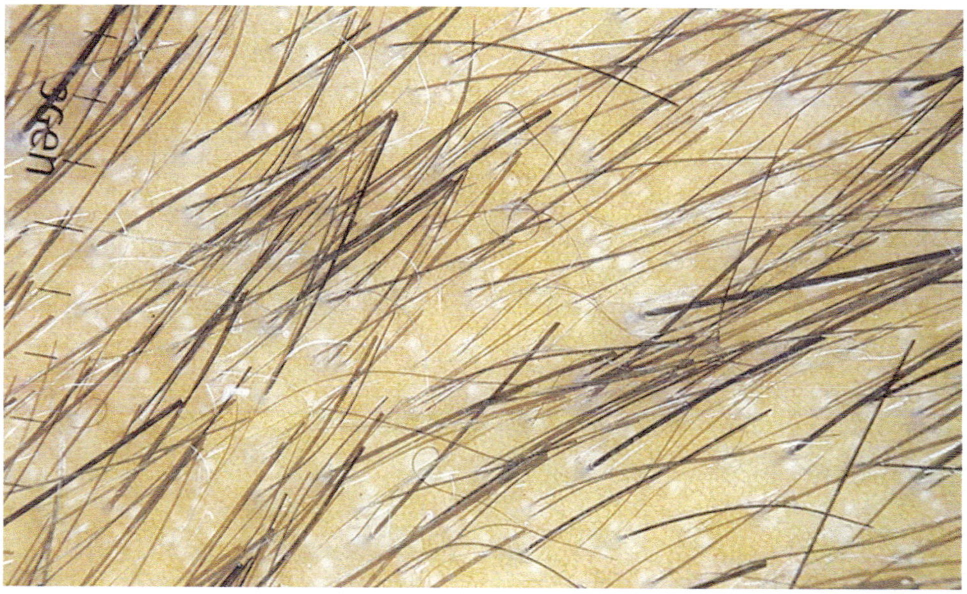

Fig. 3: Marked hair diameter diversity which is more apparent due to a recent haircut. Honeycomb pigmentation and white dots are also observed through reduced hair length.

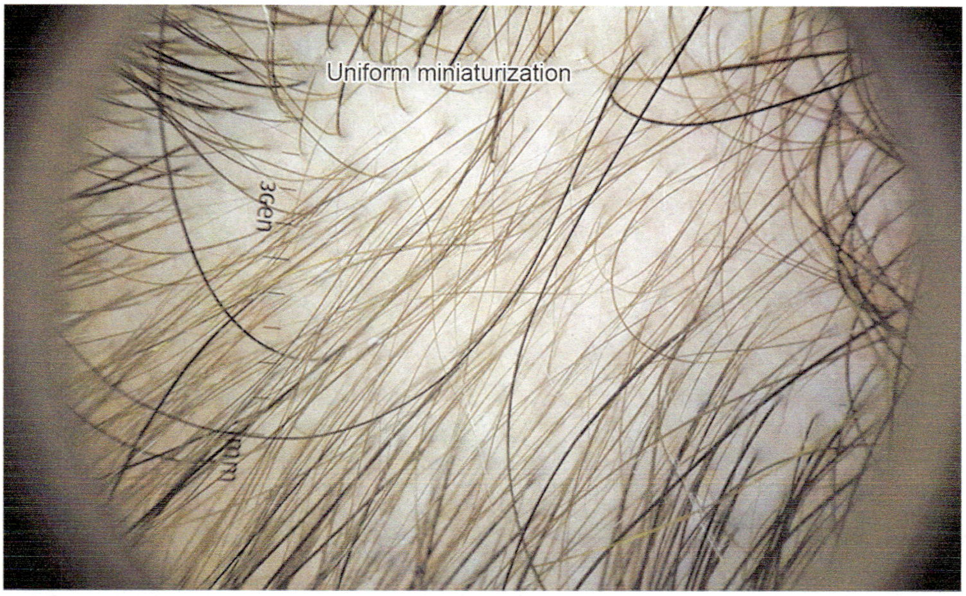

Fig. 4: Hair diameter variability can also be observed in alopecia areata. However, in alopecia areata trichoscopy shows uniform miniaturization. Note the peripheral terminal hairs surrounding the alopecic patch.

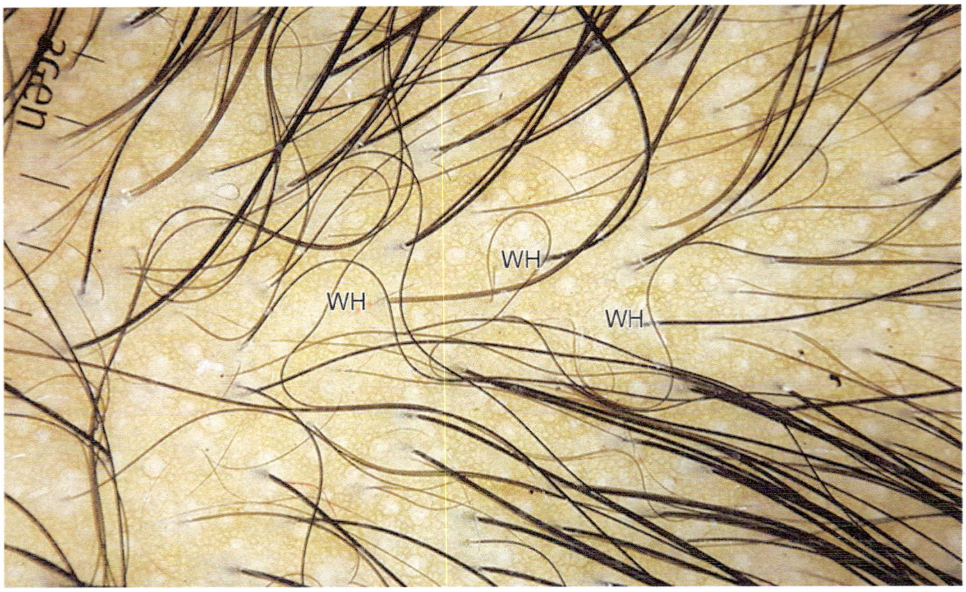

Fig. 5: Thin wavy hairs (WH)—hair diameter diversity is characterized by simultaneous presence of hairs of different diameters such as thick, thin, intermediate (WH) and vellus hairs. The diameter of WH is in between thick and thin hairs and is a result of incomplete miniaturization of hair follicles. Thin wavy hairs may also be found in *alopecia areata incognita*.[8]

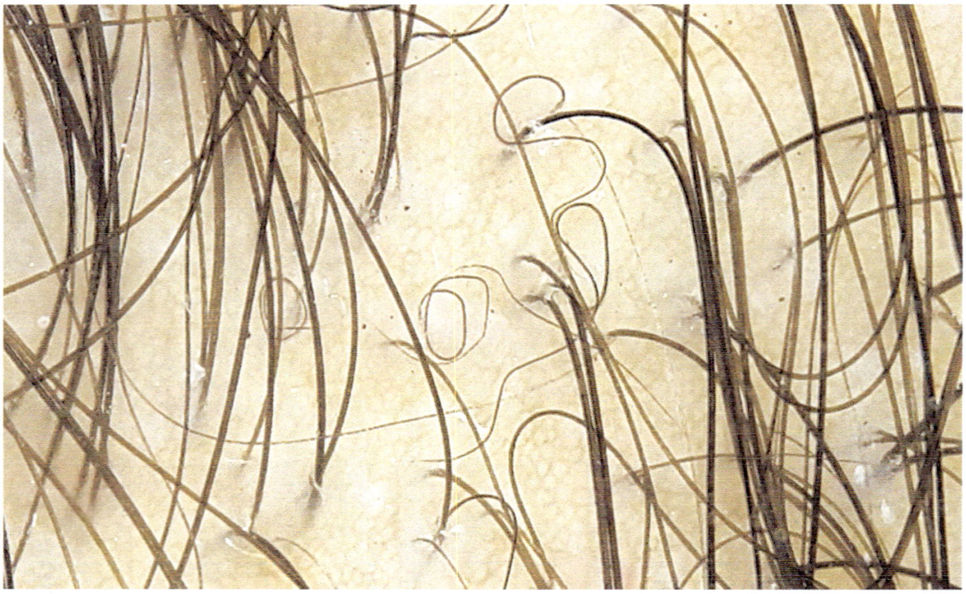

Fig. 6: Diameter of thin wavy hairs is 0.03–0.05 mm. They are thinner than terminal but thicker than vellus hairs.

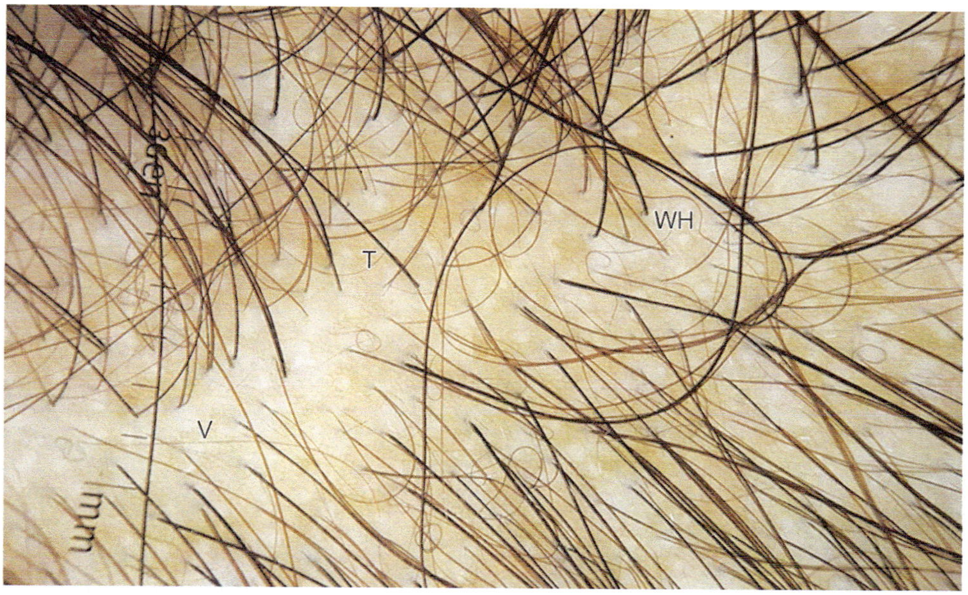

Fig. 7: This field has terminal (T), vellus (V), and thin wavy hairs (WH).

PERIPILAR SIGN

- It is seen as a brown depressed halo of approximately 1 mm diameter at the follicular emergence. It correlates with perifollicular inflammation.[9] Inui et al. hypothesized peripilar sign in Asians as a result of postinflammatory hyperpigmentation.[5]
- This sign is observed in 20–66% of patients.[5]
- This is commonly found in patients with early AGA.
- Karadog and Gulec indicated that peripilar sign is specific for AGA. <5% of hair follicle openings with brown peripilar discoloration is observed in healthy scalp.[10]
- Extensive peripilar sign is a poor prognostic factor for AGA.[8]

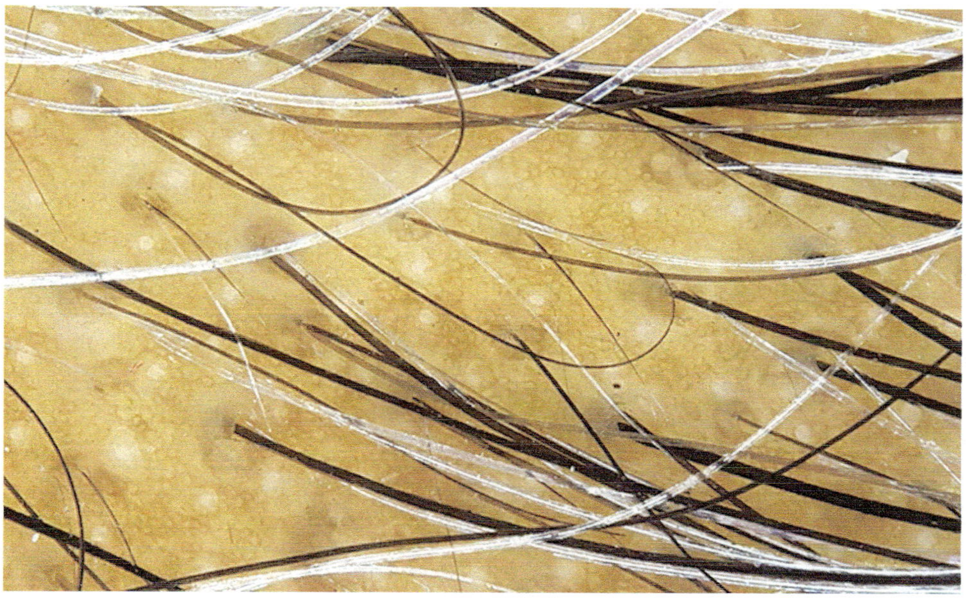

Fig. 8: Peripilar sign.

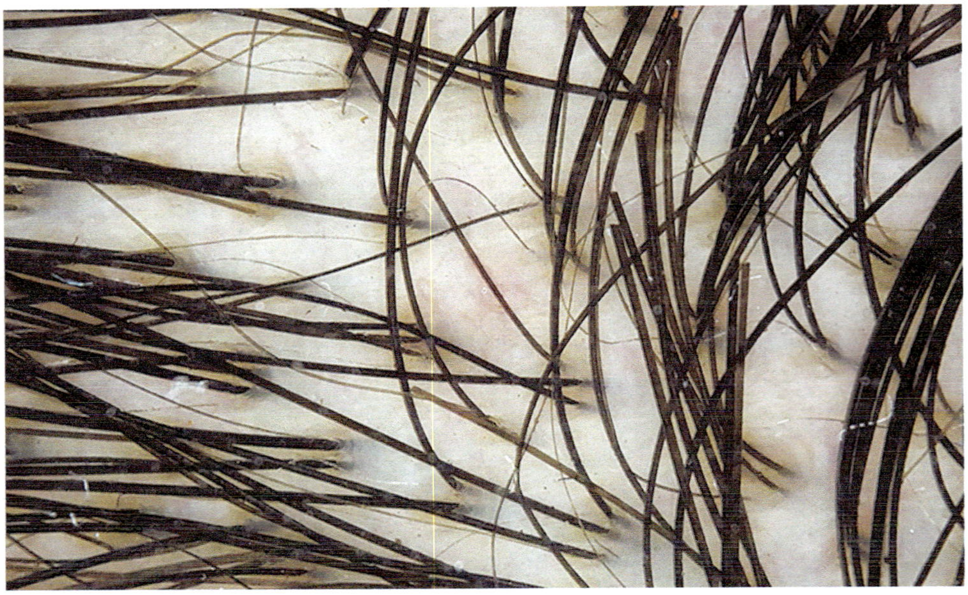

Fig. 9: Peripilar sign.

VELLUS HAIRS

- They are a sign of severe miniaturization.
- Up to 10% of normal human scalp hairs are vellus hairs. They are defined as hypopigmented, nonmedullated hairs < 30 μm thick and <3 mm long.[11,12]
- In normal population, proportion of vellus hairs are 6.15 ± 4.6%. In FPHL this proportion is 20.9 ± 12% which is much greater than in normal population.[13]

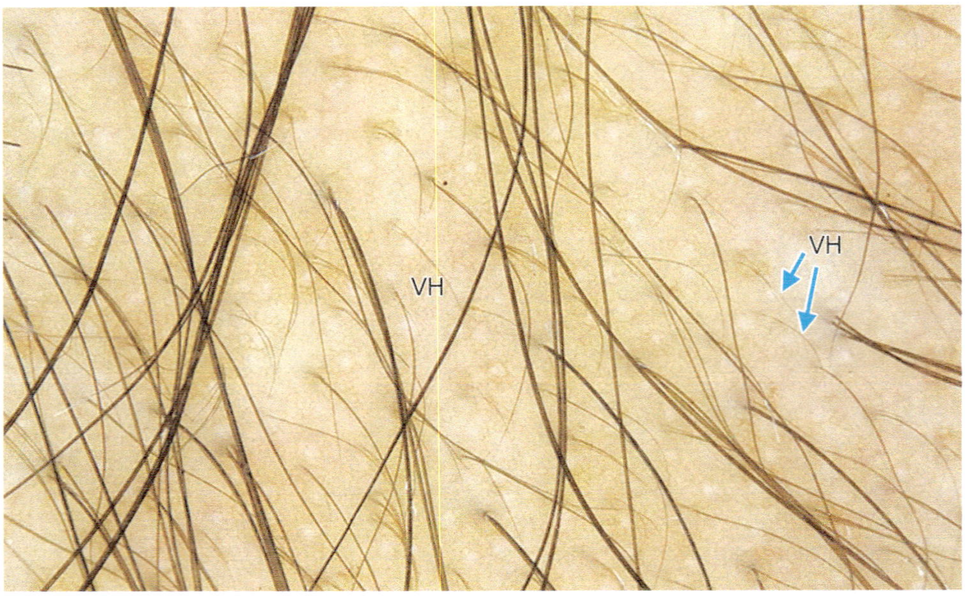

Fig. 10: Vellus hairs (VH).

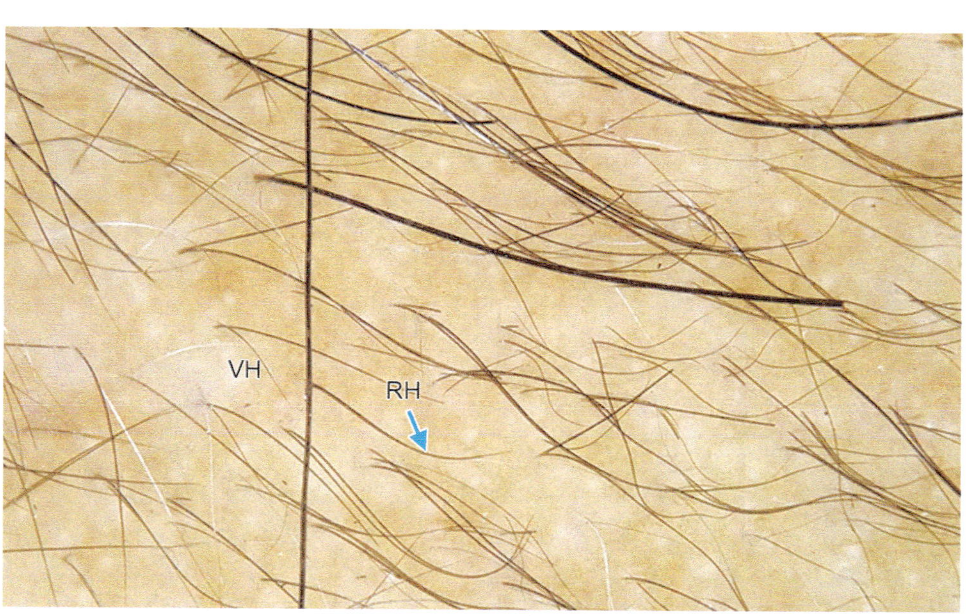

Fig. 11: Vellus hairs versus short regrowing hairs. Vellus hairs (VH) should be differentiated from regrowing hairs (RH). Regrowing hairs are short and thin, not hypopigmented, they are firm and have pointed ends. Whereas vellus hairs are hypopigmented and thin hairs.

A DECREASED NUMBER OF HAIRS PER FOLLICULAR UNIT

- It is a characteristic but nonspecific feature of AGA and FPHL.
- The normal values for the frontal area in healthy Caucasian females have been established. This is < 35% for one-hair follicular unit, 46–70% for two-hair units, and >10% for three-hair units. The respective numbers for occipital area are < 30%, 45–73%, and >10% and for temporal area, <40%, 50–75%, and >10%.[11]

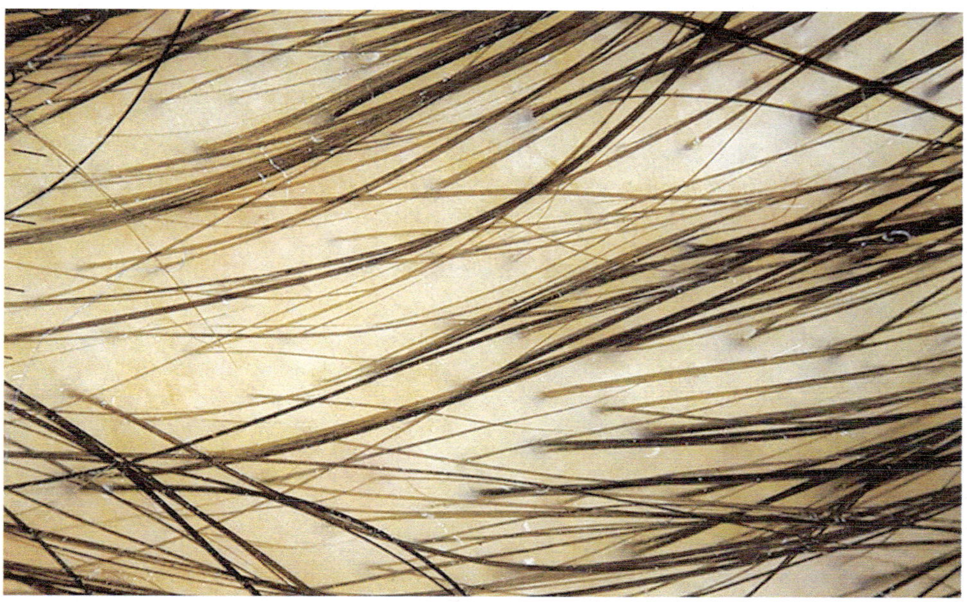

Fig. 12: Reduced number of hairs per follicular unit in androgenetic alopecia (AGA). Note hair diameter diversity.

YELLOW DOTS

- They are a feature of severe miniaturization and are more numerous in patients with severe FPHL and severe AGA.
- They correspond to follicular ostia filled with keratosebaceous material.
- They were first described in alopecia areata.
- Rudnicka et al. hypothesized that yellow dots in AGA consist mainly of sebum.[13] Yellow dots of DLE correspond to wide infundibula filled with keratotic material.[14]

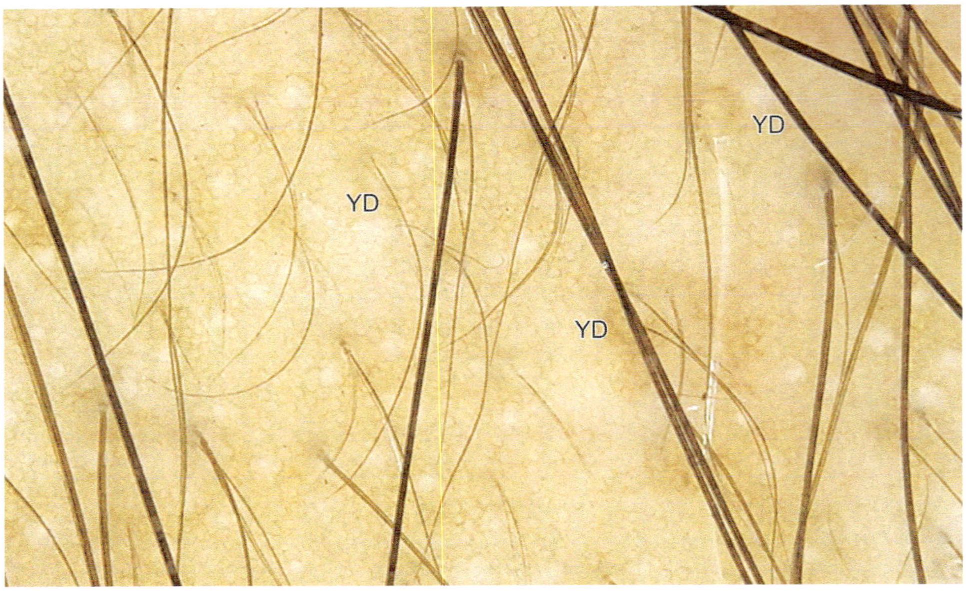

Fig. 13: Yellow dots (YD).

REFERENCES

1. Otenberg N, Finner AM, Shapiro J. Androgenetic alopecia. Endrocrinol Metab Clin North Am. 2007;36(2):379-98.
2. Olsen EA. Female pattern hair loss and its relationship to permanent/cicatricial alopecia: A new prespective. J Investig Dermatol Symp Proc. 2005;10(3):217-21.
3. Price VH. Androgenetic alopecia in women. J Investig Dermatol Symp Proc. 2003;8(1):24-7.
4. Trueb RM. Systematic approach to hair loss in women. J Dtsch Dermatol Ges. 2010;8(4):284-98.
5. Inui S, Nakajima T, Itami S. Scalp dermoscopy of androgenetic alopecia in Asian people. J Dermatol. 2009;36(2):82-5.
6. de Lacharriere O, Deloche C, Misciali C, Piraccini BM, Vincenzi C, Bastien P, et al. Hair diameter diversity: A clinical sign reflecting the follicle miniaturization. Arch Dermatol. 2001;137(5):641-6.
7. Vincenzi C, Tosti A. Nonscarring alopecias. In: Tosti A (ed). Dermoscopy of Hair and Nails, 2nd edition. New Delhi: CRC Press; 2016. pp. 29-49.
8. Rakowska A, Slowinska M, Kowalska-Oledzka E. Androgenetic alopecia. In: Rudnicka L, Olszewska M, Rakowska A (eds). Atlas of Trichoscopy. Philadelphia: Springer; 2012. pp. 231.
9. Deloche C, de Lacharriere O, Misciali C, Piraccini BM, Vincenzi C, Bastien P, et al. Histological features of peripilar signs associated with androgenetic alopecia. Arch Dermatol Res. 2004;295:422-8.
10. Karadag Kose O, Gulec AT. Clinical evaluation of alopecias using handheld dermatoscope. J Am Acad Dermatol. 2011;67:206-14.
11. Rakowska A. Trichoscopy (hair and scalp videodermoscopy) in healthy female. Method standardization and norms for measurable parameters. J Dermatol Case Rep. 2009;3(1):14-9.
12. Vogt A, McElwee KJ, Blume-Peytavi U. Biology of the hair follicle. In: Blume-peytavi U, Tosti A, Whiting D, Trueb R, editors. Hair; from basic science to clinical application. Berlin: Springer; 2008. pp. 1-22.
13. Rakowska A, Slowinska M, Kowalska-Oledzka E, Olszewska M, Rudnicka L. Dermoscopy in female androgenic alopecia: method standardization and diagnostic criteria. Int J Trichol. 2009;1(2);123-30.
14. Rudnicka L, Olszewska M, Rakowska A, Slowinska M. Trichoscopy update 2011. J Dermatol Case Rep. 2011;5(4):82-8.

ASSESSMENT IMAGE-BASED QUESTIONS

1. Brown halo around the emergence of hair follicles. (A) What is the name of this phenomenon? (B) What is its pathological correlation? (C) Name the conditions where you can find it.

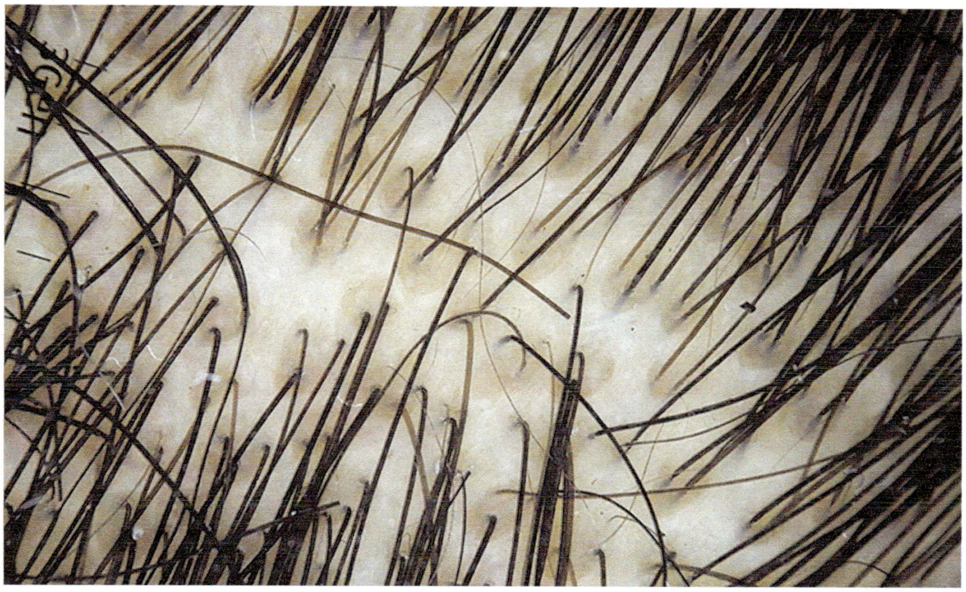

2. What is the trichoscopic finding of this field? In which condition you can find it?

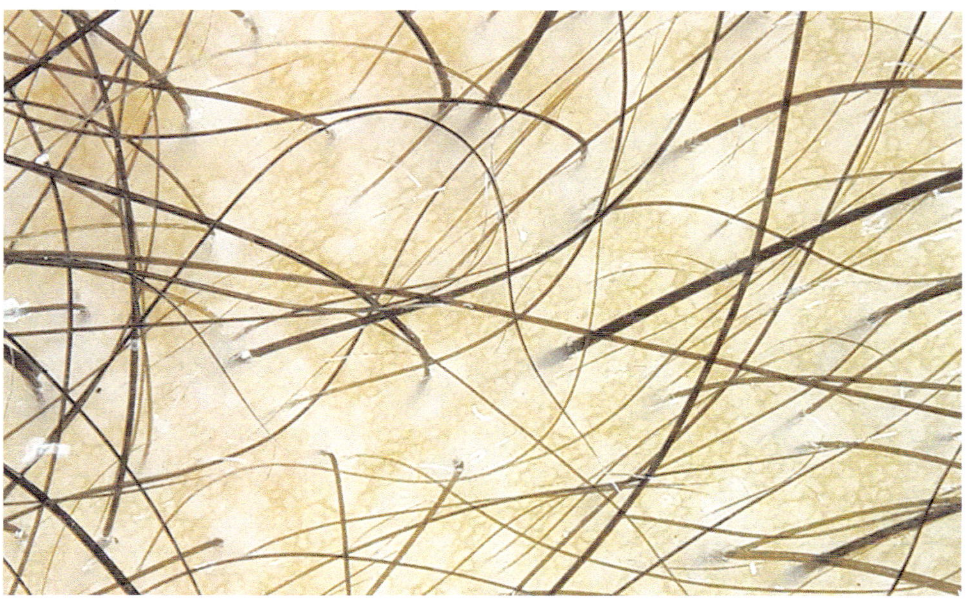

3. Red arrow points toward a thin wavy hair. Name the conditions where it may be found.

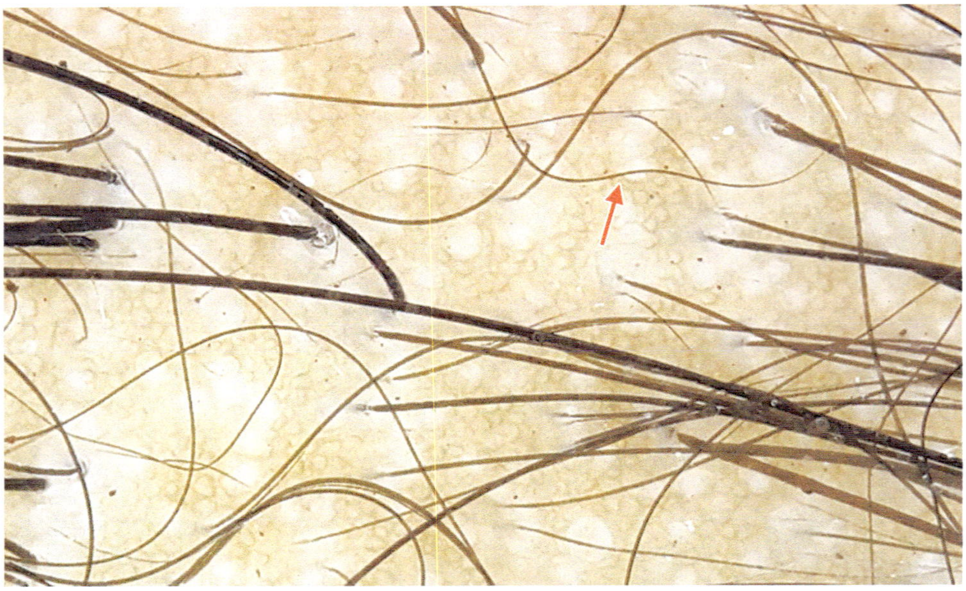

4. This trichoscopic observation is a very important distinguishing feature of AGA. What are the other trichoscopic findings of this condition?

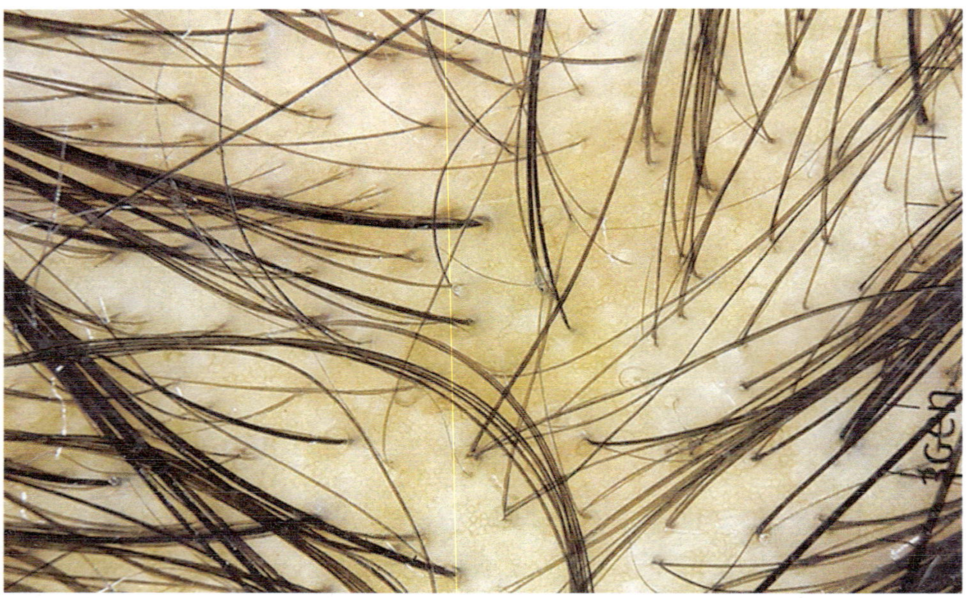

5. In this field of trichoscopic examination of AGA number of vellus hairs are increased. They are less than 30 μm in diameter and <3 mm long. They are hypopigmented and nonmedullated. What is the mechanism of vellus hair transformation from terminal hairs? Mention the percentage of normal vellus hairs.

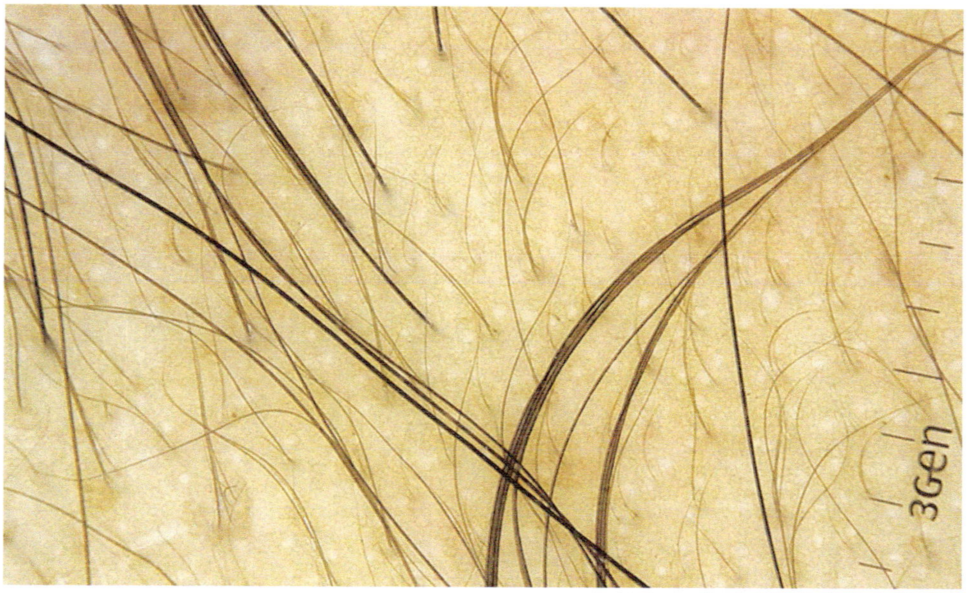

6. The proportion of single hair units are increased in AGA. Usually 1–3 hairs emerge from one follicular opening. What is the normal proportion of single hair units?

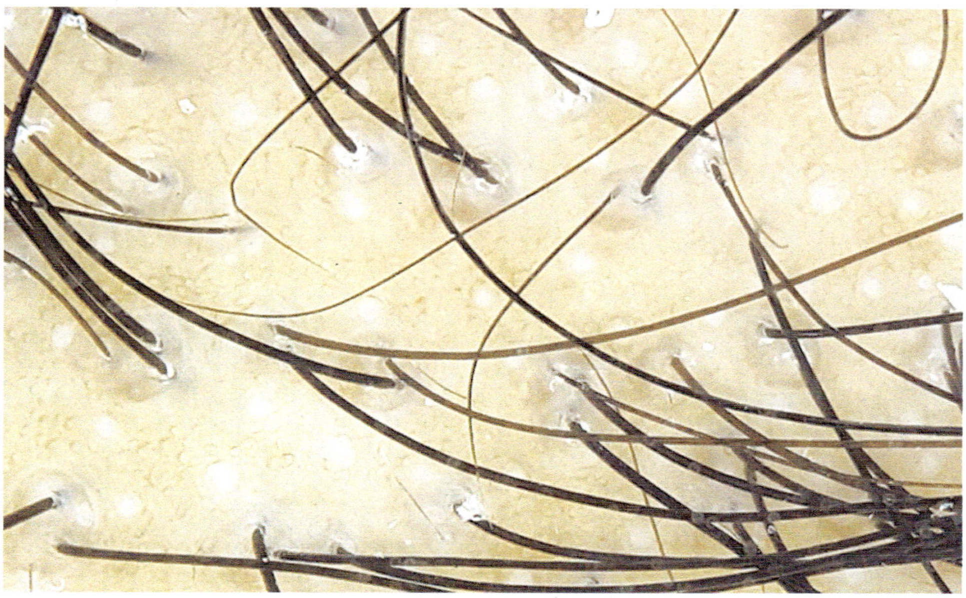

7. Yellow dots are follicular openings with keratosebaceous material. They are first described in AA and are also found in AGA. Yellow dots in AGA usually differ from those in AA; in AGA these dots are distributed irregularly and they have high variability in their size and shape. Try to locate the yellow dots in this picture.

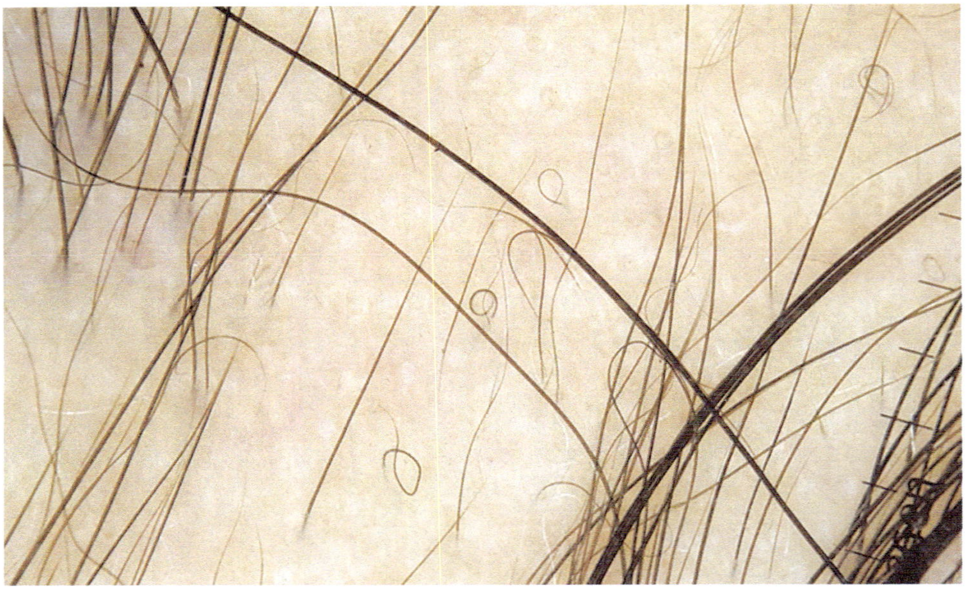

8. Clinicodermoscopically this is a case of AGA. The main trichoscopic features are hair diameter diversity, peripilar sign and yellow dots. In which area of the scalp these features are more pronounced?

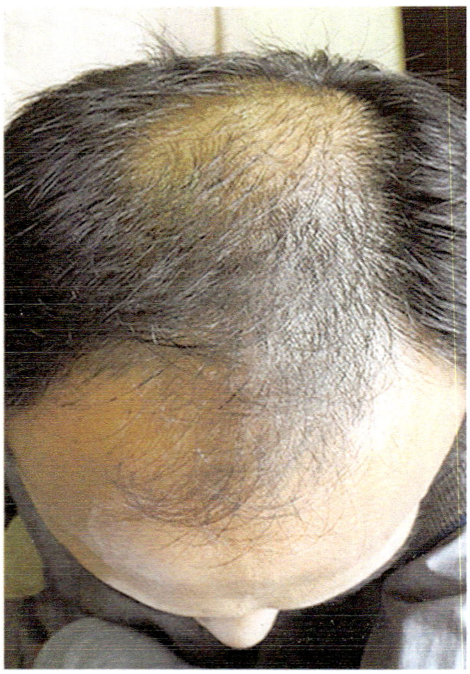

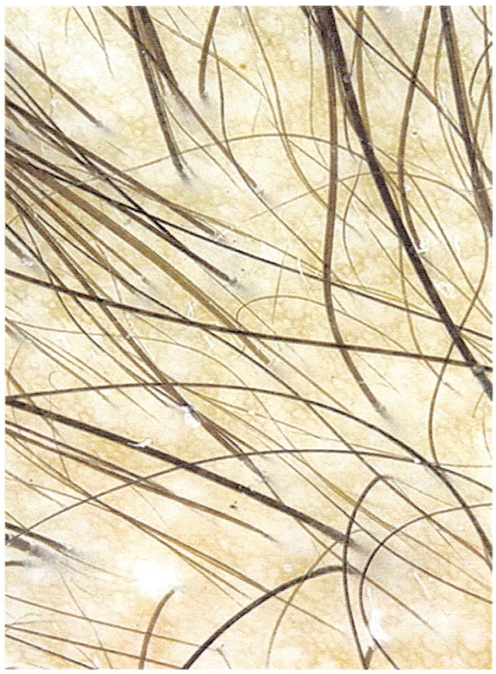

9. Arrows 1 and 2 signify which conditions?

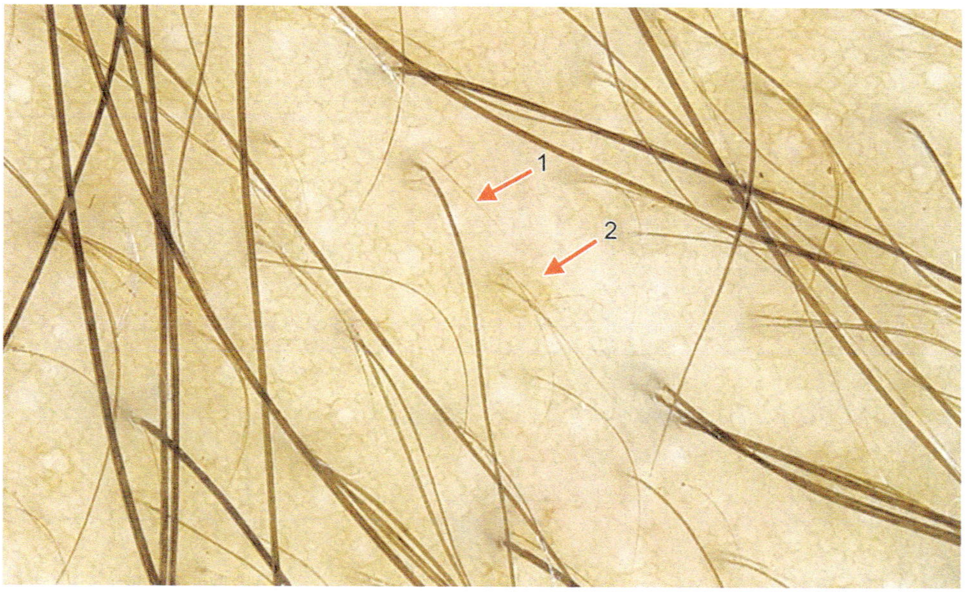

10. Arrows 1 and 2 indicate which trichoscopic features.

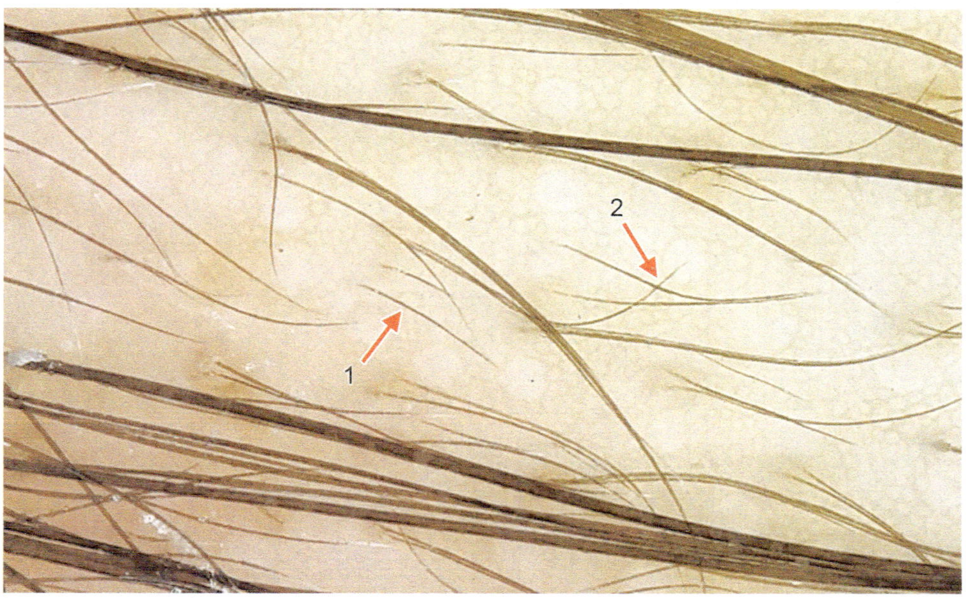

11. What are the trichoscopic features of this image?

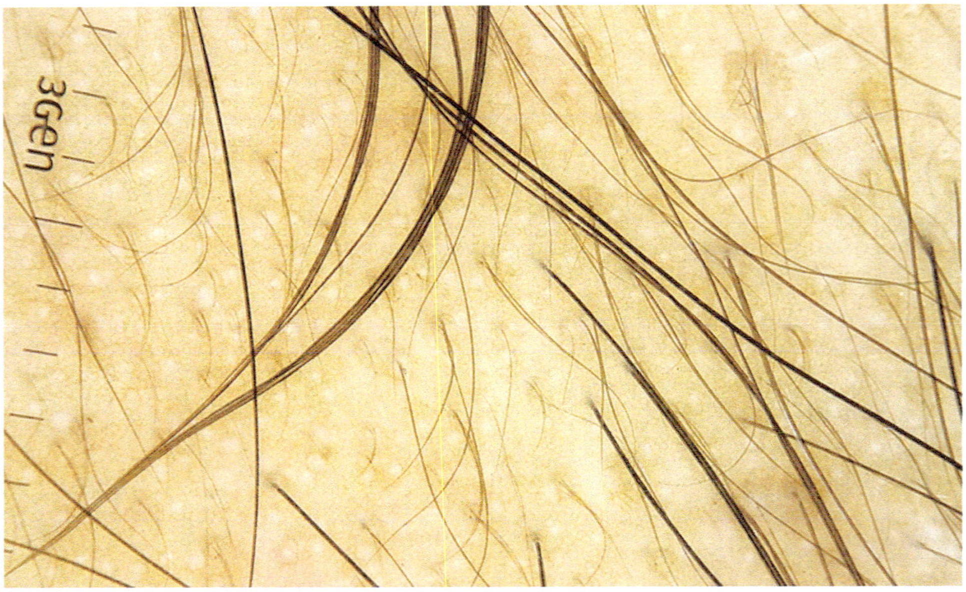

12. This trichoscopic image shows uniform miniaturization. Name the condition and its differential diagnosis.

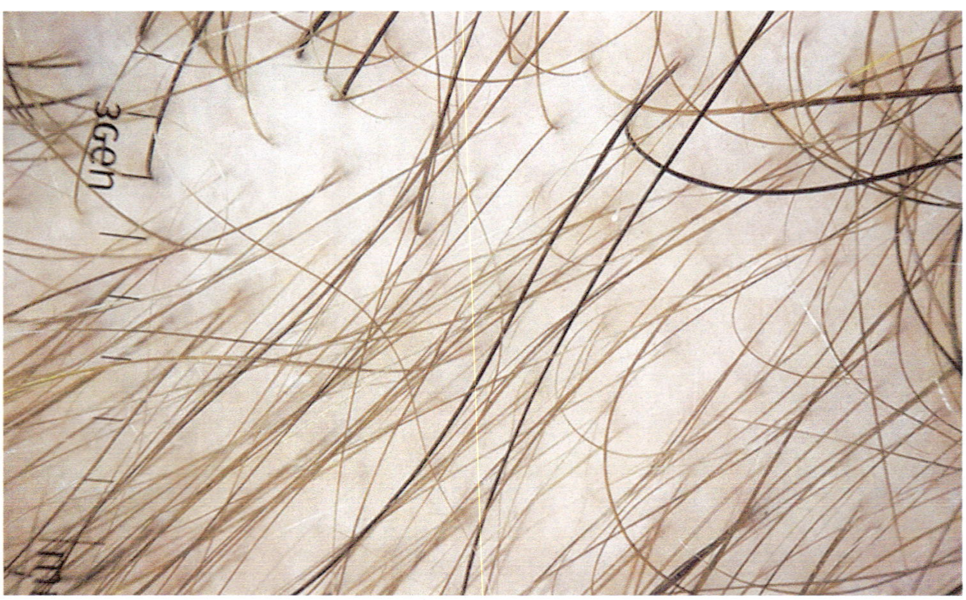

13. Thin wavy hairs are seen in this trichoscopic image. Name the conditions in which they are found.

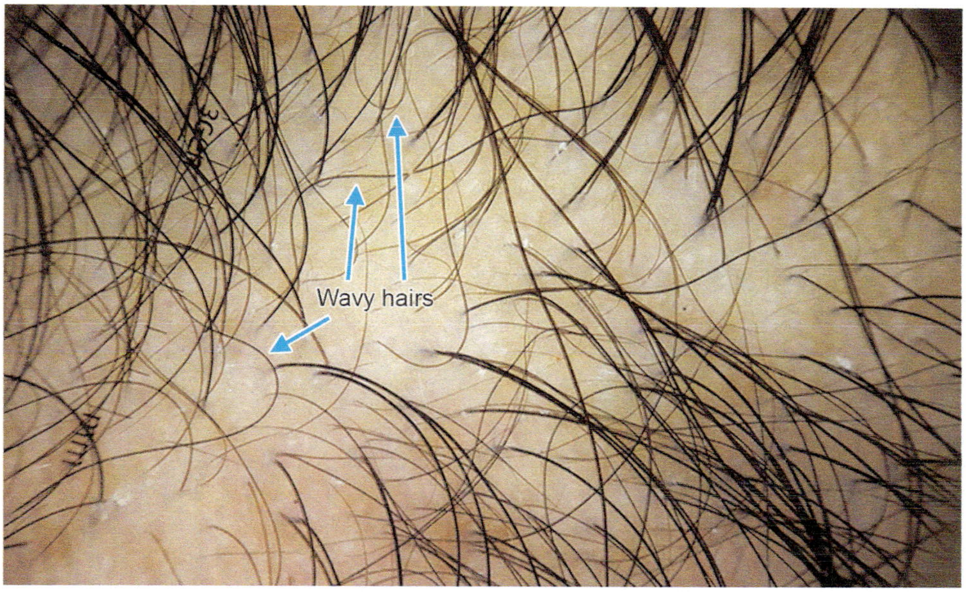

ANSWERS

1. (A) Peripilar sign; (B) Lymphocytic infiltrate around the follicle; (C) Anagen effluvium, androgenetic alopecia
2. Hair diameter diversity, androgenetic alopecia
3. AGA, Alopecia areata incognito
4. Hair diameter diversity. Peripilar sign, yellow dots
5. Miniaturization of hair due to hormonal influence. <10%
6. Up to 35%
7. 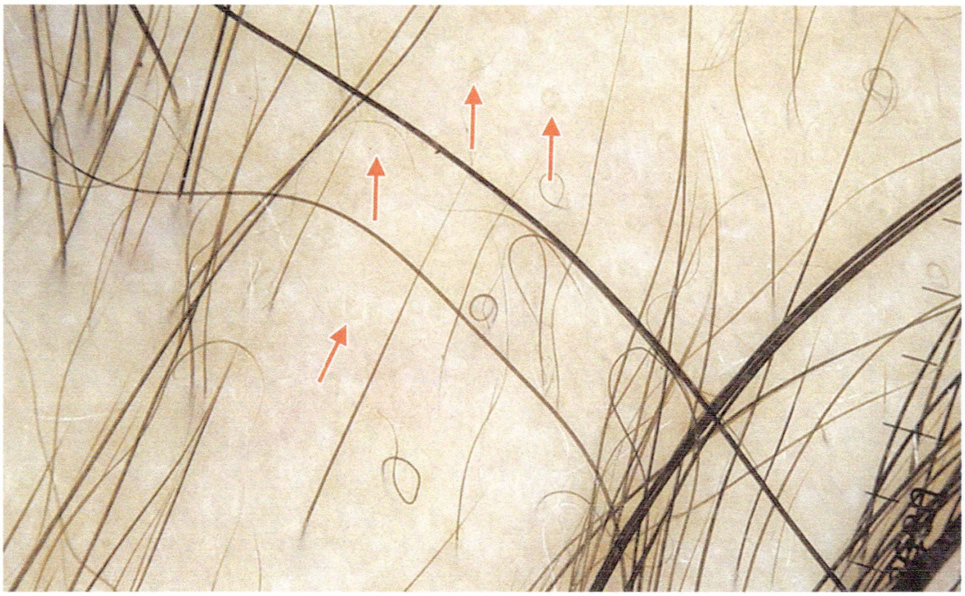
8. Frontal area
9. 1. Dark line; 2. Yellow dot
10. 1, 2. Dark line
11. Hair diameter diversity, terminal hair, vellus hair, peripilar sign, pinpoint white dots, yellow dots
12. Alopecia areata. Androgenetic alopecia, alopecia areata
13. Alopecia areata incognito, AGA

CHAPTER

10

Female Pattern Hair Loss

Subrata Malakar, Surit Malakar, Purva Mehta Movdawalla

INTRODUCTION

- Androgenetic alopecia (AGA) in female has been termed "female pattern hair loss" (FPHL) as the androgen-dependent hair loss in women has not been demonstrated adequately.[1]
- Presentation of AGA in female differs from male. Female may present with episodic or continuous shedding of hairs without any noticeable hair reduction. Diffuse thinning of the crown with no history of hair shedding may be another way of presentation of FPHL.[2]
- Majority of female are diagnosed as FPHL by thinning of the midline scalp with preservation of the frontal hair margin.[1]
- The "Christmas tree" pattern is another clue to diagnose FPHL.[3]
- AGA in male and FPHL shares the same pathogenetic pathway resulting in hair follicle miniaturization.[4-6]
- Early female AGA is difficult to diagnose without the use of trichoscopy.

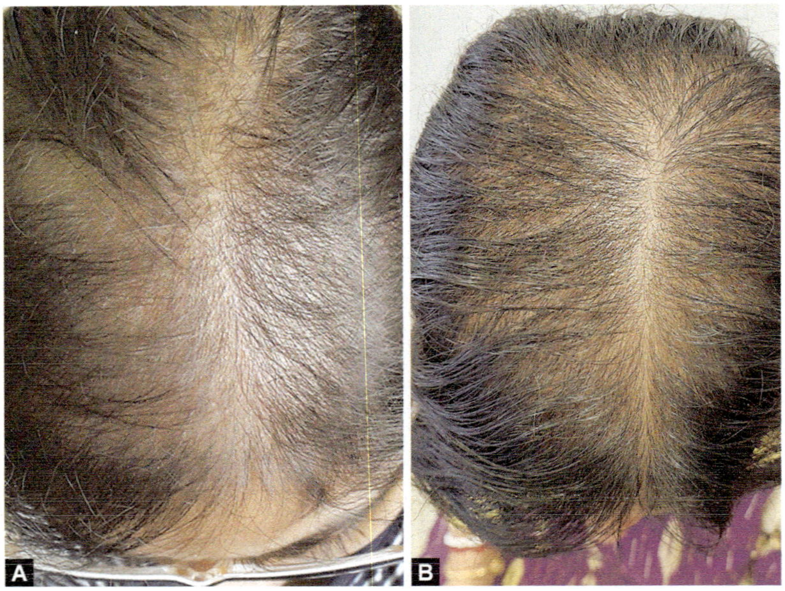

Figs. 1A and B: Female pattern hair loss.

KEY TRICHOSCOPIC FEATURES

The trichoscopic features are similar to those described for AGA and they include the following:

- Hair diameter variability > 20%
- Peripilar sign
- Yellow dots
- Short vellus hairs
- FPHL most commonly coexists with telogen effluvium (TE) which can be diagnosed trichoscopically

HAIR DIAMETER VARIABILITY

- Hair diameter variability of >20% is diagnostic of FPHL.
- Trichoscopy can differentiate FPHL from TE and is also a useful diagnostic tool to determine the coexistence of FPHL and TE.
- In severe FPHL, most follicular units contain single hair shafts.

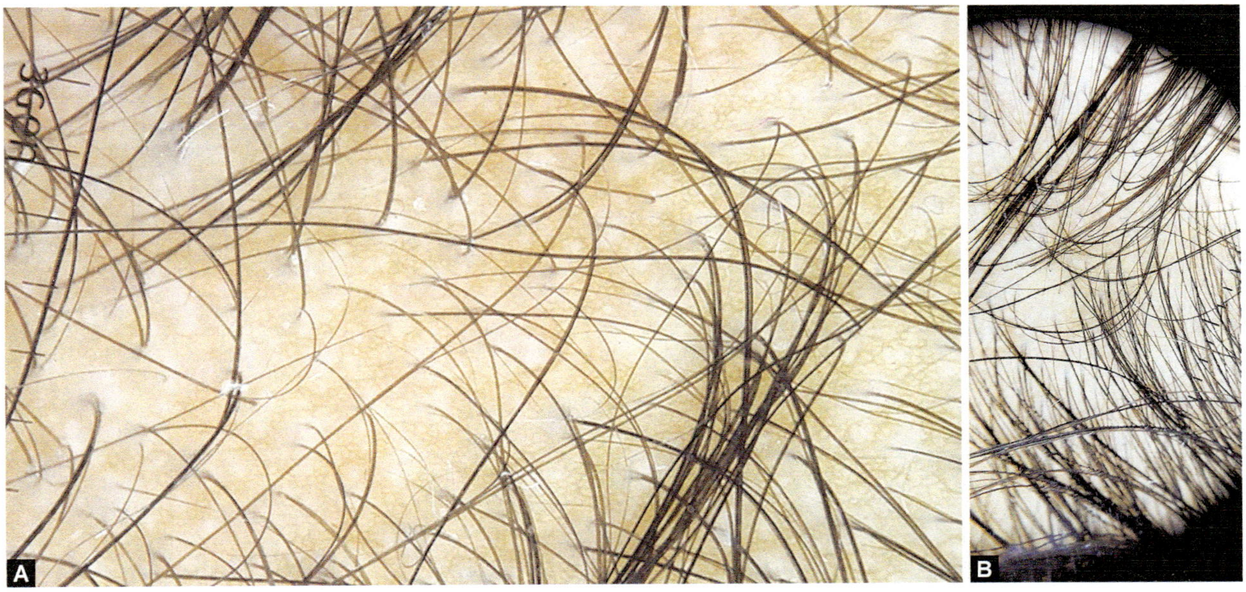

Figs. 2A and B: Hair diameter variability in a case of female pattern hair loss (FPHL).

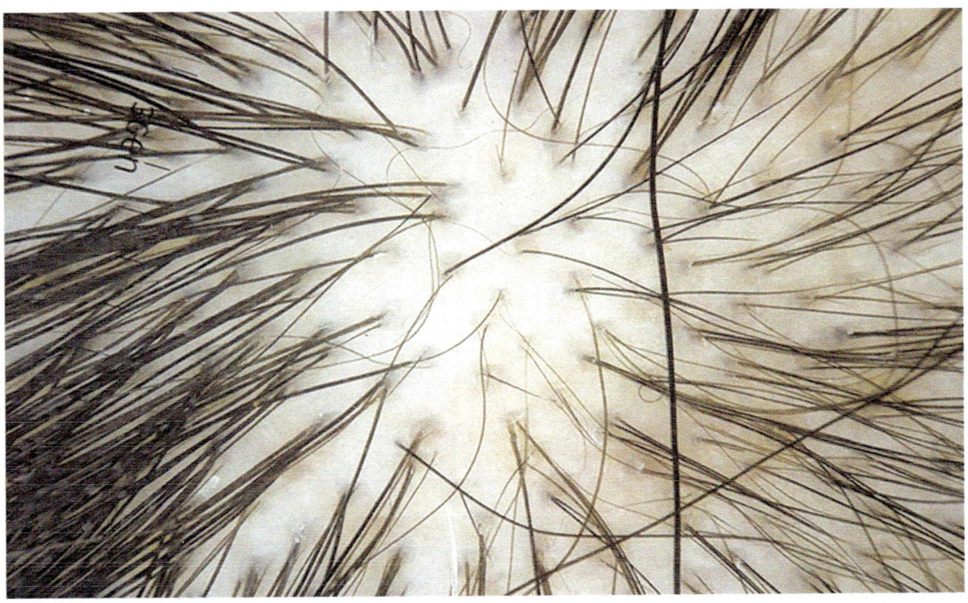

Fig. 3: Coexistence of female pattern hair loss (FPHL) and telogen effluvium. Note peripilar sign and hair diameter variability favoring diagnosis of FPHL. Telogen effluvium is diagnosed by the presence of numerous short regrowing hairs.

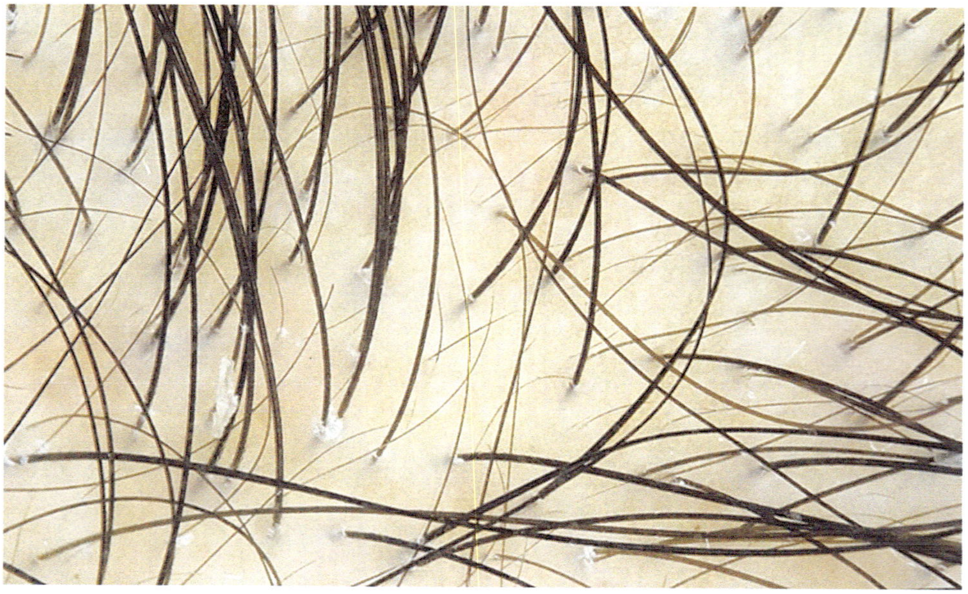

Fig. 4: Hair diameter variability and short regrowing hairs signify coexisting female pattern hair loss (FPHL) and acute telogen effluvium. Note a majority of follicular units contain single hair shafts.

PERIPILAR SIGN

- It is a brown halo of 1-mm diameter around the emergence of hair shaft.
- It corresponds to perifollicular inflammation.
- <5% of hair follicle openings with brown peripilar discoloration is observed in healthy scalp.[7]
- Extensive peripilar sign is a poor prognostic factor.[8]

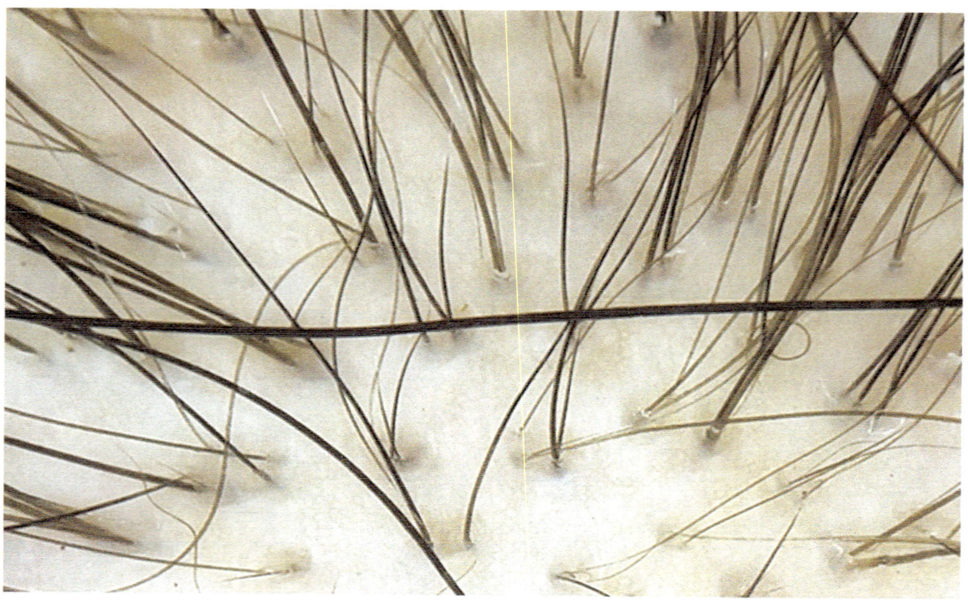

Fig. 5: Brown halo around almost all the hair shafts at their emergence. This extensive peripilar sign is believed to be a poor prognostic factor.

YELLOW DOTS

- Yellow dots does not look yellow in darker skin, rather they are whitish or in most of the circumstances are light yellow at the periphery with whitish at the center.
- In severe FPHL they are numerous.
- More than four yellow dots in four areas of frontal scalp at magnification 70 are a major criterion for diagnosis.[8]
- They are a sign of severe miniaturization.

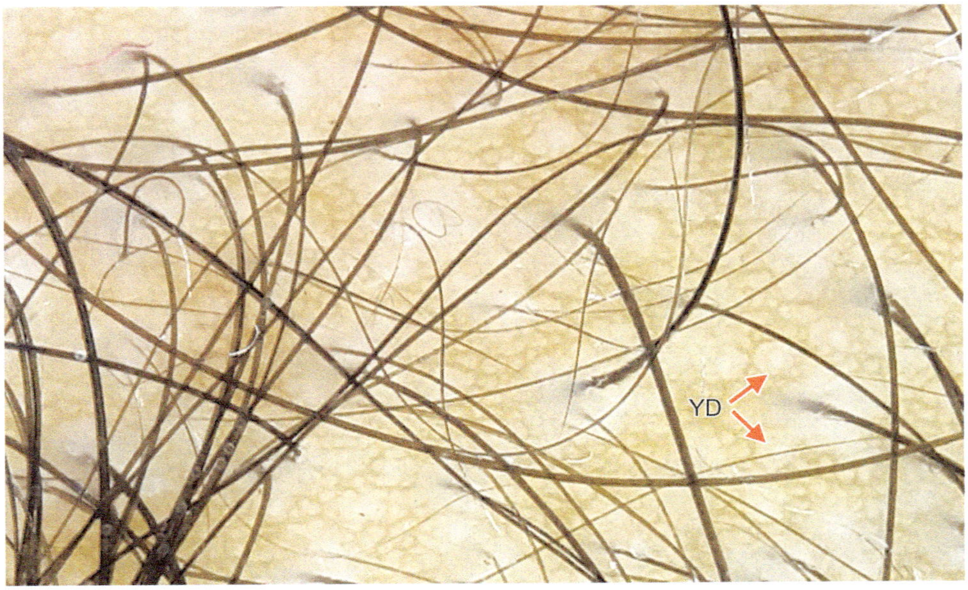

Fig. 6: Yellow dots (YD) in a case of female pattern hair loss (FPHL).

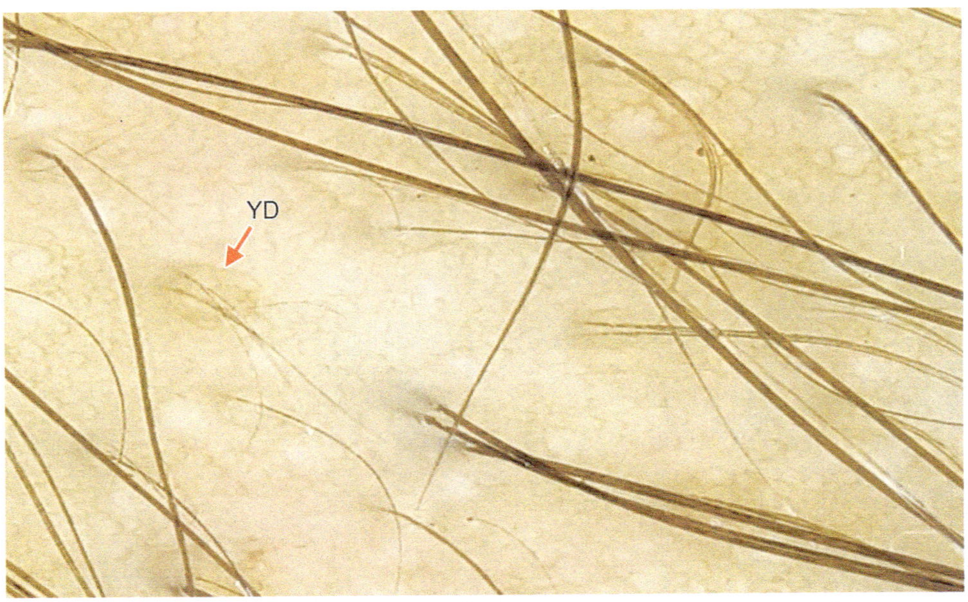

Fig. 7: One yellow dot (YD) showing miniaturization of all the hairs in a single follicular unit. More than four yards are present in the field. More than four yellow dots in four areas of frontal scalp at magnification 70 are a major criterion for diagnosis of androgenetic alopecia of both male and female.[8]

SHORT VELLUS HAIRS

- They are useful hint for the diagnosis of FPHL and are a sign of severe miniaturization.
- Presence of up to 10% vellus hairs in frontal scalp is considered normal. Beyond that or more than seven vellus hairs in frontal scalp is diagnostic for FPHL.

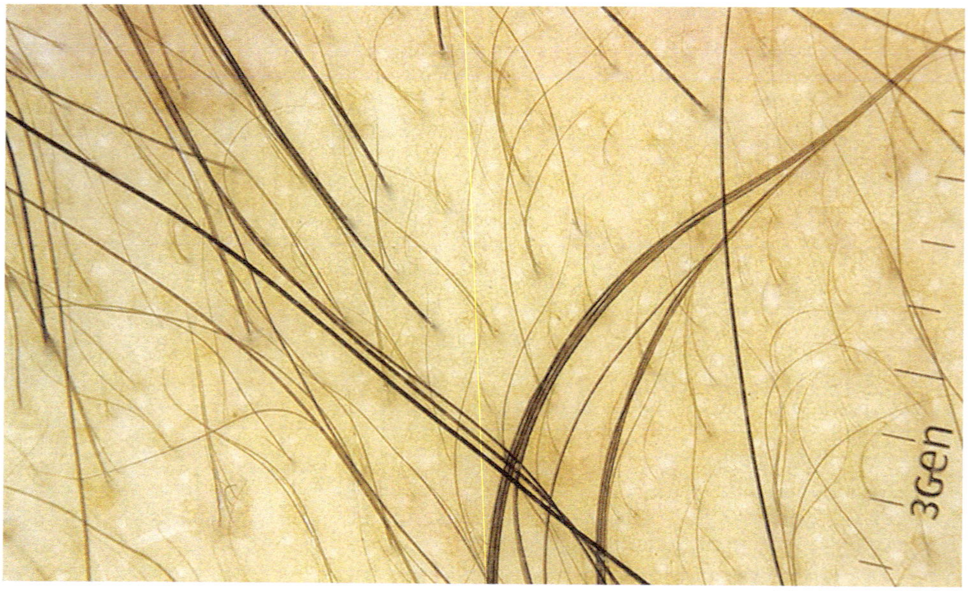

Fig. 8: Most of the follicles in the field have short vellus hairs which are a sign of severe miniaturization.

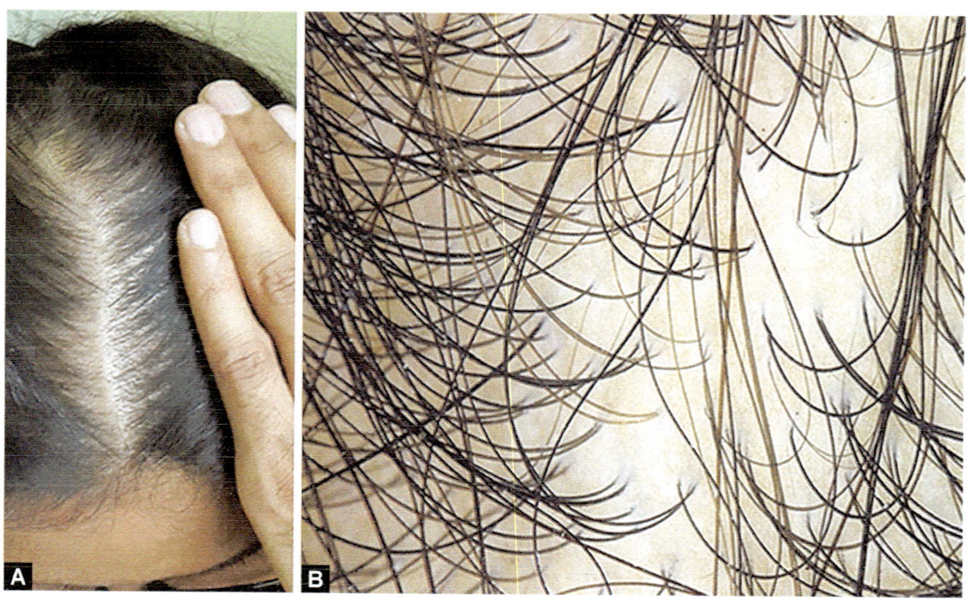

Continued

Continued

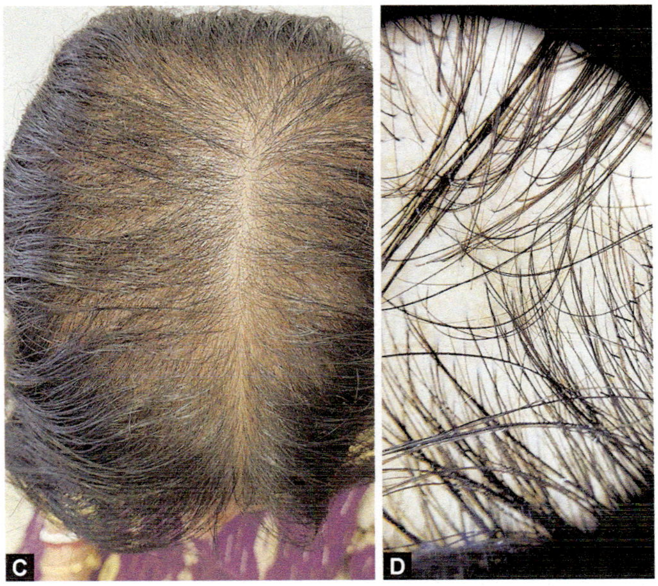

Figs. 9A to D: Female pattern hair loss. Diffuse thinning of crown with maintenance of hair line (Ludwig pattern). Trichoscopic features are similar to androgenetic alopecia (AGA) of male including hair diameter diversity and peripilar sign which are the two important criteria of diagnosis.

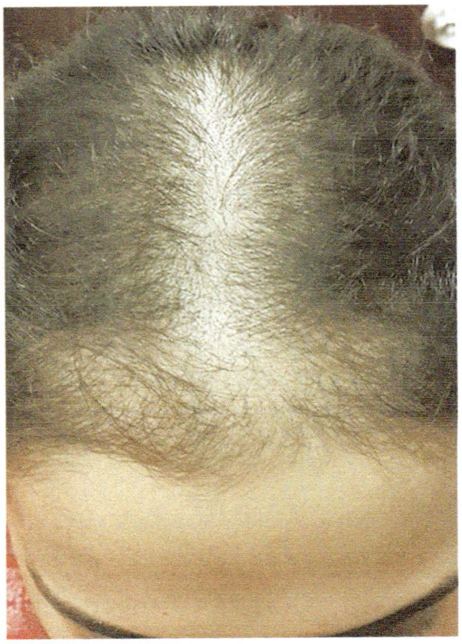

Fig. 10: Female pattern hair loss—the so called "fern tree appearance".

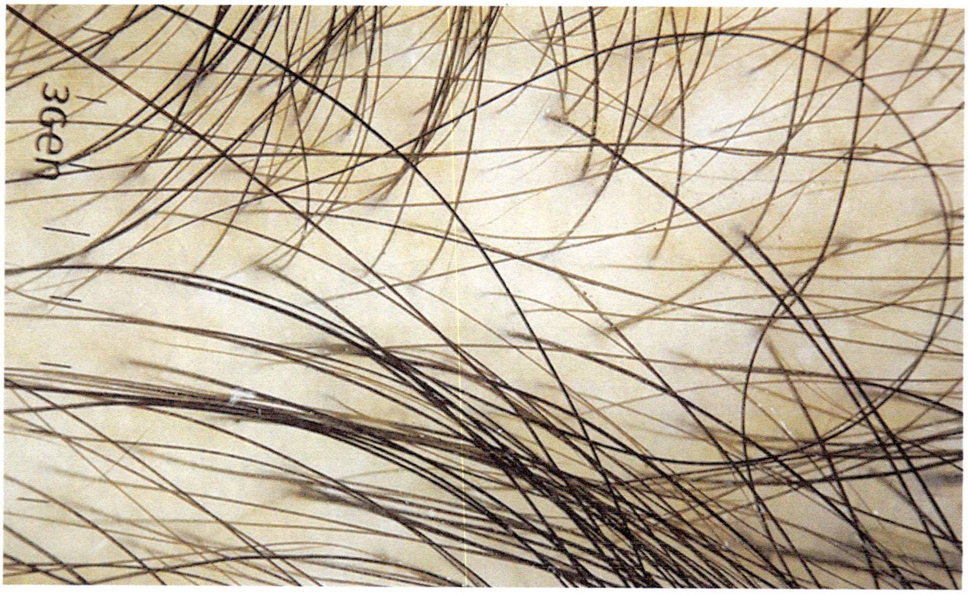

Fig. 11: FPHL showing hair diameter variability.

REFERENCES

1. Olsen EA. Female pattern hair loss. J Am Acad Dermatol. 2001;45:S70-S80.
2. Sinclair RD, Dawber RP. Androgenetic alopecia in men and women. Clinical dermatol. 2001;19:167-8.
3. Olsen EA. The midline part: an important physical clue to the clinical diagnosis of androgenetic alopecia in women. J Am Acad Dermatol. 1999;40:106-9.
4. Otenberg N, Finner AM, Shapiro J. Androgenetic alopecia. Endrocrinol Metab Clin North Am. 2007;36(2):379-98.
5. Olsen EA. Female pattern hair loss and its relationship to permanent/cicatricial alopecia: A new prespective. J Investig Dermatol Symp Proc. 2005;10(3):217-21.
6. Price VH, Androgenetic alopecia in women. J Investig Dermatol Symp Proc. 2003;8(1):24-7.
7. Karadağ Kőse O, Gűlec AT. Clinical evaluation of alopecias using handheld dermatoscope. J Am Acad Dermatol. 2011;67:206-14.
8. Rakaowska A, Slowinska K, Kowalska-Oledzka E, Olszewska M, Rudnicka L. Dermatoscopy in female androgenetic alopecia: Method standardization and diagnostic criteria. Int J Trichology. 2009;1:123-30.

ASSESSMENT IMAGE-BASED QUESTIONS

1. What do the arrows signify?

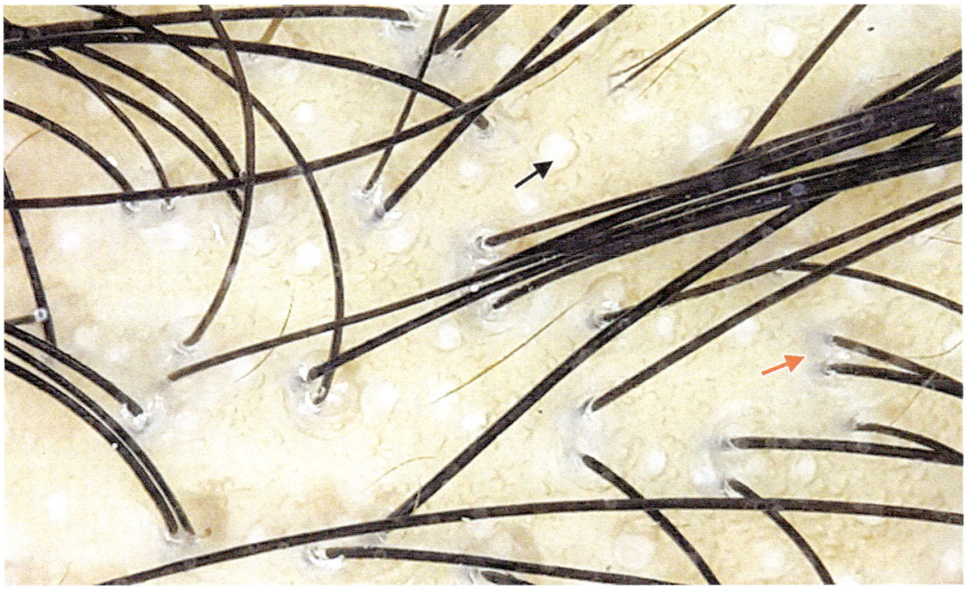

2. What do short regrowing hairs signify?

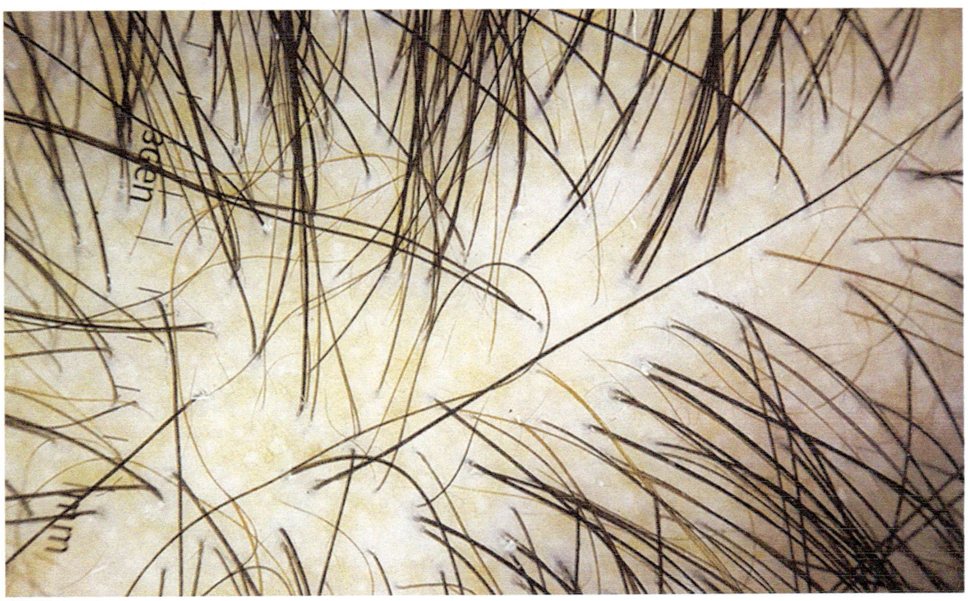

3. In which condition are thin wavy hair seen?

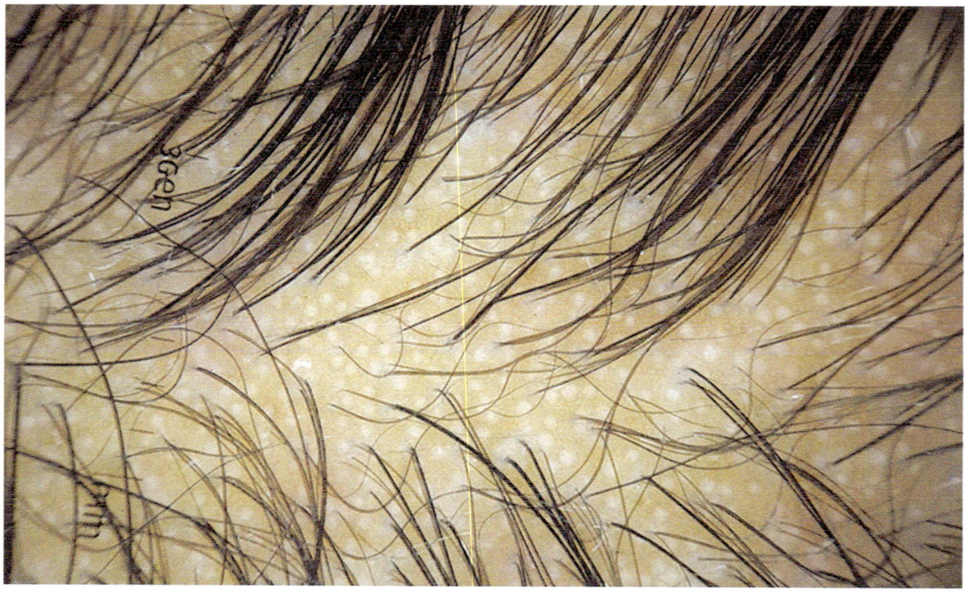

4. What do numerous pinpoint white dots signify?

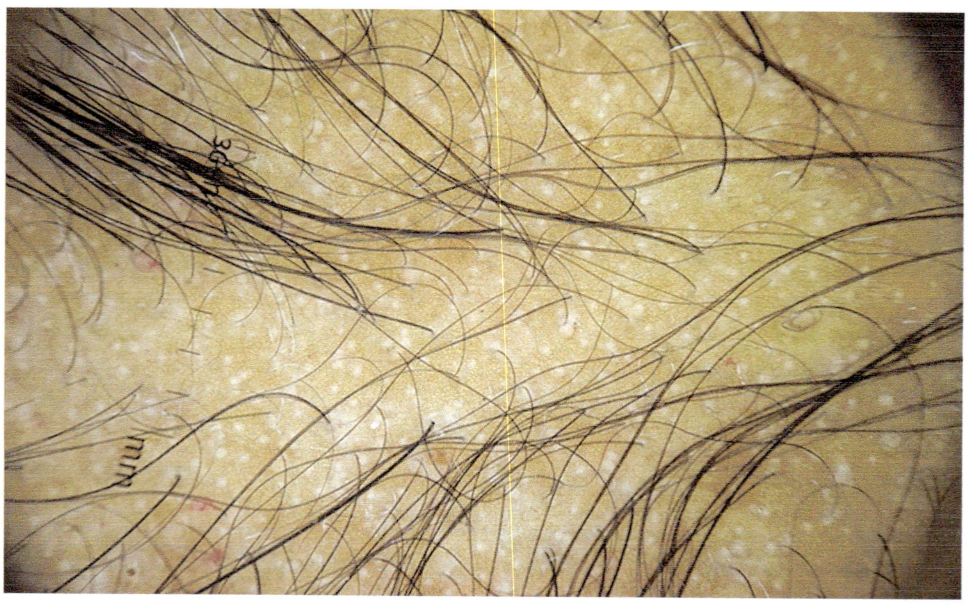

5. Clinically this is a case of FPHL. Mention the main trichoscopic features of FPHL.

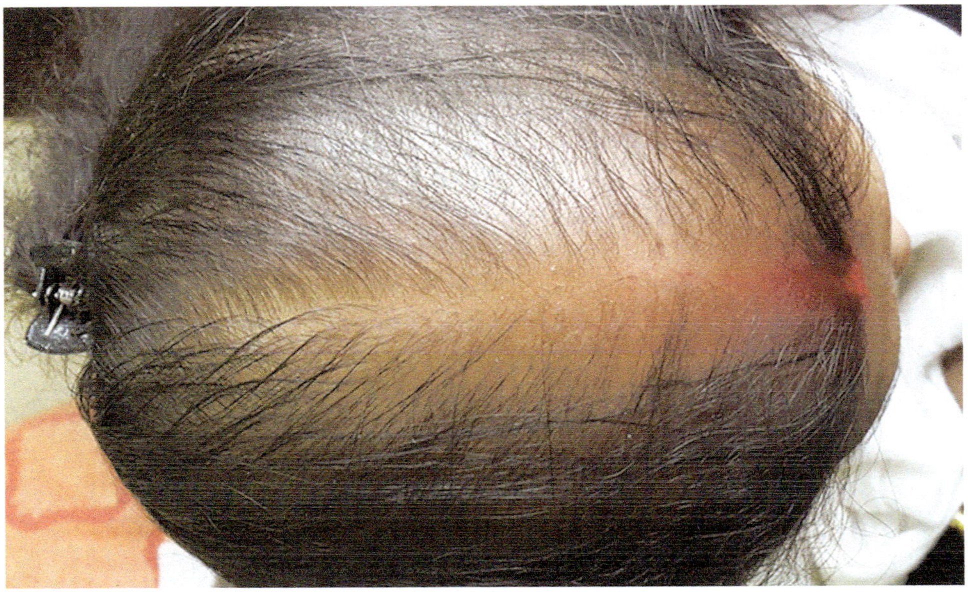

6. This is the trichoscopic image of the previous patient. Is it a case of scarring or nonscarring alopecia? Why do you think so? Identify the red patches?

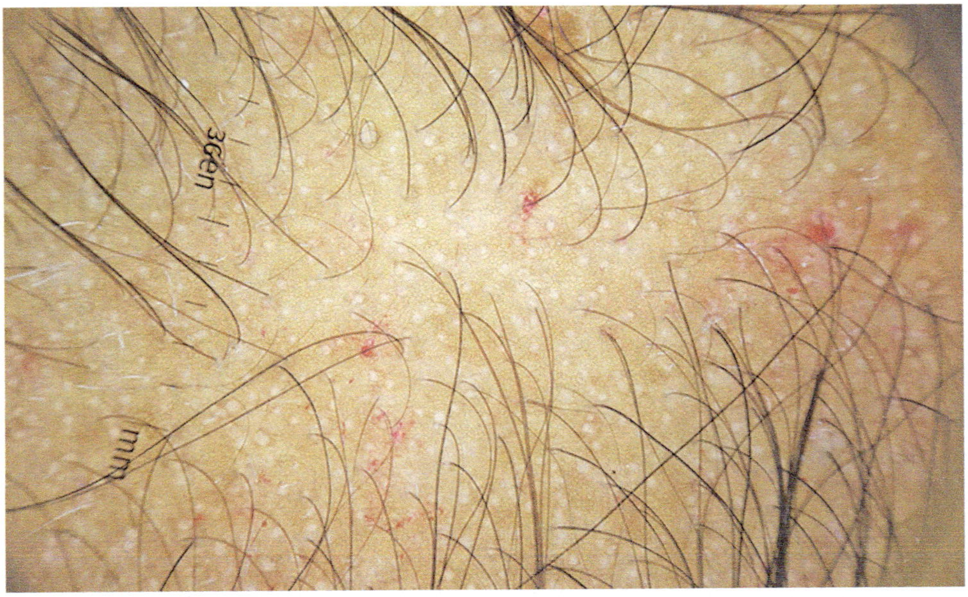

ANSWERS

1. Yellow dots
2. Telogen effluvium
3. AGA, Alopecia areata incognito
4. Non scarring alopecia
5. Hair diameter diversity, yellow dots
6. Nonscarring alopecia, pinpoint white dots, and *sindoor* application residue

CHAPTER 11A

Alopecia Areata Incognito

Subrata Malakar

INTRODUCTION

- Alopecia areata incognito (AAI) is a subtype of acute telogen effluvium (TE) that develops in patient with female androgenetic alopecia (AGA).[1]
- First described by Rebora in 1987.[2]
- It has become a matter of debate after 30 years following the initial publication because of its similarity to alopecia areata.
- Clinically, there is diffuse thinning without typical alopecic patch that is why Rebora named the condition AAI.[2]
- Commonly occurs in women, the alopecic patch may be more evident on androgen-dependent scalp. It has a good prognosis for hair regrowth.
- Pull test—telogen hairs.

KEY TRICHOSCOPIC FEATURES[3]

- Yellow dots—present in both empty follicles and follicles with emerging hair shafts.
- Short regrowing hairs—they have different lengths and shapes. A tendency to form S-shaped hairs is a common finding.
- Tadpole-like hairs—new regrowing hairs with bulging proximal end.

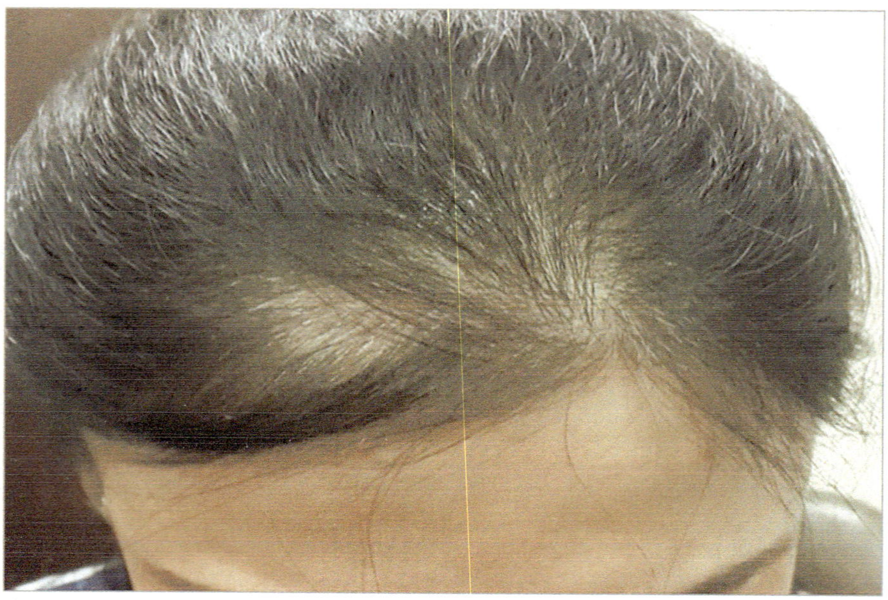

Fig. 1: Alopecia areata incognito in a middle aged lady. Acute hair loss predominantly in the frontal area and is associated with follicular miniaturization and thinning of hair shafts.

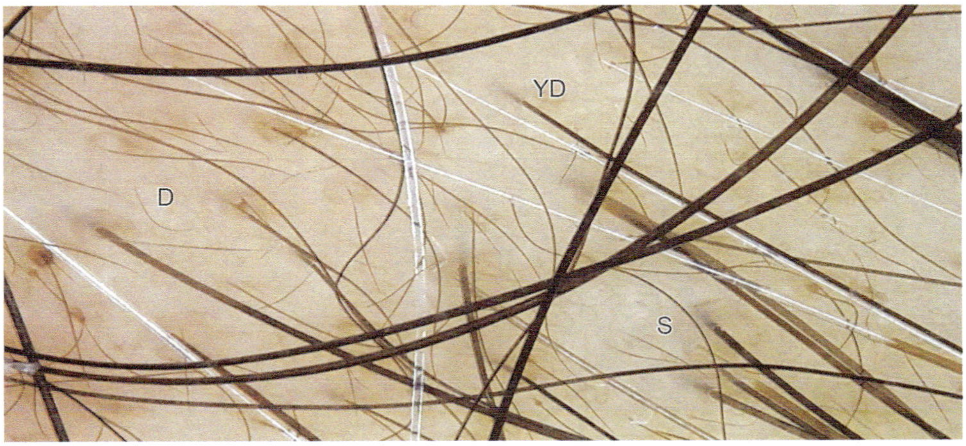

Fig. 2: Yellow dots (YD) and regrowing hairs. Regrowing hairs form different shapes such as dark lines (D) and S-shaped hairs (S).

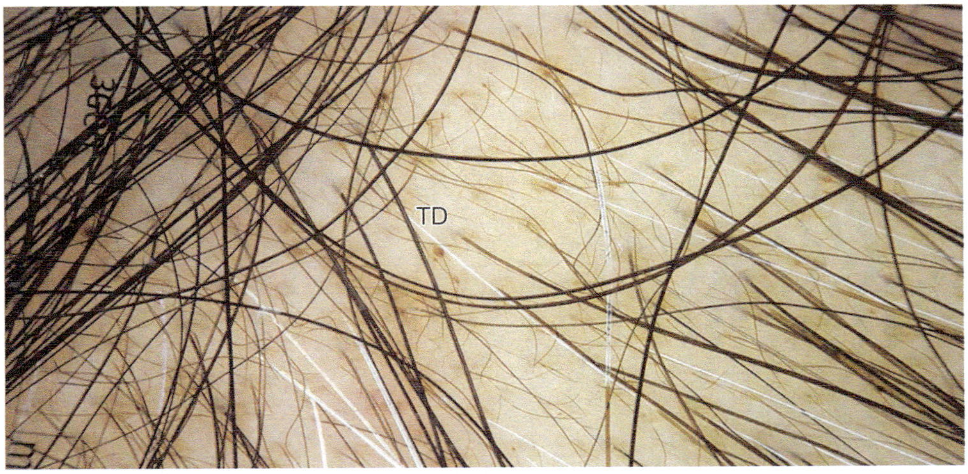

Fig. 3: Multiple shapes and lengths of regrowing hairs in the middle of the image. Tadpole-like hairs (TD) (regrowing hairs with a bulging proximal end).

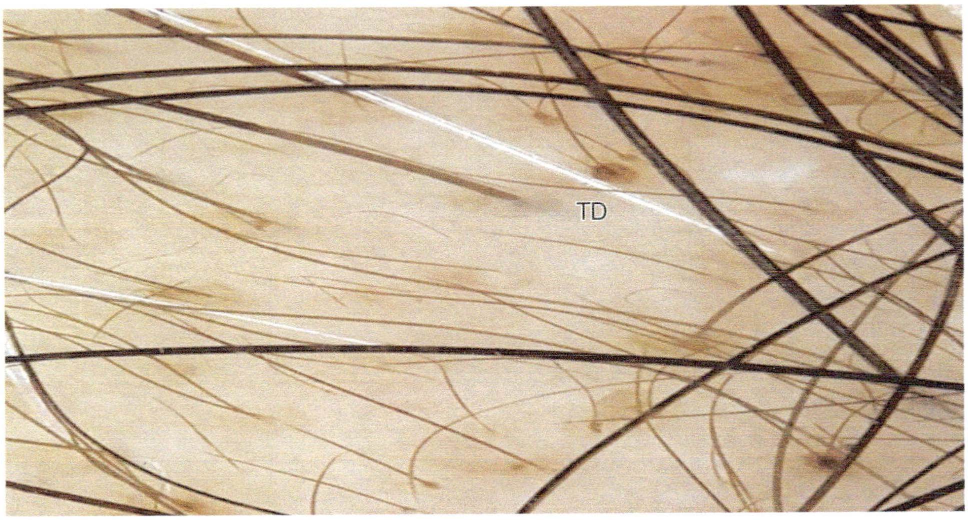

Fig. 4: Tadpole-like (TD) hairs with bulging proximal ends in regrowing hairs.

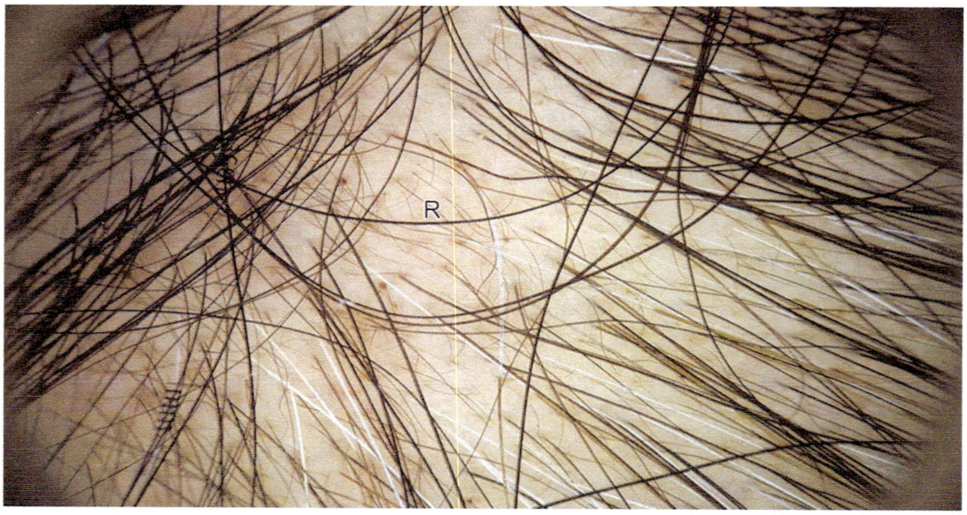

Fig. 5: Overview. Bunch of regrowing hairs (R) with different shapes and lengths. Note the presence of S-shaped hair and tadpole hairs.

REFERENCES

1. Rakowska A, Slowinska M, Kowalska-Oledzka E, Olszewska M, Czuwara J, Rudnicka L. Alopecia areata incognita:true or false? J Am Acad Dermatol. 2009:60(1):162-3.
2. Rebora A. Alopecia areata incognita: A hypothesis. Dermatologica. 1987:174(5):214-8.
3. Rakowska A, Olszewska M, Rudnicka L. Anagen effluvium. In: Rudnicka L, Olszewska M, Rakowska A (Eds). Atlas of Trichoscopy. Philadelphia: Springer; 2012. pp. 251-4.

CHAPTER

11B Alopecia Areata

Subrata Malakar

INTRODUCTION

- It is a nonscarring hair loss that can affect any hair-bearing area.
- Often asymptomatic but some patients may experience burning sensation or pruritus in the affected part.
- Alopecia areata (AA) is a T cell-mediated autoimmune disease that affects genetically predisposed individual.
- Diagnosis is usually made on clinical grounds. Scalp biopsy is rarely needed, but it can be helpful if clinical diagnosis is uncertain. After availability of dermoscopes scalp biopsy is no longer required as AA has specific features on dermoscopy.
- *Histopathology*: The most characteristic feature is peribulbar lymphocytic infiltrate typically described as "swarm of bees".

KEY TRICHOSCOPIC FEATURES OF ALOPECIA AREATA

- Black dots
- Exclamation mark hairs
- Coudability hairs
- Broken hairs
- Vellus hairs
- Yellow dots
- Pohl-Pinkus constrictions
- Zigzag hairs
- Tulip hairs
- Most common trichoscopic features of AA are yellow dots, black dots, broken hairs, coudability hairs, and clustered short vellus hairs (<10 mm).[1]
- Black dots and yellow dots correspond to disease severity.
- Black dots, broken hairs, and tapering hairs correspond to disease activity.
- Most sensitive markers are yellow dots and short vellus hairs.
- Most specific markers are black dots, broken hairs, and tapering hairs.
- Tapering hairs are marker of disease activity and severity.[2,3]

BLACK DOTS

- Black dots corresponds to hair shafts broken at scalp level.
- Presence of numerous black dots is almost diagnostic of AA and they are a sign of disease activity.
- Black dots are also seen in other nonscarring alopecias including tinea capitis, trichotillomania, and chemotherapy-induced alopecia.[4,5]
- A few isolated black dots may be present in scarring such as lichen planopilaris and frontal fibrosing alopecia.

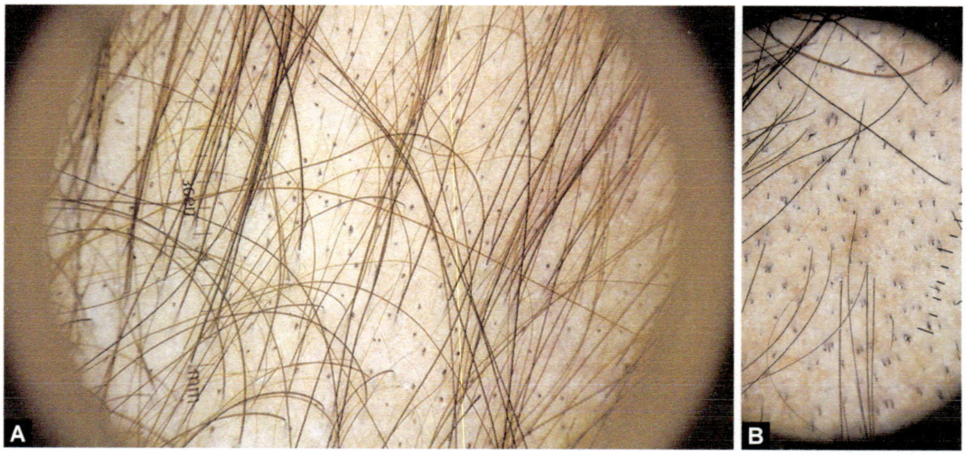

Figs. 1A and B: (A) Numerous black dots are almost diagnostic of alopecia areata (AA); (B) Numerous black dots are almost diagnostic of AA.

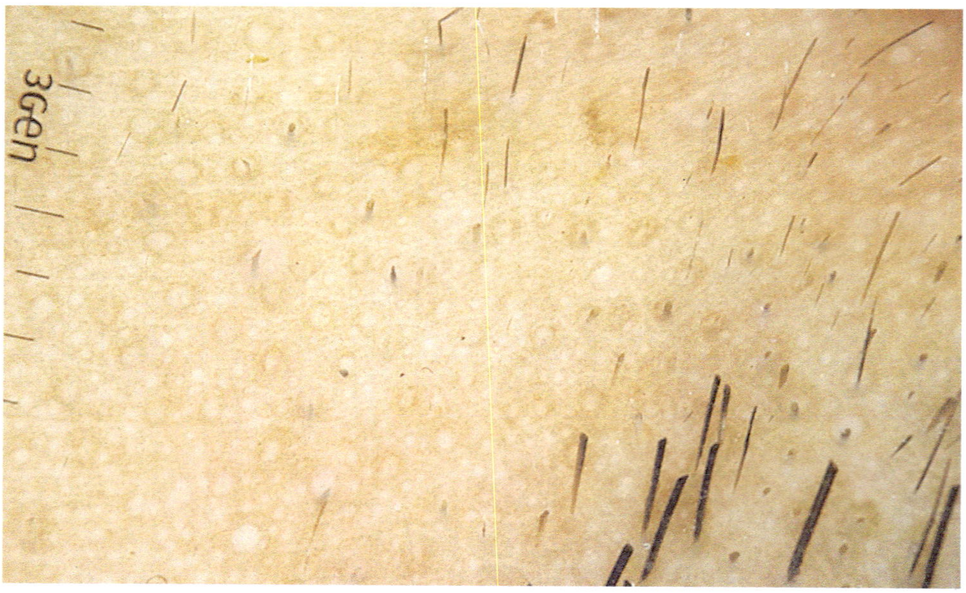

Fig. 2: Black dots, broken hairs, and exclamation mark hairs signify active alopecia areata (AA).

EXCLAMATION MARK HAIRS

- They are short hairs and are seen trichoscopically as thin and hypopigmented at the proximal end and thicker and hyperpigmented at the distal end.
- When visible to the naked eye, these hairs are more or less half inch long, whereas trichoscopic exclamation mark hairs are 1–2 mm long.
- It is mainly manifested due to the rapid transition from anagen to catagen which results in hair shaft narrowing.

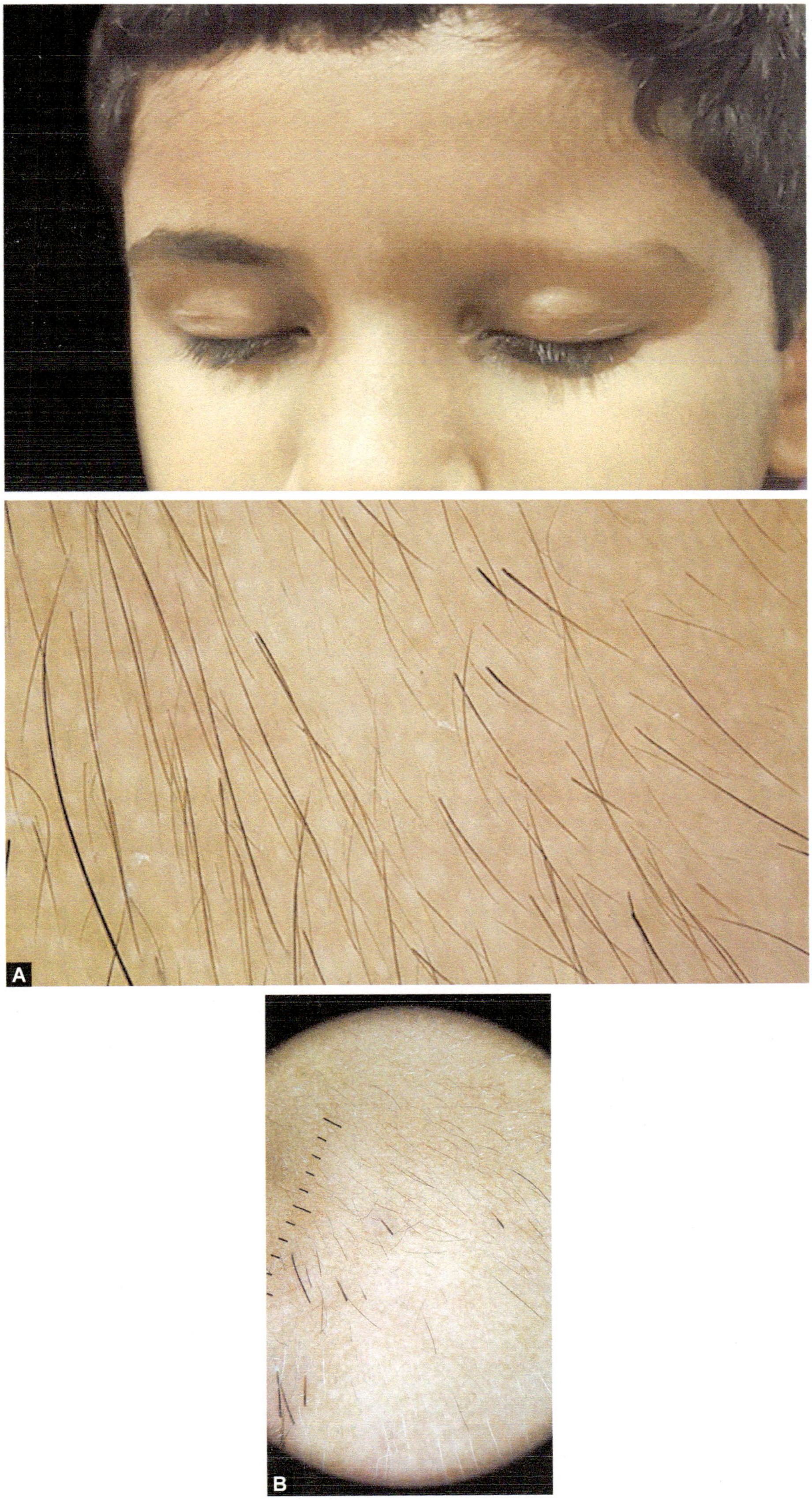

Figs. 3A and B: (A) Alopecia areata (AA) of eyebrow showing exclamation mark hairs on trichoscopy; (B) AA of eyebrow showing exclamation mark hairs on trichoscopy.

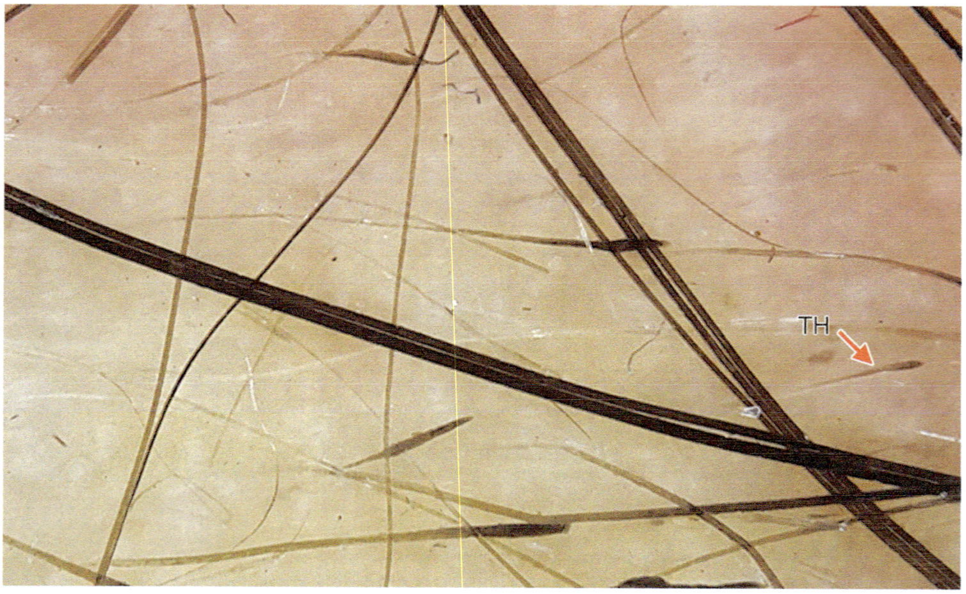

Fig. 4: Exclamation mark hairs: Tapered hairs with dark ends. Exclusively seen in alopecia areata (AA), mostly along the border of the patches. Note the presence of one tulip hair (TH) also.

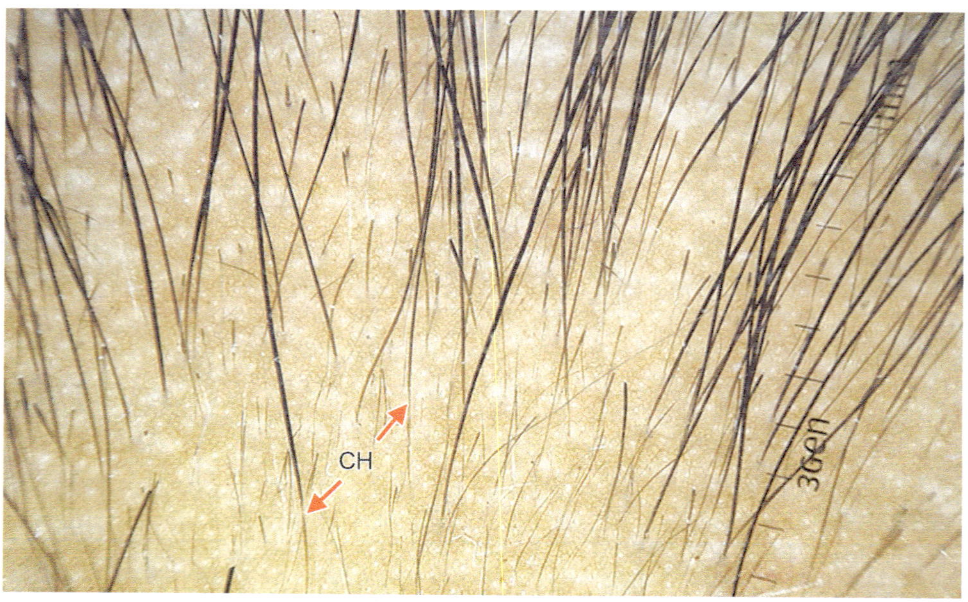

Fig. 5: Coudability hairs (CH) are hairs of normal length with a narrowed proximal hair shaft. They are mostly found in the periphery of alopecic patch.

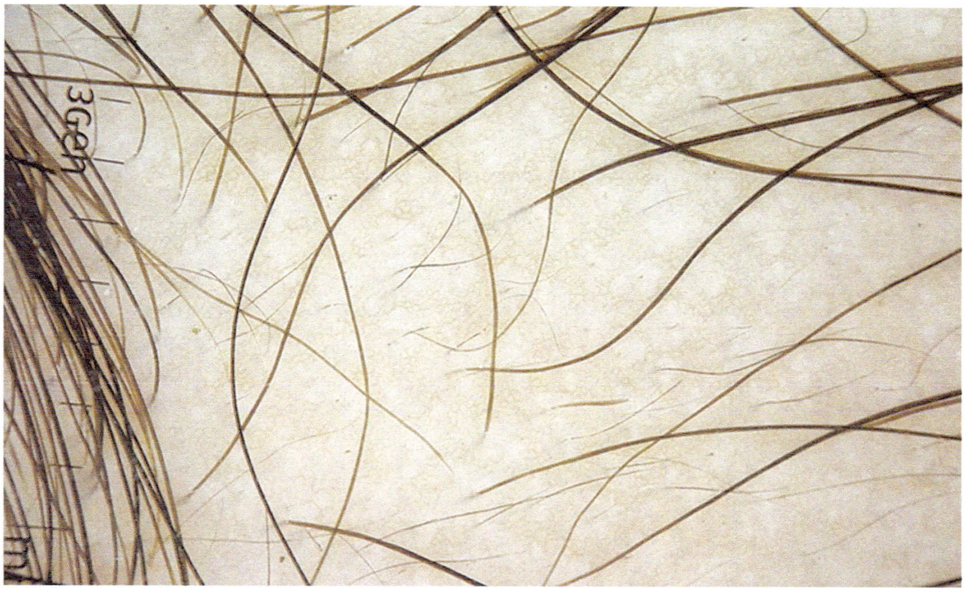

Fig. 6: In this picture regrowing hairs coexist with ongoing active disease showing exclamation mark hairs and coudability hairs.

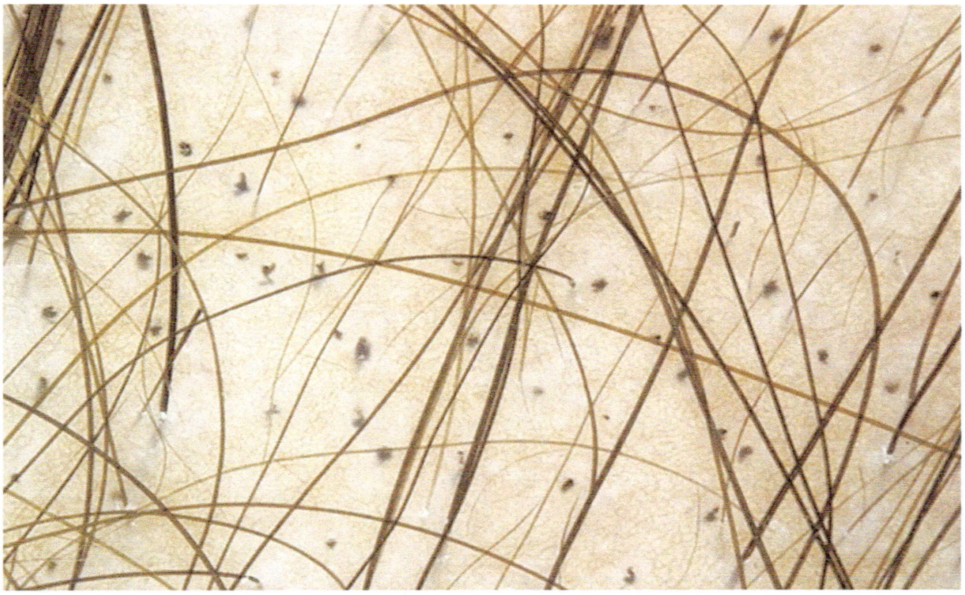

Fig. 7: Broken hairs. Hairs are broken at the same level above the scalp surface. They can also be observed in trichotillomania where the broken hairs are of different lengths.

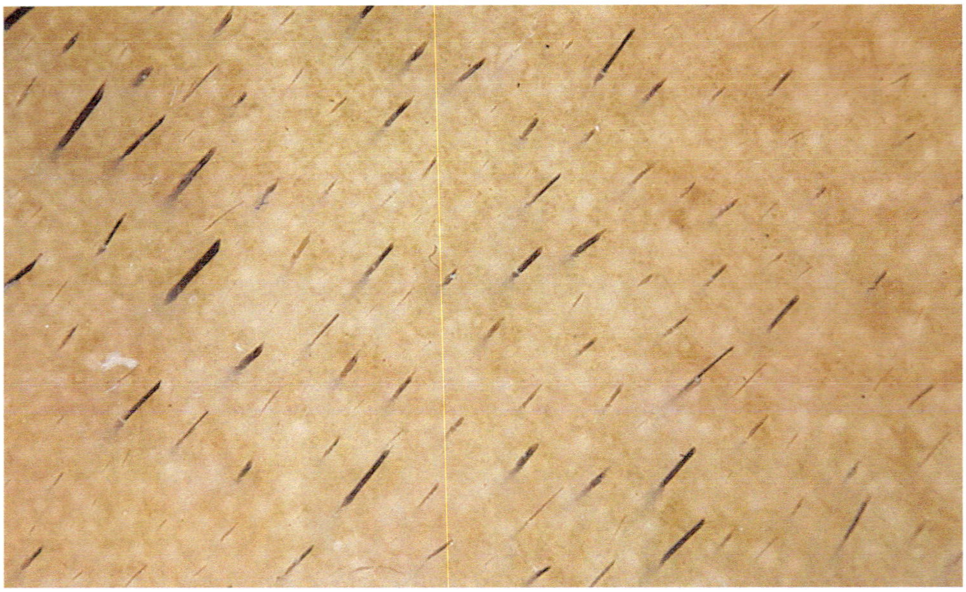

Fig. 8: Broken hairs of similar lengths seen in alopecia areata.

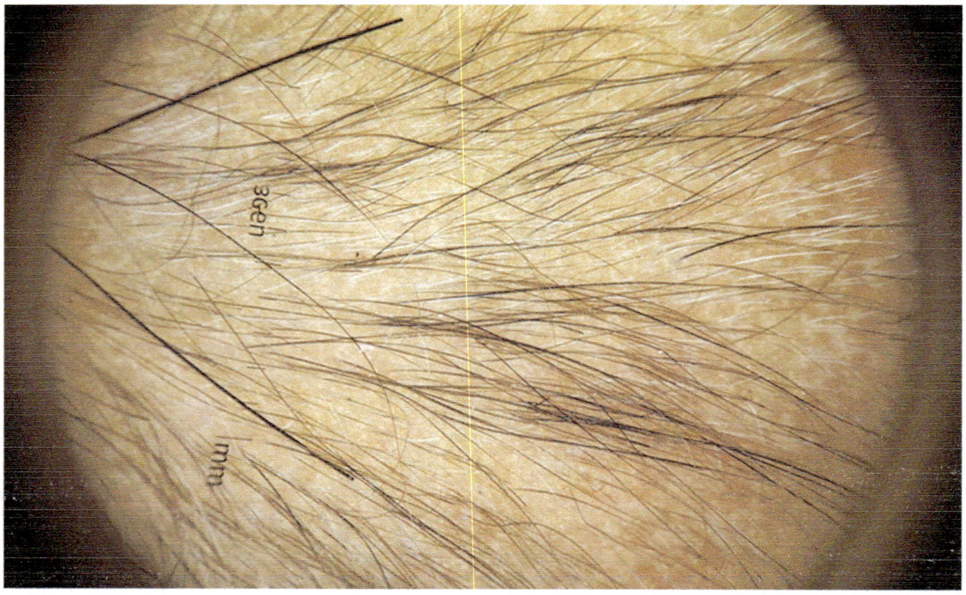

Fig. 9: Clustered vellus hairs are a common finding in alopecia areata (AA). They signify remitting stage of AA which may be white in color.[6] Vellus hairs are also seen in androgenetic alopecia (AGA) but are scattered instead of being clustered.

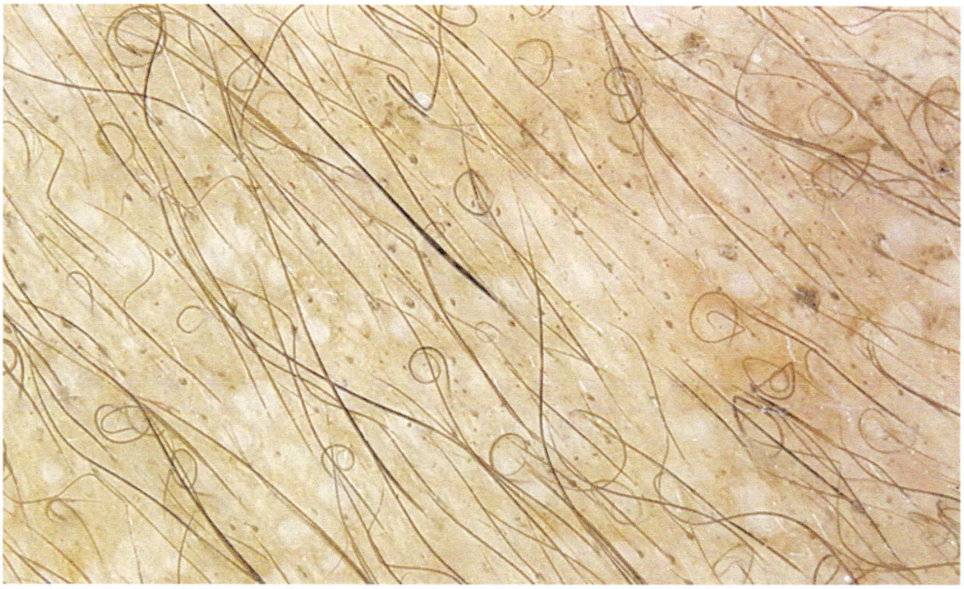

Fig. 10: Short vellus hairs may appear as circle hairs which may be a predominant feature in many cases of alopecia areata (AA). The dots in the field may be mistaken for dirty dots, but on close inspection they are produced due to the use of hair dye as concealer. Hair dye dots may be differentiated from dirty dots in that hair dye dots occupy follicular openings whereas dirty dots are not associated with follicular openings.

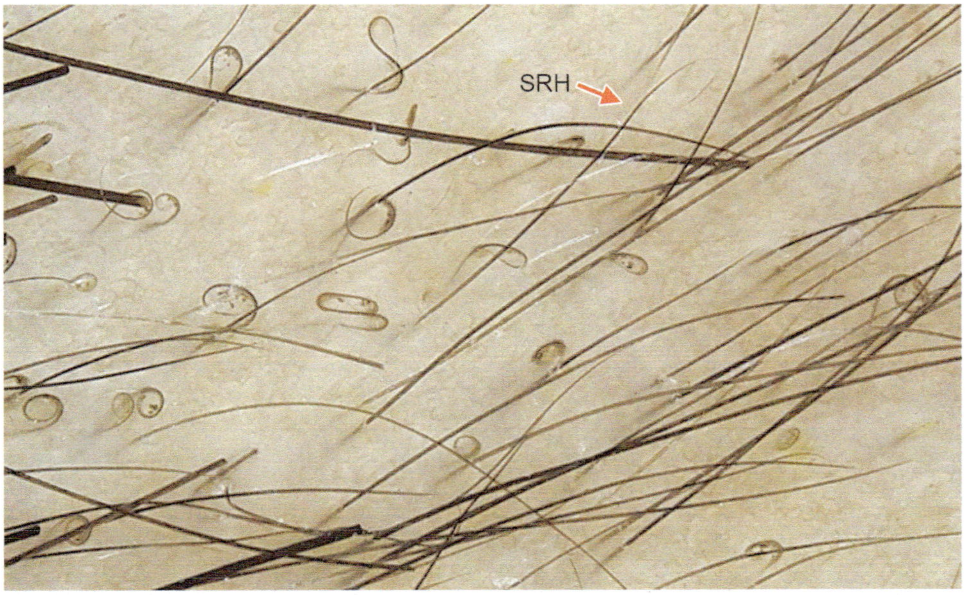

Fig. 11: Circle hairs and short regrowing hairs (SRH) in alopecia areata (AA). Short regrowing hairs have tapered end and they are black in comparison to vellus hairs which are hypopigmented.

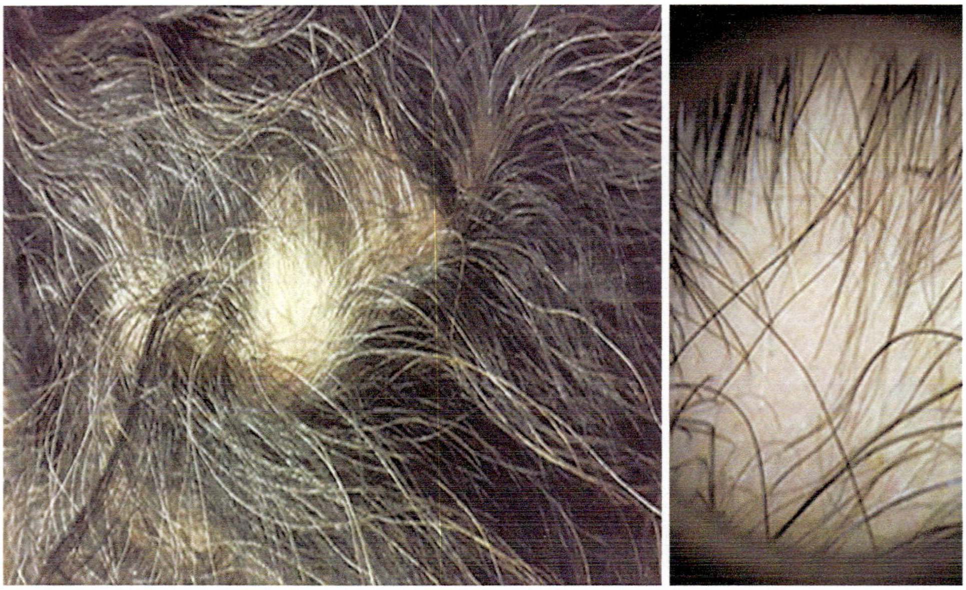

Fig. 12: A very important distinguishing feature of androgenetic alopecia (AGA) is hair diameter variability which can also be observed in alopecia areata (AA). However in contrast to AGA, AA shows uniform miniaturization instead of hair shafts with different degrees of thinning.

YELLOW DOTS

- They are rarely seen in Fitzpatrick types IV, V, and VI scalp.
- They present as round or polycyclic yellow dots.
- Yellow dots correspond on pathology to the dilated infundibulum filled with keratosebaceous material.
- Yellow dots may have no hair or may contain black dots, broken hairs, exclamation mark hairs, or miniaturized hairs.
- They are sensitive but are not specific marker because they are found in AGA, congenital hypotrichosis, etc.

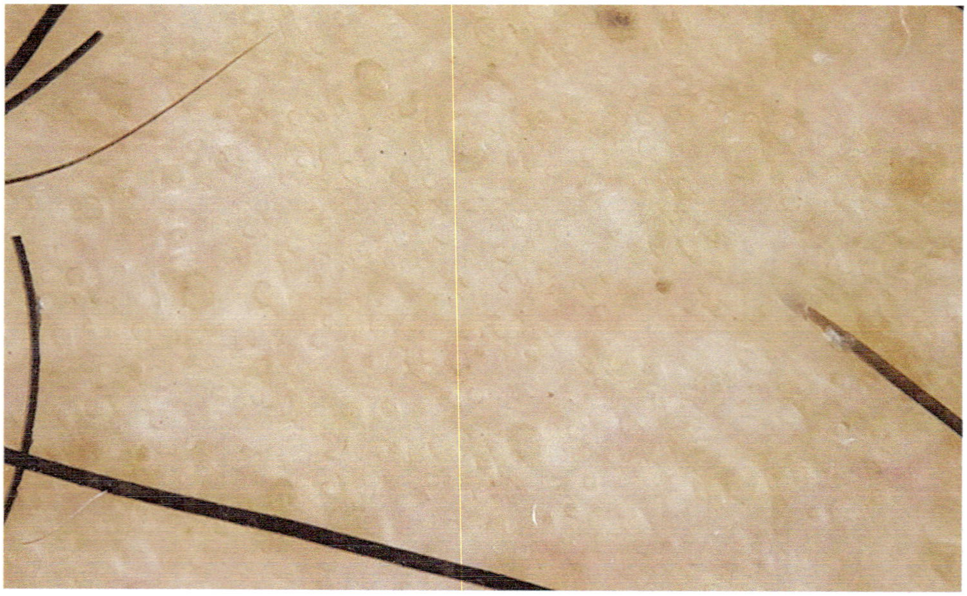

Fig. 13: The trichoscopic field is studded with yellow dots which remind us about the "Craters of moon" (author's observation). Yellow dots signify disease severity.

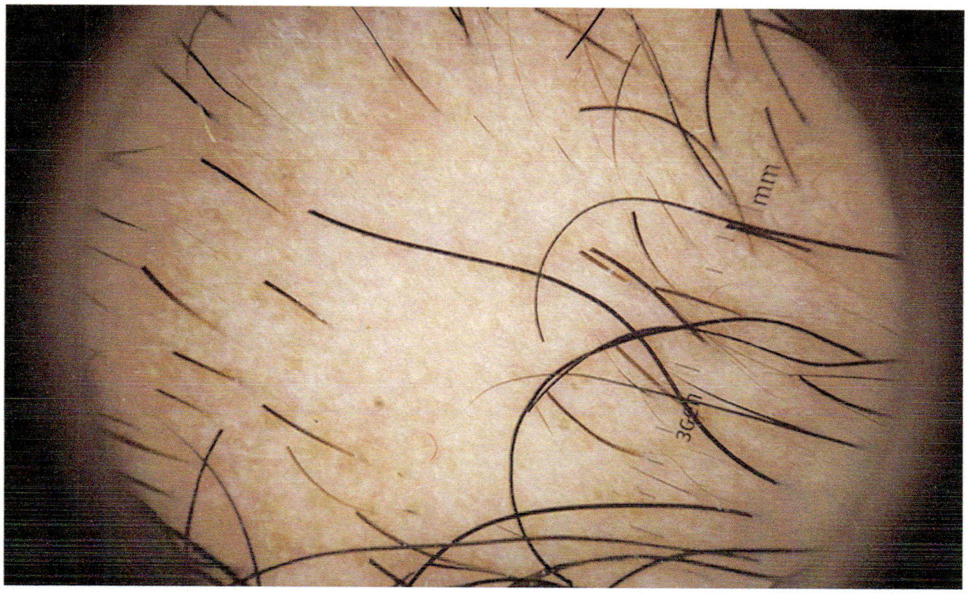

Fig. 14: Yellow dots in alopecia areata (AA). Note the presence of exclamation mark hairs. Both yellow dots and exclamation mark hair correspond to active disease.

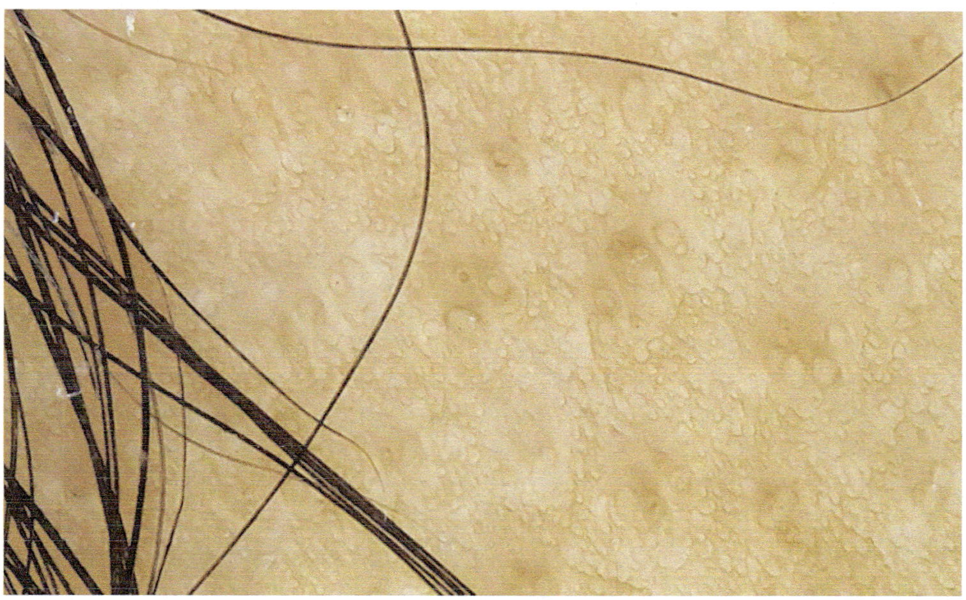

Fig. 15: A distinguishing feature of yellow dots in alopecia areata is that they are distributed almost regularly. Characteristically they are arranged in groups of two or three, sometimes four, reflecting the number of hairs per follicular unit. At the background there is honeycomb pigmentation.

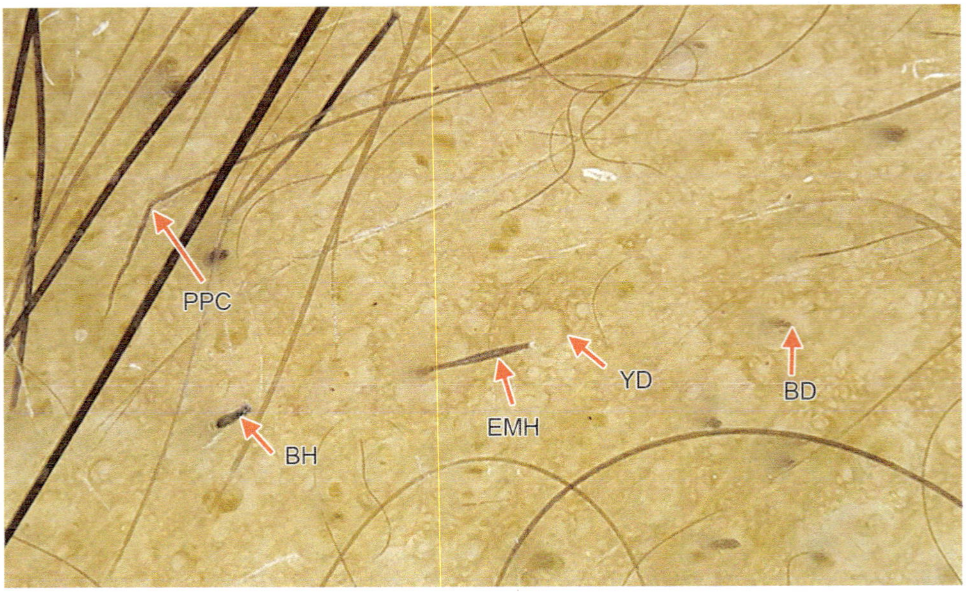

Fig. 16: Pohl–Pinkus constriction (PPC) is observed in alopecia areata (AA), scarring alopecias, localized hypotrichosis, and chemotherapy alopecia. This is a case of AA. Note also the presence of exclamation mark hair (EMH), black dots (BD), broken hairs (BH), and yellow dots (YD).

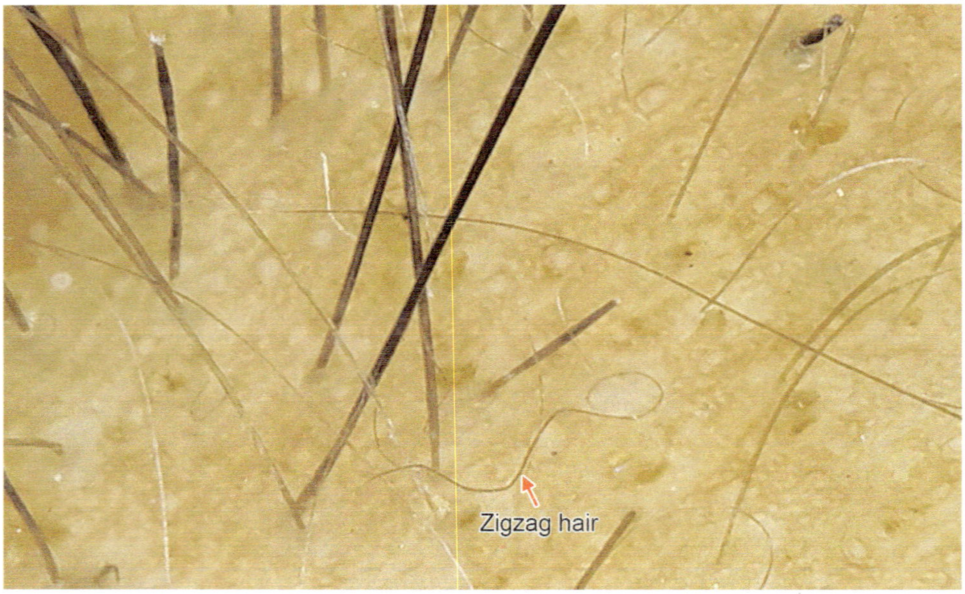

Fig. 17: Z-hairs also called zigzag hairs are formed due to focal weakening of the hair shaft. They are seen in active stage of alopecia areata (AA). Tinea capitis and trichorrhexis nodosa also show zigzag hairs. The flexures of zigzag hairs in AA are the areas of increased fragility.

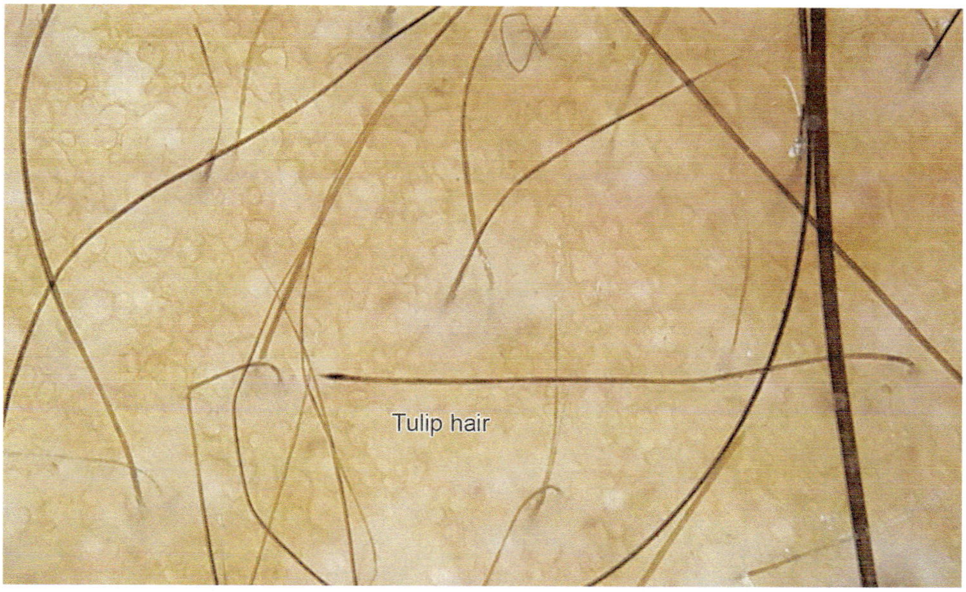

Fig. 18: Tulip hairs differ from exclamation mark hair in that they have a dark distal end with light colored hair shafts. This darker tip corresponds to an area of oblique hair rupture. Tulip hairs may also be observed in trichotillomania.

REFERENCES

1. Inui S, Nakajima T, Nakagawa K, Itami S. Clinical significance of dermatoscopy in alopecia areata: Analysis of 300 cases. Int J Dermatol. 2008;47:688-93.
2. Inui S, Nakajima T, Itami S. Coudability hairs: A revisited sign of alopecia areata assessed by trichoscopy. Clin Exp Dermatol. 2010;35:361-5.
3. Shuster S. Coudability: A new physical sign of alopecia areata. Br J Dermatol. 1984:111:629.
4. Abraham LS, Torres FN, Azulay-Abulafia L. Dermoscopic clues to istinguish trichotillomania from patchy alopecia areata. An Brass Dermatol. 2010;85:723-6.
5. Banky JP, Sheridan AT, Dawber RP. Weathering of hair in trichoteiromania. Australas J Deramatol. 2004;45:186-8.
6. Inui S, Nakajima T, Itami S. Scalp dermatoscopy of androgenetic alopecia in Asian people. J Dermatol. 2009;36:82-5.

ASSESSMENT IMAGE-BASED QUESTIONS

1. This is a case of alopecia areata. Mention its four trichoscopic features.

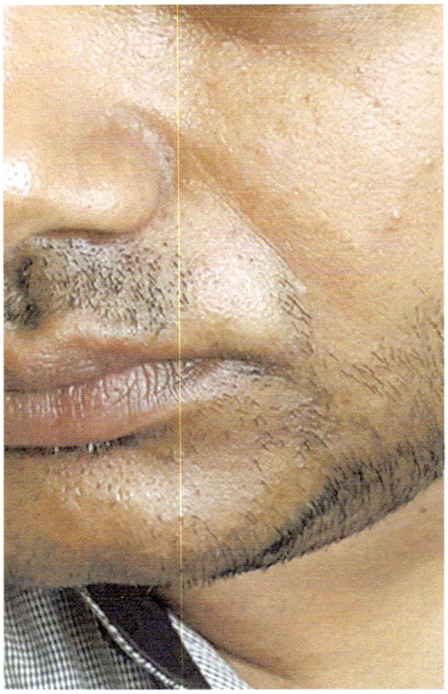

2. Mention two trichoscopic features of alopecia areata that are seen in this image.

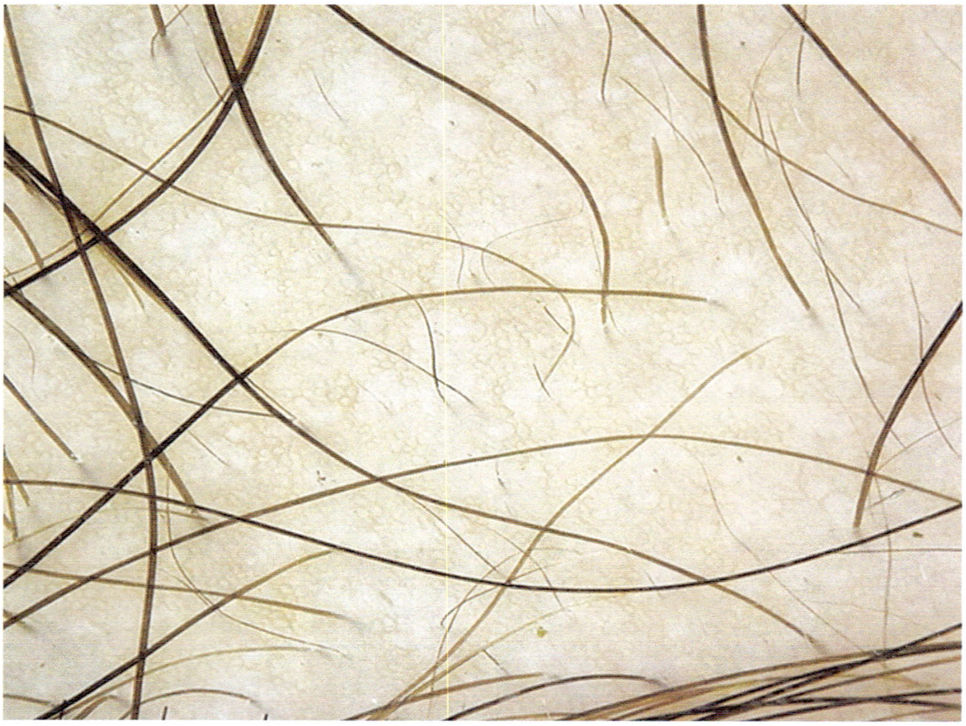

3. This is a trichoscopic picture of alopecia areata. Which feature shown here denotes disease activity? Name the other features of AA which also signify disease activity.

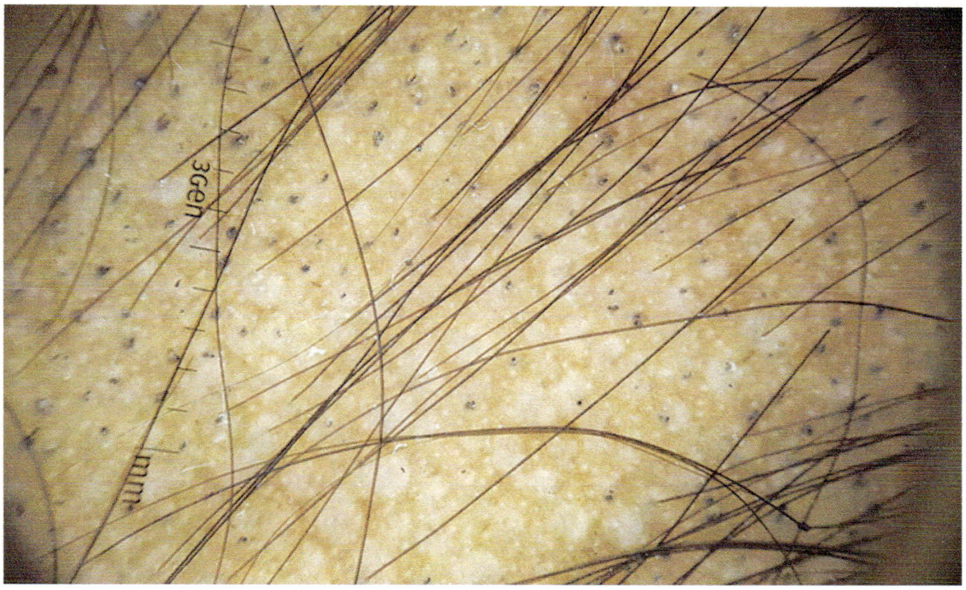

4. What do 1, 2, and 3 indicate?

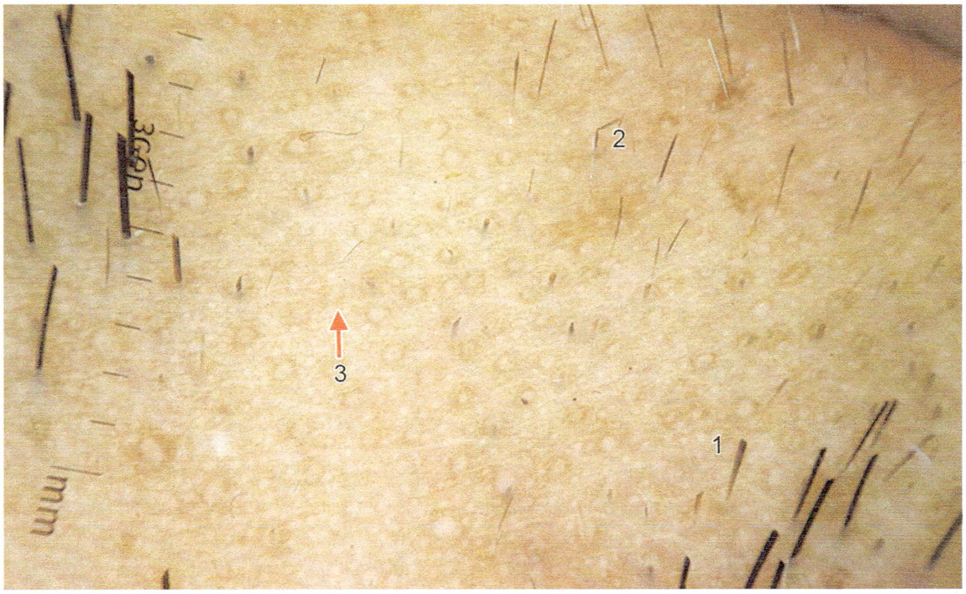

5. What do the red and black arrows signify?

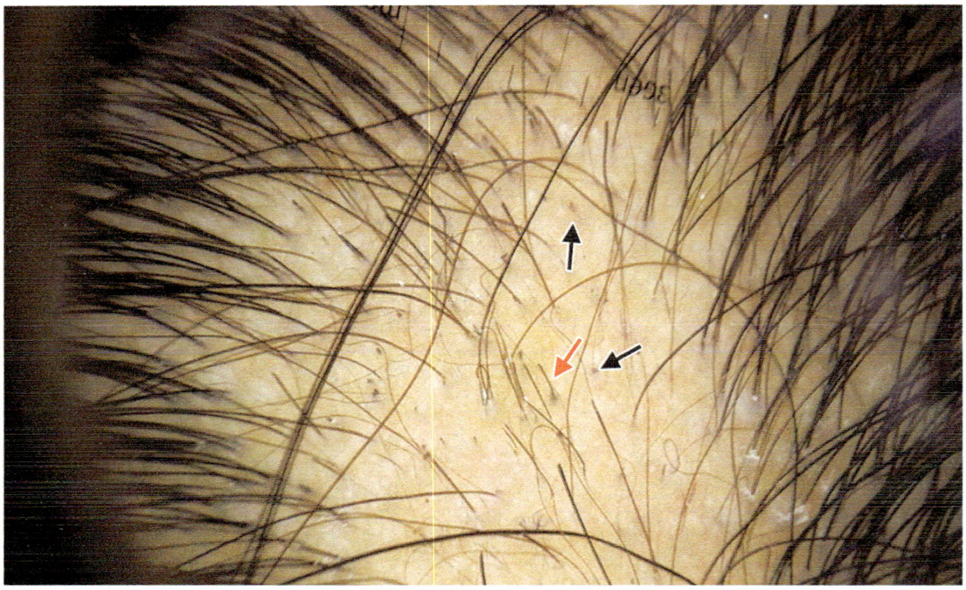

6. Which trichoscopic feature(s) of the following is true for alopecia areata: (A) exclamation mark, (B) yellow dots, (C) vellus hair, (D) all of the above.

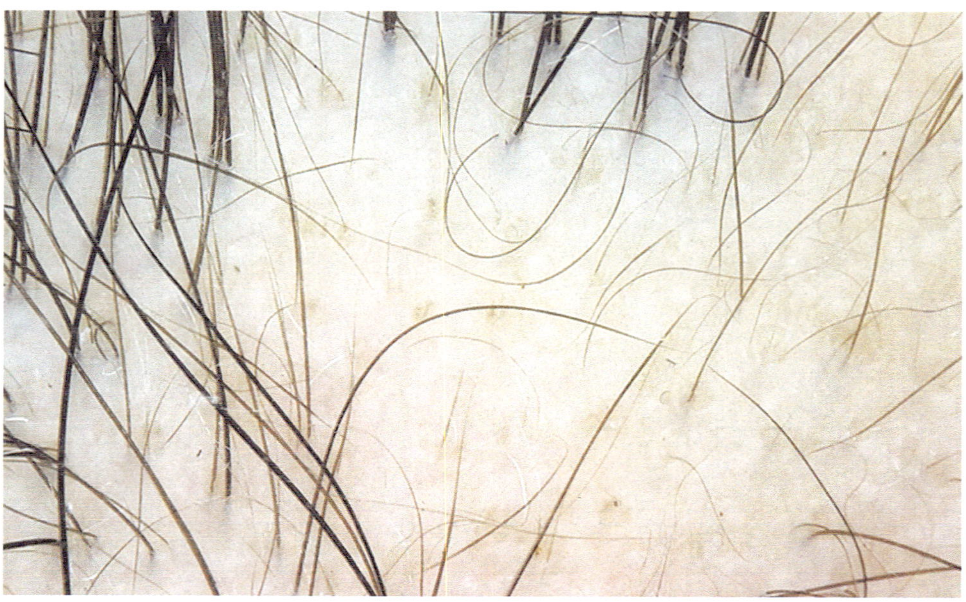

7. Will you be able to find one short hair in this image which shows both exclamation mark and Pohl-Pinkus constriction?

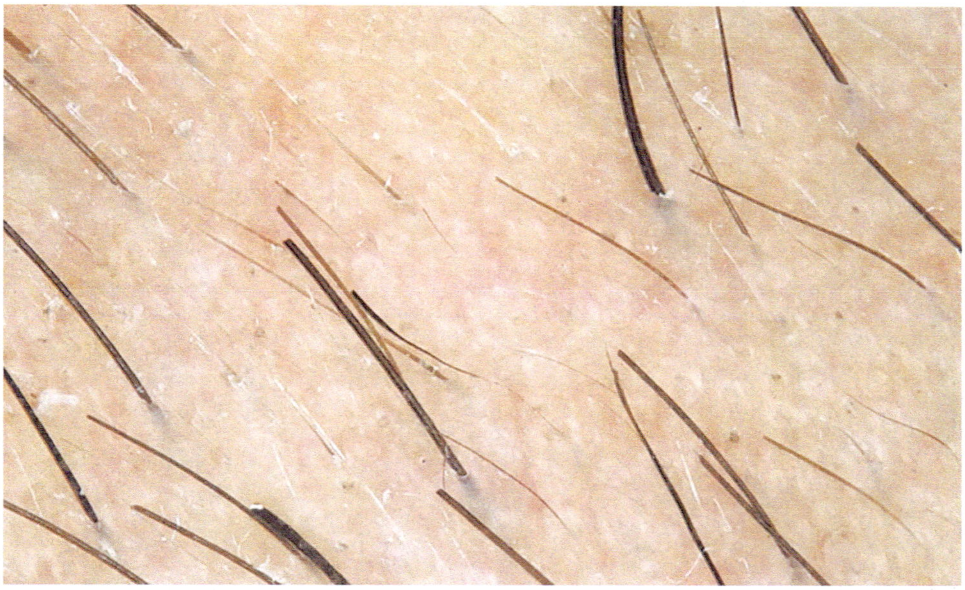

8. This trichoscopic image is full of yellow dots. Few black dots and one exclamation mark hair is also present. Name the markers of disease severity of AA. Which finding in this image is the most sensitive marker of AA?

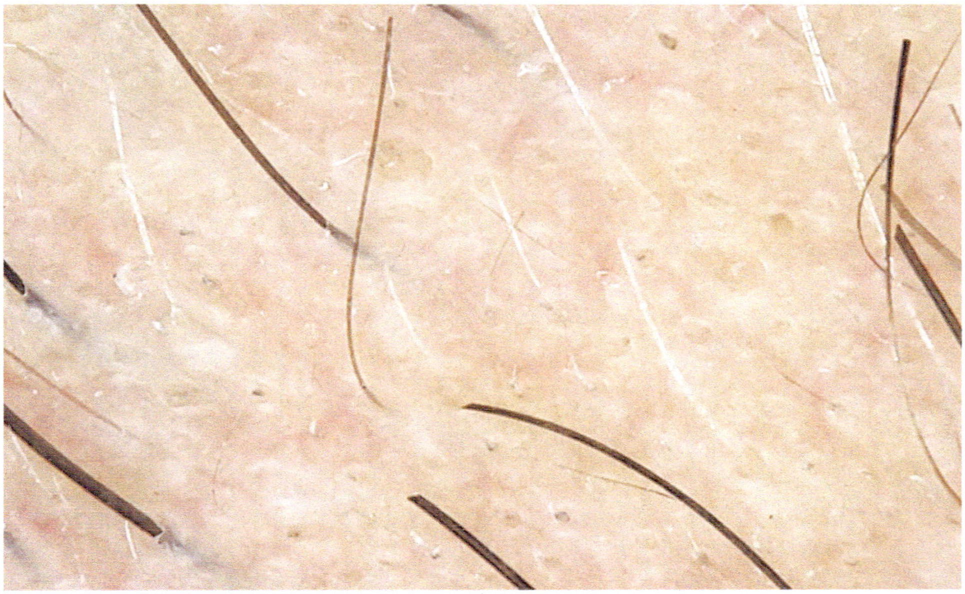

9. Extensive yellow dots are seen in this image. Are they specific markers of alopecia areata? What do they correlate histopathologically to?

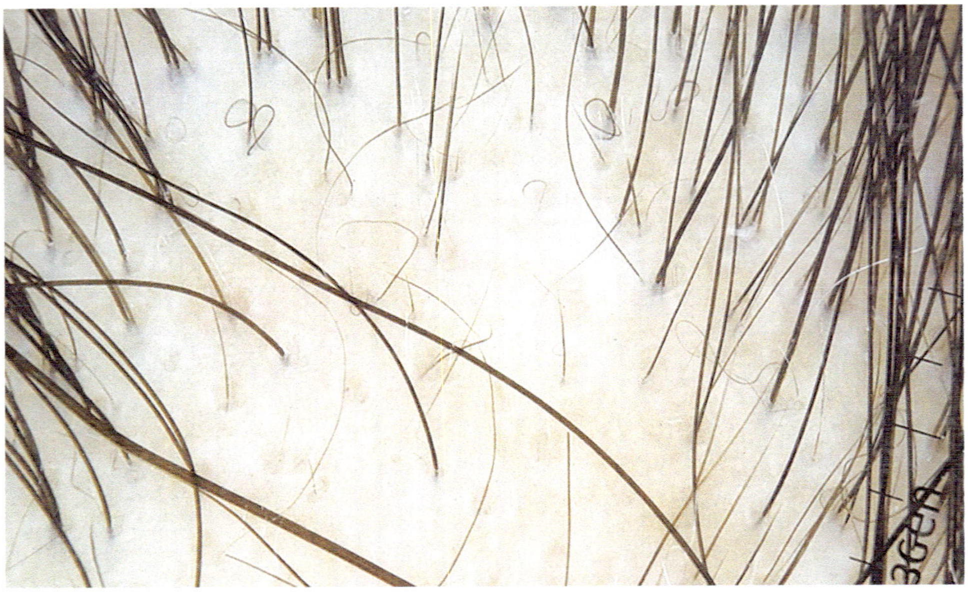

10. The numbers signify specific trichoscopic features of alopecia areata. Try to unveil them.

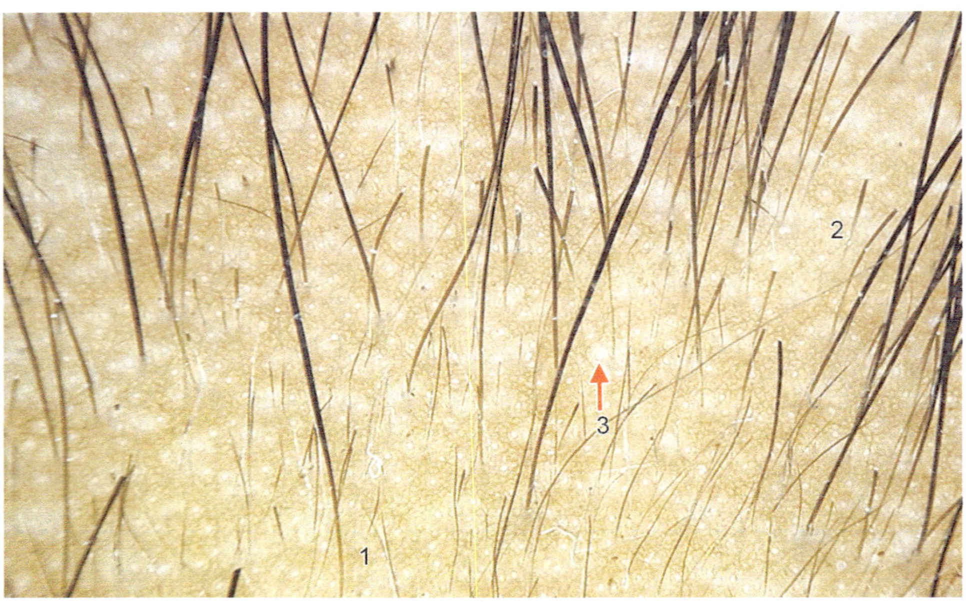

11. What do 1, 2, 3, 4, and 5 stand for?

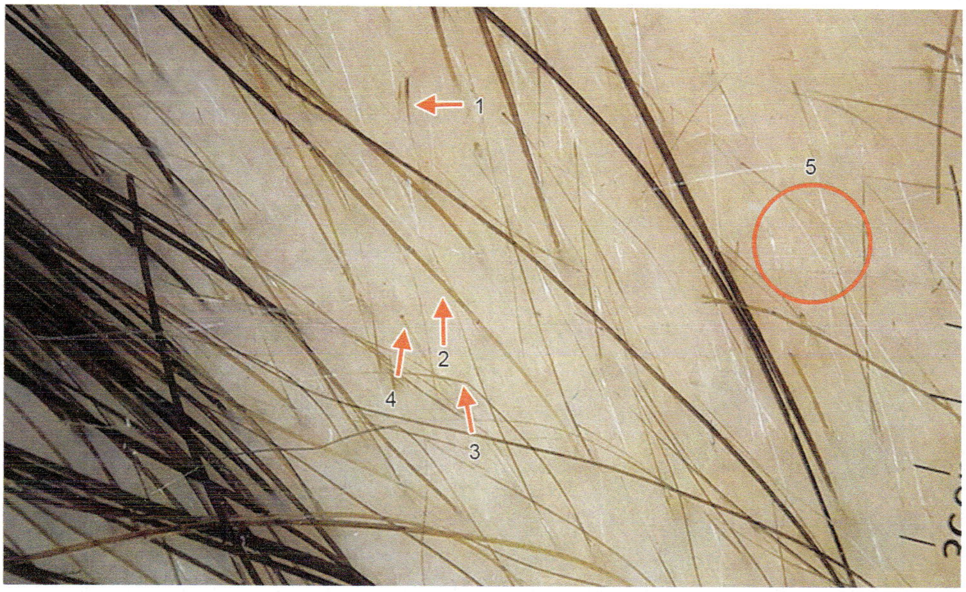

ANSWERS

1. Exclamation mark hair, yellow dots, black dots, and coudability hair
2. Exclamation mark hair, yellow dots
3. Black dots. Broken hair and tapering hair
4. (1) Exclamation mark hair; (2) Pohl–Pinkus constriction; (3) Yellow dots
5. Red arrow—broken hair, black arrow—black dots
6. (d) All of the above
7.

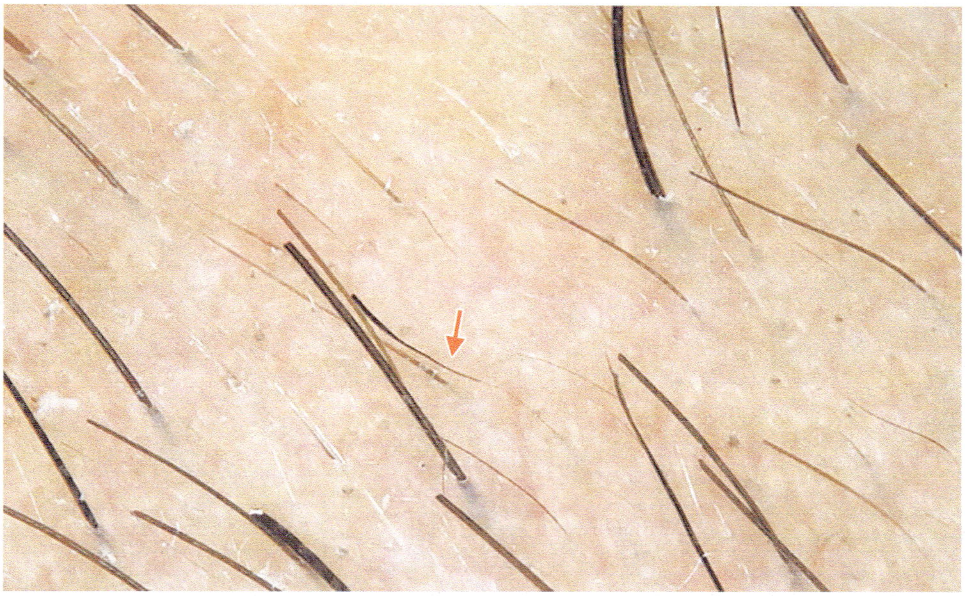

8. Yellow dots. In active and severe alopecia areata, extensive yellow dots are found resembling the "craters of moon".
9. No. They correspond to keratosebaceous material.
10. (1) Denotes coudability hair (CH); (2) Denotes exclamation mark hair (EH); (3) Denotes yellow dot (YD)

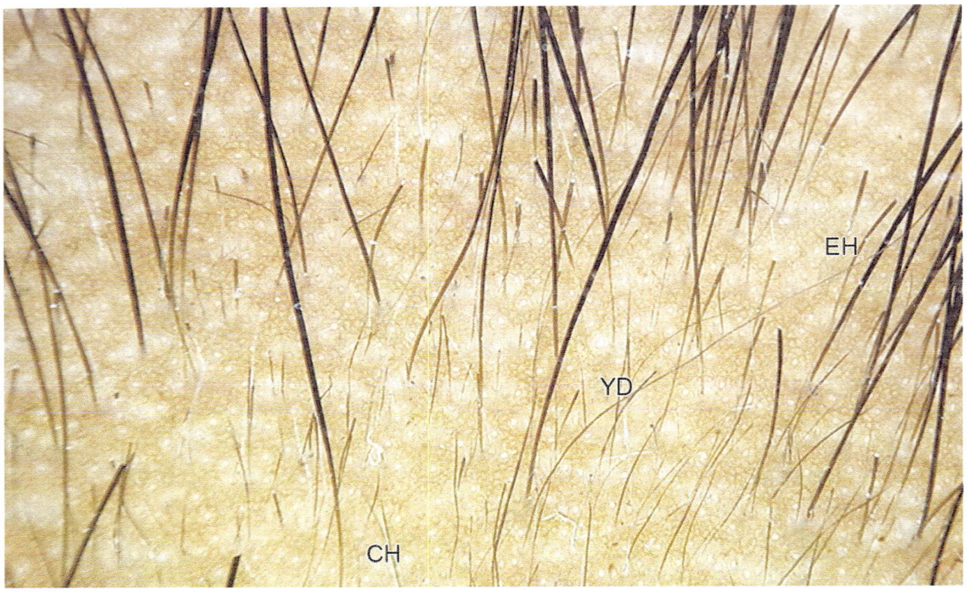

11. (1) Exclamation mark hair; (2) Coudability hair; (3) Pohl Pinkus constriction; (4) i-hair; 5. Pohl-Pinkus constriction

CHAPTER

12 Trichotillomania

Subrata Malakar

INTRODUCTION

- It is a self-induced hair loss due to repetitive pulling of one's own hair.[1,2]
- It most frequently affects children between the ages of 9 and 13 years with a female preponderance of 70–93%.[1]
- Adult-onset trichotillomania (TTM) may continue for long and is secondary to underlying psychiatric disturbances.[1]
- Clinically, there are patches of hair with varying lengths and hairless areas. Usually, the vertex is affected which gives rise to the "Friar Tuck sign".

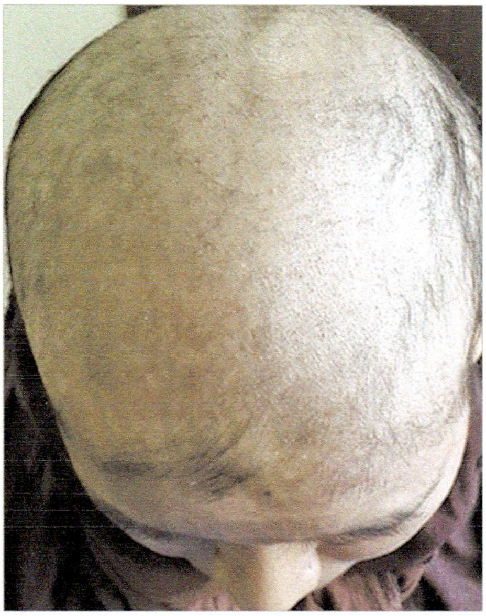

Fig. 1: A case of trichotillomania (TTM) in a 15-year-old girl. Note "Friar Tuck" sign (traditional Christian practice of shaving the midscalp area). Totally hairless area is rare as patients try to pull the long hairs only.

KEY TRICHOSCOPIC FEATURES

- Black dots, broken hairs
- Flame hairs
- Coiled hairs
- Question mark hair
- Regrowing hairs
- Short hairs with trichoptilosis (split ends)
- Hair powder
- "Mace" sign
- Tulip hairs

- "V" sign
- Block hairs
- i-hairs
- Evidence of pulling can be demonstrated by trichoscopy.
- It shows:
  - Broken hairs with a coiled tip (coiled hair or question mark hair)
  - Broken hairs of different lengths
  - Trichoptilosis, black dots, flame hairs, and hair dust
- Broken hairs and flame hairs are seen both in TTM and alopecia areata (AA). However, exclamation mark hair is not seen in TTM.
- Alopecia areata may coexist with trichotillomania[3] where AA may be the triggering factor.
- Some authors[4,5] have described exclamation mark hairs in TTM. However, it is controversial because " mace" sign described recently in TTM (authors observation, in press) mimics exclamation mark hair but with distinct differences.
- A recent study[6] showed that only two features distinguish TTM and AA.
- Exclamation mark hair is characteristic for AA.
- Coiled hair is characteristic for TTM.
- Black dots, broken hairs, and yellow dots are present in both AA and TTM.

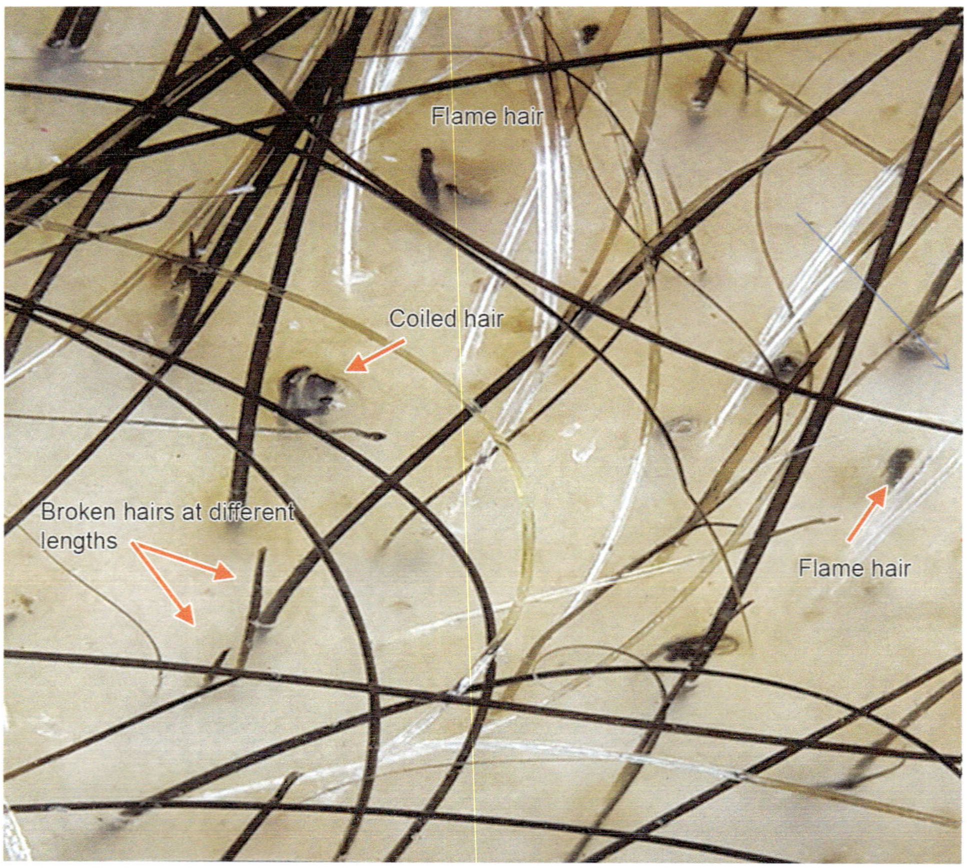

Fig. 2: Presence of multiple broken hairs at different lengths is the most frequent finding in trichotillomania. Trichoscopy shows the evidence of pulling the hair which results in flame hair, coiled hair, and broken hairs.

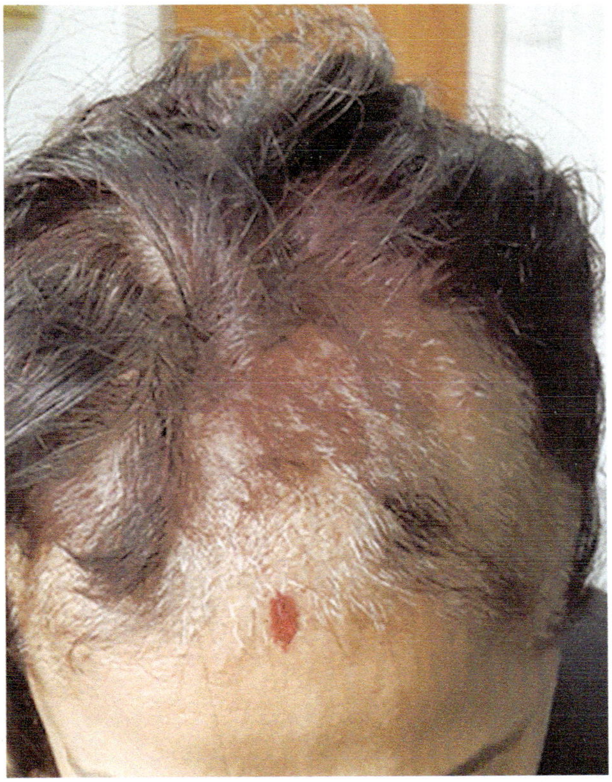

Fig. 3: A clinical picture of trichotillomania with hair of different lengths and a tendency to develop "Friar Tuck" sign.

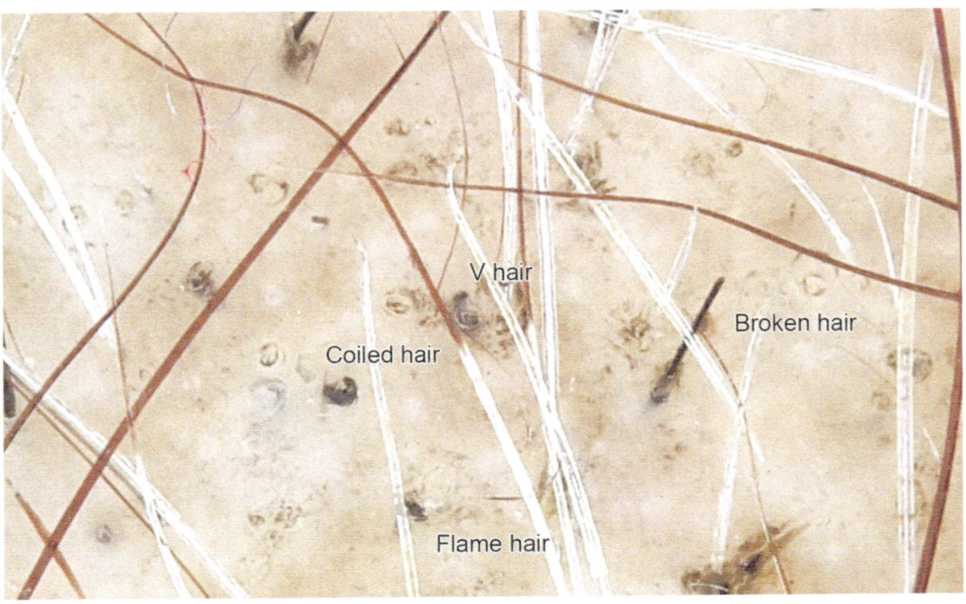

Fig. 4: Coiled hairs are highly suggestive of trichotillomania. In response to a pulling force, hair shaft breaks and the remaining fragment of hair that is fixed to the scalp contracts and coils. Partially coiled hairs are known as question mark hairs (next image).

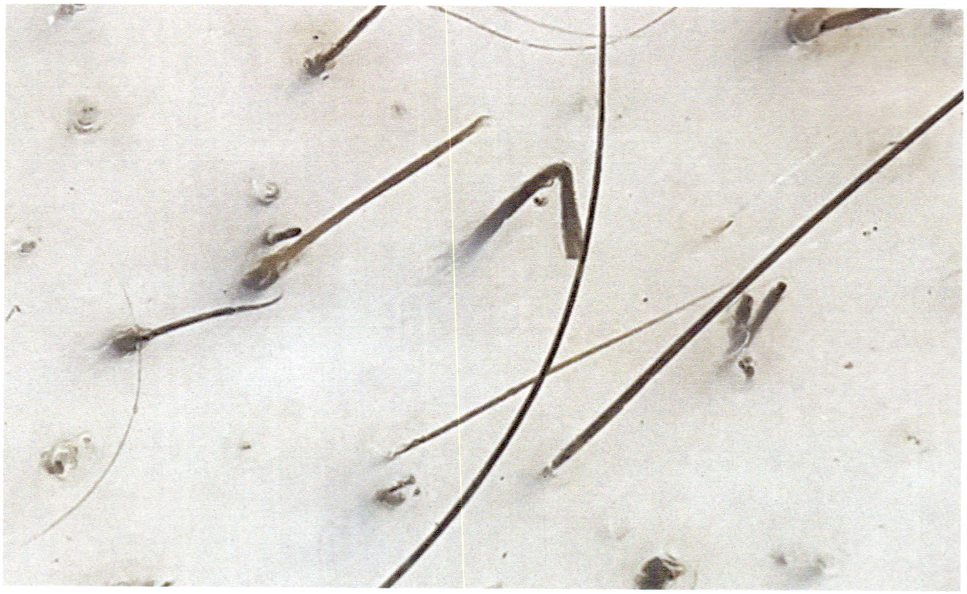

Fig. 5: Question mark hair at the center of the image. This is partially coiled hair. Note also the presence of flame hair, broken hairs, and "V" sign.

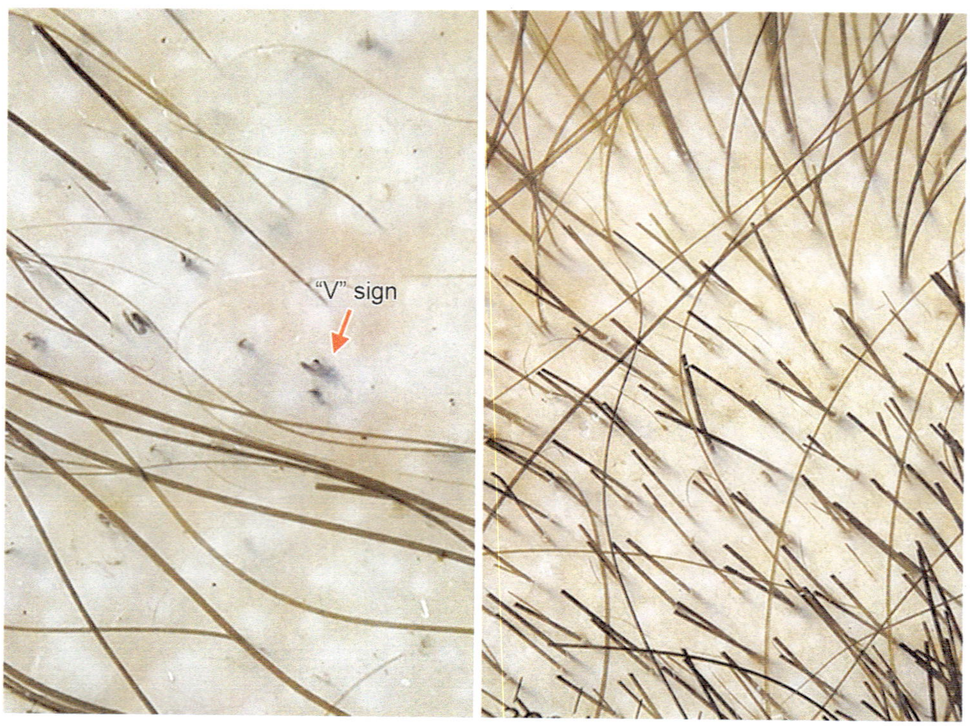

Fig. 6: "V" sign in trichotillomania. When two hairs of a follicular unit are broken at the same level it is seen as the letter "V". It should be differentiated from "V" sign seen after regrowth of shaving hairs. In the former, surrounding hairs are of normal length whereas in the latter, "V" sign is present in all regrowing hairs.

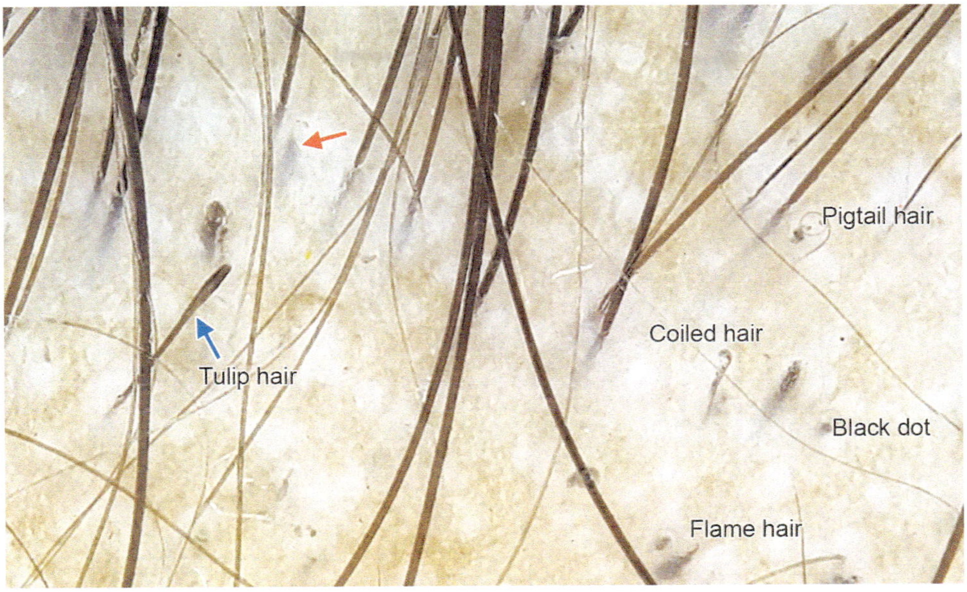

Fig. 7: This trichoscopic field shows a typical chaotic, multicomponent picture of trichotillomania (TTM). Hairs broken below the skin surface (red arrow) is seen through the epidermis. All the suggestive features of TTM such as coiled hair, flame hair, black dot, and broken hair are visible. Pigtail hair, marker of regrowing hair is also present. Tulip hair is hair with a dark tip. It is a nonspecific feature of TTM, alopecia areata (AA), and traction alopecia and is observed in this image.

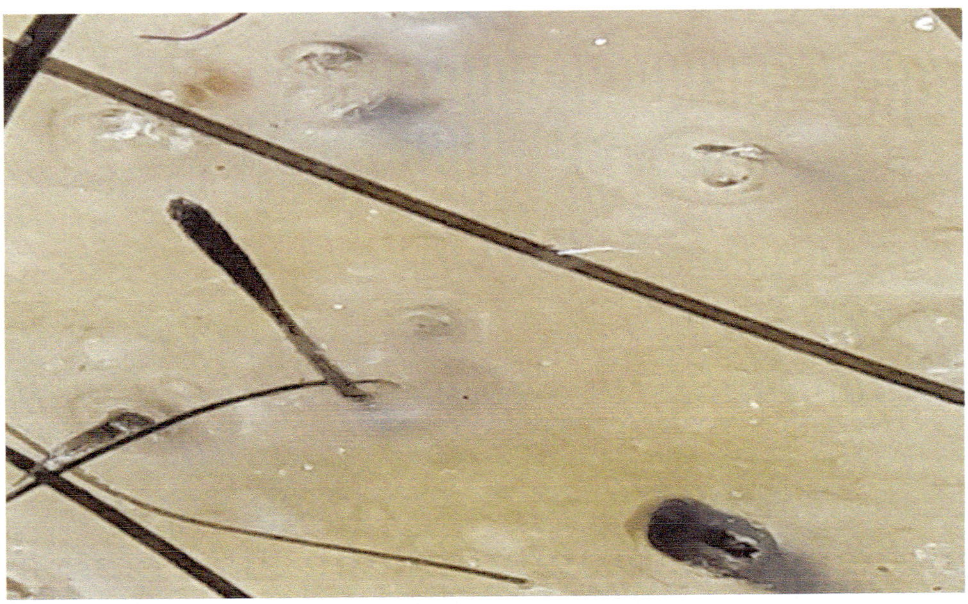

Fig. 8: "Mace" sign is a recently described sign (author's observation) in active trichotillomania (TTM). Exclamation mark is its closest differential diagnosis where the short hair shaft is hypopigmented in its lower part and hyperpigmented in its upper part. The hair shaft in "mace" sign is hyperpigmented throughout its entire length and the upper half is not as smooth as exclamation mark hair; it being rather rough in texture due to pulling and playing with the hair in TTM.

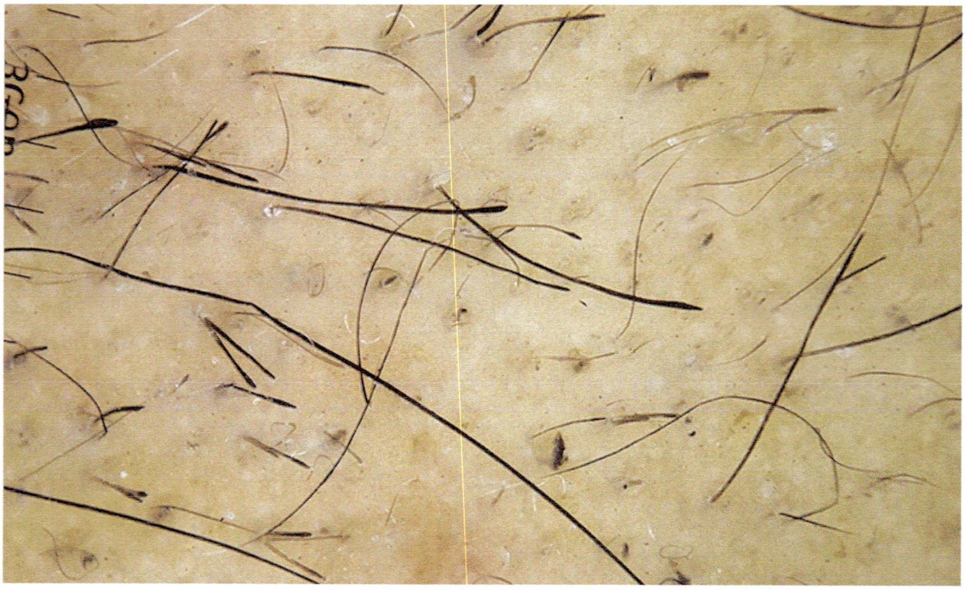

Fig. 9: Extensive "mace" sign.

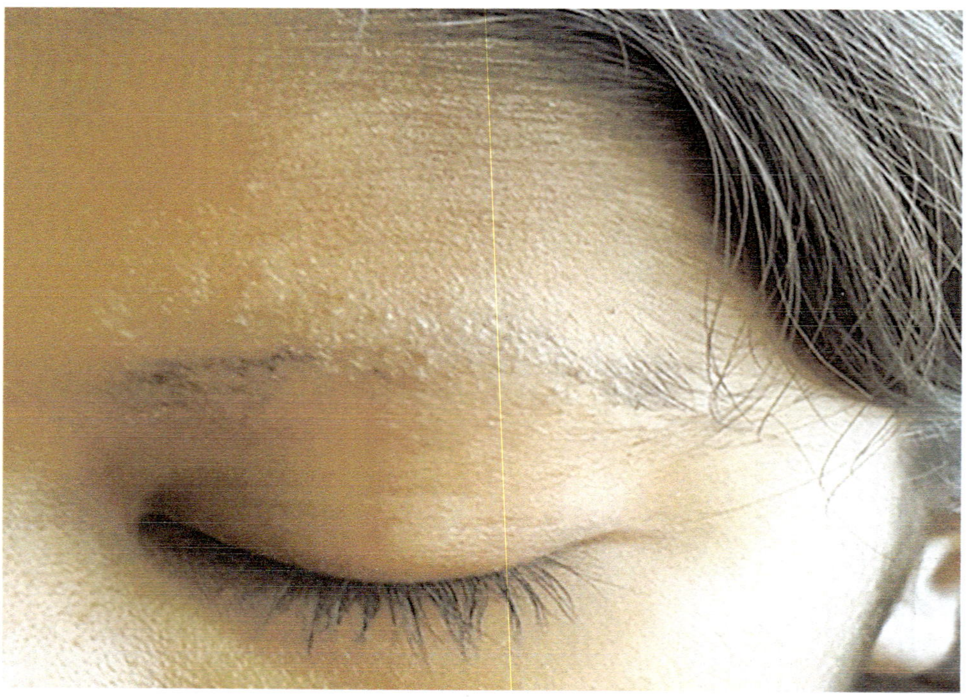

Fig. 10: Trichotillomania (TTM) of eyebrow in an 18-year-old girl.

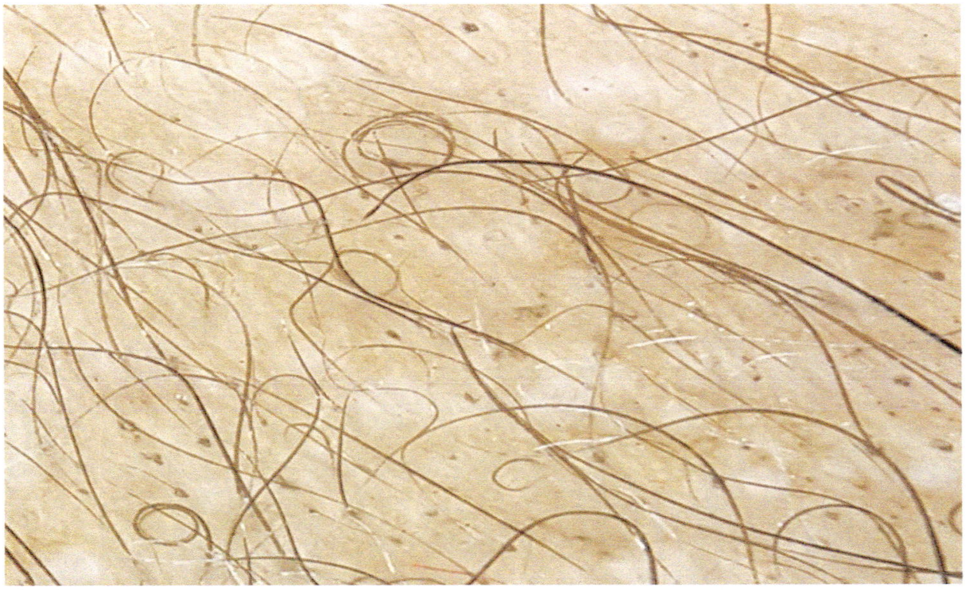

Fig. 11: Regrowing pigtail hairs and black dots in trichotillomania (TTM) of eyebrow. Note black residues of hair dyes used to camouflage the alopecic patch of TTM.

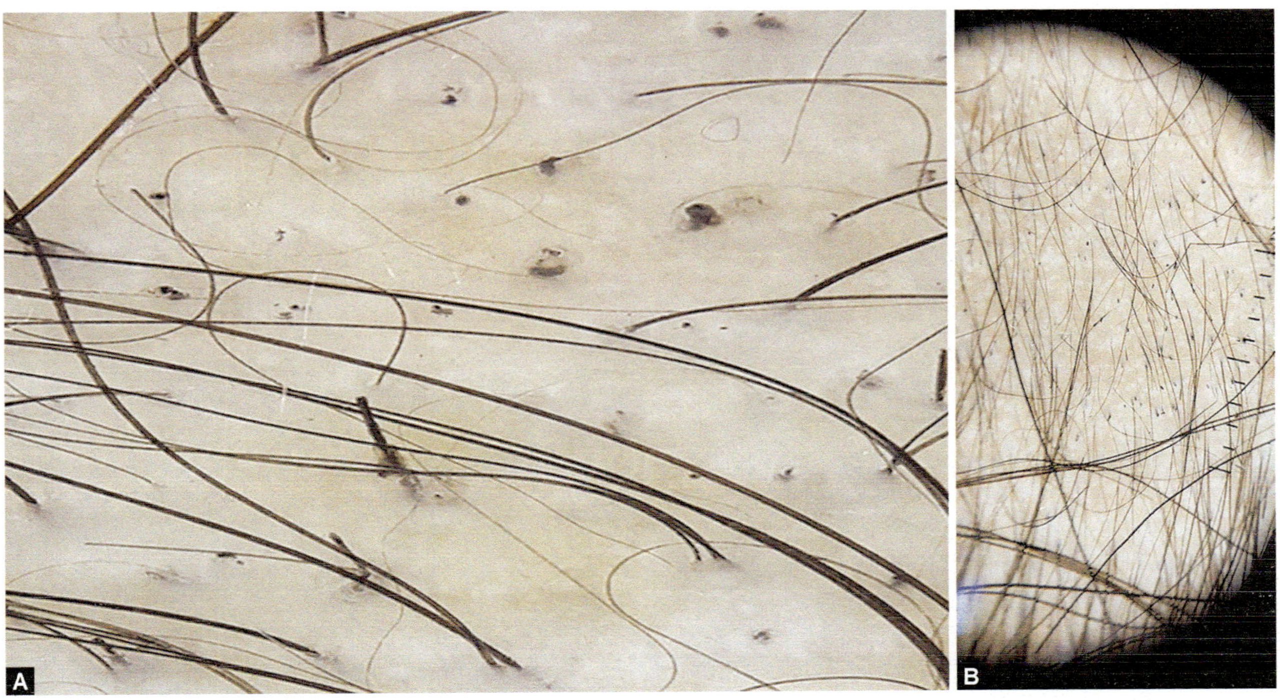

Figs. 12A and B: Multiple hairs broken at different lengths showing extreme variability in morphology. Hair broken below the skin surface is seen through the epidermis; it is a result of the mechanical force used to pull hair. (B) Multiple hairs broken at different lengths showing extreme variability in morphology. Hair broken below the skin surface is seen through the epidermis; it is a result of the mechanical force used to pull hair.

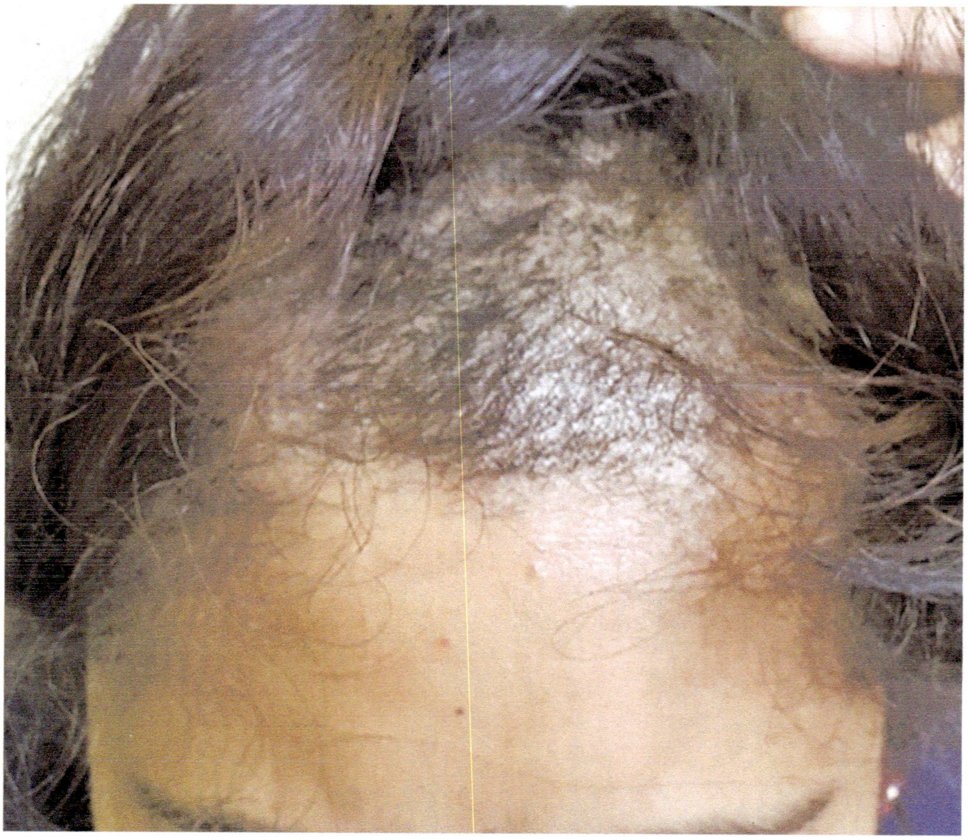

Fig. 13: Decreased hair density and irregular hair length. In this case of trichotillomania, hair pulling is limited mainly to the range of her right hand. The left side of scalp is spared.

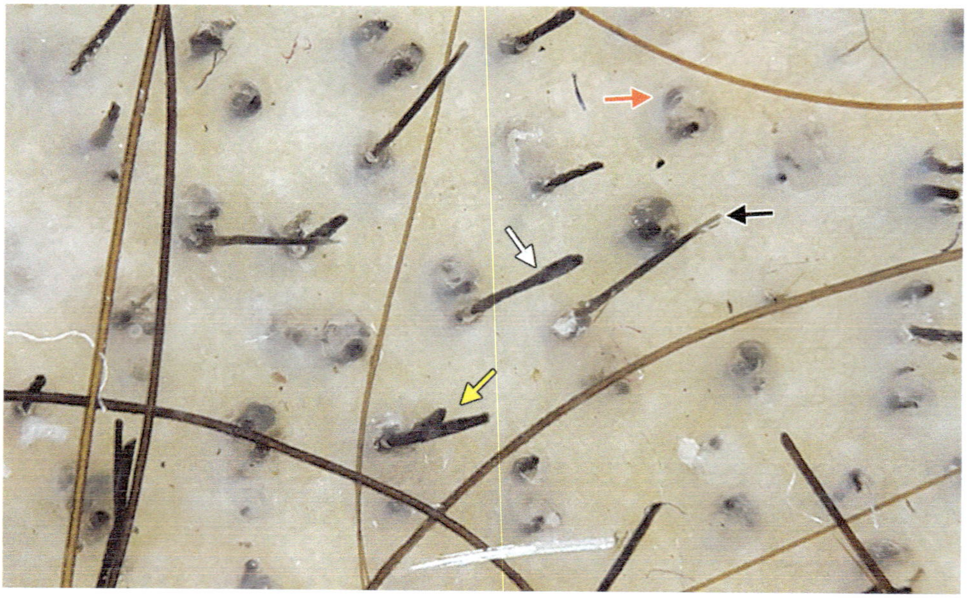

Fig. 14: Red arrow: Hair broken below the skin surface, black arrow: trichoptilosis, yellow arrow: broken hairs at different lengths, and white arrow: "mace" sign.

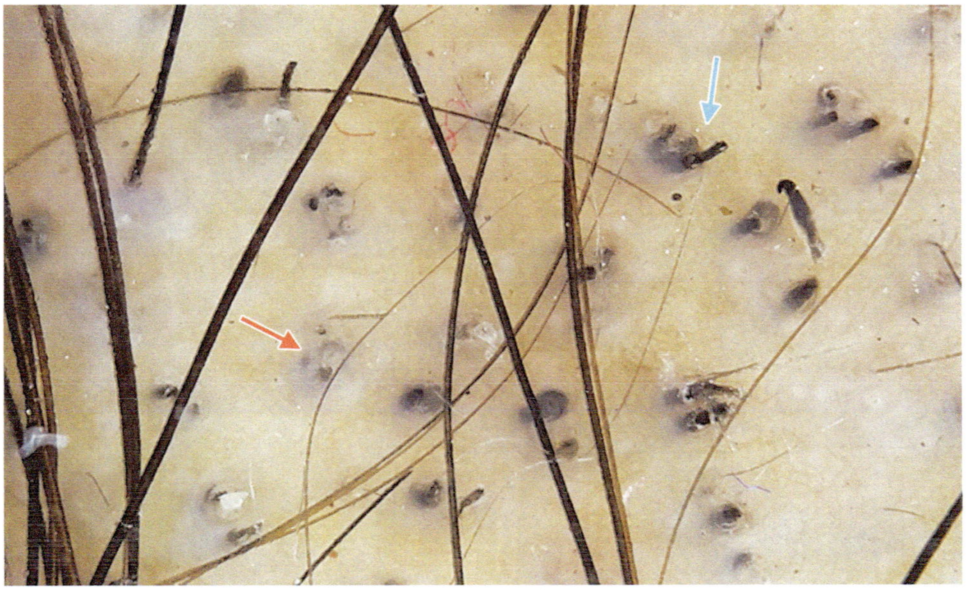

Fig. 15: Every broken hair has a different length and morphology. Red arrow: hairs broken below the skin surface, blue arrow: broken hairs of a follicular unit showing different height and morphology.

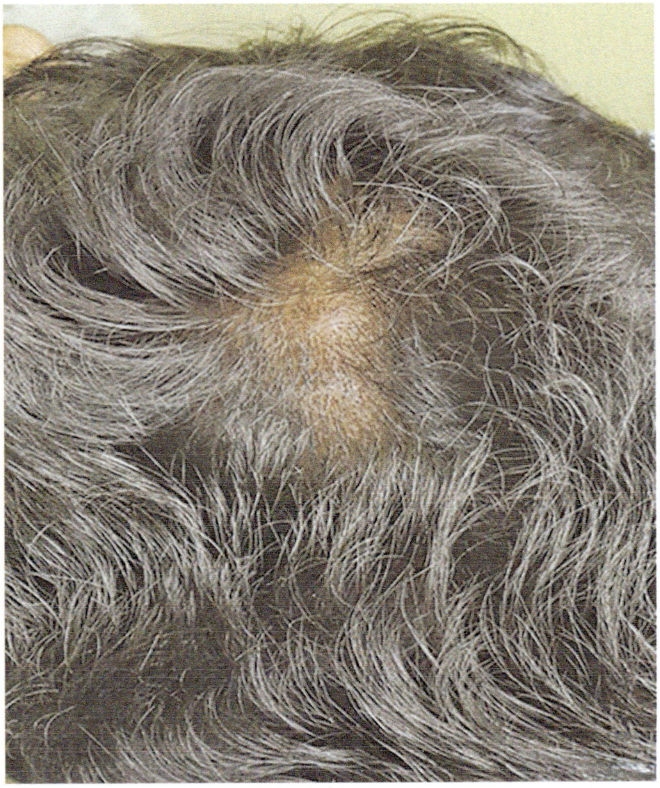

Fig. 16: A case of trichotillomania masquerading alopecia areata (AA). It can be confirmed by trichoscopy

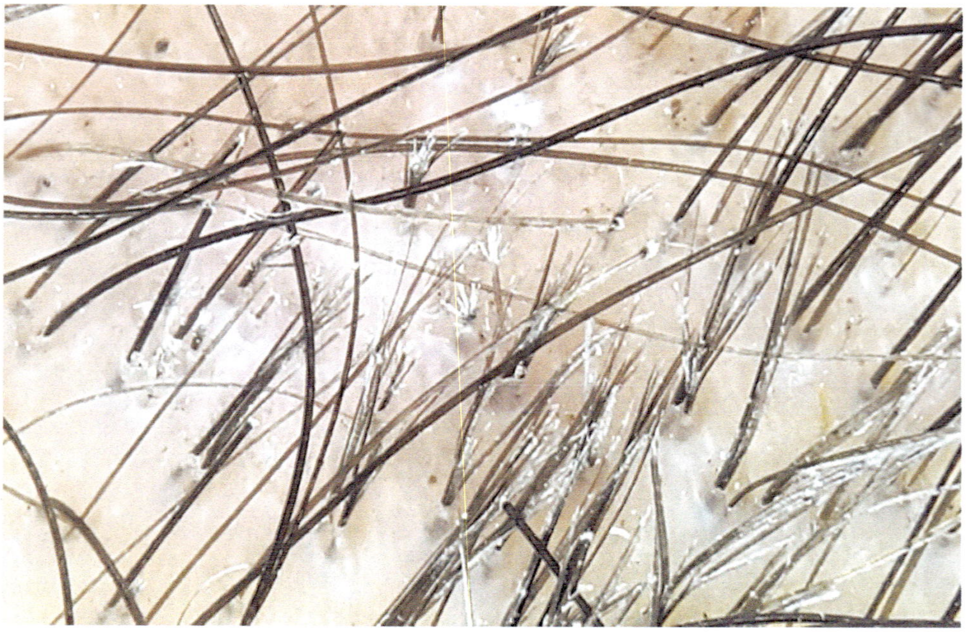

Fig. 17: Extensive broom hairs indicate the case as trichotillomania.

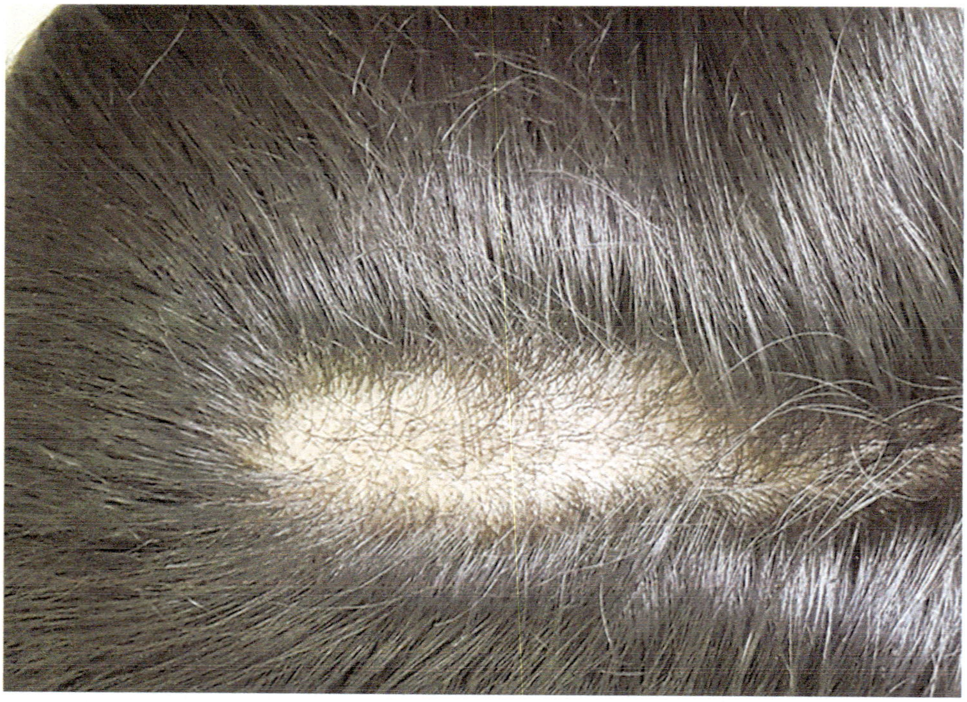

Fig. 18: Another case of trichotillomania which mimics alopecia areata. Observe the trichoscopic features in the next image.

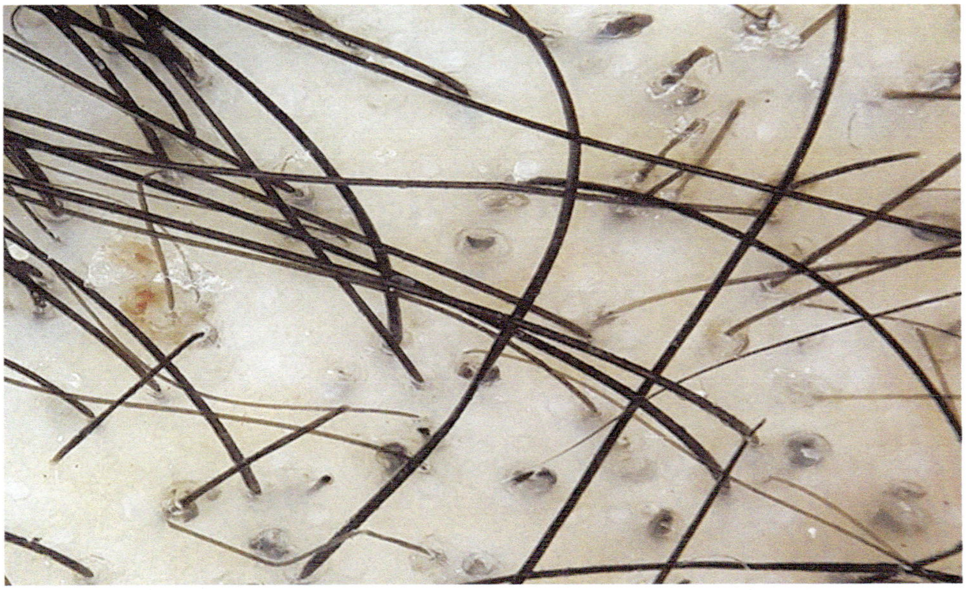

Fig. 19: This is the trichoscopic image of the previous patient. Flame hairs and multiple broken hairs at different lengths are seen.

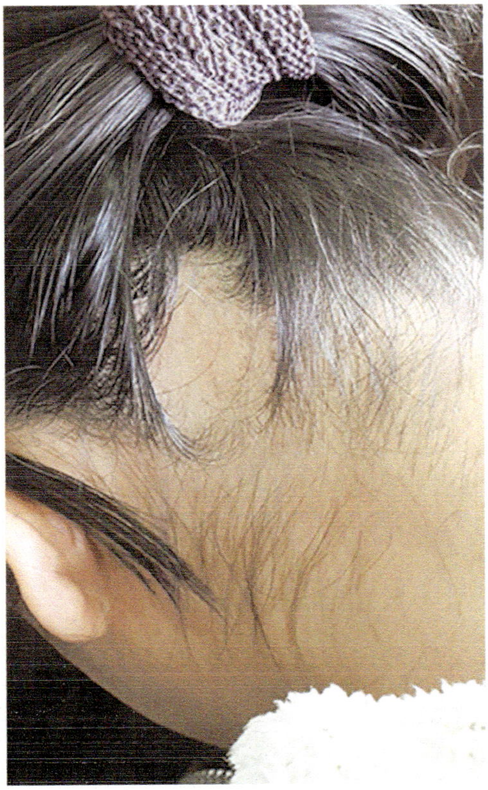

Fig. 20: Clinical diagnosis is alopecia areata. But after trichoscopic findings diagnosis is revised. Please check the features in the next image.

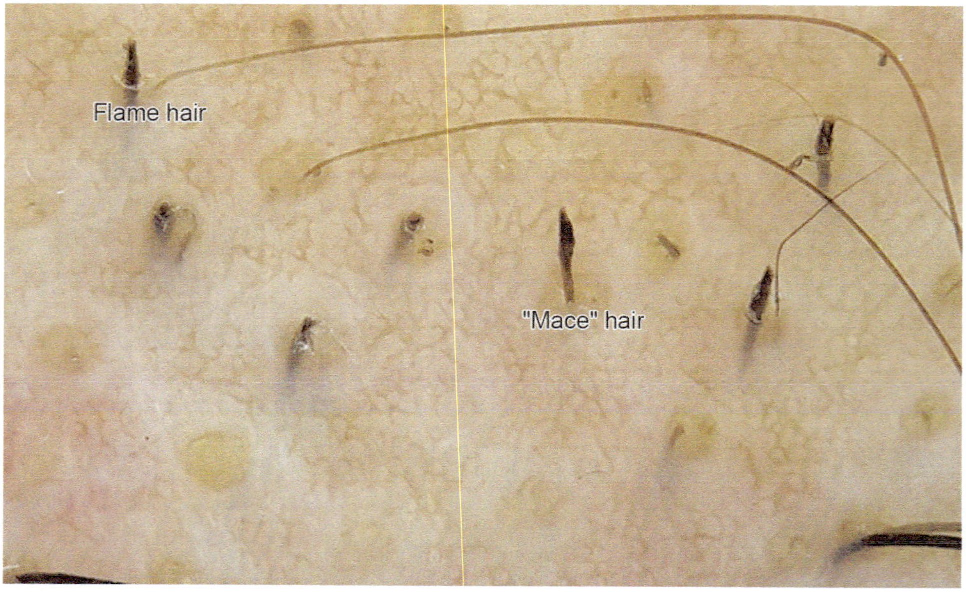

Fig. 21: The image has no features of alopecia areata but flame hairs and "mace" hair are clearly observed.

REFERENCES

1. Sah DE, Koo J, Price VH. Trichotillomania. Dermatol Ther. 2008;21(1):13-21.
2. Hautmann G, Hercogova J, Lotti T. Trichotillomania. J Am Acad Dermatol. 2002;46(6):807-21;quiz 22-6.
3. Sah DE, Koo J, Price VH. Trichotillomania. Dermatol Ther. 2008:21(1):13-21.
4. Ihm CW, Han JH. Diagnostic value of exclamation mark hairs. Dermatology. 1993;186(2):99-102.
5. Rudnica L, Olszewska M, Rakowska A, Slowinska M. Trichoscopy update 2011. J Dermatol Case Rep. 2011;5(4):82-8.
6. Cerullo L, Vincenzi C, Fabbrocini G, et al. Scalp dermoscopy in the diagnosis of trichotillomania. Int J Dermatol. In press.

ASSESSMENT IMAGE-BASED QUESTIONS

1. (A) Friar Tuck sign in a case of trichotillomania (TTM). It is the Christian practice of shaving the midscalp hair leaving a peripheral rim of hairs unshaved.

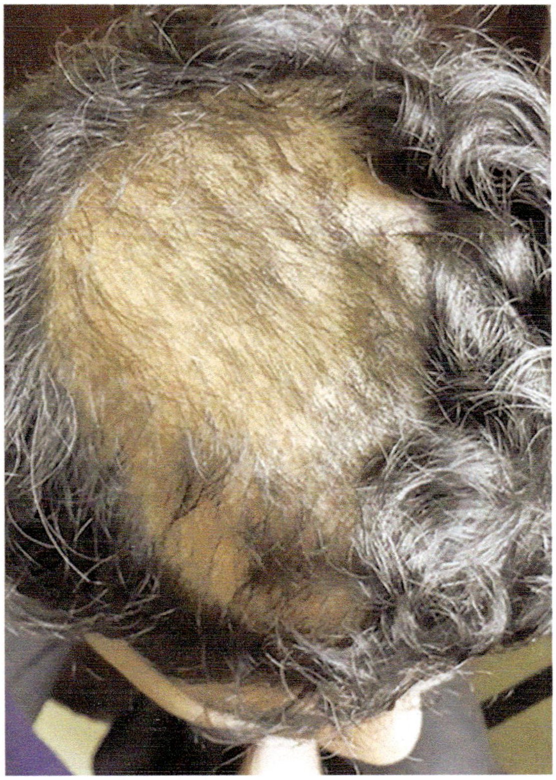

(B) Trichoscopy of the previous patient shows the following features. What do a, b, c, and d denote?

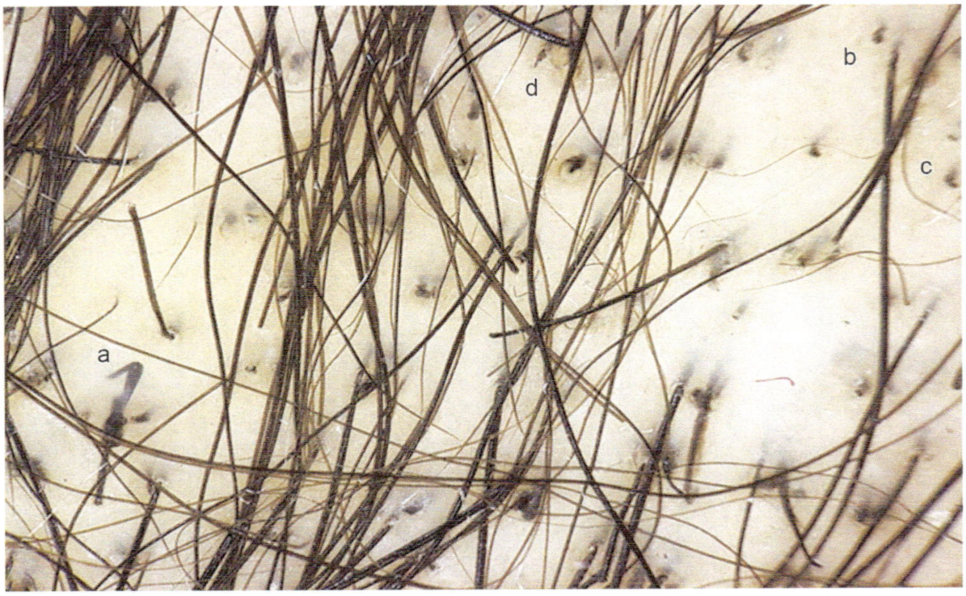

2. (A) Friar Tuck sign in another case of trichotillomania (TTM).

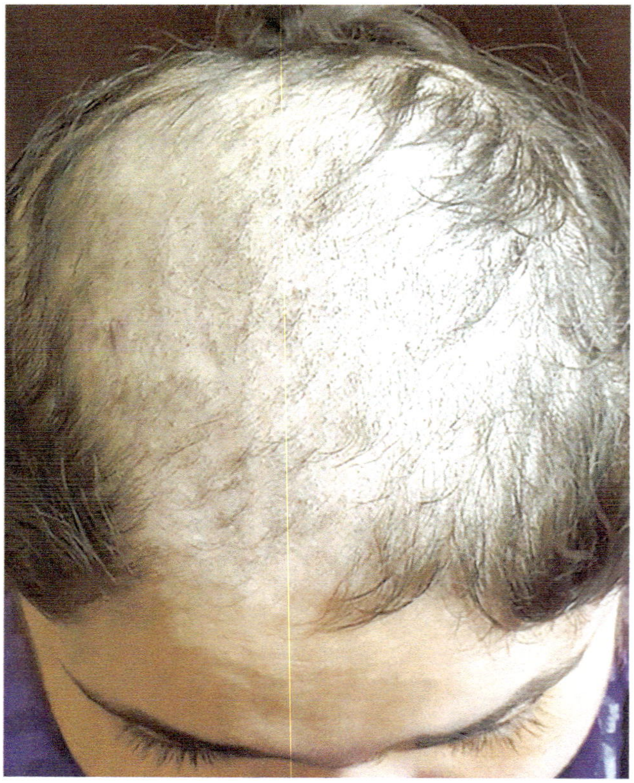

(B) Trichoscopy of the previous image shows the following. What do a, b, and c stand for?

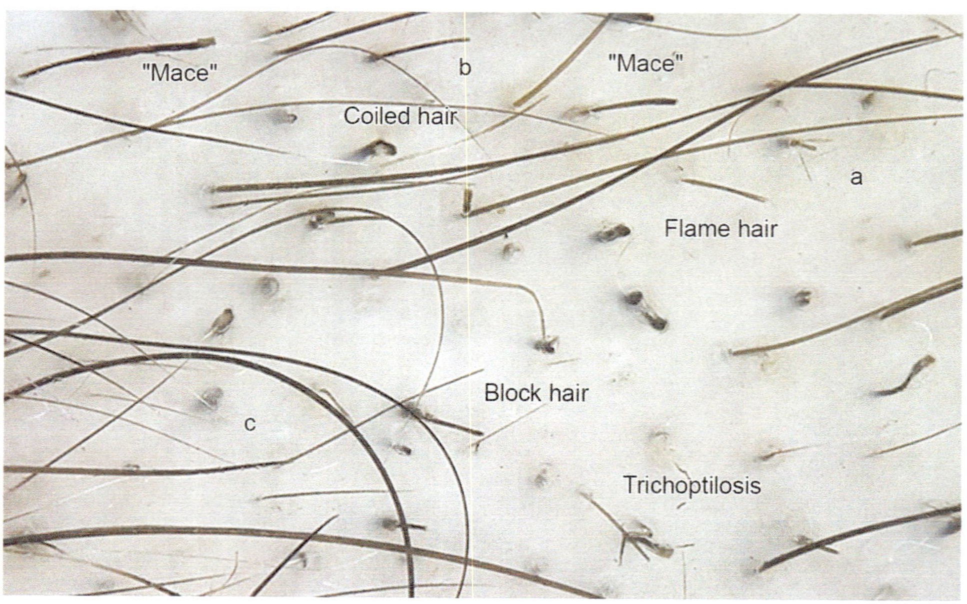

3. Mention three trichoscopic features of TTM seen in this image.

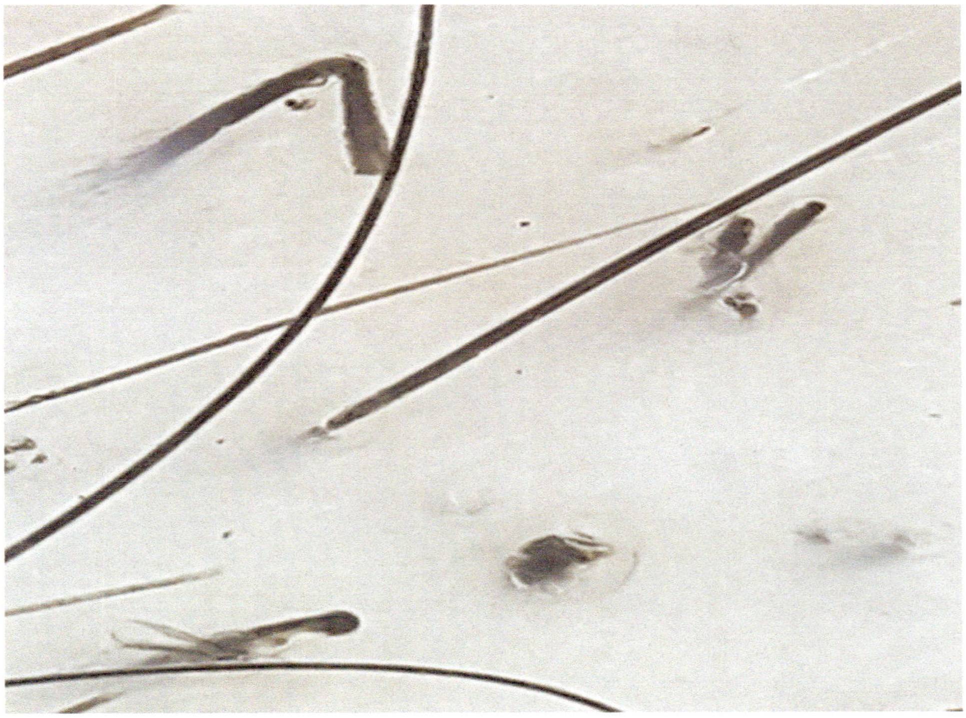

4. (A) Complete hairless areas in TTM are rare as patients tend to pull the long hairs only.

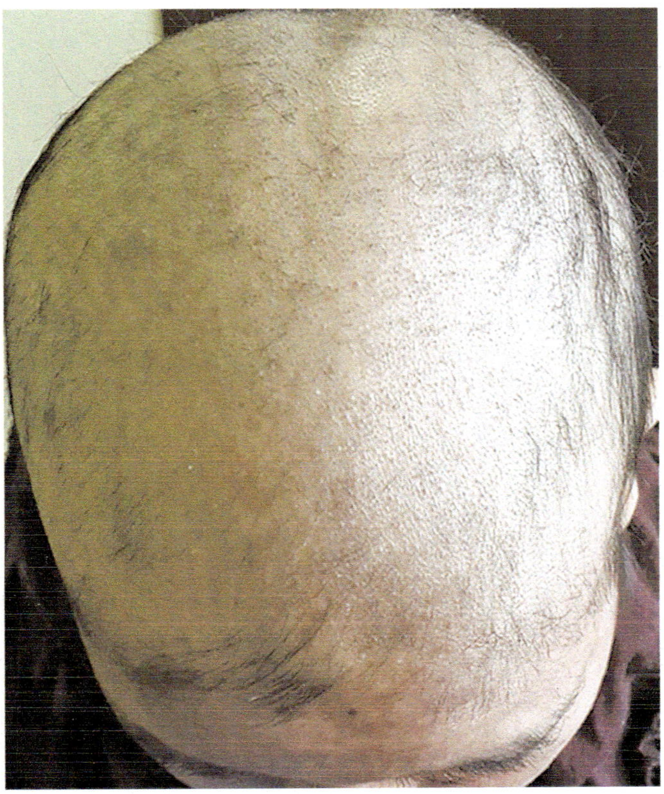

(B) Trichoscopy of the previous patient shows multiple "mace" hairs (M) and coiled hair (CH). What do "a" and "b" indicate?

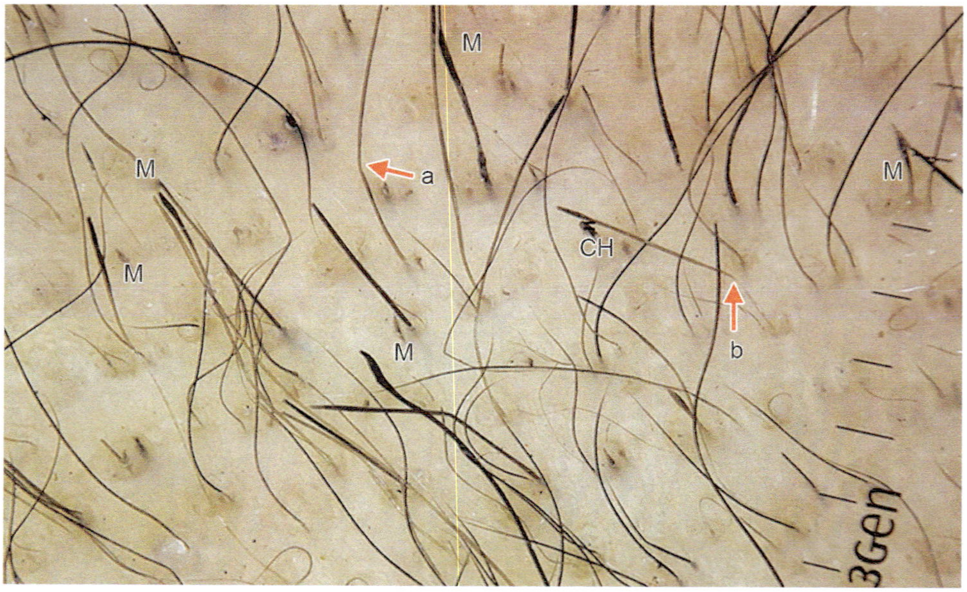

5. Extensive "mace" hairs in a case of trichotillomania. Indicate "a" and "b".

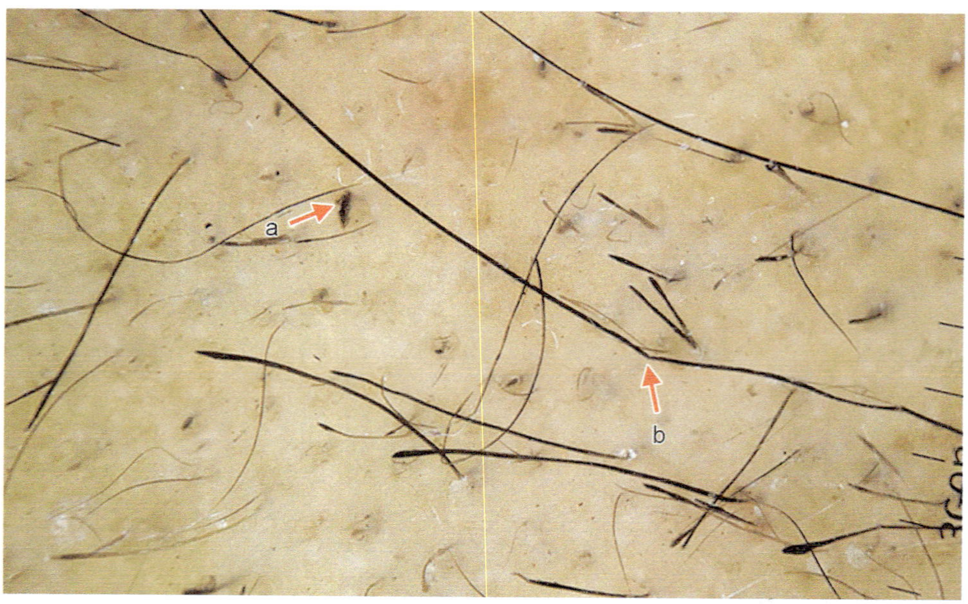

6. (A) Hair pulling in TTM most commonly involves the scalp resulting in irregular patches of hair loss. The affected areas are not completely bald but show hairs of different lengths.

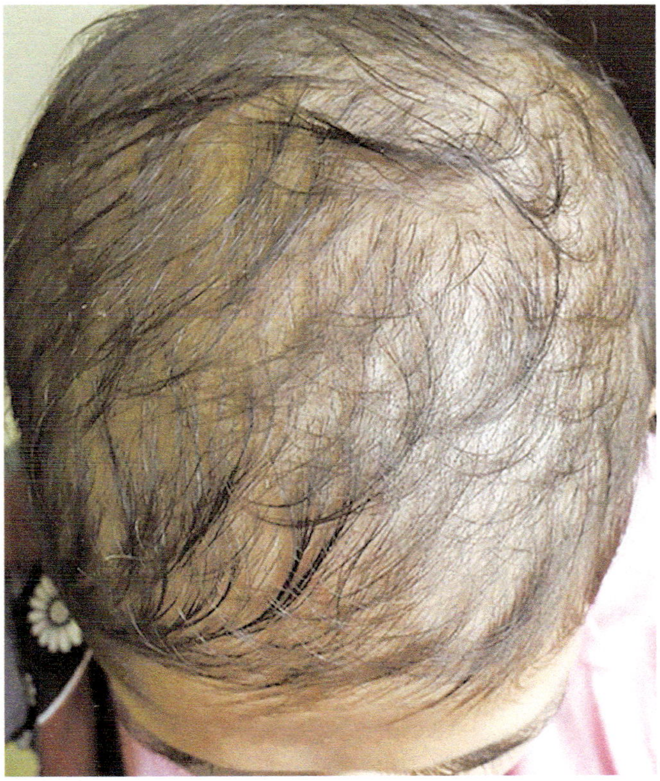

(B) Mention three features of TTM seen in the image.

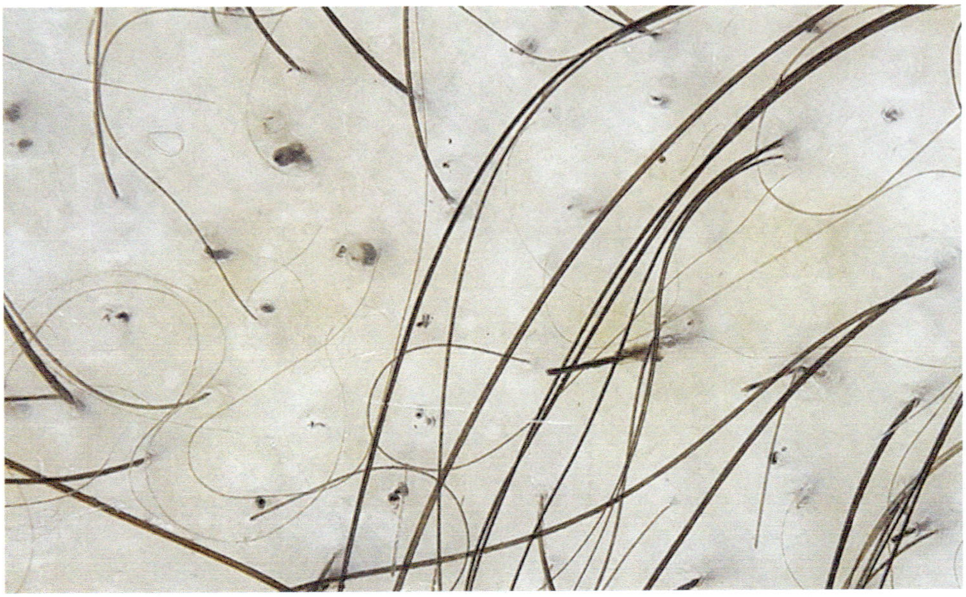

7. What is the clinical differential diagnosis of this patchy alopecia?

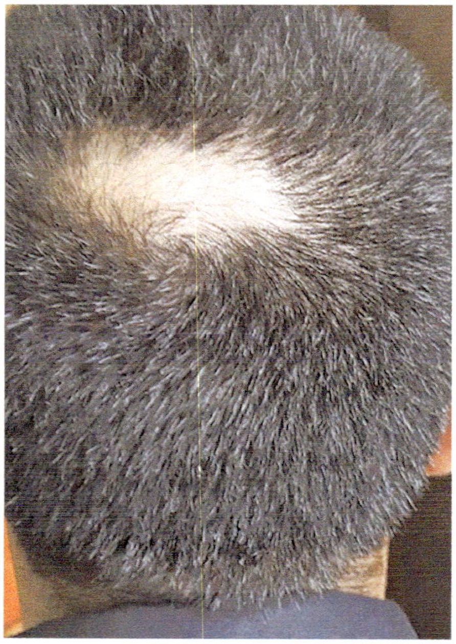

8. Trichoscopy of the previous patient shows "mace" hair, flame hair, and broken hairs. Observe few black hair-like particles in the interfollicular space, the diameter of which are less than hair shafts. What are those hair-like particles?

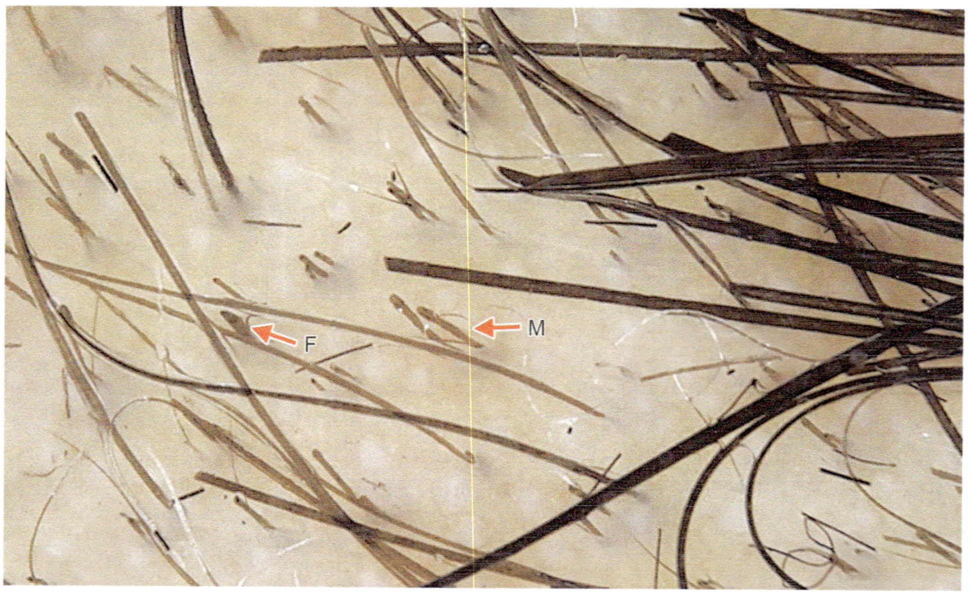

ANSWERS

1. (B) a: question mark hair, b and c: coiled hair, d: flame hair
2. (B) a: trichoptilosis, b: broken hair, c: flame hair
3. Question mark hair, flame hair, and "v" sign.
4. (B) Pohl-Pinkus constrictions
5. a: flame hair, b: Pohl-Pinkus constriction
6. (B) Flame hair, broken hair and black dots
7. Alopecia areata, androgenetic alopecia
8. Cosmetic hair fibers

CHAPTER 13

Traction Alopecia

Subrata Malakar

INTRODUCTION

- It is a traumatic hair loss due to severe pulling of scalp hair. The pulling of hairs usually results from hairstyling practices.[1] The most common hairstyling practices are ponytails, dreadlocks, and clips on hair extensions and turbans.
- Scarring alopecia most commonly affects the marginal scalp when it is termed marginal traction alopecia. Uncommonly tractional alopecia may affect other areas of the scalp.
- The clinical course of tractional alopecia progresses from early stage nonscarring to scarring alopecia with prolonged traction.
- Trichoscopy is useful in distinguishing traction alopecia from other causes of alopecias. It shows hair casts around the hair shafts at the margin of the patches where it is seen as cylindrical casts that envelop the proximal portion of the hair shaft.[2]

KEY TRICHOSCOPIC FEATURES

- *Early stage*: Hair casts around hair shafts at the periphery of the lesions.
- *Late stage*: Decreased hair density, predominance of single-hair follicular units, white dots lacking follicular openings.

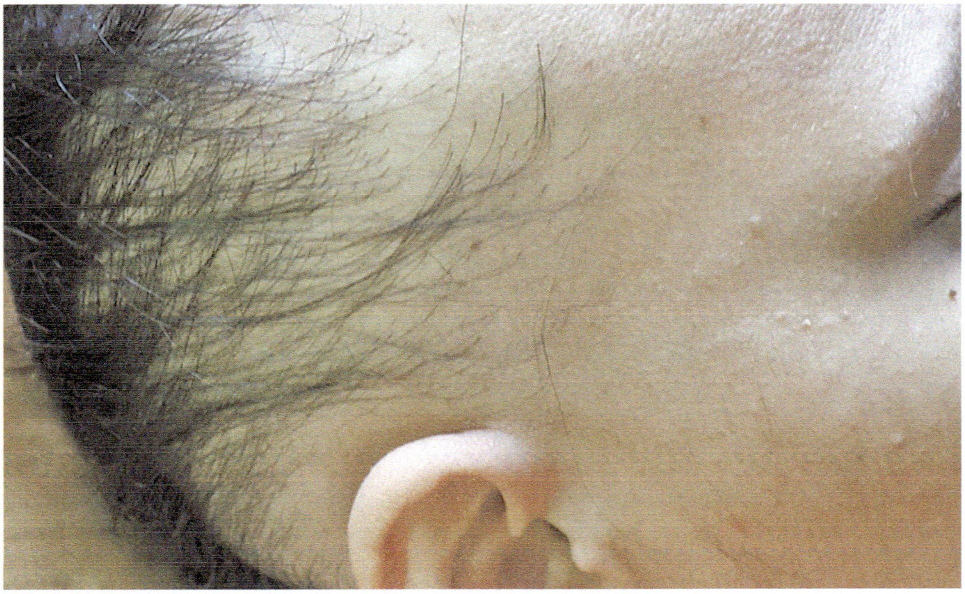

Fig. 1: Marginal traction alopecia due to long-standing hair pull resulting from ponytail hairstyle practices.

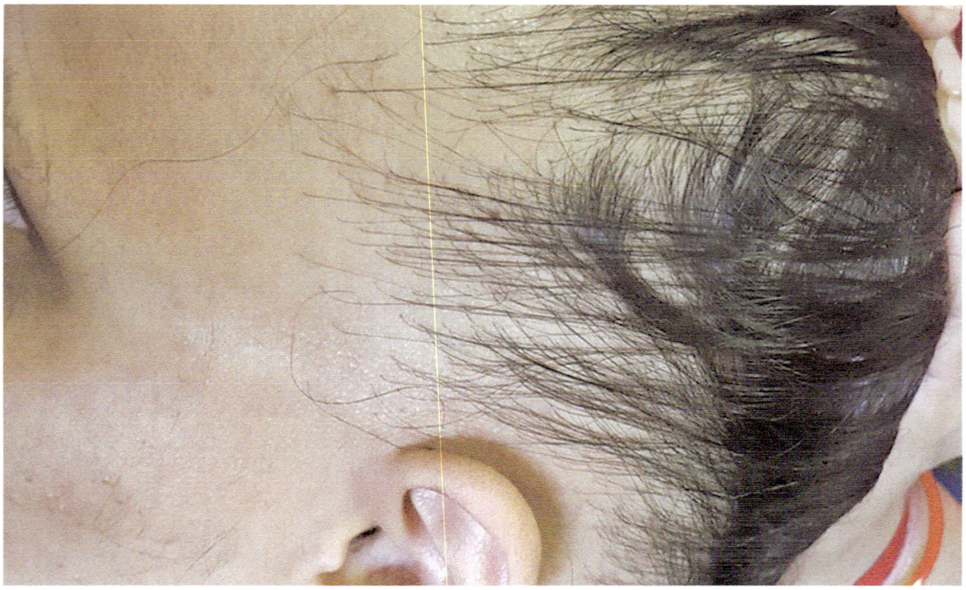

Fig. 2: Same patient, left lateral view.

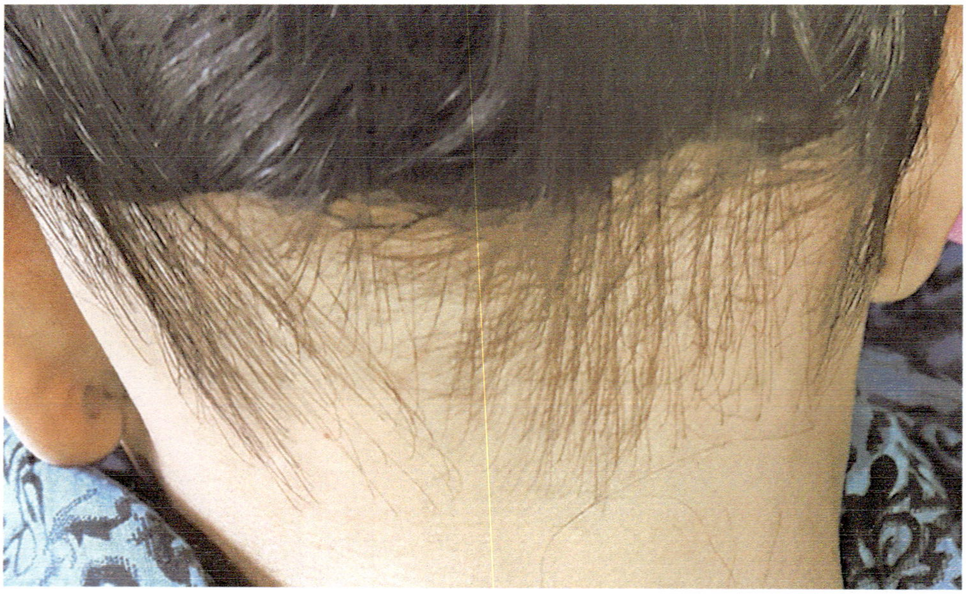

Fig. 3: Same patient, view from behind, showing marginal traction alopecia involving the lower occiput.

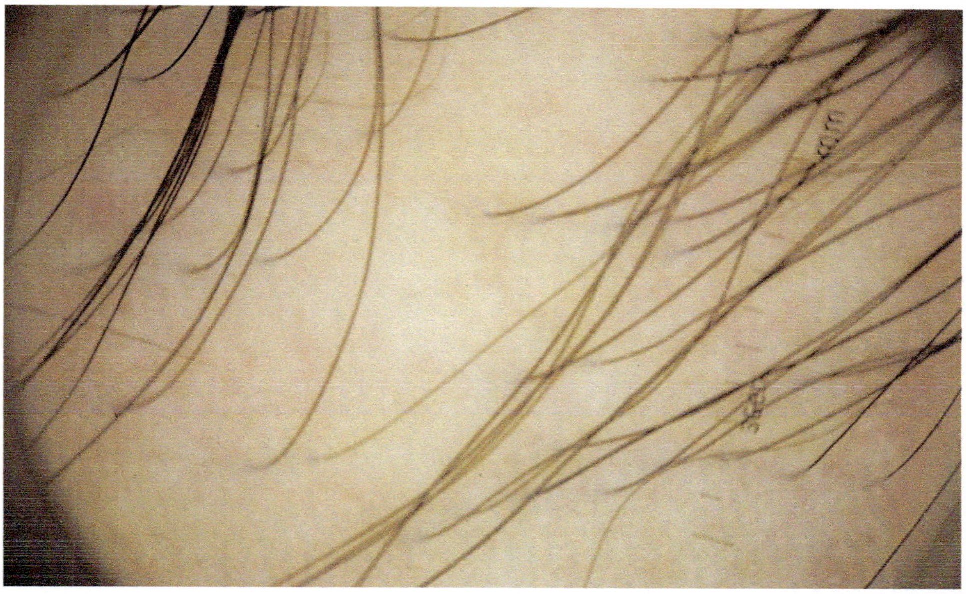

Fig. 4: Low hair density, mostly single-hair follicular units, and absence of follicular openings. This is a late-stage marginal traction alopecia.

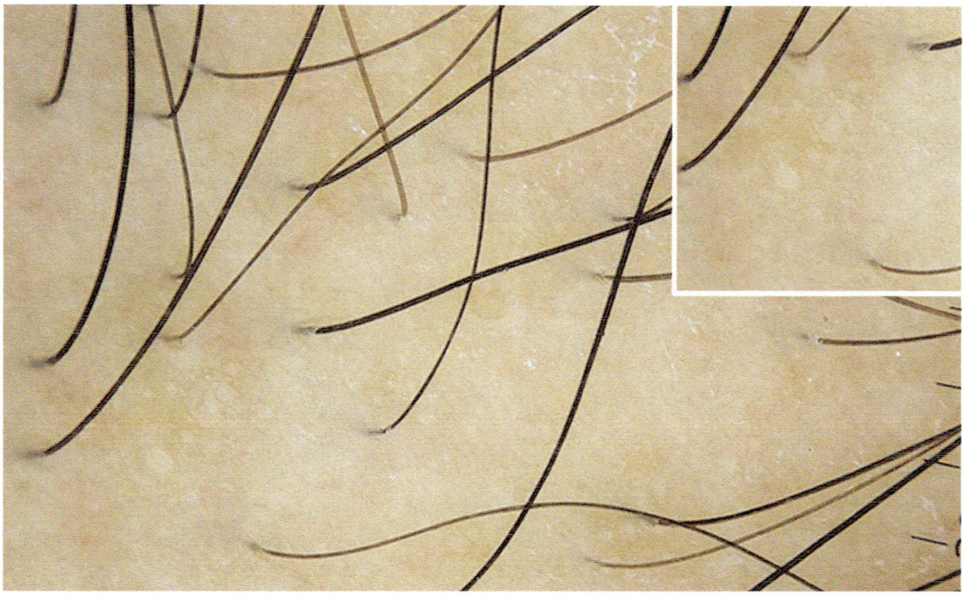

Fig. 5: Fibrotic white dots (see inset) resulting from perifollicular fibrosis are seen in the late-stage marginal traction alopecia. All the hairs in the field are single-hair follicular units. Note the white dots are coalescing to form white patches.

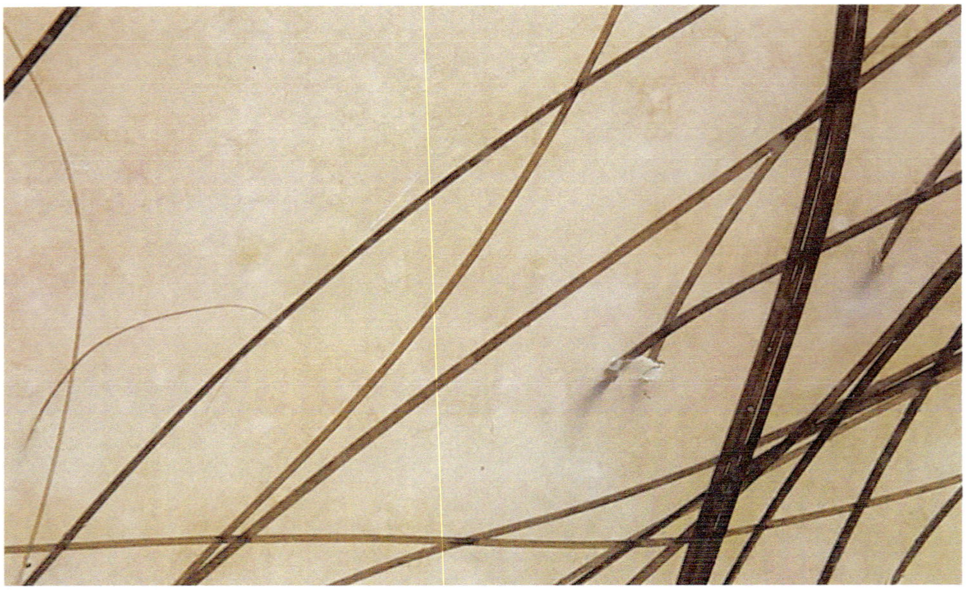

Fig. 6: Hair cast around two hair are visible at the margin of the patch. Though cylindrical hair casts are early signs of traction alopecia, it may be observed rarely in the final stage. These hair casts are freely movable along the hair shaft.

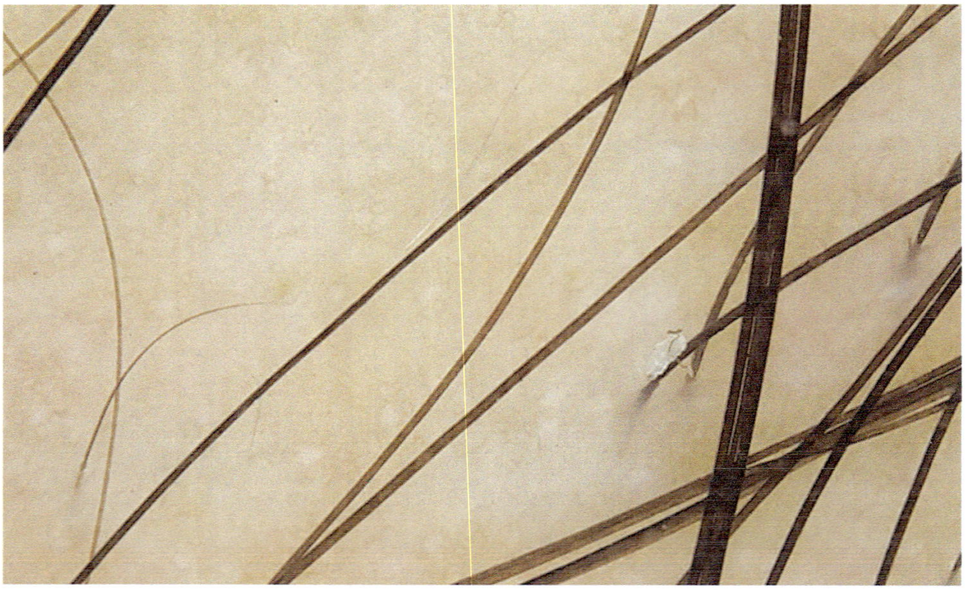

Fig. 7: The main differential diagnosis of advanced traction alopecia is lichen planopilaris that differs from cicatricial traction alopecia in its prominent perifollicular scaling and erythema.

REFERENCES

1. Hantash BM, Schwartz RA. Traction alopecia in children. Cutis. 2003;71(1):18-20.
2. Zhu WY, Xia MY, Wu JH, et al. Hair casts: A clinical and electron microscopic study. Pediatric Dermatol. 1990;7:270-4.

CHAPTER

14 Telogen Effluvium

Subrata Malakar, Purva Mehta Movdawalla, Surit Malakar

INTRODUCTION

- Telogen effluvium (TE) is defined as sudden generalized shedding of telogen hairs few months after an acute systemic stressful episode.
- It may be triggered by internal or external factors which cause a large number of hairs to enter the telogen phase at a time. Telogen hairs start shedding after 3–4 months of exposure to triggering factors. These factors include various physical and psychological trauma, medications such as beta-blockers and retinoids, and ultraviolet exposure.[1-7]
- Chronic TE is characterized by a diffuse loss of telogen hairs continuing for >6 months. Hair loss is usually associated with progressive hair thinning.[7,8]
- Diagnostic aids for acute and chronic TE are histopathology and trichogram along with a history and examination to identify the cause of TE.[9]
- Coexistence of TE and female pattern hair loss (FPHL) is very frequent.

ACUTE TELOGEN EFFLUVIUM

- Acute hair shedding with or without thinning of scalp hairs.
- Pull test is positive (telogen hairs on microscopy).
- *Trichoscopy*: Empty follicles and short regrowing hairs.
- Trichoscopy is not useful because it does not show any specific features.

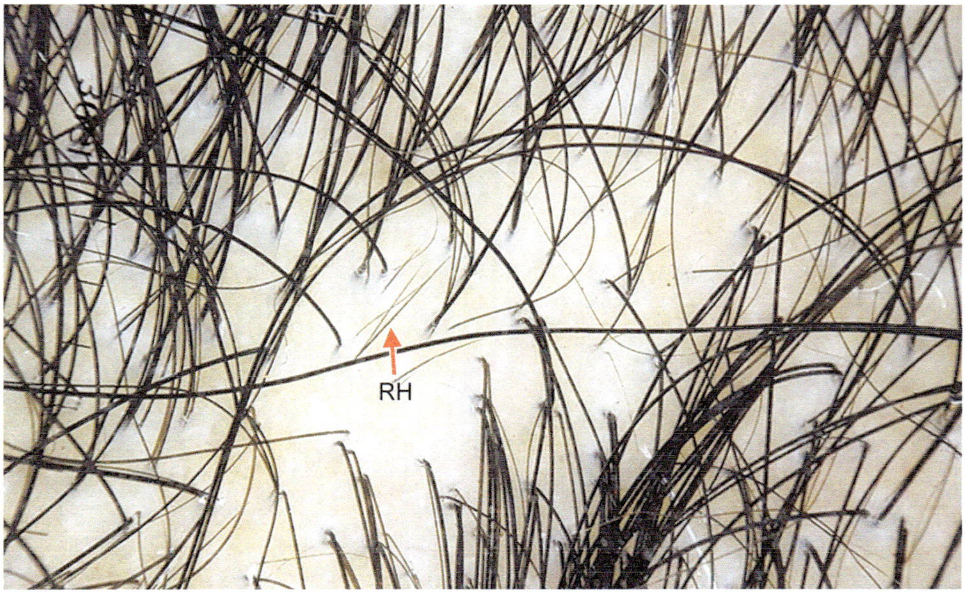

Fig. 1: Acute telogen effluvium (TE). Many upright regrowing hairs (RH) at the center of the image.

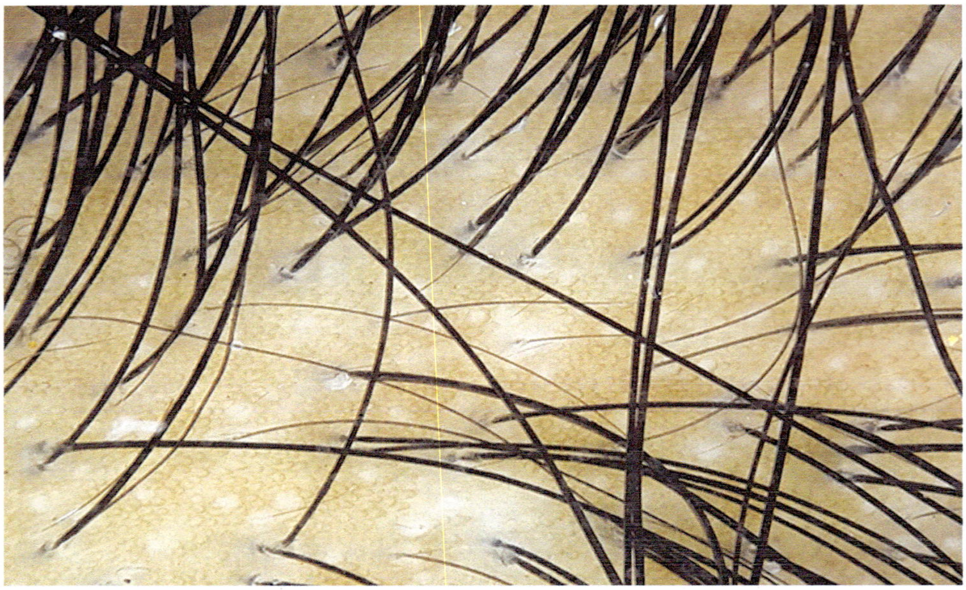

Fig. 2: Acute telogen effluvium (TE). Presence of many upright regrowing hairs is characteristic of acute TE. Presence of thick terminal hairs goes in favor of acute TE, whereas in chronic TE, terminal hairs tend to become thinner. This image also has empty follicles.

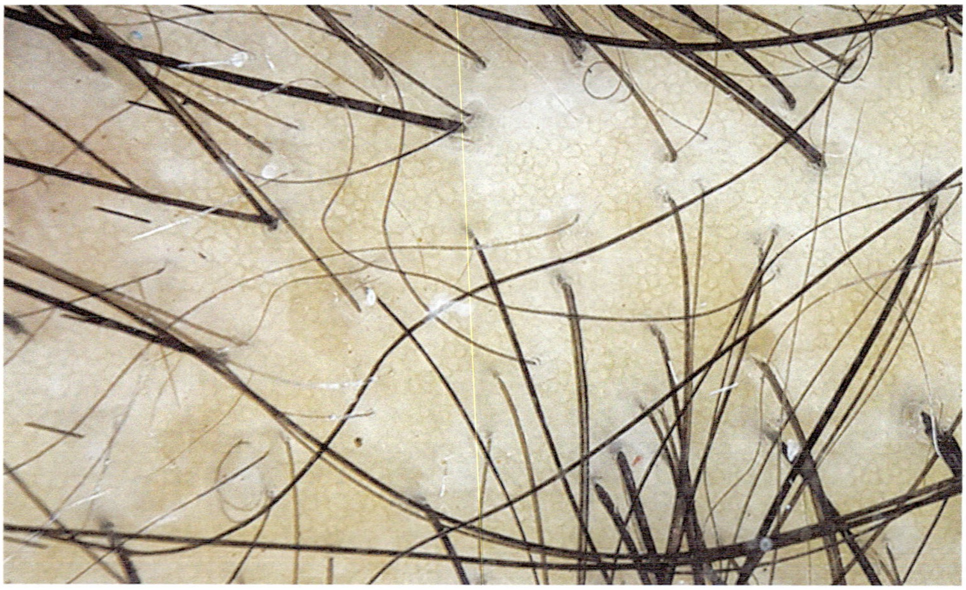

Fig. 3: Another case of acute telogen effluvium showing short regrowing hairs.

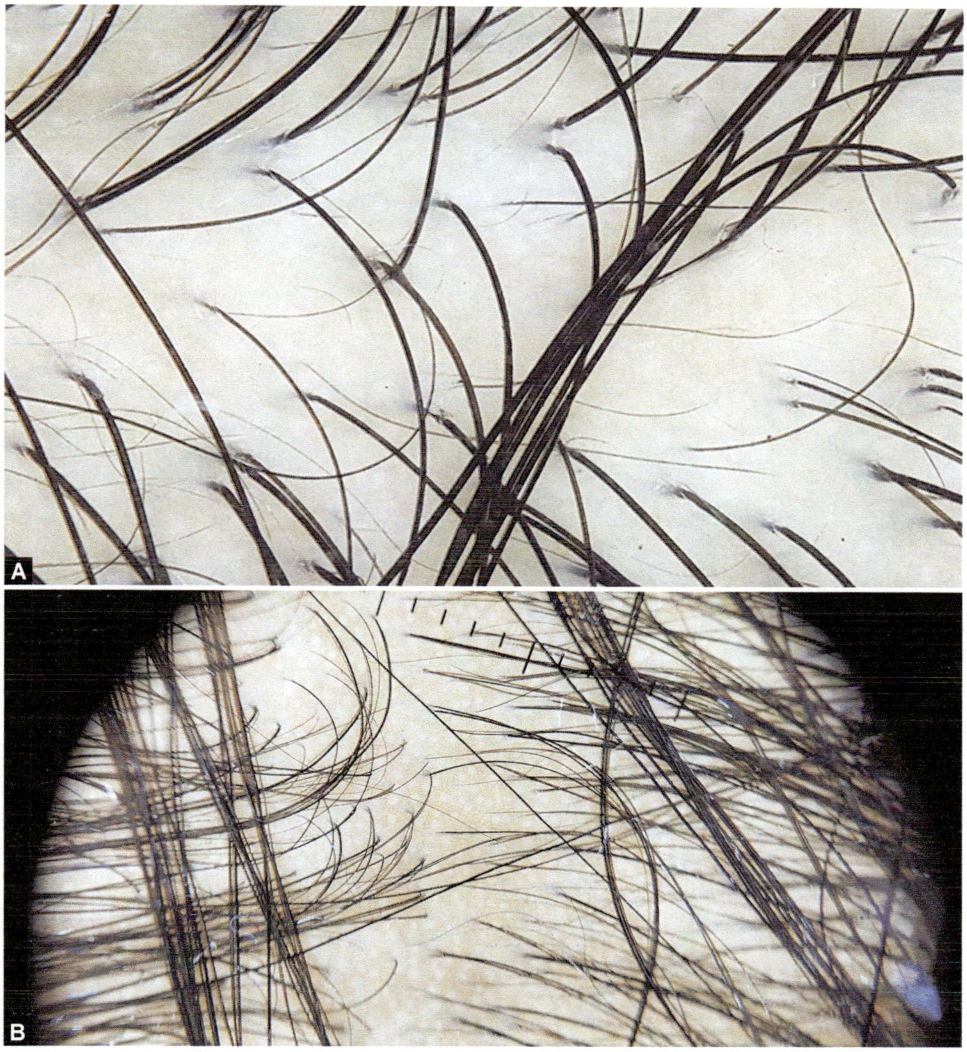

Figs. 4A and B: (A) This image shows the predominance of single-hair units and a marked decrease of follicular units with three or four hairs. Numerous upright regrowing hairs are visible. (B) The predominance of single-hair units and a marked decrease of follicular units with three or four hairs. Numerous upright regrowing hairs are visible.

CHRONIC TELOGEN EFFLUVIUM[10]

- Chronic TE is defined as abrupt onset of generalized hair shedding of the scalp for >6 months.
- Hair-thinning and bitemporal recession are present.
- Pull test is negative.
- Diagnosis is based on exclusion rather than specific diagnostic criteria.
- On dermoscopy, absence of hair diameter variability of <20% and short regrowing hairs.

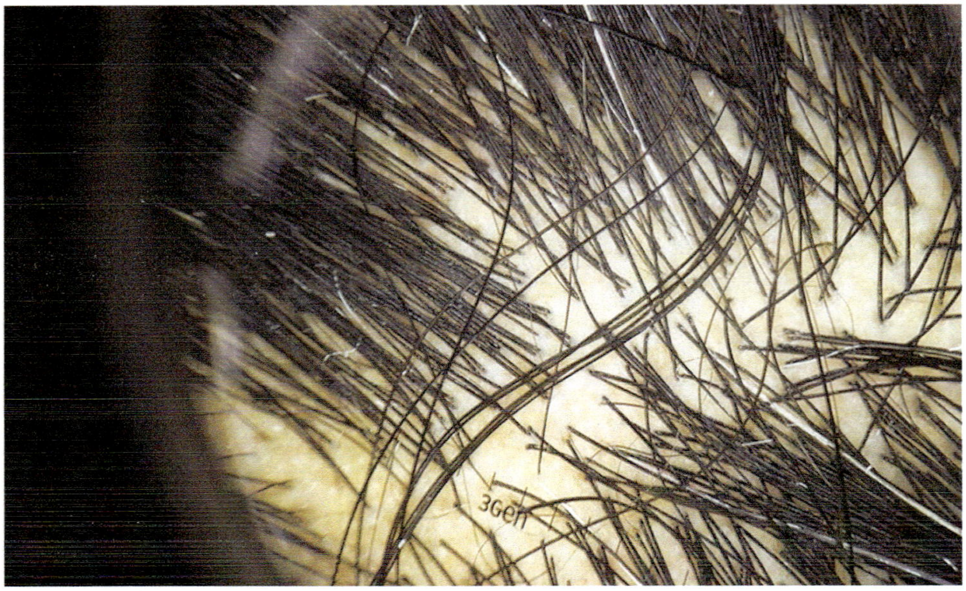

Fig. 5: Diagnosis of chronic telogen effluvium is based on exclusion rather than specific criteria. A critical feature is the presence of less than 20% hair diameter diversity.

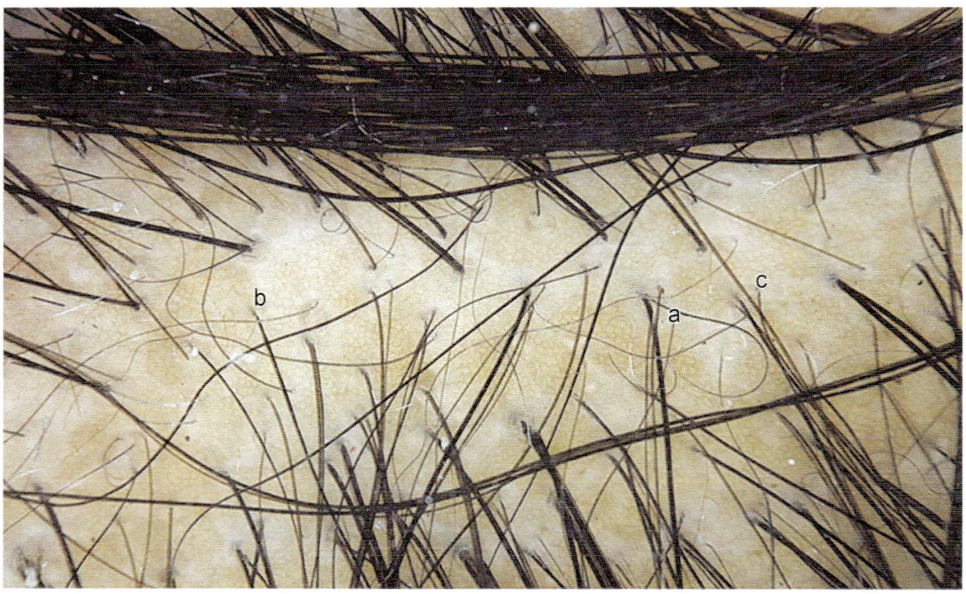

Fig. 6: Trichoscopic features of this image are: (a) empty follicles, (b) peripilar sign, and (c) regrowing hairs. In chronic telogen effluvium, the terminal hairs tend to become thinner over the years.

REFERENCES

1. Trueb RM. Systemic approach to hair loss in women. J Dtsch Dermatol Ges. 2010;8(4):284-98.
2. Mounsey AL, Reed SW. Diagnosing and treating hair loss. Am Fam Physician. 2009;80(4):356-62.
3. Durusoy C, Ozenli Y, Adiguzel A, Budakoglu IY, Tugal O, Arikan S, et al. The role of psychological factors and serum zinc, folate and vitamin B12 levels in the aetiology of trichodynia: a case control study. Clin exp Dermatol. 2009;34(7):789-92.
4. Katz KA, Cotsarelis G, Gupta R, Seykora JT. Teloen effluvium associated with dopamine agonist primiprexole in a 55-year-old women with Parkinson's disease. J Am Acad Dermatol. 2006;55(5 Suppl):S103-4.
5. Patrizi A, Savoia F, Negosanti F, Posar A, Santucci M, Neri I. Telogen effluvium caused by magnesium valproate and lamotrigine. Acta Dermatol Venereol. 2005;85(1):77-8.
6. Pirracini BM, van Neste DJ. Telogen effluvium after allergic contact dermatitis of the scalp. Arch Dermatol. 2001;137(2):187-90.
7. Harrison S, Sinclair R. Telogen effluvium. Clin Exp Dermatol. 2002;27(5):389-95.
8. Chen W, Yang CC, Todorova A, Al Khuzaei S, Chiu HC, Worret WI, et al. Hair loss in elderly women. Eur J Dermatol. 2010;20(2):145-51.
9. Olszewska M, Warszawik O, Rakowska A, Słowińska M, Rudnicka L. Method of hair loss evaluation in patients with endocrine disorders. Endokrynol Pol. 2010;61(4):406-11.
10. Whiting DA. Chronic telogen effluvium: Increased scalp hair shedding in middle- aged women. J Am Acad Dermatol. 1996;35:899-906.

ASSESSMENT IMAGE-BASED QUESTION

1. Upright regrowing hair is a feature of acute TE. What are the other trichoscopic features of acute TE? Is there any specific trichoscopic sign of chronic TE?

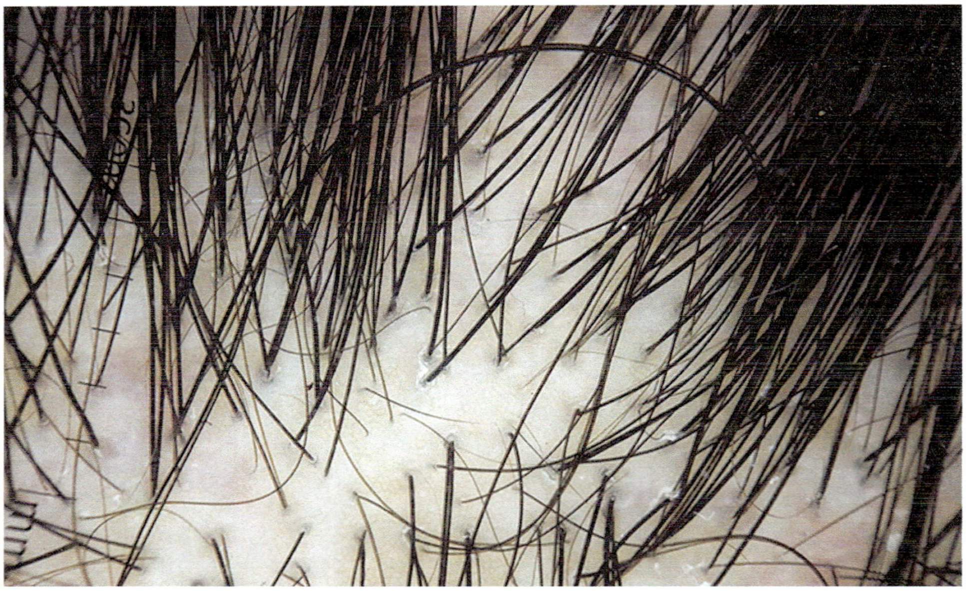

ANSWER

1. Empty follicles. No specific trichoscopic features in chronic TE. In chronic TE, absence of hair diameter variability of less than 20% and short regrowing hairs are seen.

CHAPTER

15

Anagen Effluvium

Subrata Malakar, Barnali Chowdhury

INTRODUCTION

- It is diffuse hair loss in the anagen phase of hair cycle.
- It occurs most commonly when mitotic and metabolic activity of the hair follicle is suppressed by a cytotoxic drug.[1,2]
- Anagen hair loss is usually observed postchemotherapy, it can also be observed with noncytotoxic agents such as acitretin,[3-5] postradiotherapy,[6] and smoking.[7]
- Anagen effluvium (AE) is also seen in conditions like loose anagen syndrome and short anagen syndrome.
- Loose anagen syndrome is characterized by weak attachment of the anagen hairs to the follicle.[8,9]
- Short anagen syndrome is diagnosed when hairs are pulled out easily and painlessly and the anagen phase is extremely short. Hairs fall out before they grow longer than 3–6 cm.[8,9]

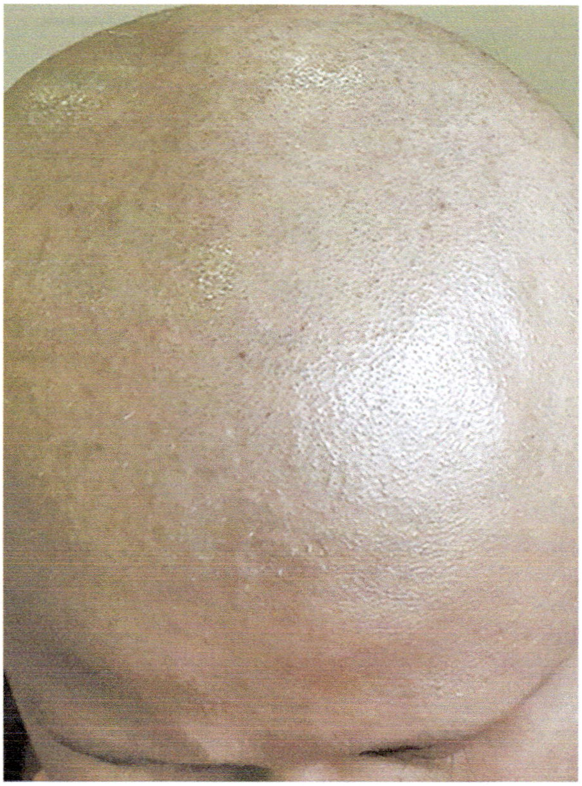

Fig. 1: The onset of chemotherapy alopecia is seen approximately 1–3 weeks after the initial dose of chemotherapy.[1] Incidence of anagen effluvium following chemotherapy is 65%. Combination chemotherapy produces more severe hair loss compared with monotherapy.[3]

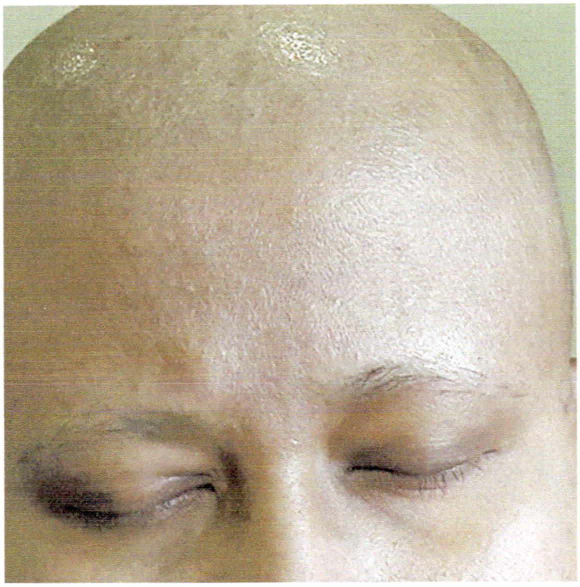

Fig. 2: Chemotherapy alopecia involves almost all of the scalp hairs, eyebrows and also eyelashes.

KEY TRICHOSCOPIC FEATURES

- Black dots
- Monilethrix-like hairs
- Yellow dots
- Flame hairs
- Tapering hairs, e.g., exclamation mark hairs and coudability hairs
- Changes in the hair shaft color
- Peripilar sign
- Tulip hair-like structure (author's observation)
- Dystrophic hair (author's observation)
- Circle hair (author's observation)

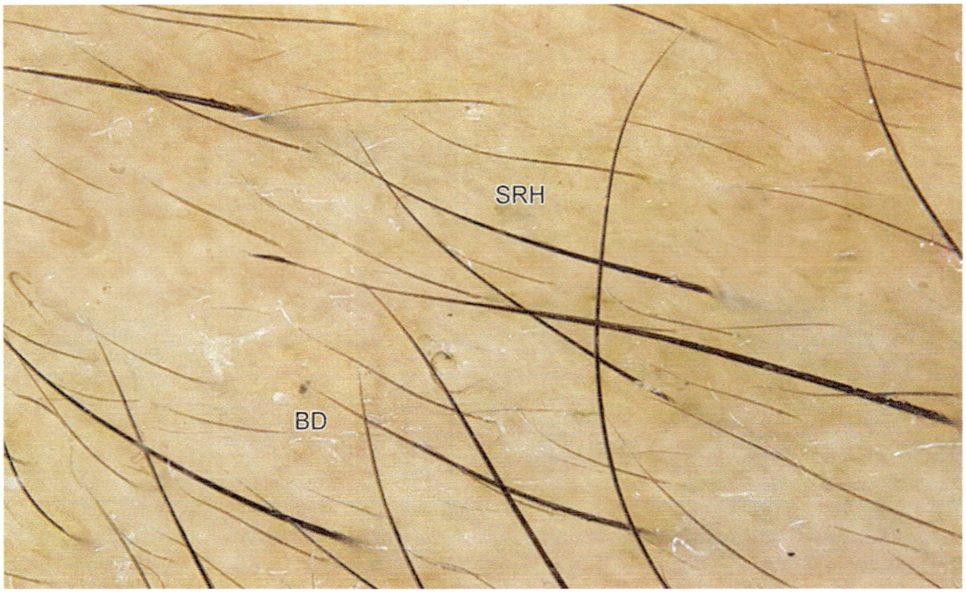

Fig. 3: Within a few weeks after the chemotherapy is stopped, the hair follicles resume their activity and the hair starts regrowing. Numerous short regrowing hairs (SRH) are seen in the field after chemotherapy is over. A few black dots (BD) are also is visible.

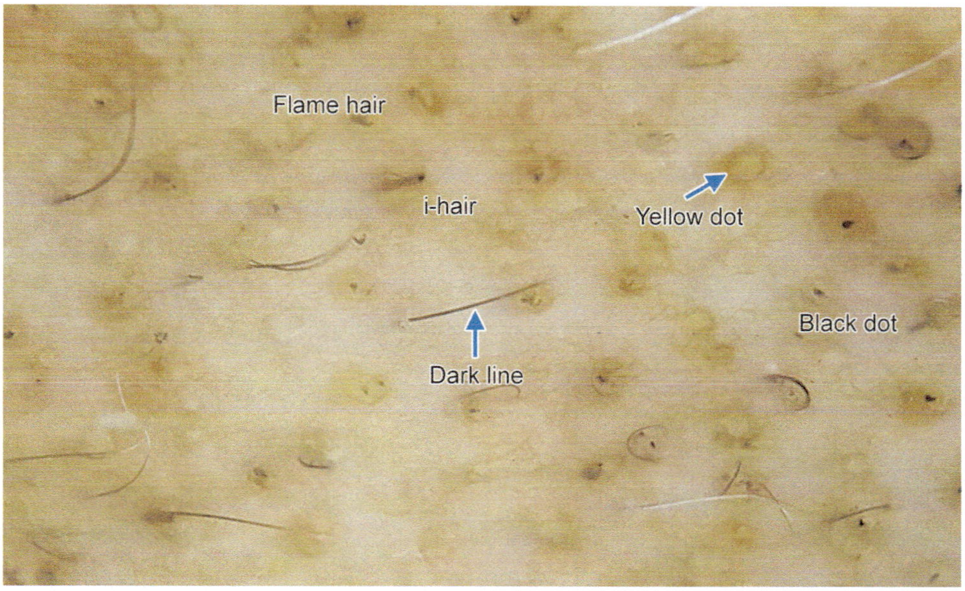

Fig. 4: Chemotherapy-induced alopecia showing the above trichoscopic features.

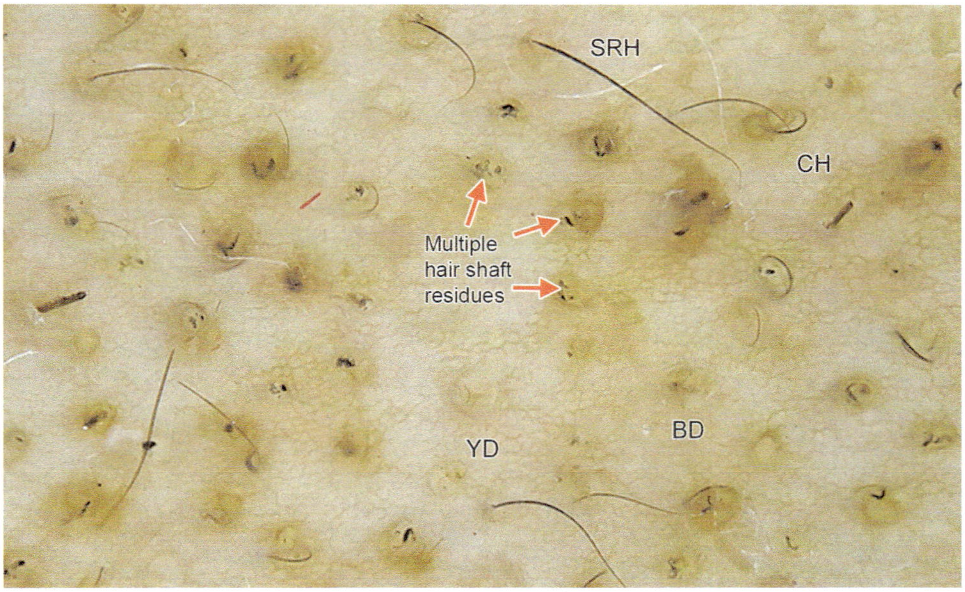

Fig. 5: Multiple hair shaft residues. Other features in this image are yellow dots (YD), black dots (BD), short regrowing hairs (SRH), and circle hairs (CH).

- Tulip hair-like structure after resumption of follicular activity (author's observation). Tulip hair is thin at its proximal part and has a light-colored shaft with dark tip. This dark tip corresponds to an area of oblique hair rupture.[10] However, in tulip hair-like structure, the proximal part of hair has normal color and thickness; above which there is an acute constriction and hair becomes narrow ending as a dark tip. Probably this tip is the area of oblique hair fracture. We hypothesize the genesis of the tulip hair-like structure in the following way—the distal part corresponds to the time when chemotherapy was induced; whereas the portion of the hair distal to the tip has broken and fallen off leaving a tulip like tip. The proximal normal shaft corresponds to the time when chemotherapy was stopped and the follicle resumed its activity when the shaft thickens again.

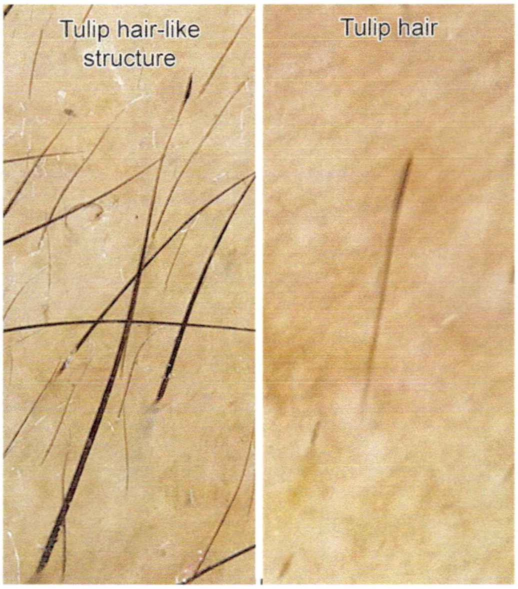

Fig. 6: Comparison of tulip hair-like structure with tulip hair (author's observation).

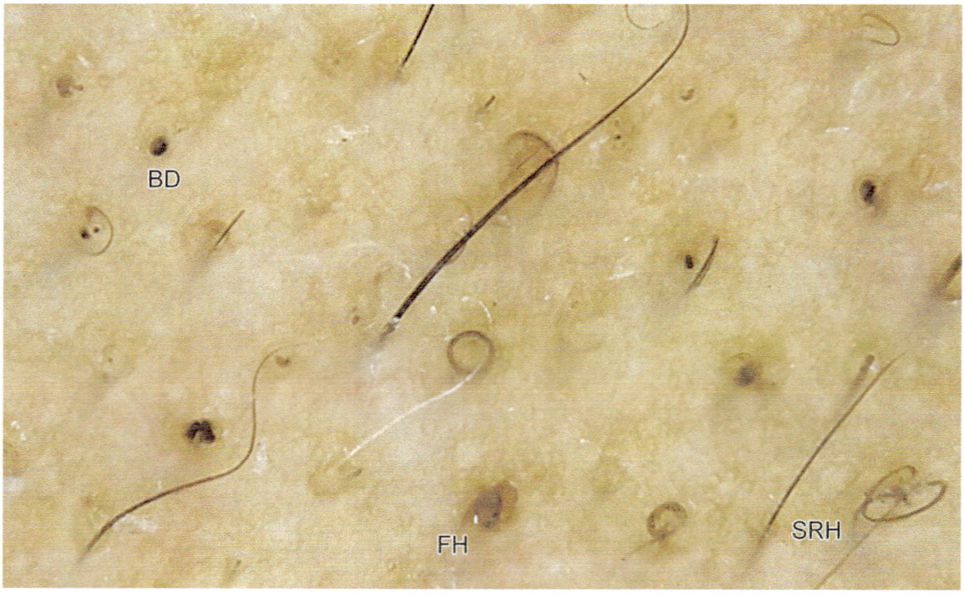

Fig. 7: Circle hairs, which are a common trichoscopic feature of body hair abnormalities can also be frequently seen in chemotherapy alopecia.

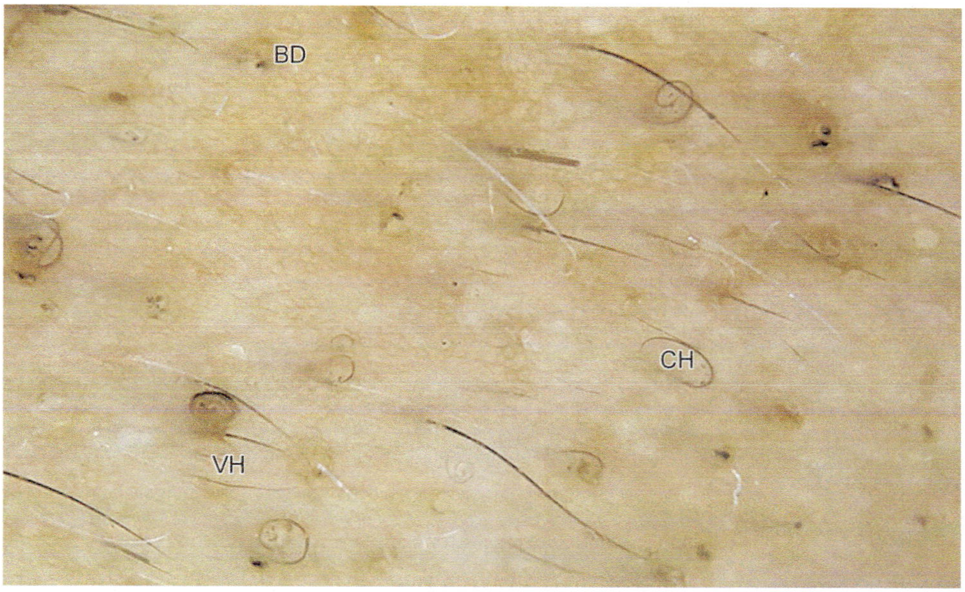

Fig. 8: In chemotherapy alopecia, the mitotic activity of the hair follicle is quickly suppressed. The hair shafts become thinner and then break. If it breaks at the scalp level black dots are formed. After the drug has been stopped the follicle resumes its activity soon and the hairs regrow. In this field, black dots as well as regrowing hairs are present simultaneously.

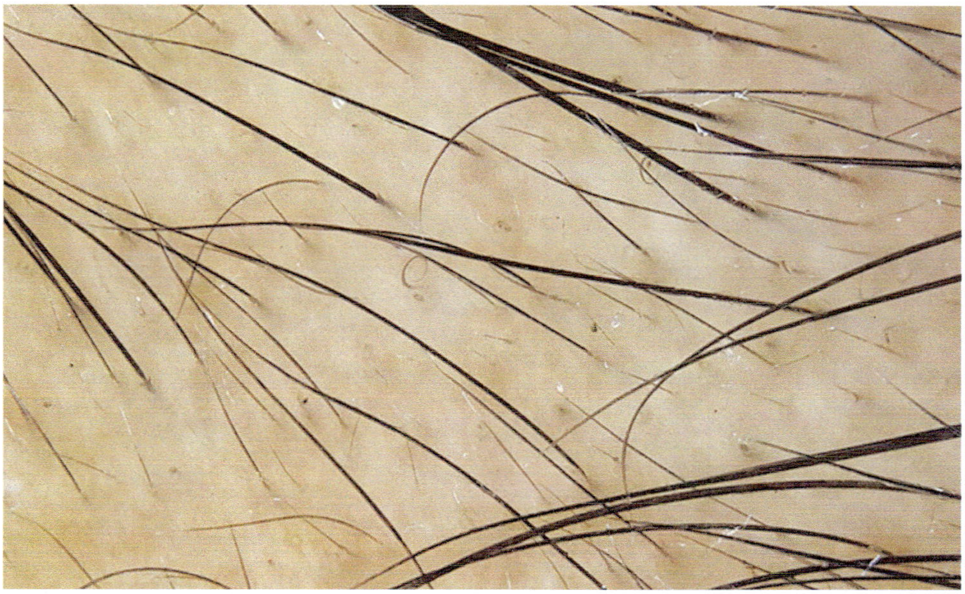

Fig. 9: Numerous regrowing hairs indicate that chemotherapy has been stopped 3 weeks back.

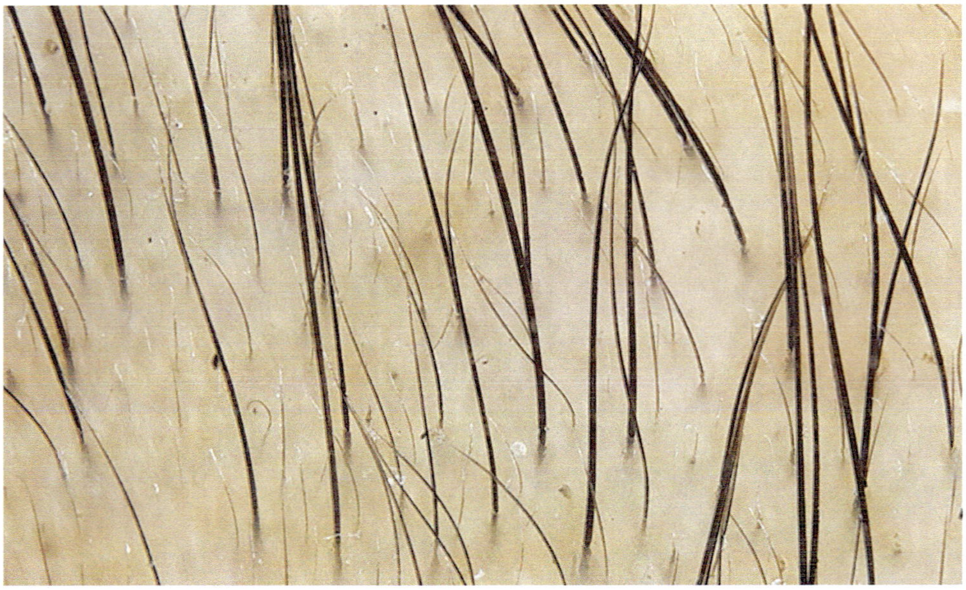

Fig. 10: Numerous short regrowing hairs are seen along with normal hairs. Normal hairs have uniform shape and thickness but mostly they are single-hair follicular units.

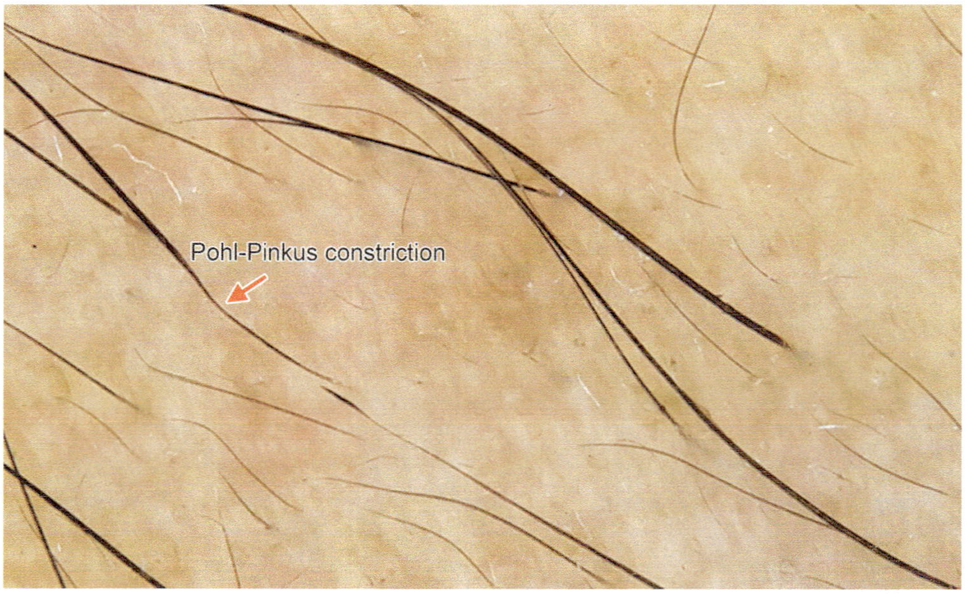

Fig. 11: After chemotherapy, hair is fractured at the scalp level leaving behind black dots. But with lower doses, there may be just segmental thinning instead of fracture of the hair shaft, resulting in Pohl-Pinkus constriction.

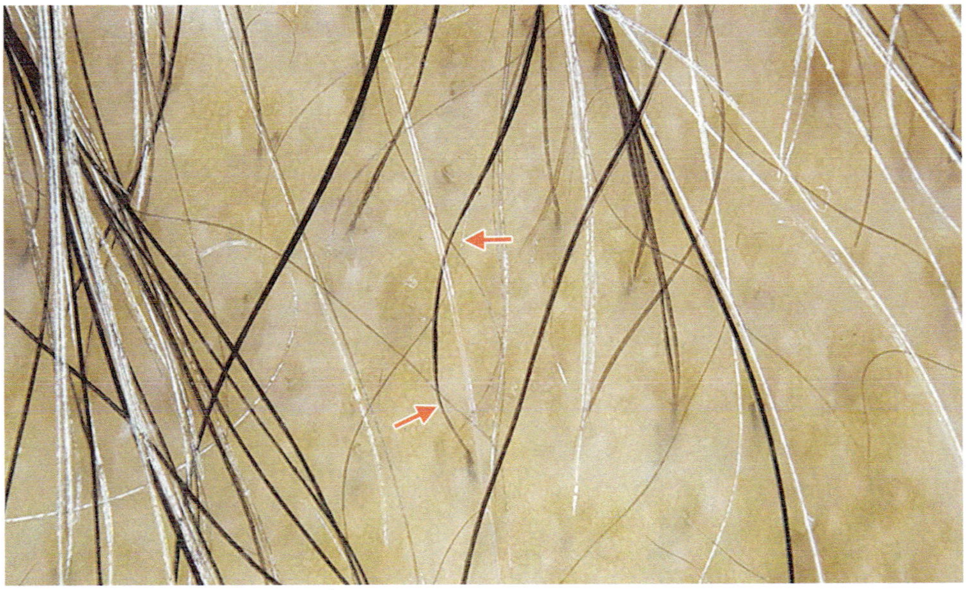

Fig. 12: Multiple Pohl-Pinkus constrictions (arrows).

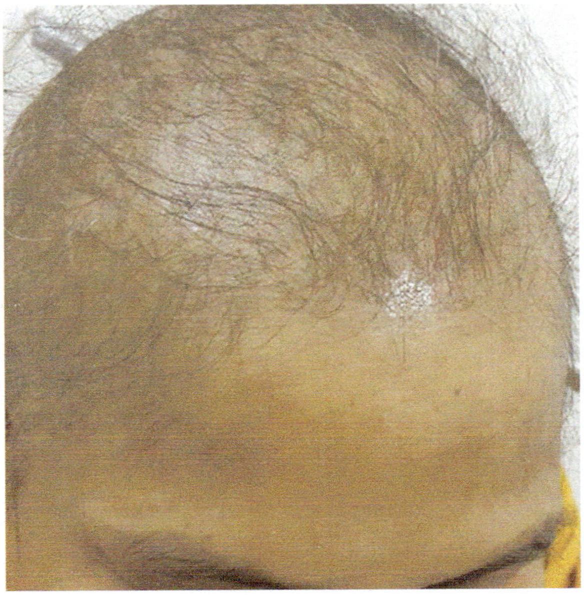

Fig. 13: Another patient on chemotherapy. Note all the hairs have not been affected. Postchemotherapy hair loss shows high variability depending on the agent used.

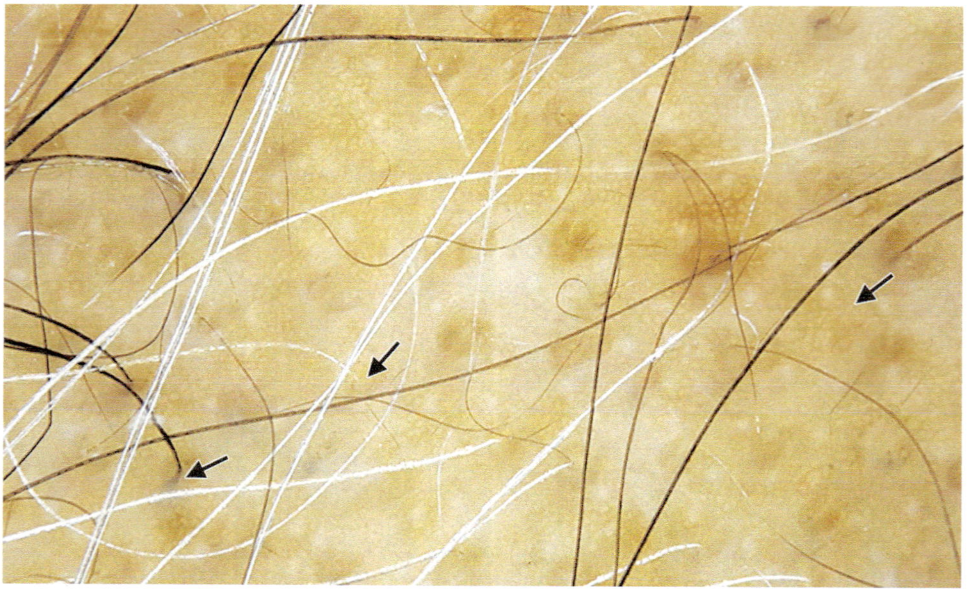

Fig. 14: Extensive peripilar sign in a case of postchemotherapy alopecia.[11]

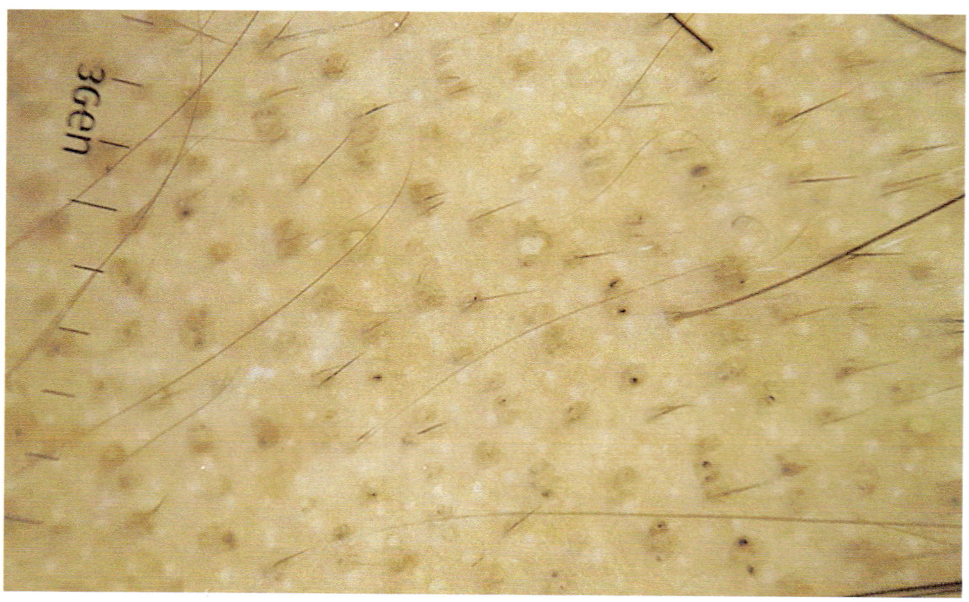

Fig. 15: This field is full of yellow dots many of which show regrowing hairs. Note also the presence of pinpoint white dots indicating nonscarring alopecia.

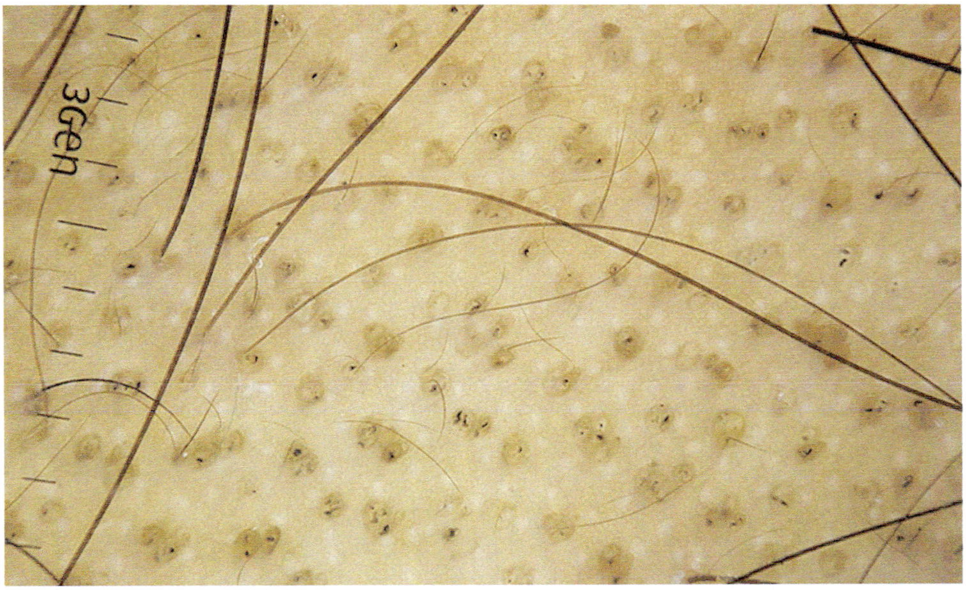

Fig. 16: Some hair follicles may escape the effect of chemotherapy; this field shows some of them as single-hair units which have uniform color and thickness. Numerous yellow dots and black dots are also markedly visible.

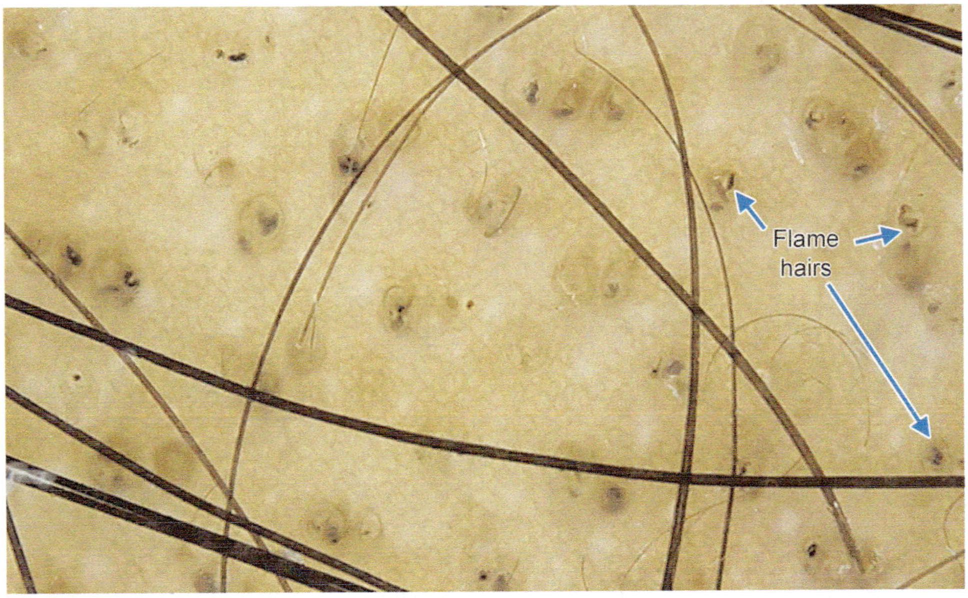

Fig. 17: Flame hairs are common trichoscopic finding of chemotherapy alopecia.

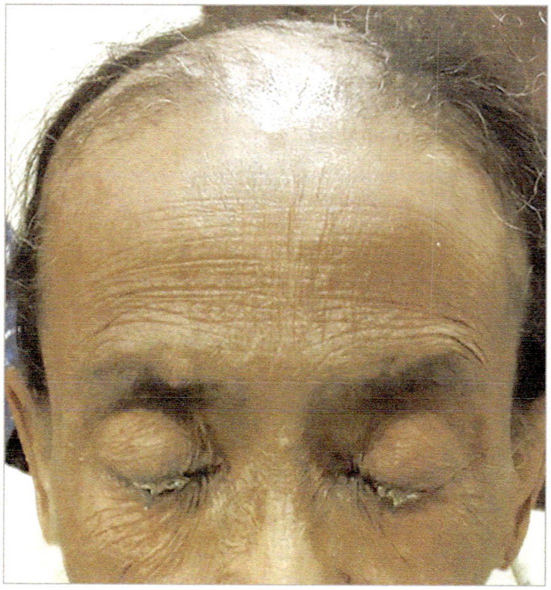

Fig. 18: A patient who has undergone chemotherapy for lung carcinoma.

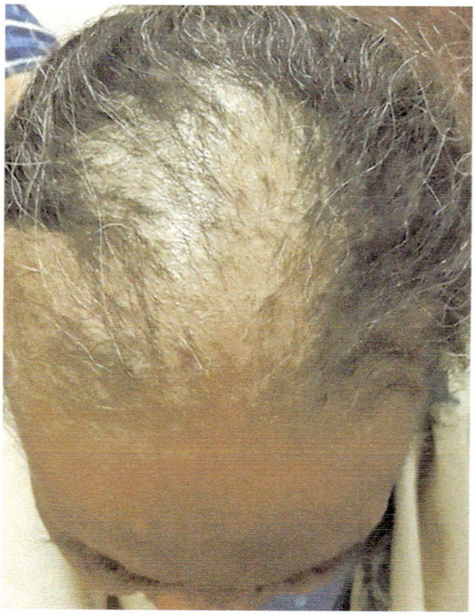

Fig. 19: The degree of loss of hair postchemotherapy depends upon the agent.

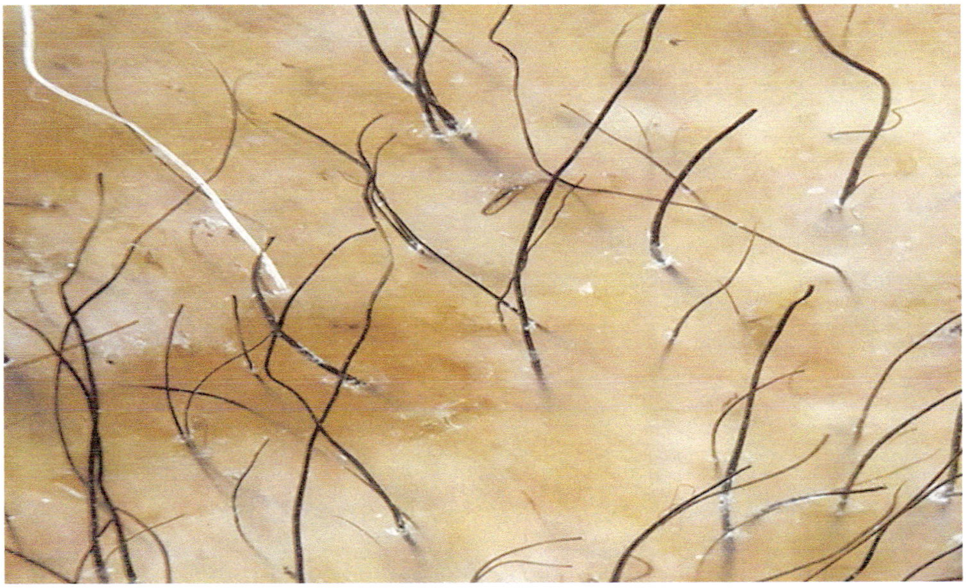

Fig. 20: Lone dystrophic hair in the same patient suggesting severe dystrophy in the anagen phase of the hair cycle.

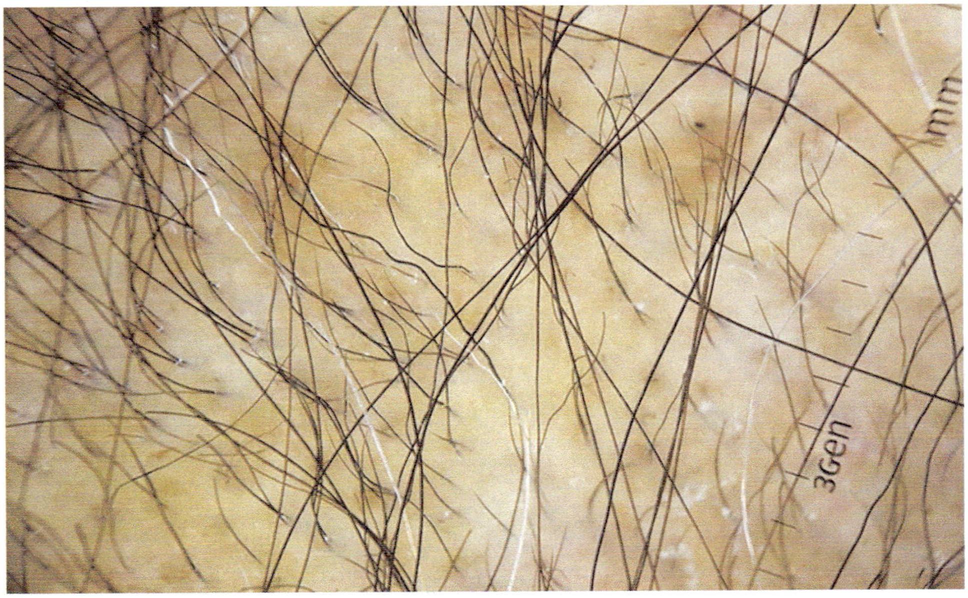

Fig. 21: Almost all the hair follicles contain single hairs. All the hairs in the field are dystrophic.

RADIOTHERAPY ALOPECIA

INTRODUCTION

- Anagen effluvium can occur as a single patch of nonscarring alopecia or as diffuse alopecia.
- Radiotherapy may also cause scarring alopecia depending on dosage and duration.
- Short-term exposure to 300–600 Gy of irradiation causes temporary alopecia.

KEY TRICHOSCOPIC FEATURES

- Black dots
- Yellow dots
- Flame hairs
- Pohl-Pinkus constrictions

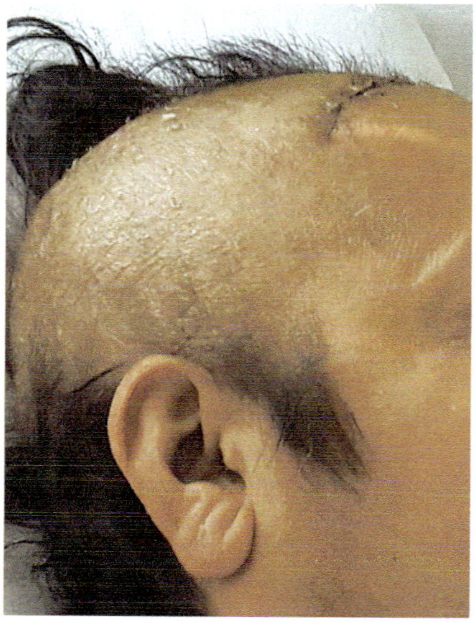

Fig. 22: Anagen effluvium (nonscarring alopecia) in a patient who received radiotherapy for primary central nervous system (CNS) lymphoma.

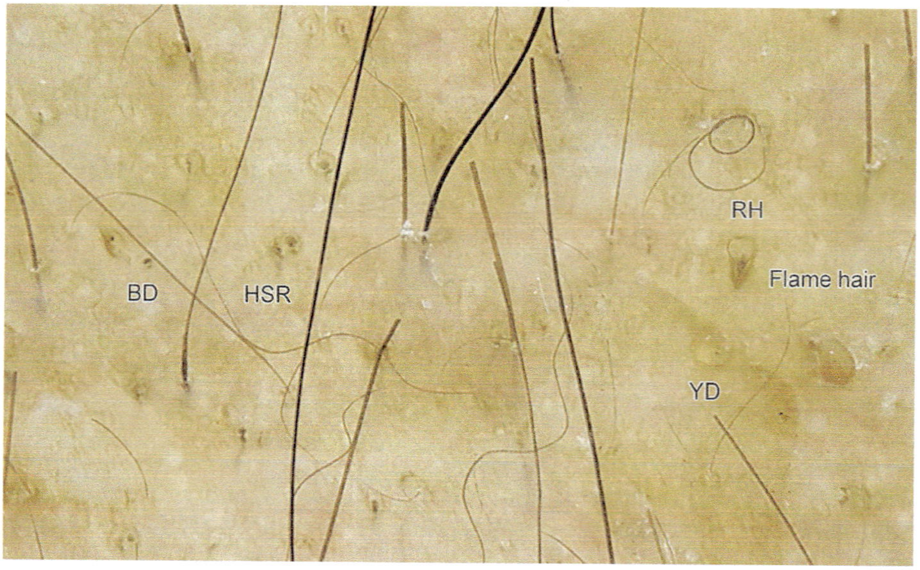

Fig. 23: Postradiotherapy trichoscopic image showing black dots (BD), regrowing hairs (RH), flame hairs, yellow dots (YD), and hair shaft residues (HSR).

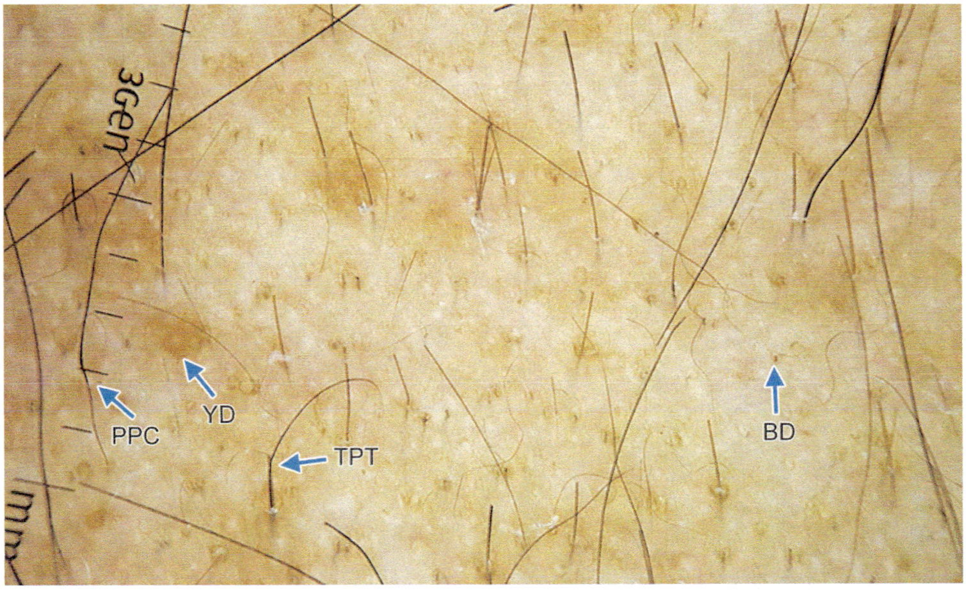

Fig. 24: This image shows black dot (BD), Pohl-Pinkus constrictions (PPC), yellow dots (YD), and trichoptilosis (TPT).

REFERENCES

1. Trueb RM. Chemotherapy-induced alopecia. Curr Opin Support Palliat Care. 2010;4(4):281-4.
2. Ramos-e-Silva M, Chaves Azevedo-e-Silva M, Carneiro SC. Hair, nail, pigment changes in major systemic disease. Clin Dermatol. 2008;26(3):296-305.
3. Tosti A, Pazzaglia M. Drug reactions affecting hair: diagnosis. Dermatol Clin. 2007;25(2):223-31,vii.
4. Piraccini BM, lorizzo M, Rech G, Tosti A. Drug induced hair disorders. Curr Drug Saf. 2006:1(3):301-5.
5. Trueb RM. Systemic approach to hair loss in women. J Dtsch Dermatol Ges. 2010:8(4):284-98.
6. Severs GA, Griffin T, Werner-Wasik M. Cicatricial alopecia secondary to radiation therapy: Case report and review of the literature. Cutis. 2008:81(2):147-53.
7. D, Agostini F, Balansky R, Pesce C, Fiallo P, Lubet RA, Kelloff GJ, et al. Induction of alopecia in mice exposed to cigarette smoke. Toxicol Lett. 2000:114(1-3):117-23.
8. Dhurat RP, Deshpande DJ. Loose anagen hair syndrome. Int J Trichol. 2010;2(2):96-100.
9. Tosti A, Piraccini BM. Loose anagen hair syndrome and loose anagen hair. Arch Dermatol. 2002;138(4):521-2.
10. Rakowska A, Olszewska M, Rudnicka L. Anagen effluvium. In: Rudnicka L, Olszewska M, Rakowska A, (Eds). Atlas of Trichoscopy. Philadelphia: Springer; 2012. pp. 247.
11. Malakar S, Mehta P, Malakar. Trichoscopy in Anagen Effluvium: Extensive peripilar sign. Dermatol Online. 2017;8(4):493-4.

ASSESSMENT IMAGE-BASED QUESTIONS

1. This is a trichoscopic image of chemotherapy alopecia. Mention four main features seen here. When is the onset of this type of anagen alopecia? When does the hair follicle resume its activity?

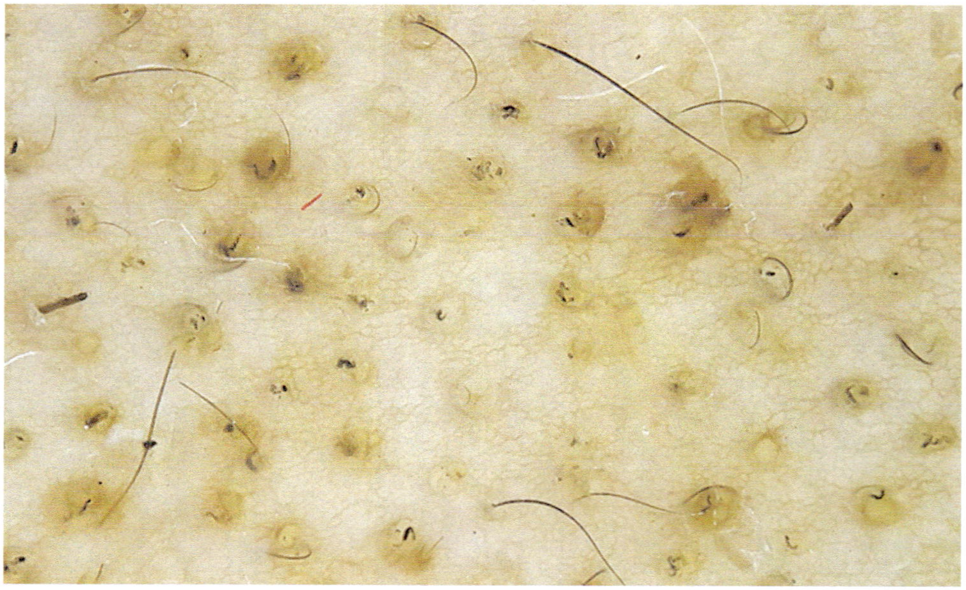

2. What do 1, 2, 3, and 4 signify?

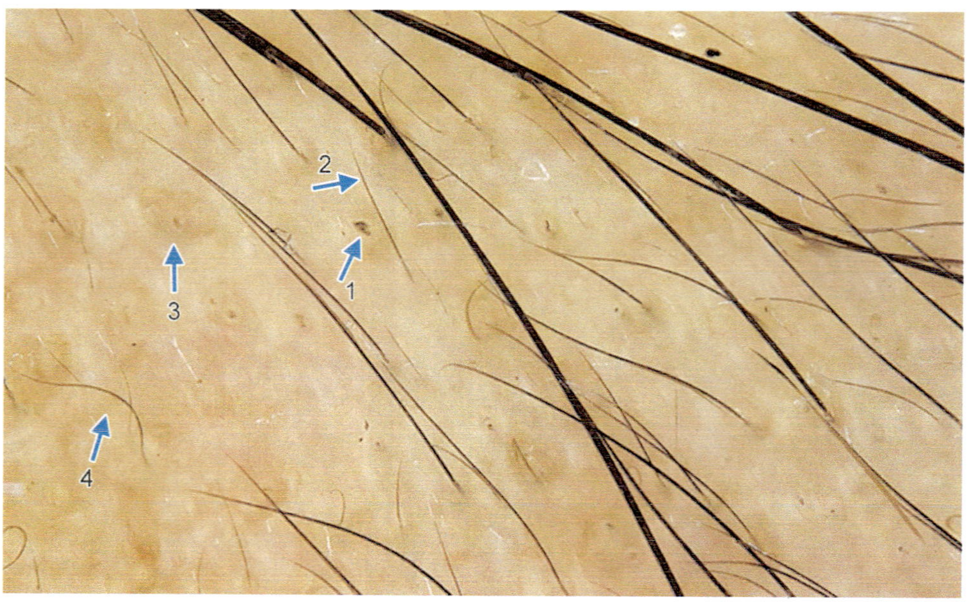

3. The image shows lone dystrophic hairs. Name two conditions where lone dystrophic hairs are found.

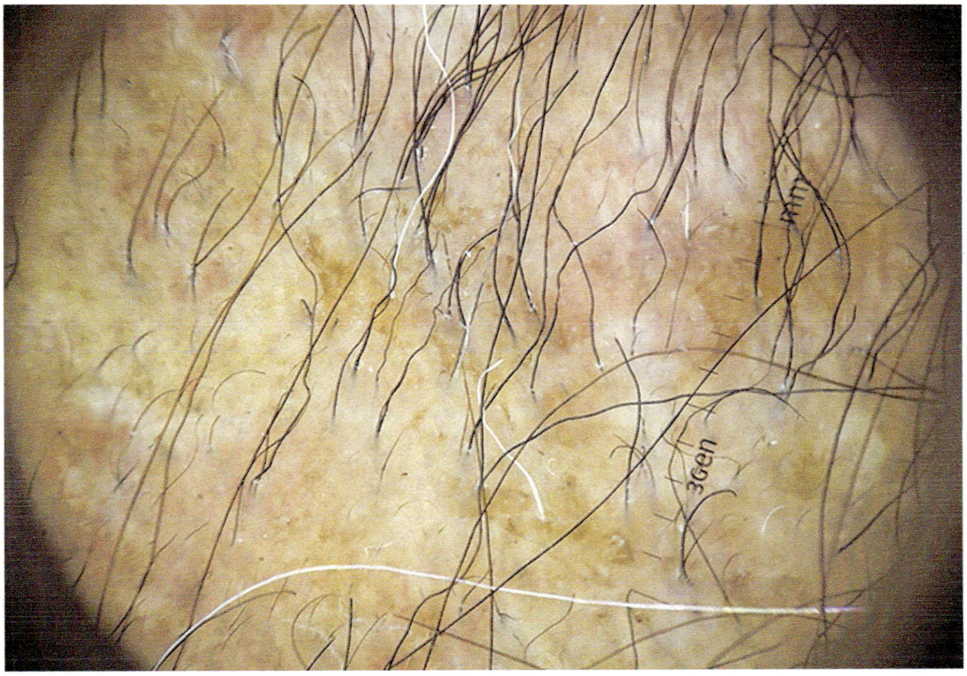

4. Peripilar sign is demonstrated in this image. Name two other conditions where peripilar sign is seen.

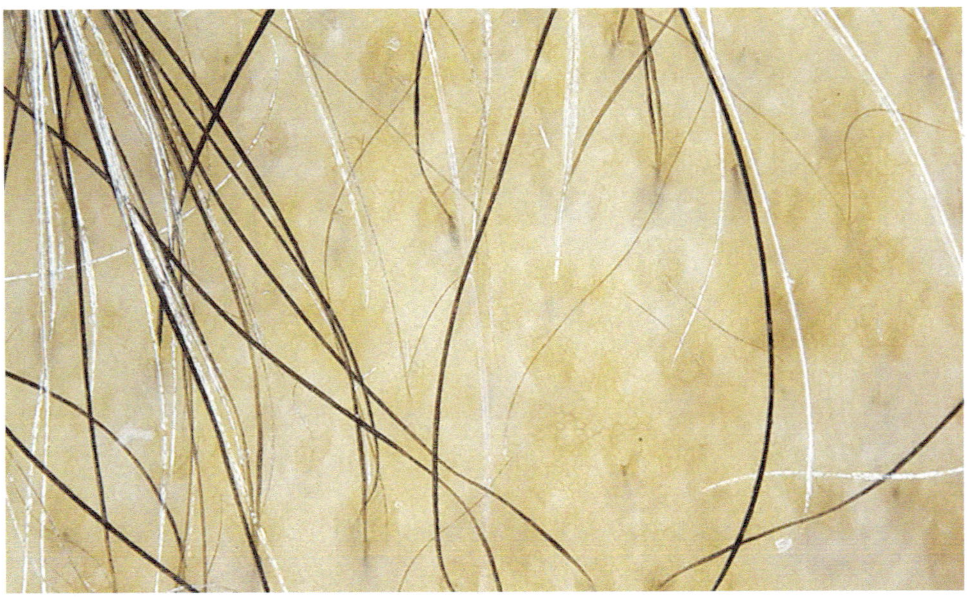

ANSWERS

1. Broken hair, black dots, yellow dots, dark lines. Three weeks after starting chemotherapy. Three weeks after stopping chemotherapy.
2. (1) Black dot; (2) Dark line; (3) Yellow dot; (4) Dark line
3. Anagen effluvium, and lichen planopilaris
4. Androgenetic alopecia, and anagen effluvium

7

SECTION

Scarring Alopecias

CHAPTER

16

Lichen Planopilaris

Subrata Malakar, Surit Malakar

INTRODUCTION

- Frequently a disease of middle-aged women, lichen planopilaris (LPP) is the most common cause of cicatricial alopecia where the hair loss is associated with scalp itching. More active the disease, more severe is the itching.[1,2]
- Multiple irregular areas of scarring alopecia associated with scalp itching, perifollicular erythema, and sometimes papules around the emergence of hair shafts are the important signs of LPP.[3]
- Though slowly progressive, extensive alopecia is the usual outcome.

KEY TRICHOSCOPIC FEATURES[4]

- Absence of follicular openings
- Absence of vellus hair
- Fibrotic white patches
- Blue-gray dots in a target pattern around the hair follicles
- Scalp erythema
- Broken hairs
- Presence of a group of two-thirds hairs surrounded by peripilar casts should raise the suspicion of LPP; sometimes a cast surrounds a tuft of 4 or 5 hairs.[5]
- The target pattern corresponds histopathologically to melanophages in the papillary dermis and is a sign of pigmentary incontinence confined to the hair follicles.

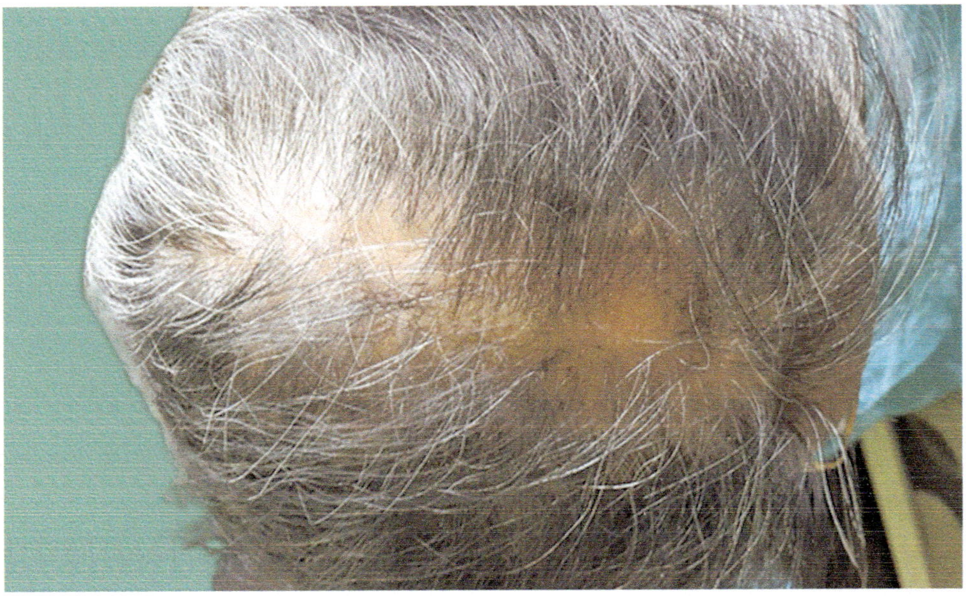

Fig. 1: Multiple irregular areas of scarring alopecia, associated with scalp itching in a case of lichen planopilaris.

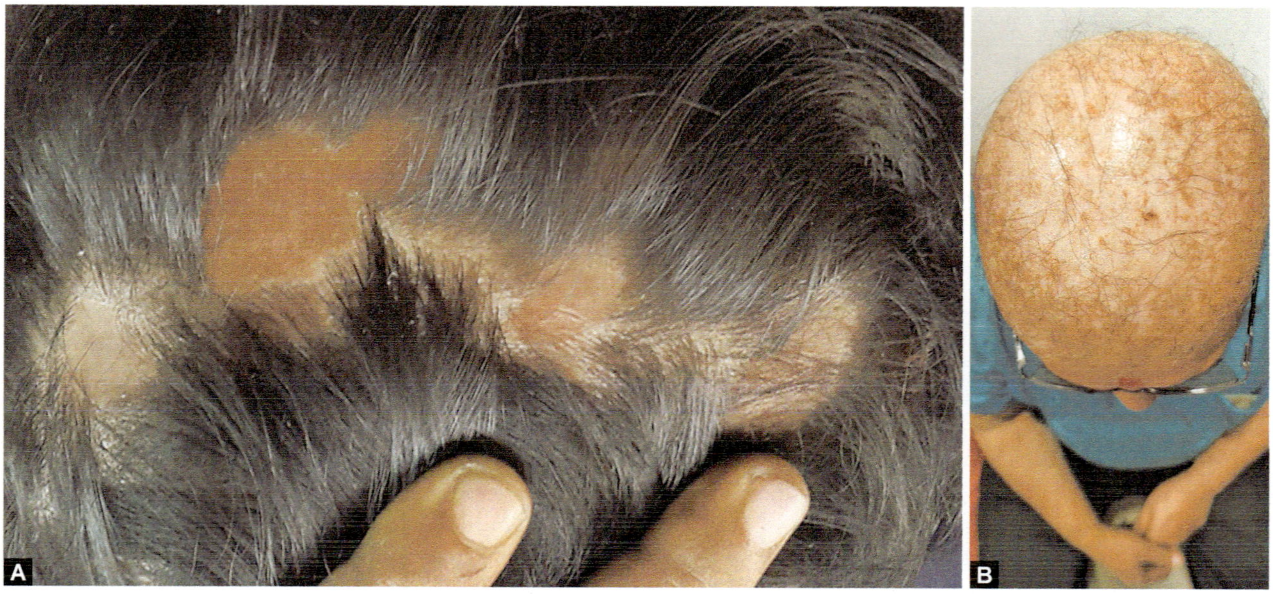

Figs. 2A and B: (A) Late stage of lichen planopilaris (LPP); (B) Late stage of LPP.

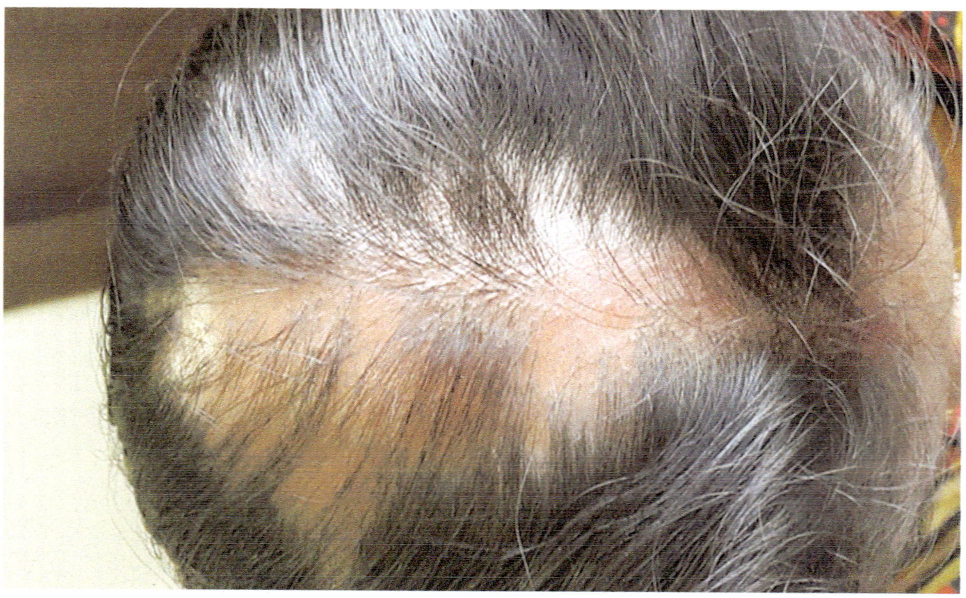

Fig. 3: The most common cause of scarring alopecia is lichen planopilaris. The disease activity correlates with severity of scalp itching.

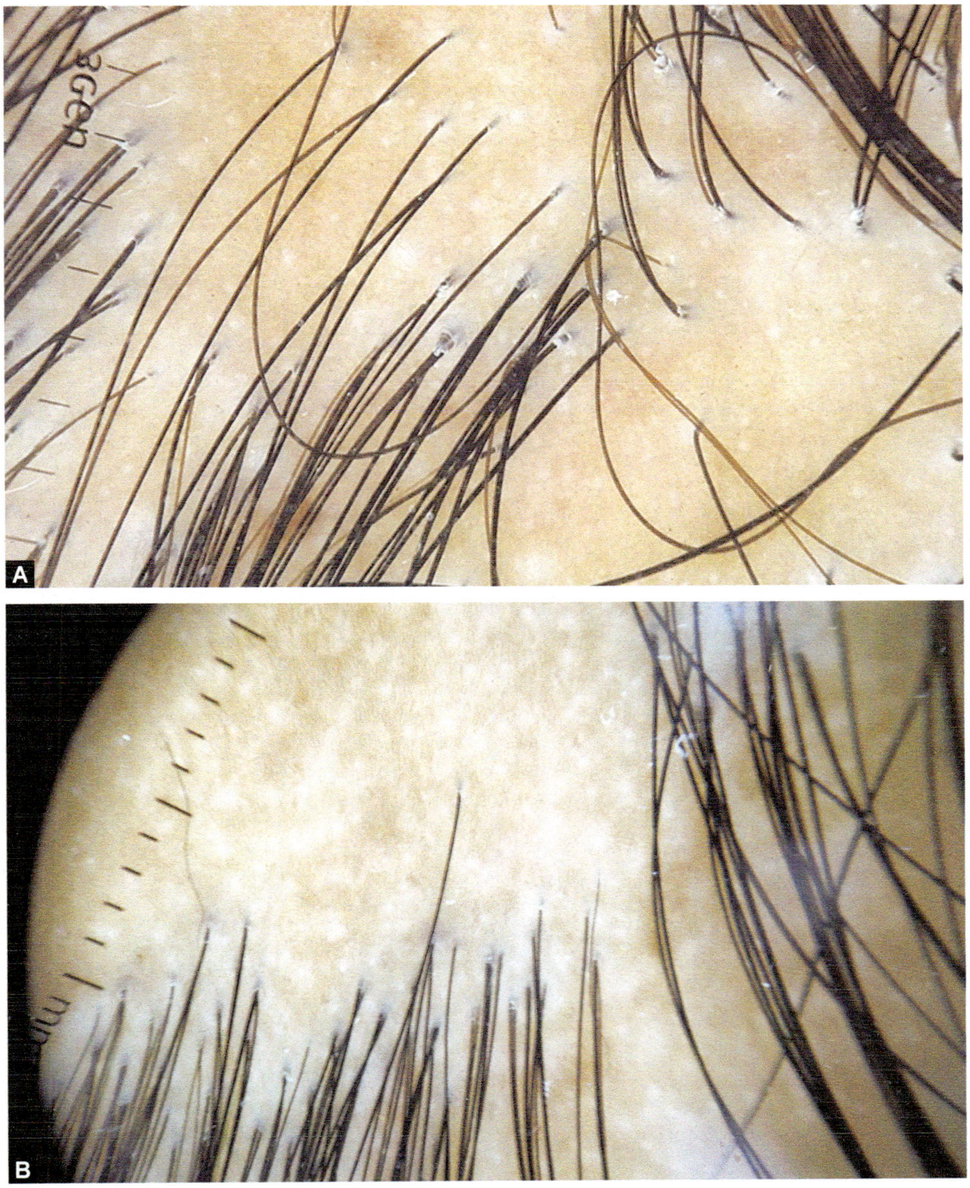

Figs. 4A and B: (A) Early disease: Thin casts surrounding groups of 2–3 hairs at their emergence. There is loss of follicular openings. Vellus hairs are absent. (B) Early disease: Thin casts surrounding groups of two to three hairs at their emergence. There is loss of follicular openings. Vellus hairs are absent.

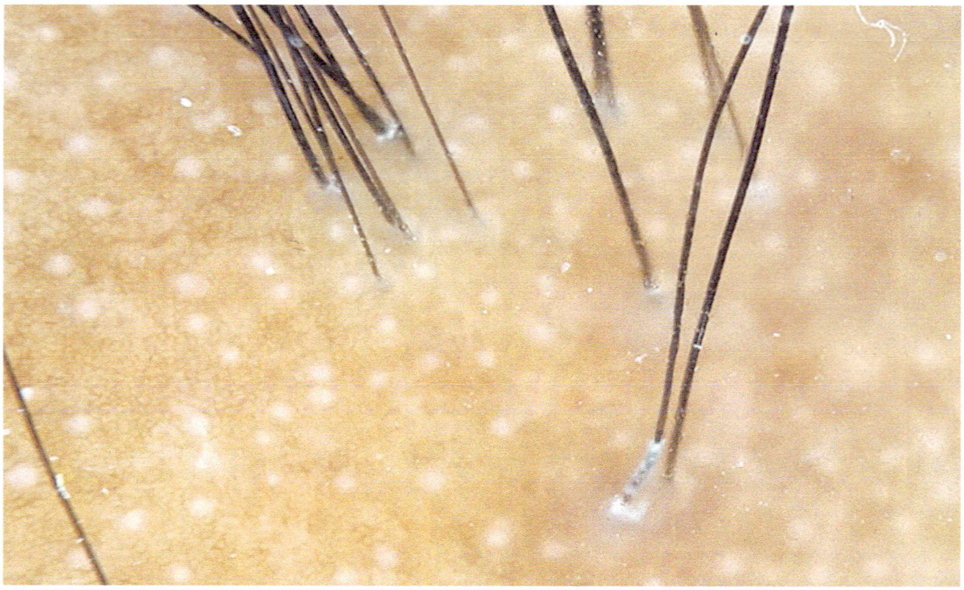

Fig. 5: A hallmark of lichen planopilaris (LPP) is perifollicular collar-like scaling. Scales form silver-white tubular structures usually reaching a few millimeters above the scalp surface. This corresponds to the changes in the outer hair follicle root sheath resulting in excessive perifollicular scaling.

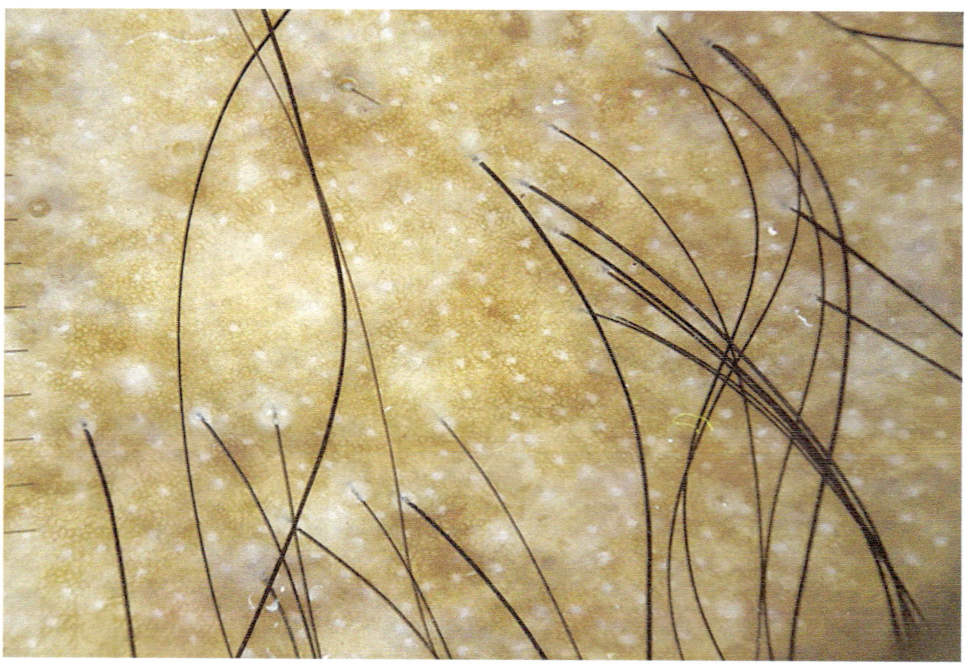

Fig. 6: Classic lichen planopilaris (LPP) in dark skin type shows pinpoint white dots in the background of honeycomb pigmented network forming a "starry sky" pattern.

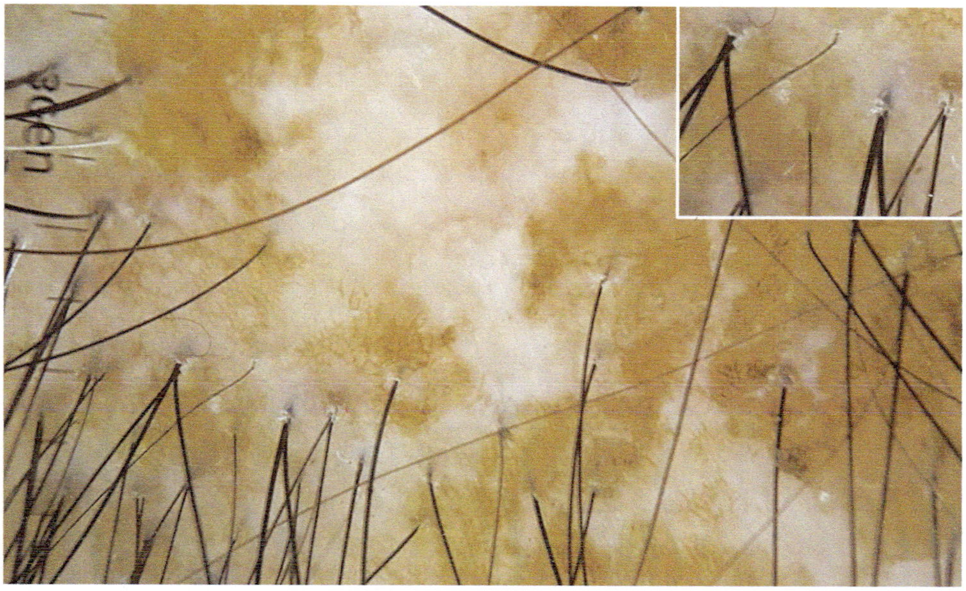

Fig. 7: Trichoscopic features of lichen planopilaris (LPP) showing cicatricial white patches, absence of follicular openings, and peripilar casts (inset) around groups of two and three hairs.

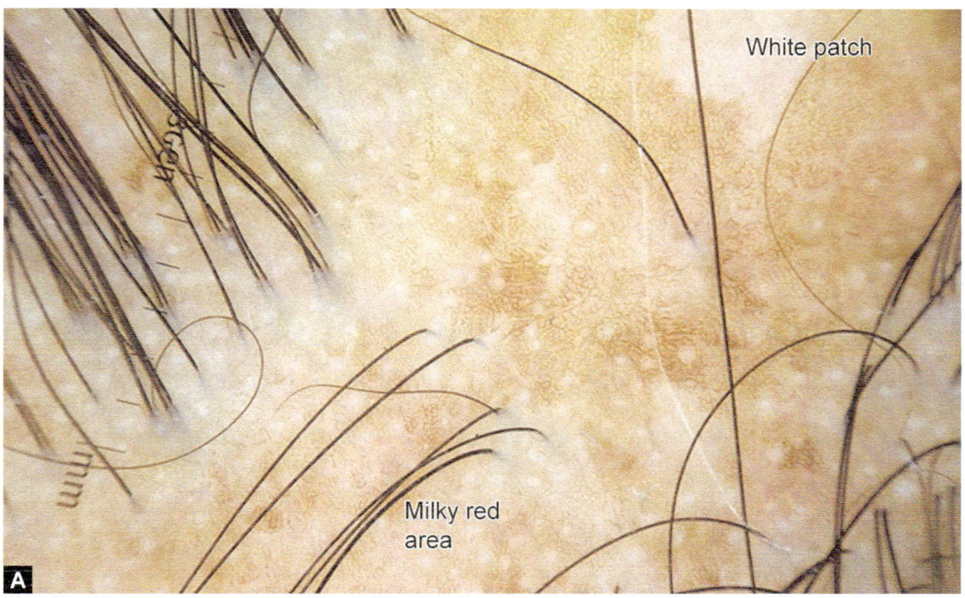

Continued

Continued

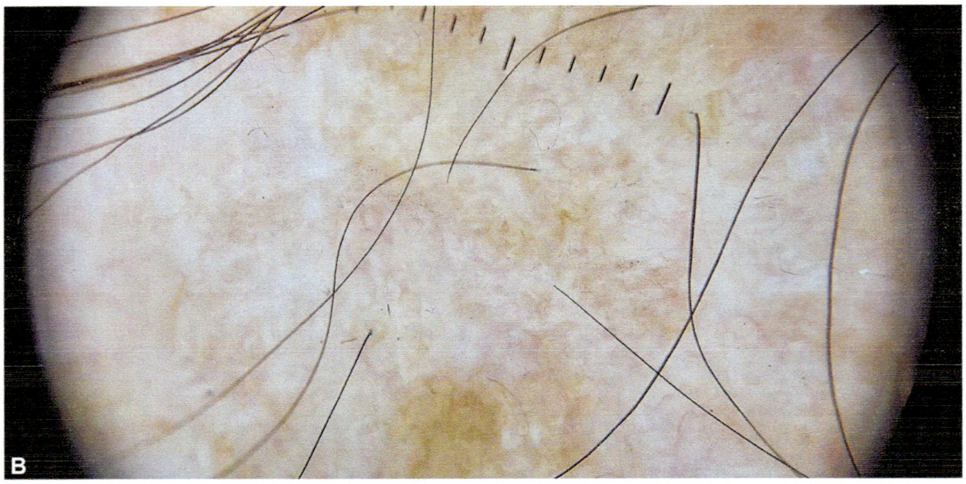

Figs. 8A and B: In lichen planopilaris (LPP), white dots merge as the disease progresses. They form white and milky red areas that lack follicular openings corresponding to fibrosis. Milky red areas are fibrosis of recent onset and it fades over time and changes to white patches. (B) In LPP, white dots merge as the disease progresses. They form white and milky red areas that lack follicular openings corresponding to fibrosis. Milky red areas are fibrosis of recent onset and it fades over time and changes to white patches

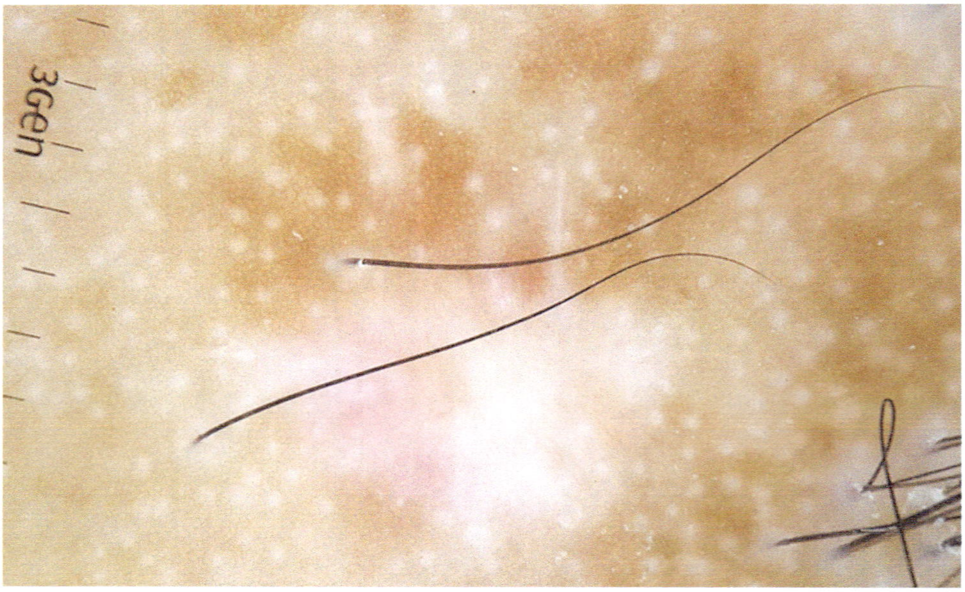

Fig. 9: This image is a demonstration of milky red area changing to white patch in the course of LPP. Milky red area corresponds to fibrosis of recent onset which fades gradually and changes to white patch. Note the presence of two lonely hairs in the field. Lonely hairs are also frequently observed in frontal fibrosing alopecia (FFA).

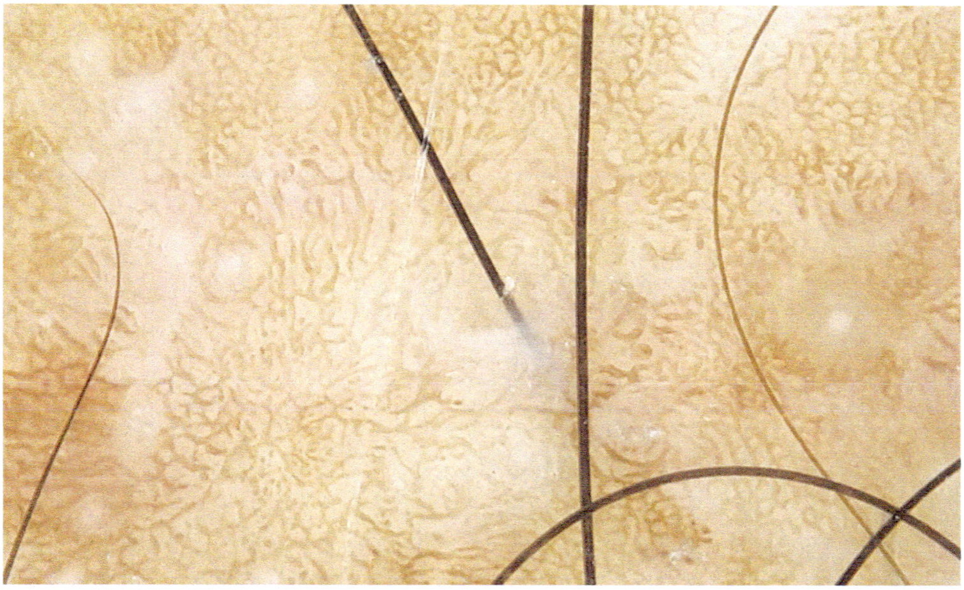

Fig. 10: White dots are of two types. Pinpoint white dots and fibrotic white dots. This is an example of fibrotic white dots. In the left side of the image fibrotic white dots are seen merging to form white patch. At the center of the image, the white halo surrounding the lone hair corresponds to perifollicular fibrosis. If the process continues, the hair follicle is replaced by fibrotic tissue.

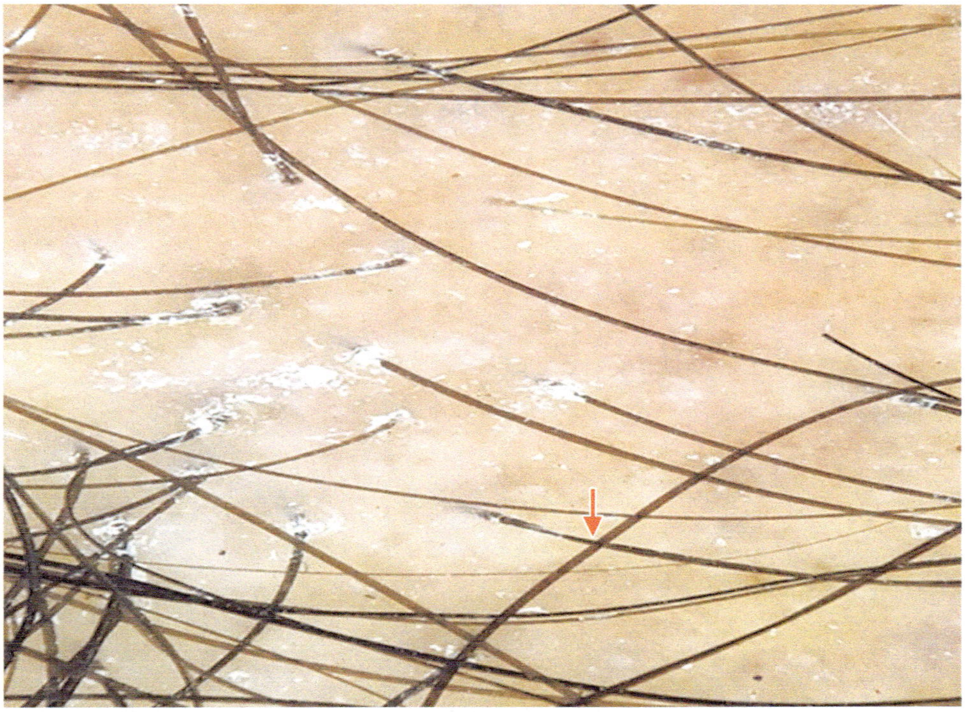

Fig. 11: Case of lichen planopilaris (LPP) showing pili torti (arrow), peripilar casts, absence of vellus hairs, scalp erythema, and absence of follicular opening.

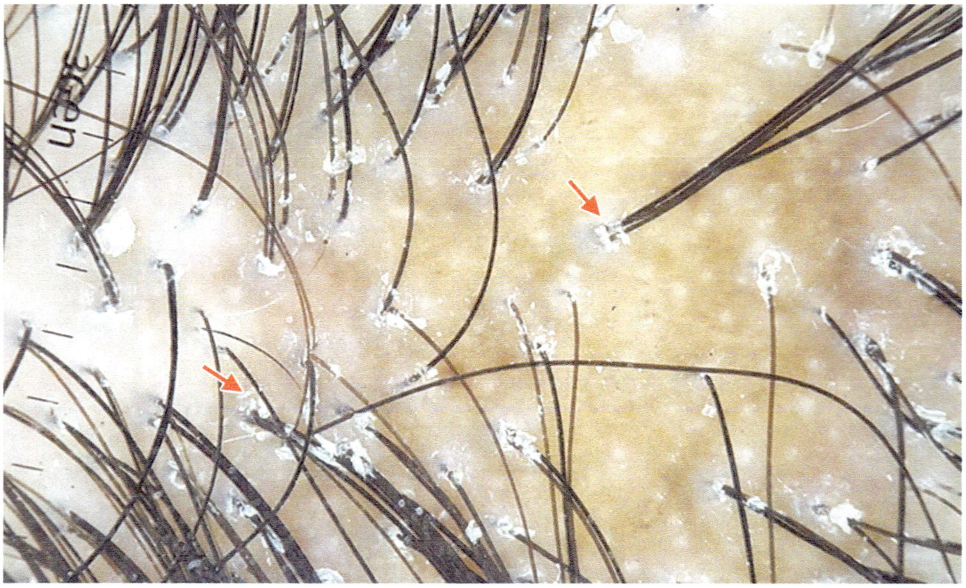

Fig. 12: Trichoscopic image showing peripilar casts surrounding tufts of four to five hairs (red arrows), peri- and interfollicular blue-gray dots and patches. Tufted hairs are seen in only 5% of patients with lichen planopilaris (LPP). Tufted hairs are also observed in folliculitis decalvans. They can be differentiated by the color of the scales. In LPP, the hair tufts have silver-white scales whereas they are yellowish in folliculitis decalvans.

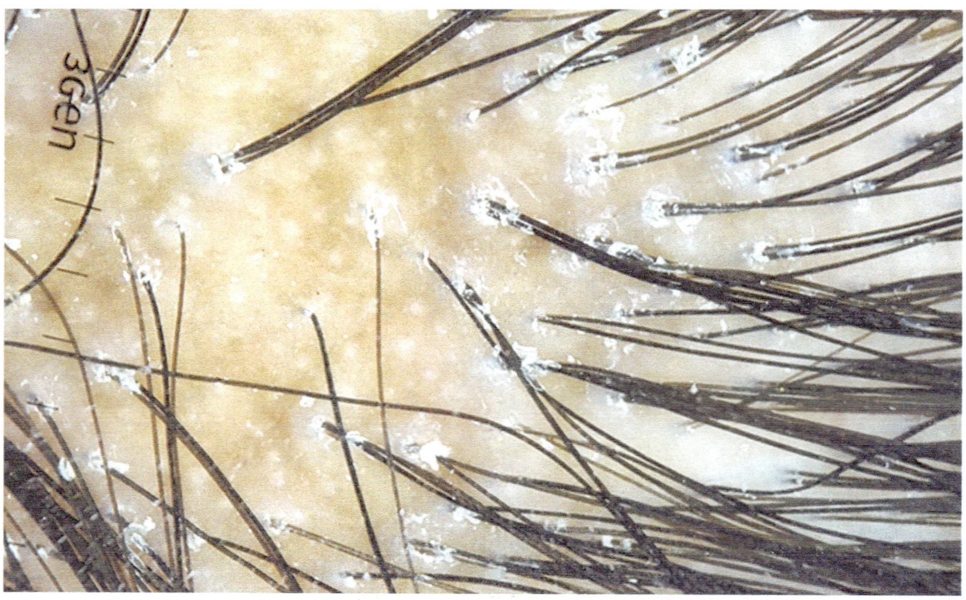

Fig. 13: Highly active disease: Note the thick peripilar casts which surround most of the hair shafts at its emergence, erythema and blue-gray patches. Note: Cast surrounding tuft of four to five hairs.

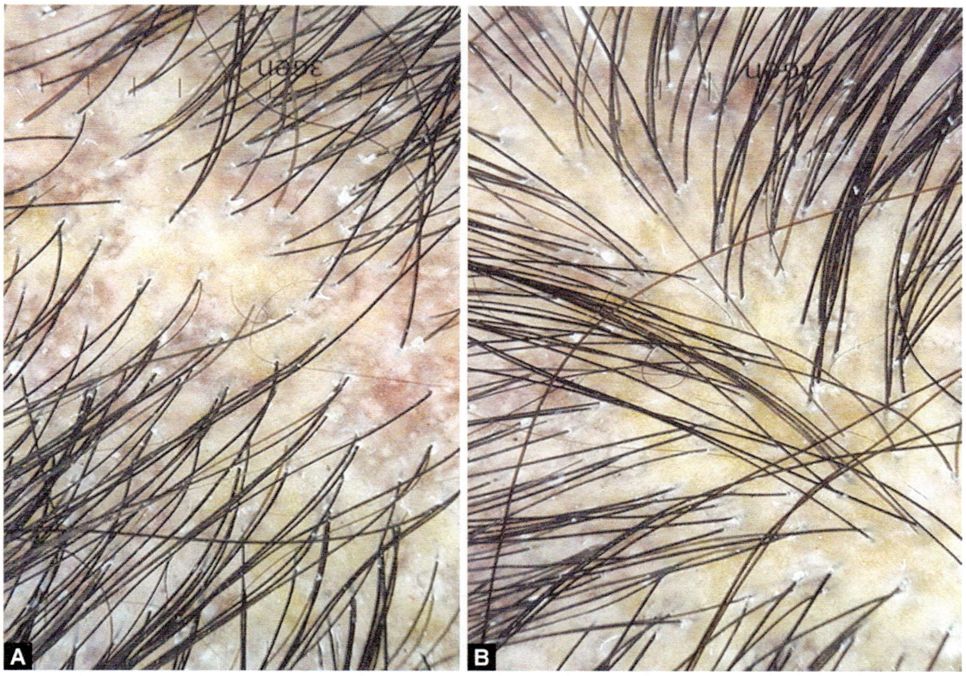

Figs. 14A and B: Trichoscopy helps to follow-up the treatment response. (A) Erythema, peripilar scaling and blue-gray patches indicate highly active disease. (B) Visible improvement of lichen planopilaris showing much less erythema and scaling after treatment which can be appreciated by trichoscope.

REFERENCES

1. Duque-Estrada B, Tamler C, Sodre CT, Barcaui CB, Pereira FB. Dermoscopy patterns of cicatricial alopecia resulting from discoid lupus erythematous and lichen planopilaris. An Bras Dermatol. 2010;2:40-5.
2. Tosti A. Primary scarring alopecias. In: Tosti A (Ed). Dermoscopy of the Hair and Nails, 2nd edition. Philadelphia: Springer; 2016. pp. 68.
3. Tosti A. Primary scarring alopecias. In: Tosti A (Ed). Dermoscopy of the Hair and Nails, 2nd edition. Philadelphia: Springer; 2016. pp. 50.
4. Inui S, Nakajima T, Shono F, Itami S. Dry dermatoscopy in clinical treatment of alopecia areata. J Dermatol. 2007;34:635-9.
5. Tosti A. Dermoscopy of the Hair and Nails, 2nd edition: Philadelphia: Springer; 2016:51.

CHAPTER

17

Frontal Fibrosing Alopecia

Subrata Malakar

INTRODUCTION

Frontal fibrosing alopecia (FFA) is a clinical variant of lichen planopilaris (LPP) which commonly affects postmenopausal women and is characterized by progressive symmetric band of hair loss on the frontal and temporal region of the scalp. Patchy or total alopecia of the eyebrows may be present.

KEY TRICHOSCOPIC FEATURES[1-4]

- Absence of follicular openings
- Absence of vellus hair
- Minor perifollicular scaling
- Perifollicular erythema is a characteristic feature of FFA
- Lonely hairs
- Pili torti
- The trichoscopic and pathologic features of both FFA and LPP may be indistinguishable which include absence of follicular openings, cicatricial white patches, peripilar casts, blue-gray dots, and perifollicular erythema.[5]
- Peripilar casts are better appreciated with dry dermoscopy.
- Peripilar casts consist of concentrically arranged layers of scales, but in FFA they can be very thin.
- Perifollicular erythema is a characteristic feature of FFA though it may not always be evident on trichoscopy.
- Blue-gray dots arranged in a target pattern around the follicular ostia can be seen in LPP but not in discoid lupus erythematosus (DLE).
- Lonely hair sign may be seen in the receding frontal margin or preauricular area and presents as standalone hair.
- However, this sign is not specific, it is also seen in lupus, follicular keratosis spinulosa decalvans, central centrifugal alopecia and alopecia mucinous, and LPP.[6]

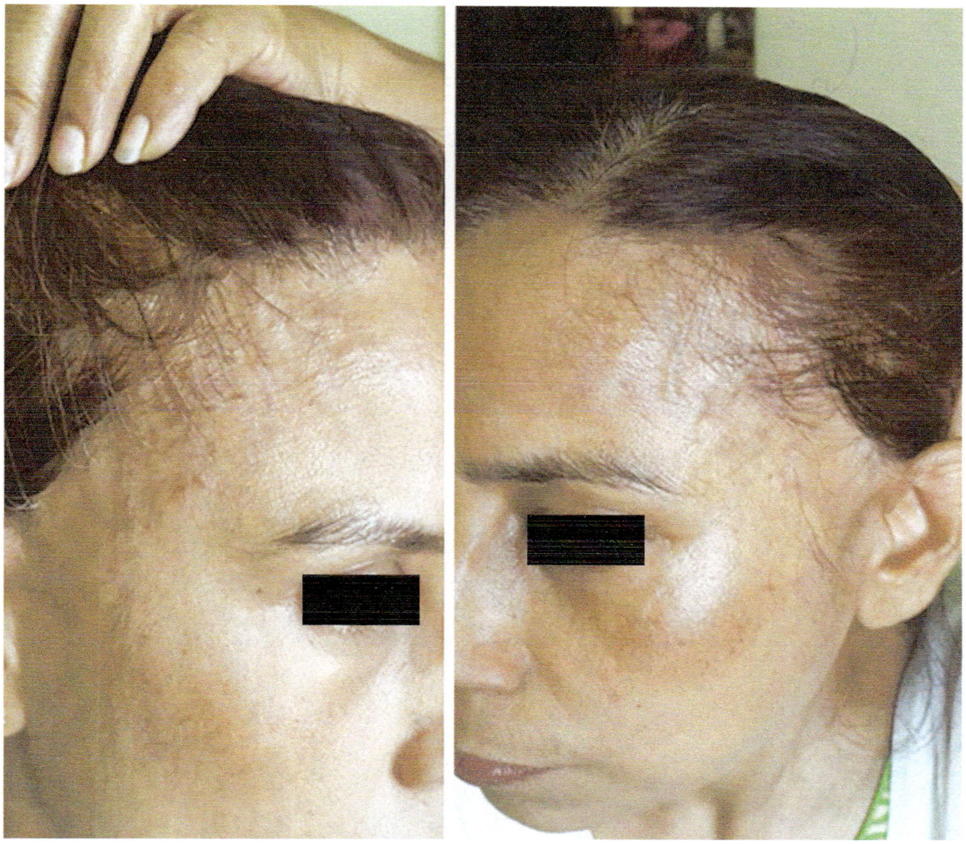

Fig. 1: Frontal fibrosing alopecia showing progressive recession and band like frontal-temporal alopecia in a postmenopausal woman. Characteristically eyebrow loss starts at the lateral third and rarely progresses to its total loss.

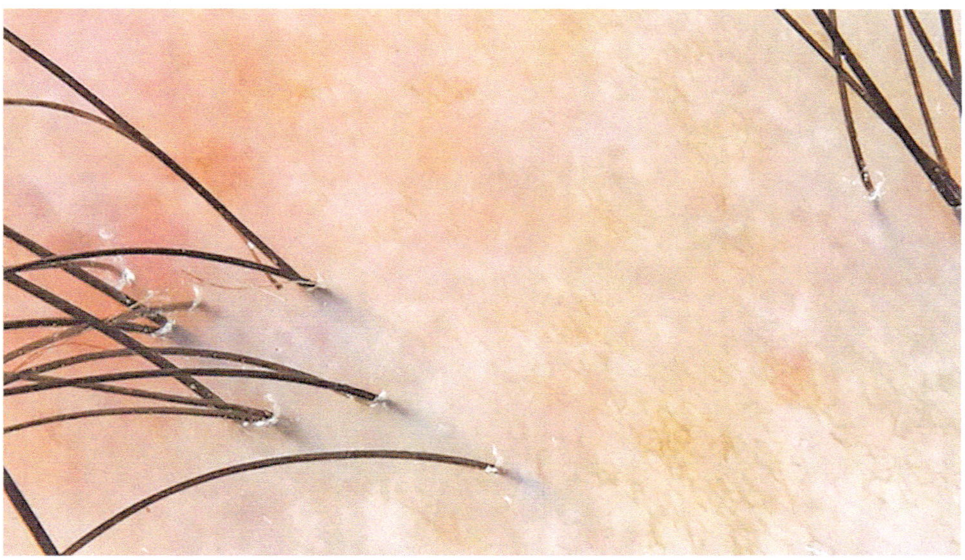

Fig. 2: Frontal fibrosing alopecia absence of follicular openings, absence of vellus hair, minor peripilar scaling, and perifollicular erythema. There is a strong predominance of single-hair units at the hair bearing margin.

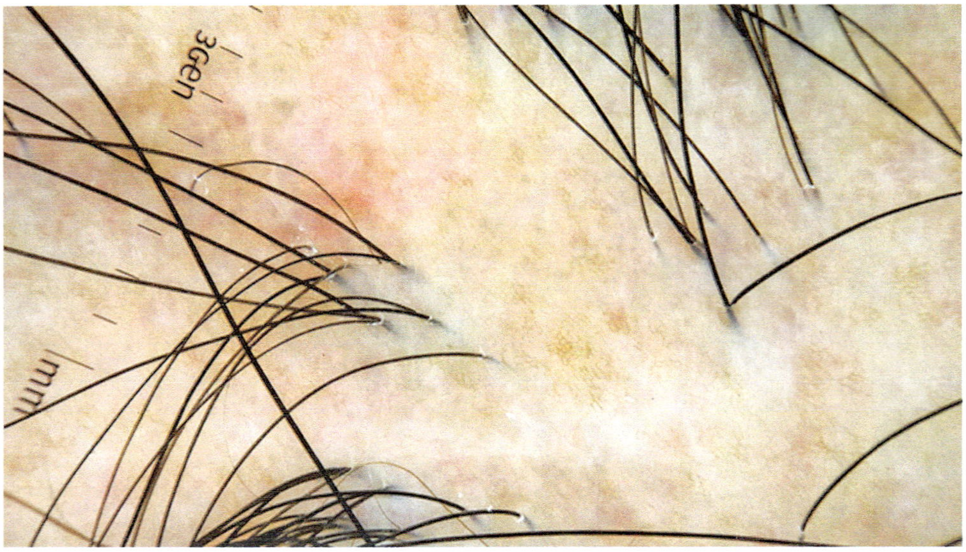

Fig. 3: Background color. It is usually ivory-beige or ivory white or rarely ivory pink. In lichen planopilaris and other scarring alopecias, the background color is white or milky red. Note minor perifollicular scale.

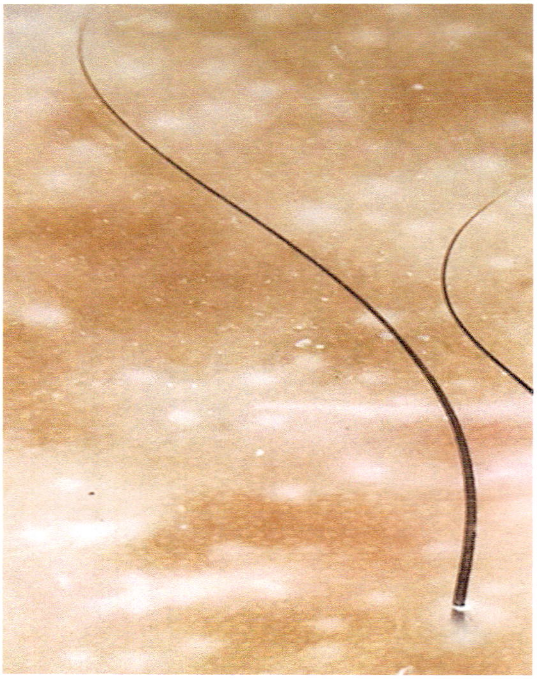

Fig. 4: Lonely hair and ivory pink background. Fibrotic white dots are coalescing to form white patch. Clinical clue to the diagnosis of Frontal fibrosing alopecia is "lonely hair". Lonely hair is few centimeter long that has been associated with perifollicular scaling. They are also found in lichen planopilaris and other scarring alopecias.

REFERENCES

1. Tosti A. Dermatoscopy of Hair and Scalp Disorders. London: Informa Healthcare: 2007.
2. Duque-Estrada B, Tamler C, Sodre CT, Barcaui CB, Pereira FB. Dermoscopy patterns of cicatricial alopecia resulting from discoid lupus erythematosus and lichen planopilaris. An Bras Dermatol. 2010;2:179-83.
3. Inui S, Nakajima T, Shono F, Itami S. Dermoscopic findings in frontal fibrosing alopecia: report of four cases. Int J Dermatol. 2008;47:796-9.
4. Rubegni P, Mandato F, Fimiani M. Frontal fibrosing alopecia: Role of dermoscopy in differential diagnosis. Case Rep Dermatol. 2010,2:40-5.
5. Tosti A. Primary scarring alopecias. In: Tosti A (ed). Dermoscopy of the Hair and Nails, 2nd edition. Philadelphia: Springer; 2016. pp. 53.
6. Camacho FM. Lonely hair sign: Not specific for frontal fibrosing alopecia. Arch Dermatol. 2012;148(10):1208-9.

CHAPTER

18 Discoid Lupus Erythematosus

Subrata Malakar, Samipa S Mukherjee, Surit Malakar

INTRODUCTION

- Discoid lupus erythematosus (DLE) on the scalp is usually associated with the DLE of face and other exposed parts of the body such as beard, v-area of neck, upper back, and ears.
- Examination of scalp reveals atrophic alopecic patches. The affected area may be edematous in the initial stage and is often associated with follicular plugging, erythema, scaling, and telangiectasia. The patch may look white due to loss of pigment and fibrosis due to scarring.

KEY TRICHOSCOPIC FEATURES[1]

- Loss of pigmentation and disruption of honeycomb pattern
- Follicular keratotic plugs
- Red dots
- Giant irregular capillaries (thick arborizing vessels)
- Peri-and interfollicular blue-gray dots
- Loss of follicular openings, a common trichoscopic feature of all the scarring alopecias, is also present in DLE.

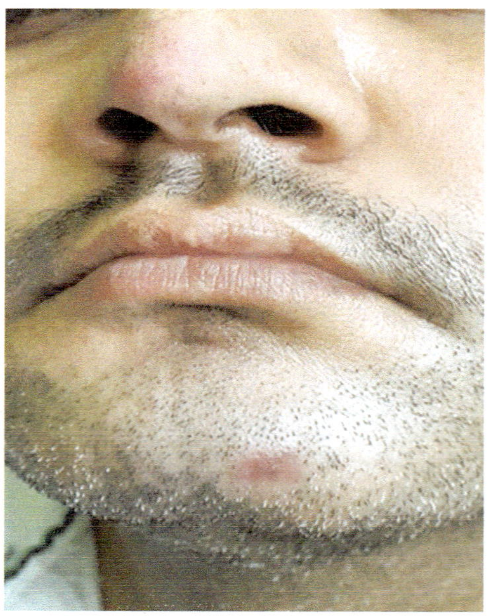

Fig 1: An erythematous and atrophic, early patch of discoid lupus erythematosus (DLE) over the chin area.

- The specific features of DLE include keratotic plugs, enlarged branching vessels, and red dots.
- The other features of DLE are peri-and interfollicular blue-gray dots, disruption of honeycomb pigment, and loss of pigment.[2]

- Follicular plugging relates to keratin material occluding the dilated infundibular openings and the plugs protrude from the scalp.
- Enlarged and tortuous branching vessels are a common feature of DLE.
- Red dots are a helpful trichoscopic marker for active DLE which are regularly distributed around the follicular ostia. Red dots correspond to follicular openings surrounded by dilated vessels. If treated early hair regrowth may be achieved from the areas with red dots.[3]
- Blue-gray dots in peri- and interfollicular areas may be present in a speckled pattern.[3] They correspond to melanophages in the papillary dermis and are frequently seen.

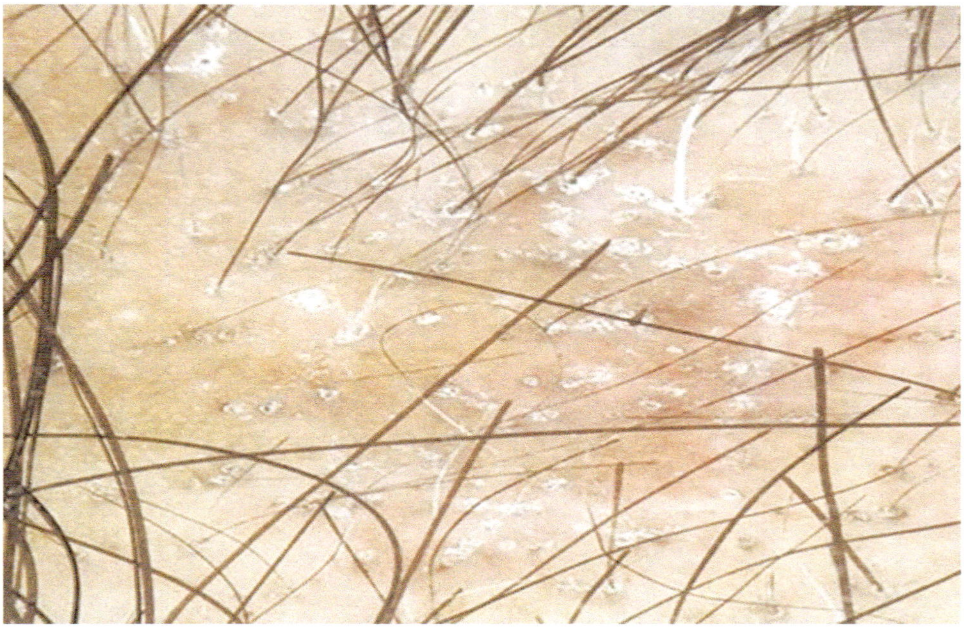

Fig. 2: Early trichoscopic change of a discoid lupus erythematosus (DLE) patch: Disruption of honeycomb pattern and keratotic follicular plugs.

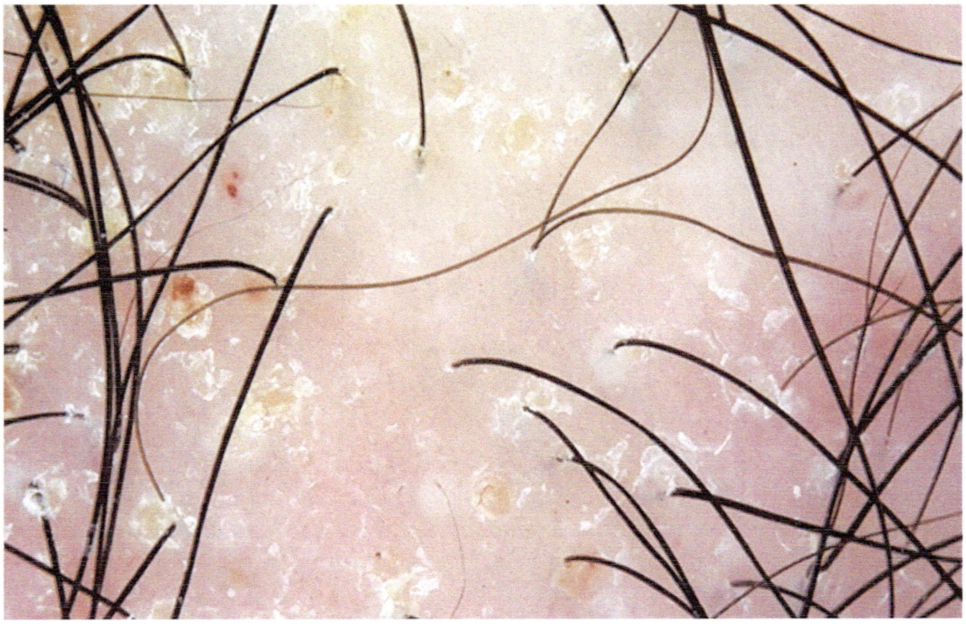

Fig. 3: Discoid lupus erythematosus (DLE): Loss of pigment and prominent keratotic follicular plugs.

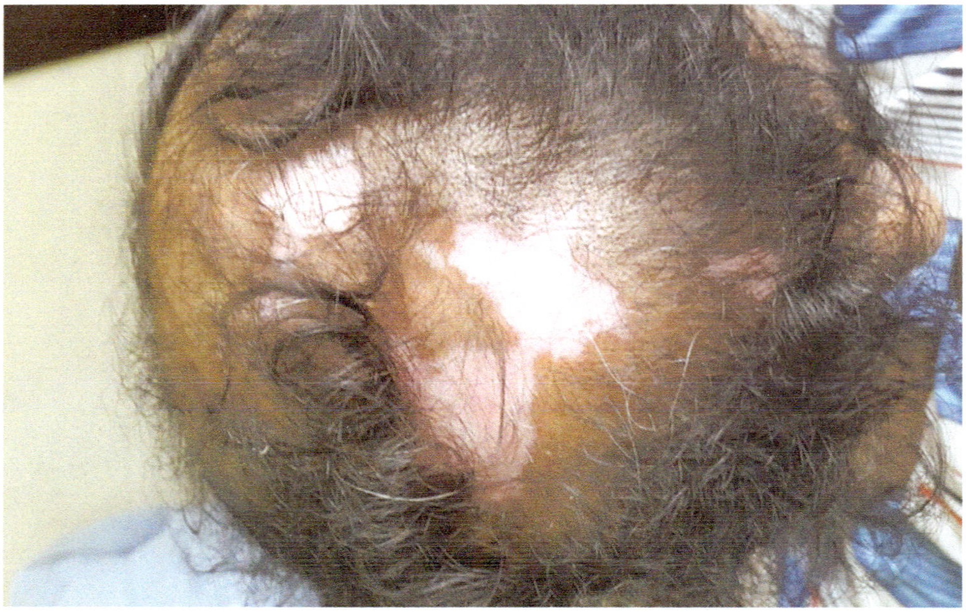

Fig. 4: Longstanding discoid lupus erythematosus (DLE) with atrophic patch and depigmentation. The trichoscopic features depend upon disease activity or inactivity.

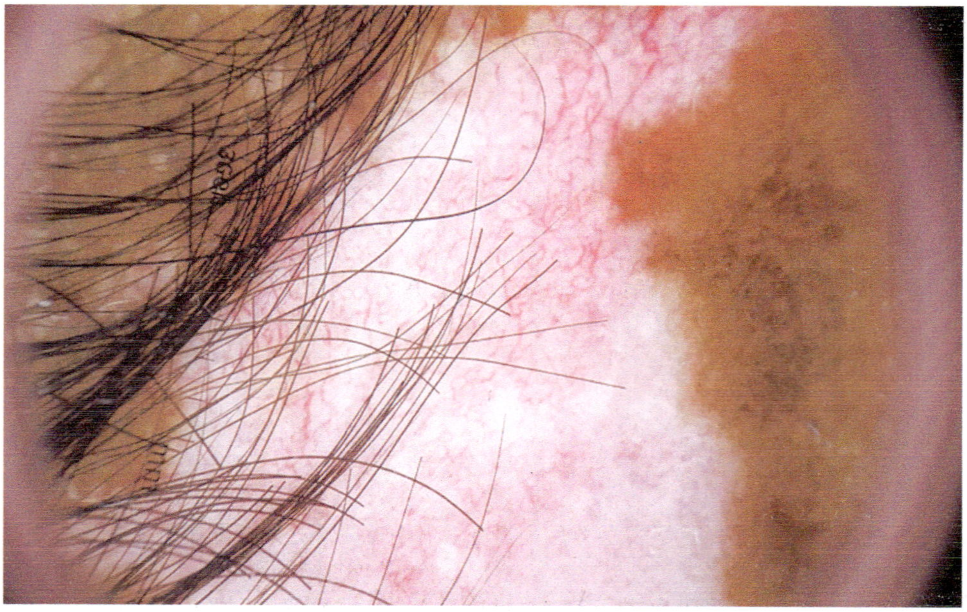

Fig. 5: Thick arborizing vessels in a case of discoid lupus erythematosus (DLE). Thin arborizing vessels are seen in healthy individuals, whereas thick arborizing vessels are also seen in basal cell carcinoma. Thick arborizing vessels can be differentiated from thinner ones by "vessel-hair" test.

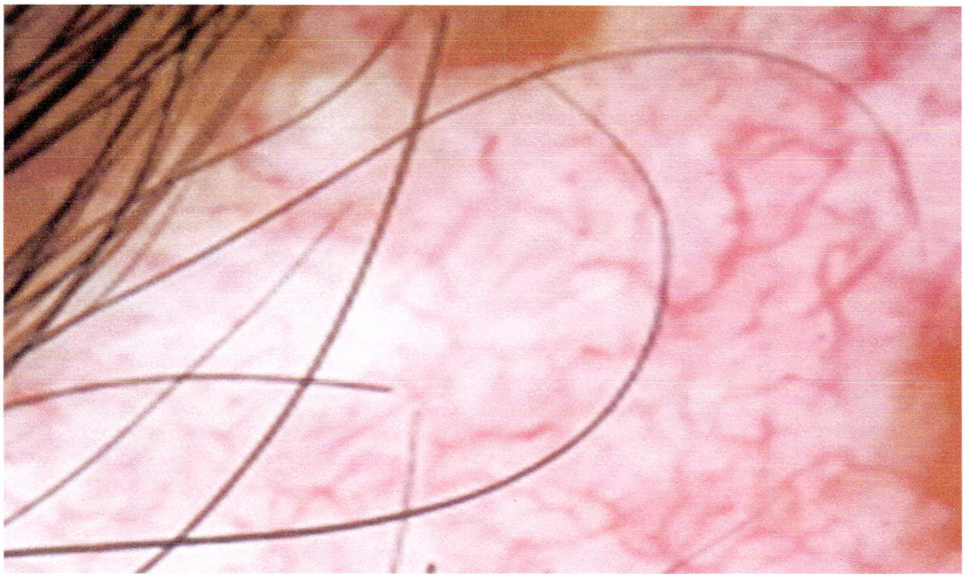

Fig. 6: Vessel-hair test:[4] The test compares thickness of blood vessel with that of hair shaft. This is how the comparison takes place—diameter of thin arborizing vessels are < 50 μ, diameter of thick arborizing vessels are > 100 μ, thickness of most of the hair shafts are 50–100 μ. Thus, the vessels which are thicker than hair shaft are thick arborizing blood vessels. The vessels in the image are thick arborizing vessels in comparison to the hair shafts and are a trichoscopic feature of discoid lupus erythematosus (DLE).

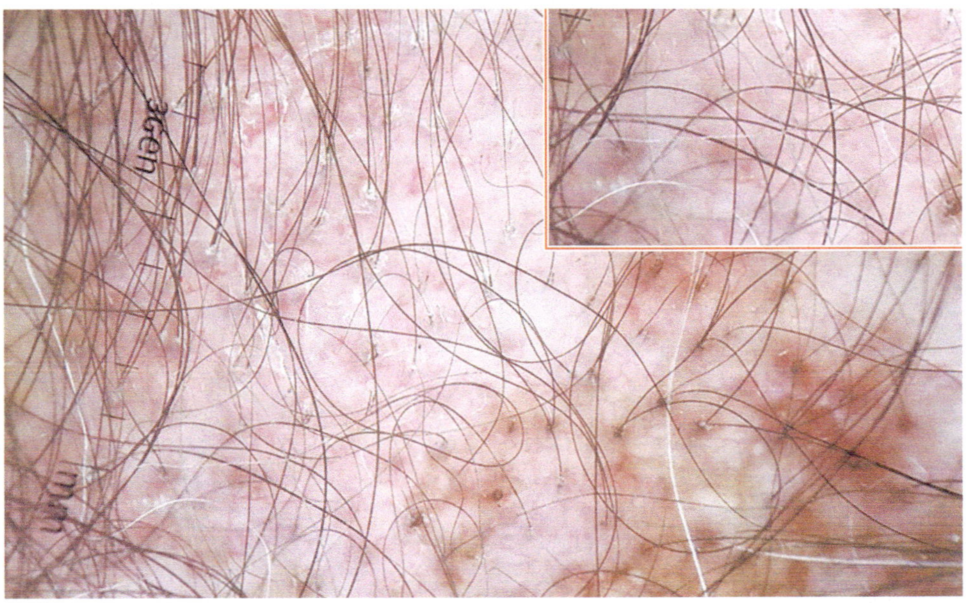

Fig. 7: The image shows loss of pigment, disruption of honeycomb pattern, keratotic follicular plugs, peri- and interfollicular blue-gray dots, red dots (inset). Red dots correspond to follicular openings surrounded by dilated vessels.

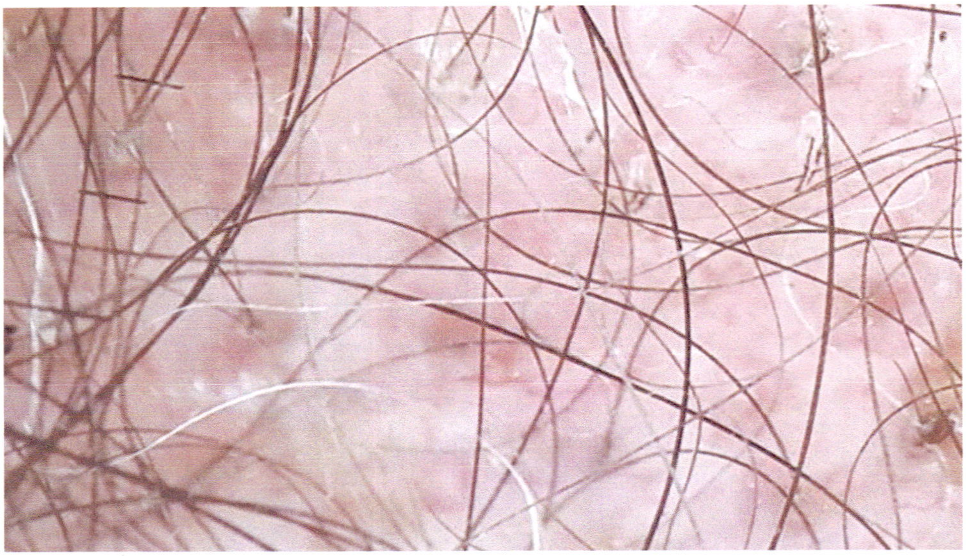

Fig. 8: Magnified image of red dots seen in discoid lupus erythematosus (DLE). A characteristic feature of active DLE, red dots are considered as a good prognostic factor for hair regrowth.[1]

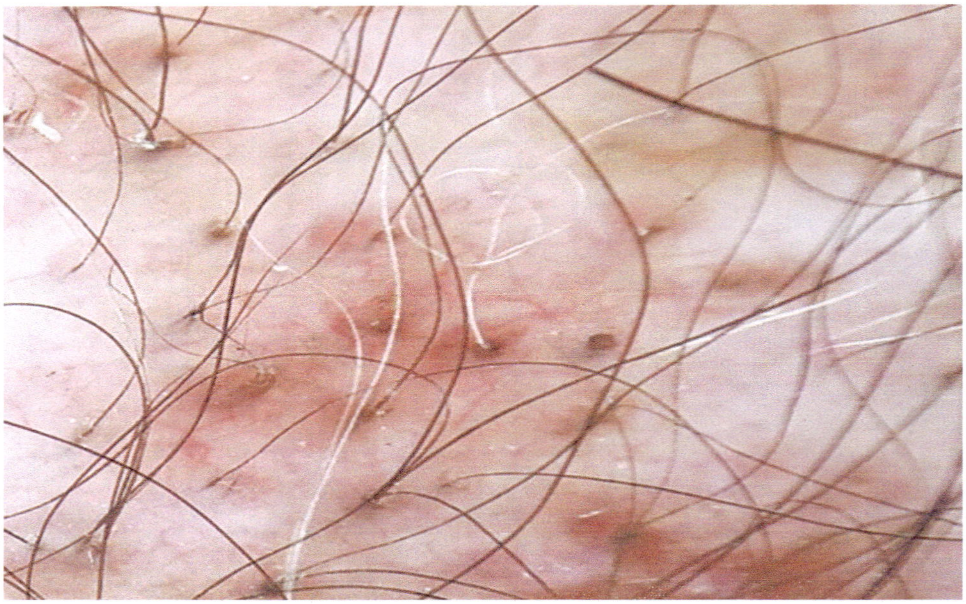

Fig. 9: Blue-gray dots in a speckled pattern. In discoid lupus erythematosus (DLE) they correspond histopathologically to pigment incontinence in the papillary dermis of follicular and interfollicular areas.[3]

REFERENCES

1. Tosti A, Torres F, Misciali C, Vincenzi C, Starace M, Miteva M, et al. Follicular red dots: a novel dermoscopic pattern observed in scalp discoid lupus erythematous. Arch Dermatol. 2009;145:1406-9.
2. Tosti A. Primary Scarring Alopecias. In: Tosti A (ed). Dermoscopy of the Hair and Nails, 2nd edition. Philadelphia: Springer 2016. pp. 5.
3. Duque-Estrada B, Tamler C, Sodre CT, Barcaui CB, Pereira FB. Dermoscopy patterns of cicatricial alopecia resulting from discoid lupus erythematous and lichen planopilaris. An Bras Dermatol. 2010;85(2):179-83.
4. Rudnica L, Olszewska M, Rakowska A, Slowinska M. Trichoscopy update 2011. J Dermatol Case Rep. 2011;5(4):82-8.

CHAPTER

19

Acne Keloidalis Nuchae

Subrata Malakar, Purva Mehta Movdawalla, Priya Diwaker

INTRODUCTION

- It is a chronic inflammatory condition of the occipital scalp and posterior neck where recurrent papular and pustular lesions occur leading to hairless keloidal plaques and scarring alopecia.
- The disease may begin with an injury during a close cut or during close shaving. An association with obesity and metabolic syndrome has also been implicated.

KEY TRICHOSCOPIC FEATURES

- Tufted hairs
- Broken hairs
- Ingrown hairs
- Dermoscopy shows tufting of hairs and peripilar casts.
- Broken hairs have also been described. Whitish areas are also found.[1]

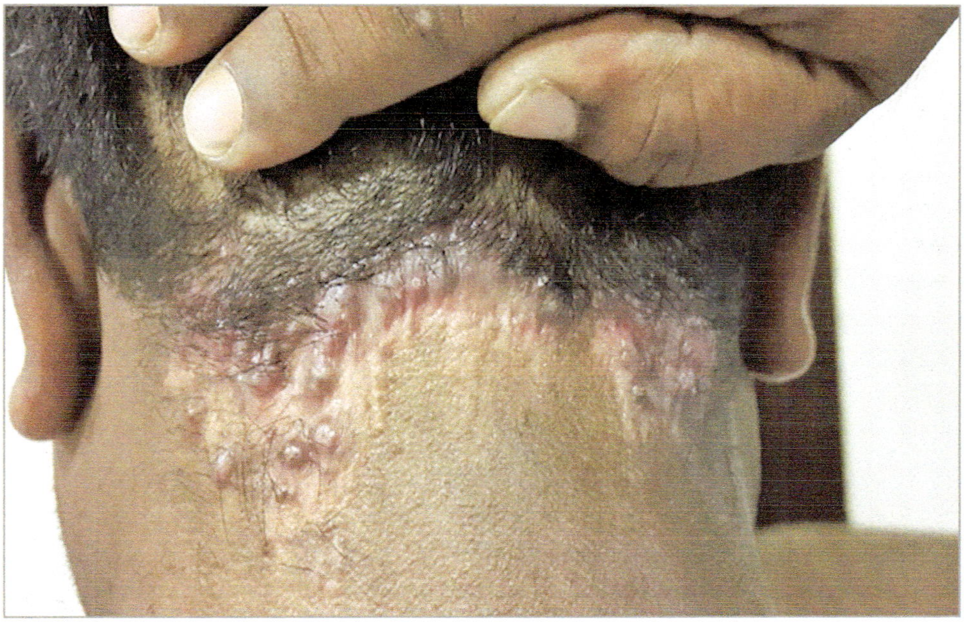

Fig. 1: Papulonodules and pustules producing scars in a case of acne keloidalis nuchae.

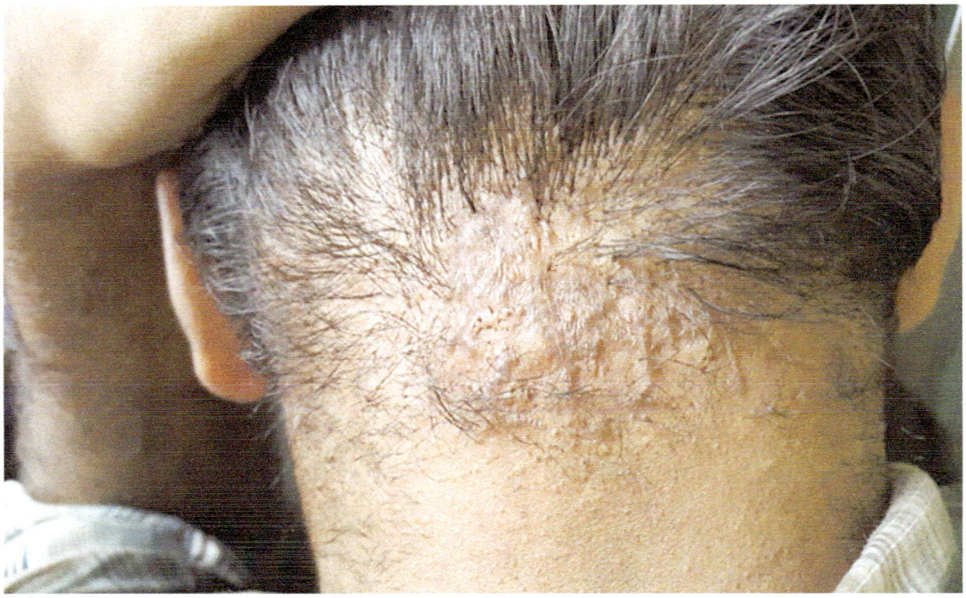

Fig. 2: Acne keloidalis nuchae resulting in scarring alopecia.

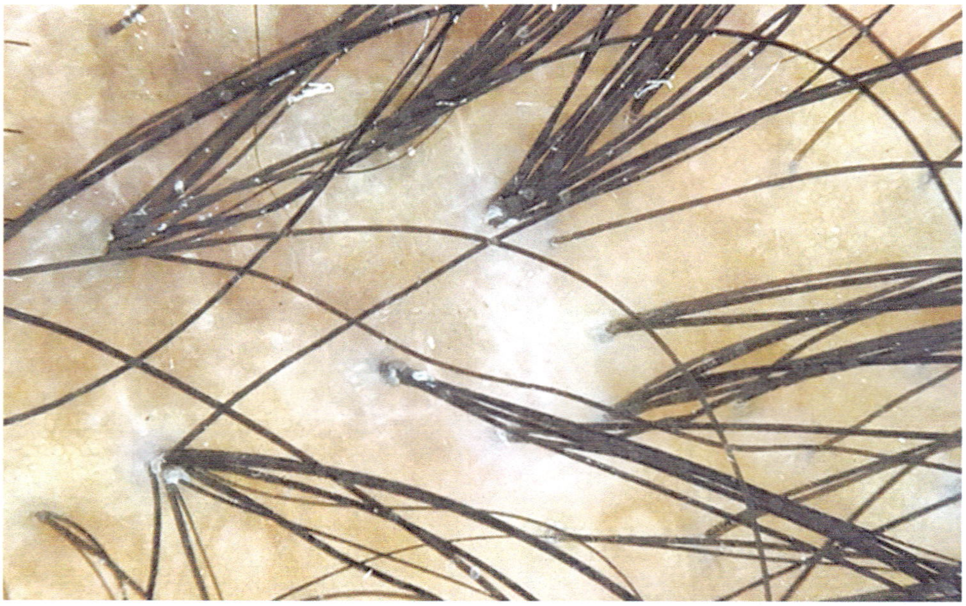

Fig. 3: Trichoscopic image of previous picture showing tufted hairs (several hairs emerge from one dilated follicular opening) and peripilar casts. Whitish areas are also visible which represent dermal fibrosis.

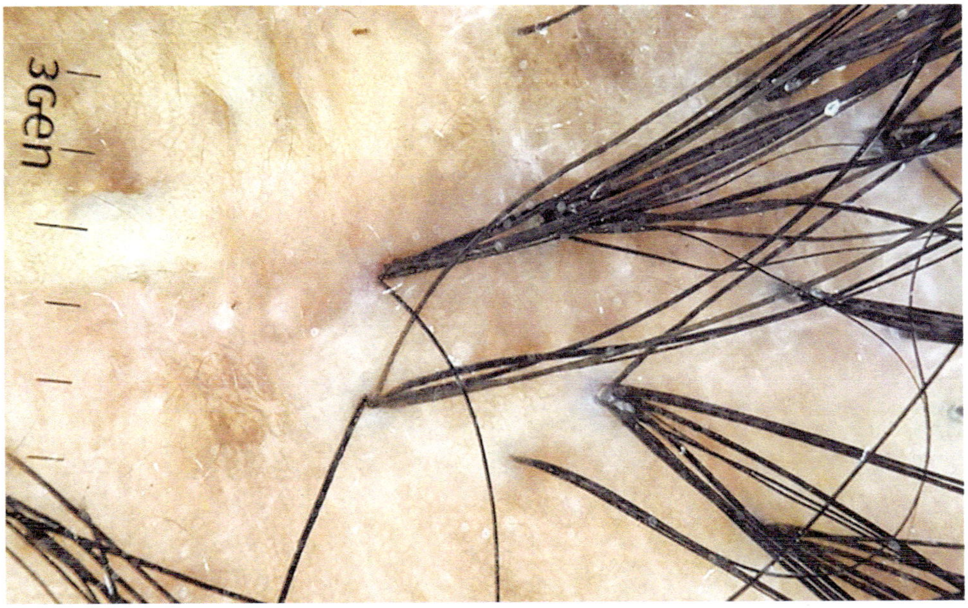

Fig. 4: Tufted hairs of five to six emerged from a single follicle.

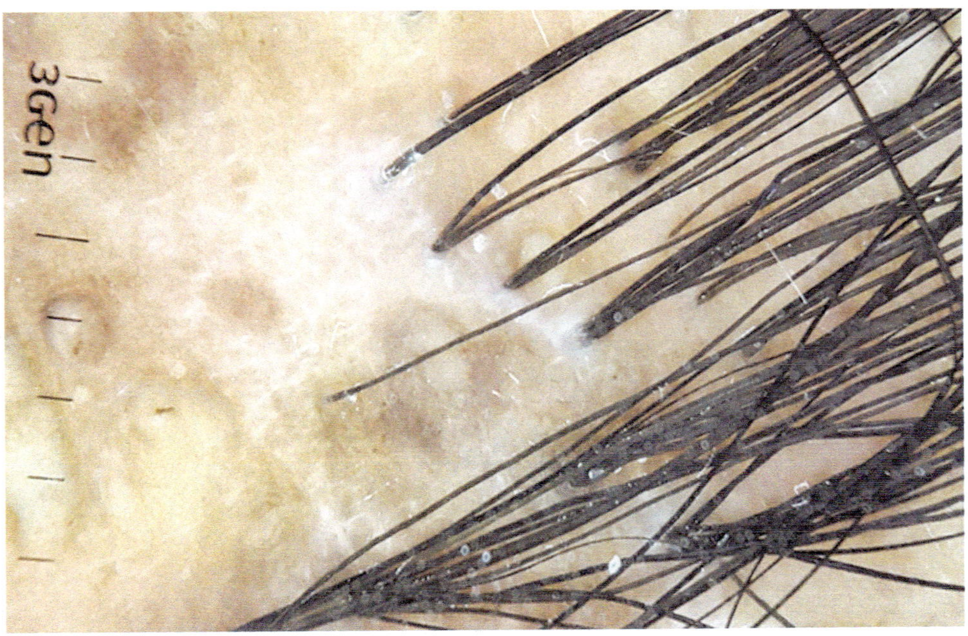

Fig. 5: Whitish area represents cicatricial alopecia which is a common feature of acne keloidalis nuchae. The trichoscopic field is full of tufted hairs.

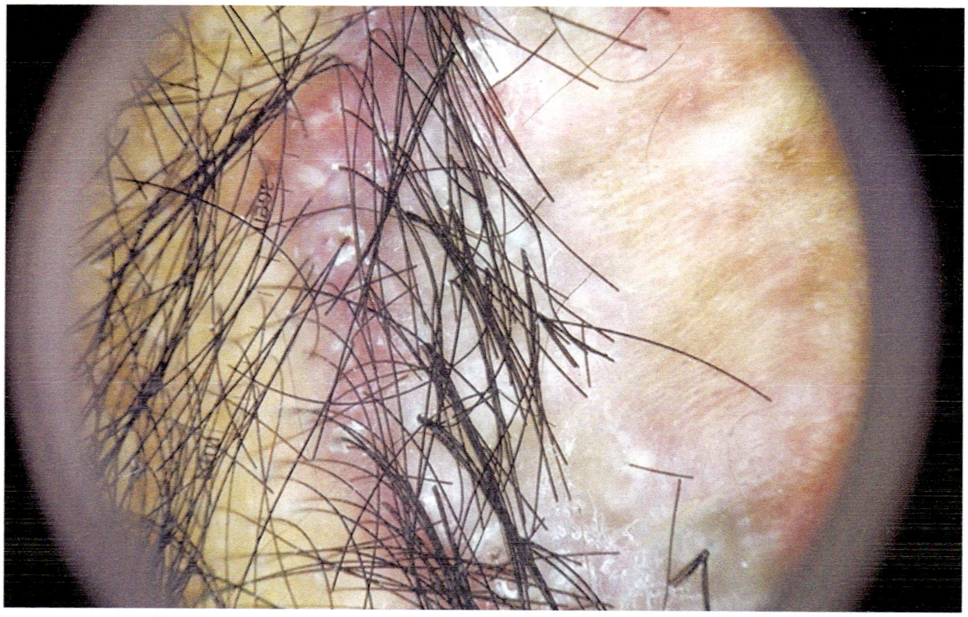

Fig. 6: A trichoscopic overview showing tufted hair and peripilar casts.

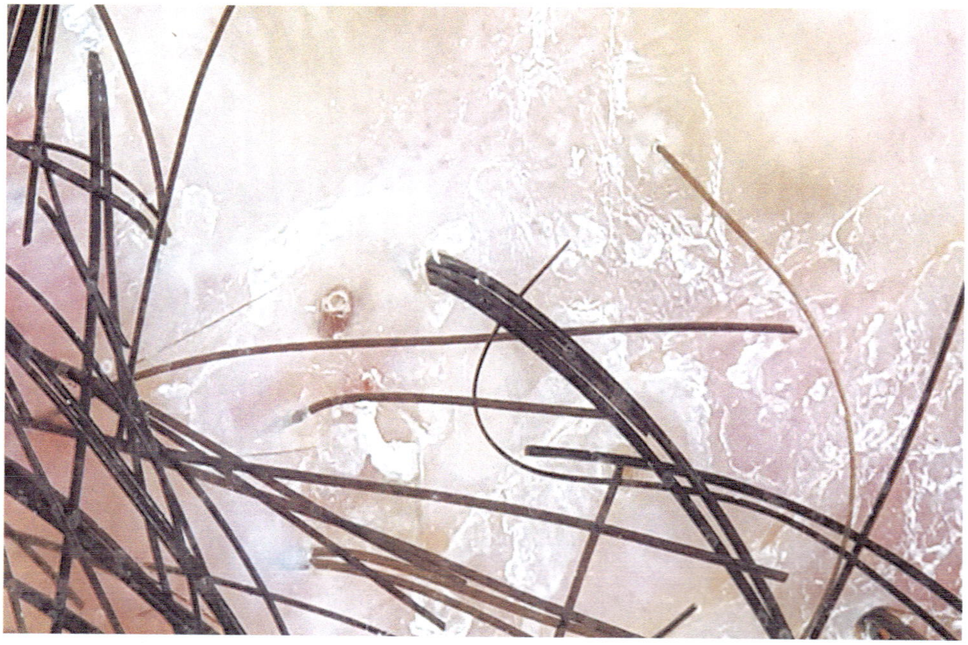

Fig. 7: Whitish scar like area with tufted hairs.

REFERENCE

1. Tosti A. Primary Scarring Alopecias. In: Tosti A (Ed). Dermoscopy of the Hair and Nails, 2nd edition: Philadelphia: Springer; 2016. pp. 65.

CHAPTER

20

Central Centrifugal Cicatricial Alopecia

Subrata Malakar

INTRODUCTION

- Central centrifugal cicatricial alopecia (CCCA) is a form of alopecia of the central scalp that extends centrifugally and is one of the common forms of scarring alopecia seen in dark skinned individuals.
- Hair loss typically starts at the central scalp and extends outward in a progressive manner.
- The exact cause of CCCA is unknown, however, the proposed causative factors are hair care practices such as hot comb, relaxers, and tight extensions, are implicated.
- Fungal infections, autoimmune diseases, etc., may also be responsible in some patients.

KEY TRICHOSCOPIC FEATURES

- Preserved honeycomb pattern
- Irregularly distributed white dots
- Irregular white patches
- Sparse terminal hairs emerging as single hairs or groups of two hairs
- Peripilar white-gray halo—highly specific and sensitive for CCCA in all clinical stages[1]
- Asterisk-like brown patches[2]
- Broken hairs
- Peripilar scales and erythema
- Dermoscopy of CCCA showed a preserved honeycomb pattern though in some patients, it may show interruptions and variations in the density of the brown color; in these patients brown asterisk like blotches are present which probably corresponds to postinflammatory hyperpigmentation.
- Peripilar gray-white halo around the emergence of the hairs is both a specific and a sensitive sign of CCCA. It correlates with lamellar fibrosis which destroys the normal melanization in the outer root sheath.
- Pin-point white dots are irregularly distributed.
- Irregular white patches corresponding to follicular scarring are scattered between the dots.
- Broken hairs are sometimes found. Recently, it was suggested as a sign of occult CCCA.[3]

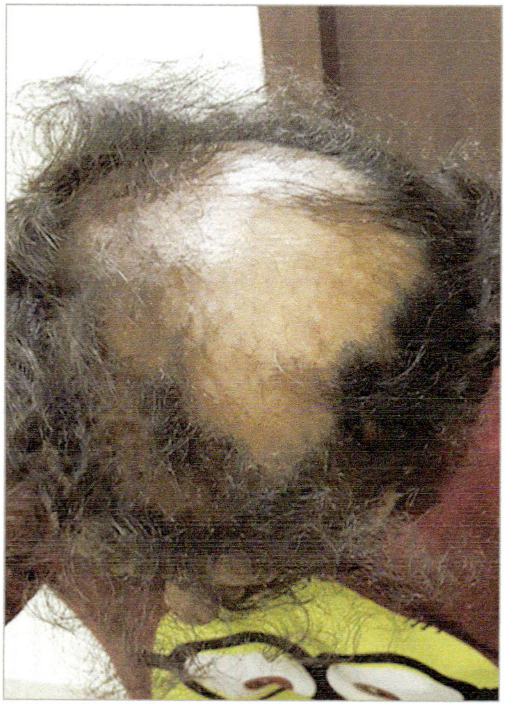

Fig. 1: Clinical image of central centrifugal cicatricial alopecia (CCCA). The disease presents with alopecia of the central scalp which extends peripherally. It occurs in all races and is believed to be multifactorial in origin.

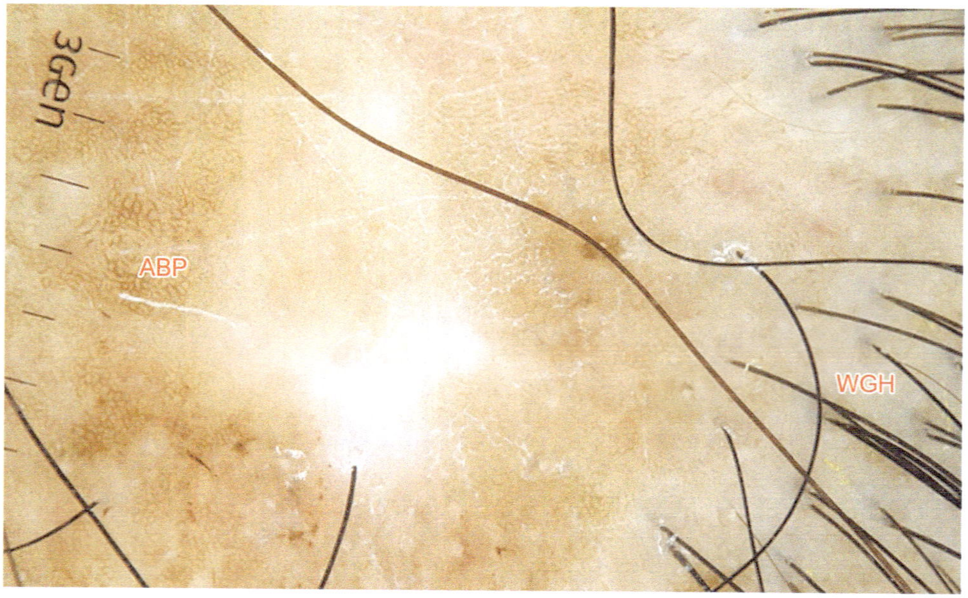

Fig. 2: White patches, disrupted honeycomb pattern at the periphery, minor peripilar scales, asterisk like brown patches (ABP), and white-gray halo (WGH) around the emergence of the hair shaft.

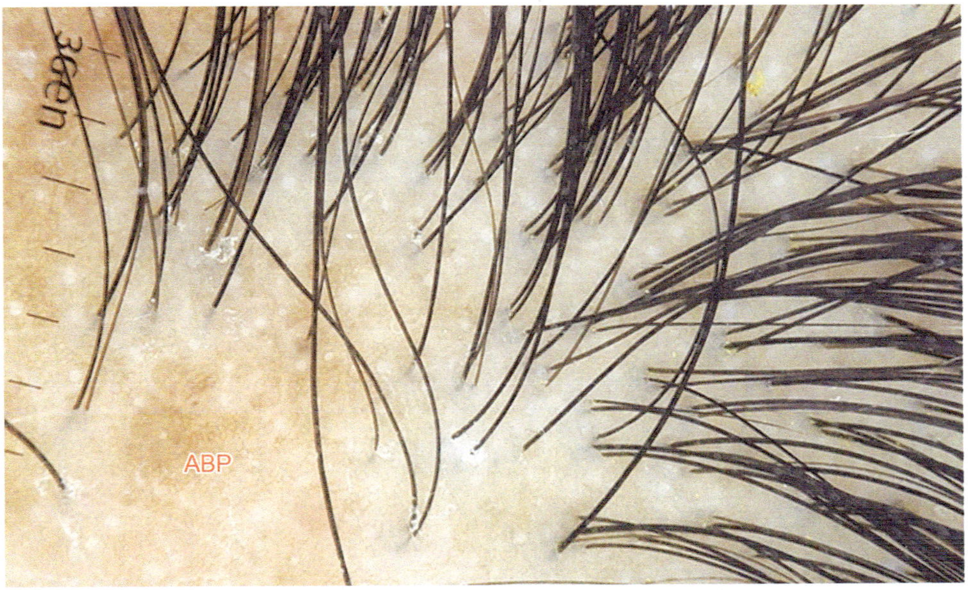

Fig. 3: The image is taken from the border of the alopecic patch of central centrifugal cicatricial alopecia (CCCA) which shows small peripilar scale, white dots and asterisk like brown patch (ABP).

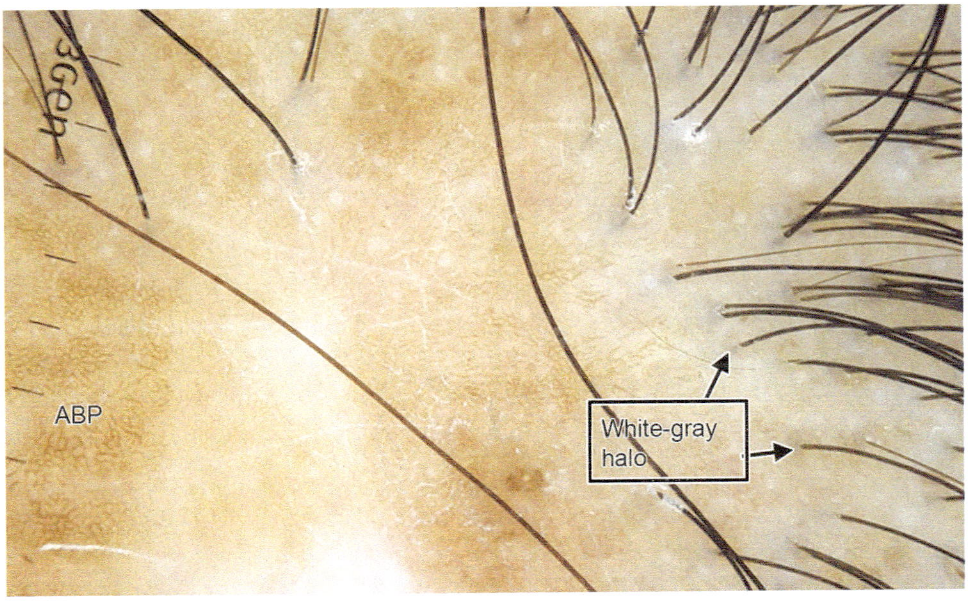

Fig. 4: White-gray halo surrounding the hairs, asterisk like brown patch (ABP), white patch and white-gray halo.

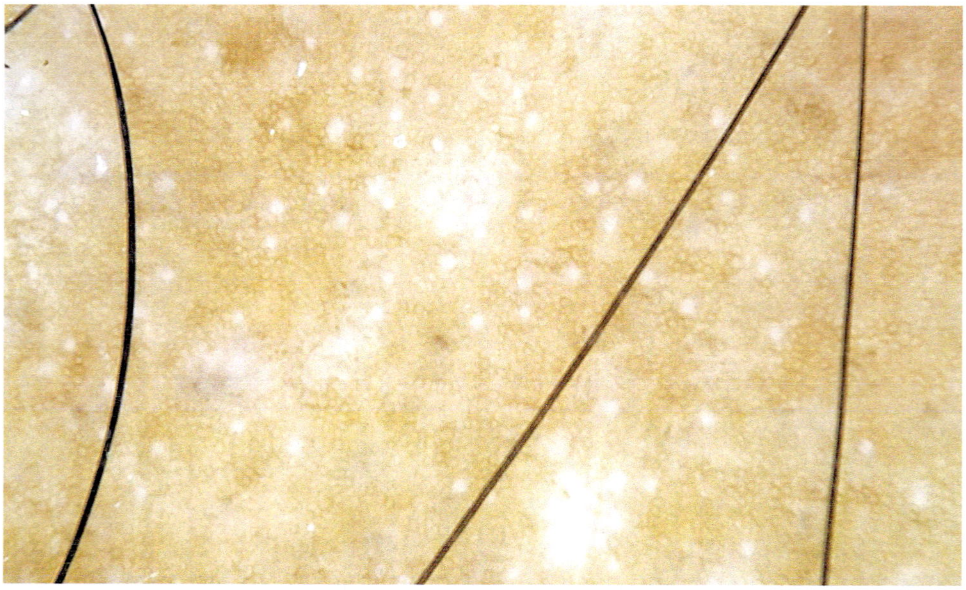

Fig. 5: Central centrifugal cicatricial alopecia (CCCA): White dots (fibrotic) and small white patches dispersed across the field. Honeycomb pigmentation is preserved.

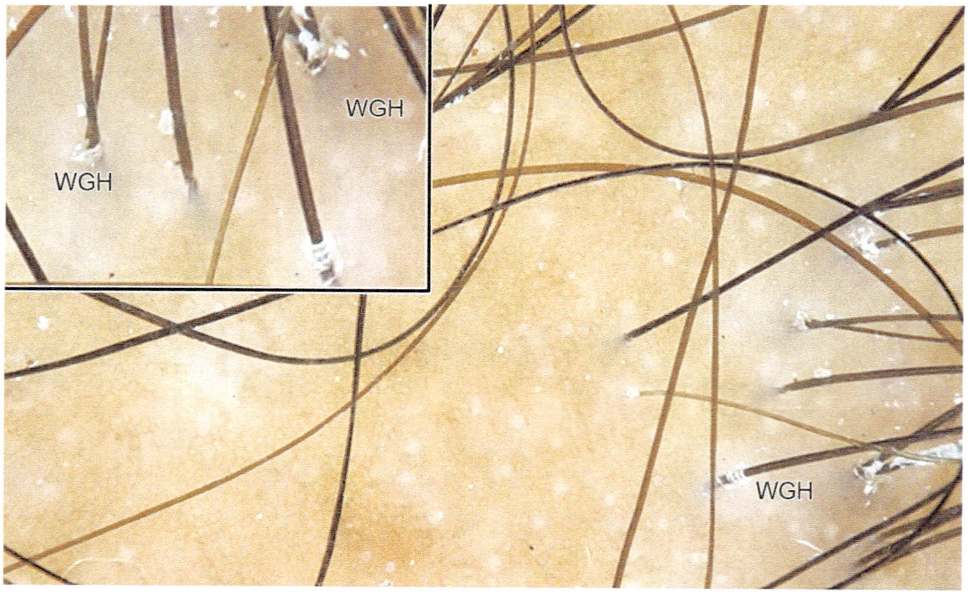

Fig. 6: Fibrotic white dots and patches, sparse hairs, mild peripilar scales, and white-gray halo (WGH) around the emergence of hair shaft. On histopathology, the peripilar white halos correlate with the follicular ostia of both terminal and vellus follicle surrounded by perifollicular fibrosis. The halo is white gray because the lamellar fibrosis obscures and destroys the normal melanization in the outer root sheath.

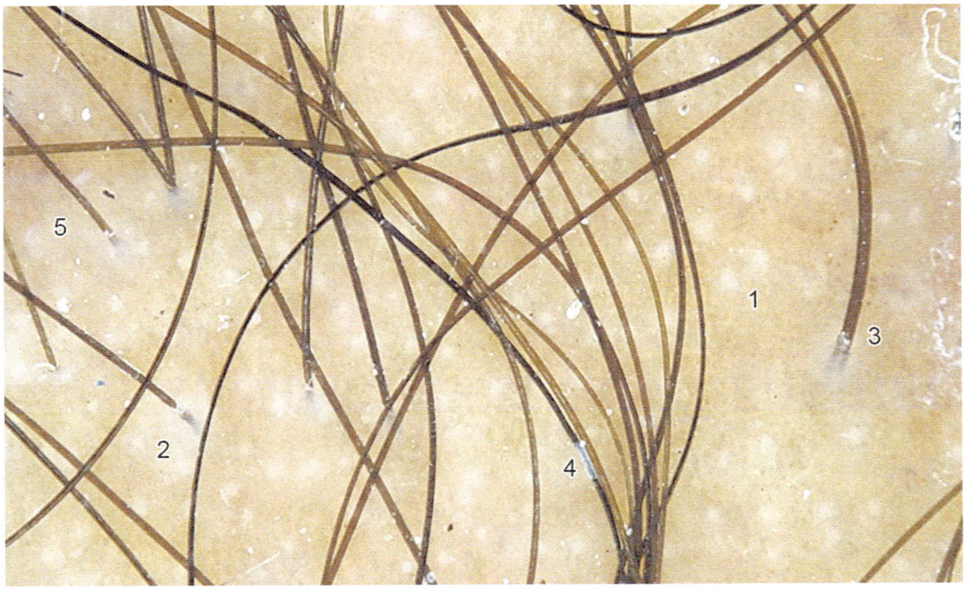

Fig. 7: This is a beautiful image showing genesis of features of scarring alopecia. (1) fibrotic white dots corresponding to fibrosis of the hair follicles, (2) perifollicular fibrosis. If the process progresses further whole of the follicle will be replaced by fibrosis and the hair will be lost permanently, (3) minor perifollicular scaling, (4) perifollicular cast, (5) fibrotic dots coalescing to form a white patch. The above features are common to all the primary lymphocytic scarring alopecias.

REFERENCES

1. Miteva M, Tosti A. Dermatoscopic features of central centrifugal cicatricial alopecia. J Am Dermatol. 2014;71(3):443-9.
2. Summers P, Kyei A, Bergfeld W. Central centrifugal cicatricial alopecia an approach to diagnosis and management. Int J Dermatol. 2011;50:1457-64.
3. Miteva M, Tosti A. Dermatoscopic features of central centrifugal cicatricial alopecia. J Am Acad Dermatol. 2014;415-31.

CHAPTER 21

Folliculitis Decalvans

Subrata Malakar

INTRODUCTION

- Folliculitis decalvans (FD) is a neutrophilic primary cicatricial alopecia characterized by multiple recurrent papulopustular lesions that result in cicatricial alopecia.
- Typically there is centrifugal progression and diffuse thick scales may be the presenting sign.

KEY TRICHOSCOPIC FEATURES[1]

- Tufts of six or more hairs emerging from same ostia is almost diagnostic.
- Hair casts
- Dilated and coiled capillaries
- Perifollicular pustules and scaling
- Starburst sign

- The characteristic trichoscopic finding is tufting of hairs that include six or more hairs emerging together from a single ostia.
- Perifollicular pustules are seen in active FD.
- Thick white scales are present both in the inter- and perifollicular area.
- Coiled and dilated capillary loops are suggestive of diagnosis of FD.[2]
- At the base of hair tufts, a starburst pattern is formed which is known as starburst sign. This is formed by a band of yellowish scales and perifollicular epidermal hyperplasia.[3]

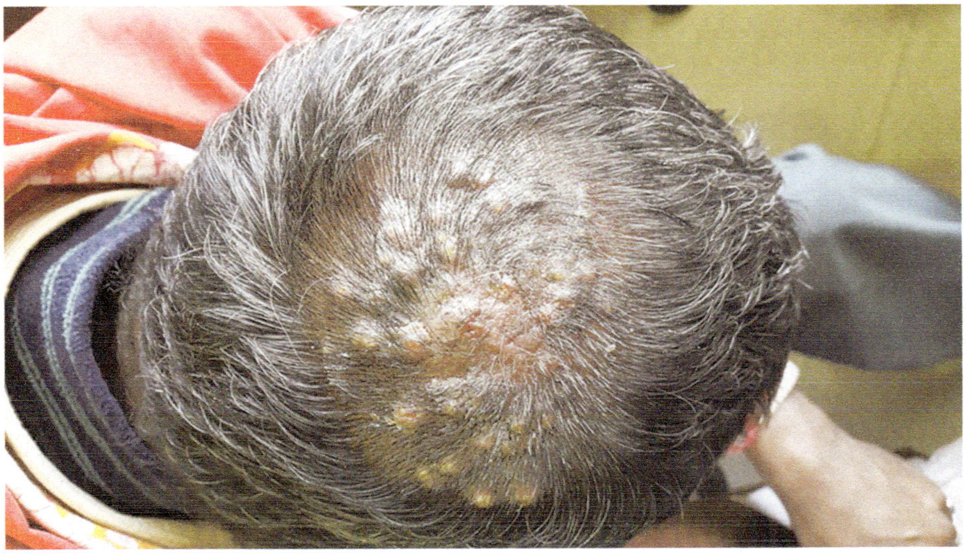

Fig. 1: Folliculitis decalvans predominantly affects the vertex and occipital areas of the scalp. Prominent features are dilated follicular openings with a tendency to tufting. The active phase in this image is depicted by follicular pustules, erythema, and yellow gray scales. Scalp pain, itching, and burning sensation are the symptoms.

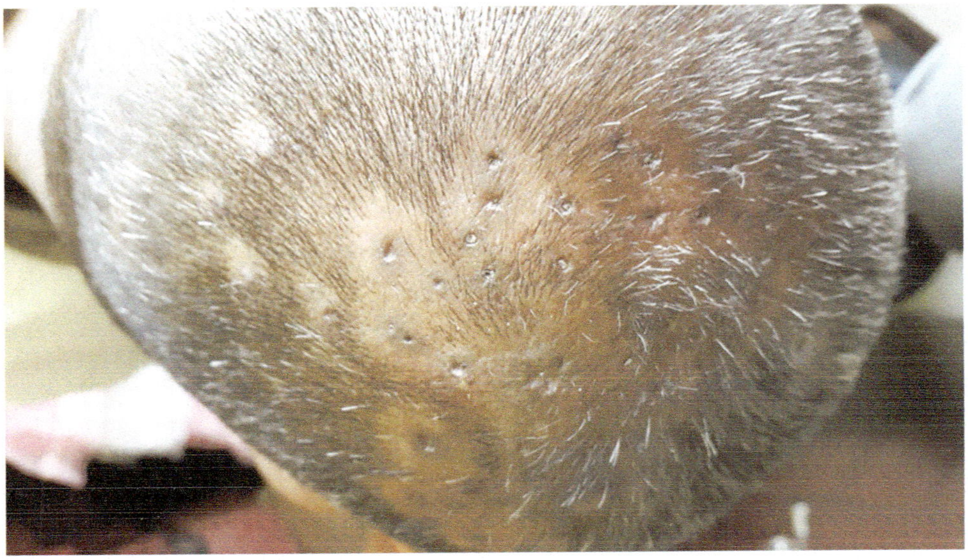

Fig. 2: In long-standing cases, cicatricial alopecia develops.

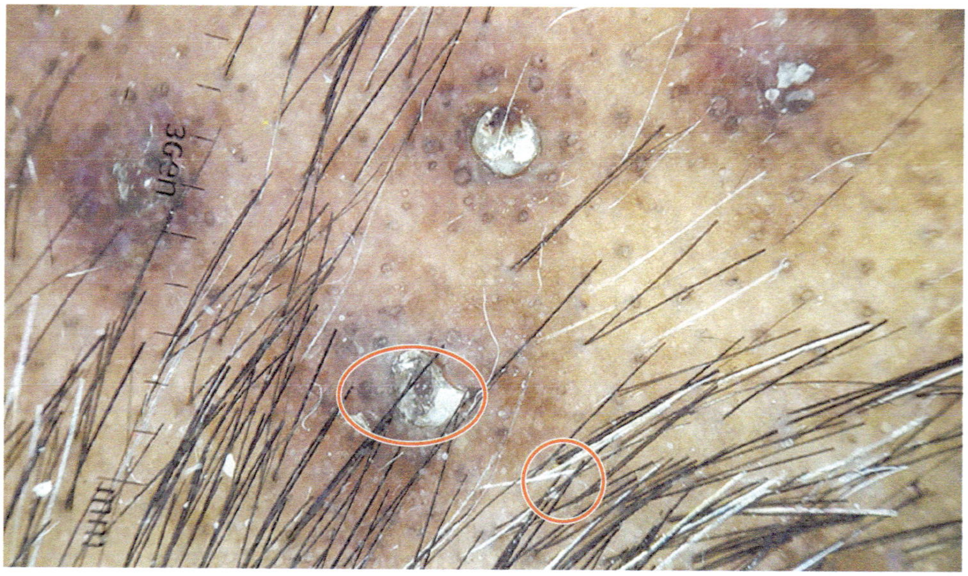

Fig. 3: Tufting of hair, yellowish tubular scaling with collar formation seen on trichoscopy.

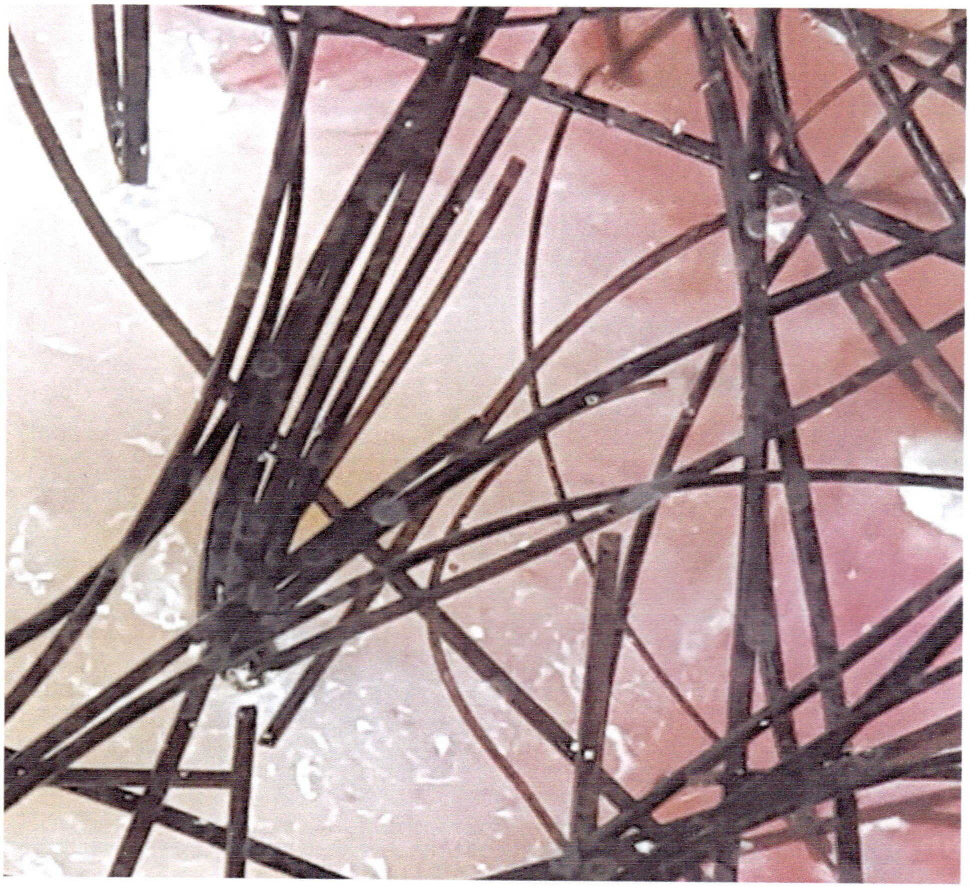

Fig. 4: Hair tufts in a case of folliculitis decalvans.

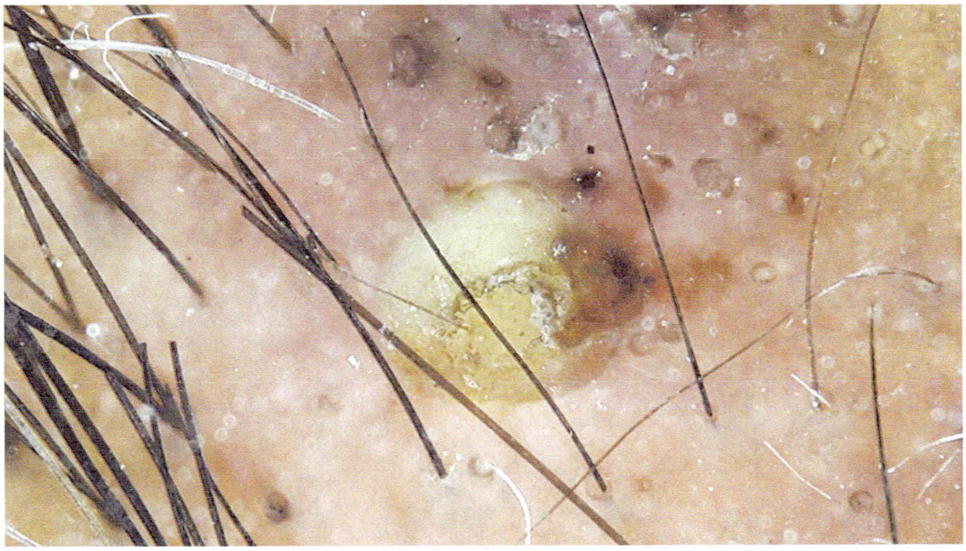

Fig. 5: At the onset of disease activity, formation of a yellowish pustule is seen around the hair follicle.

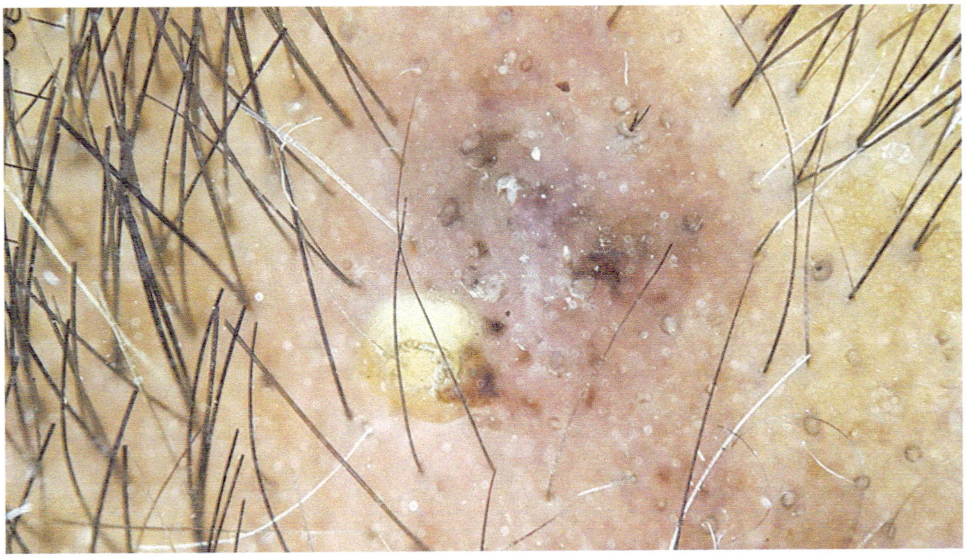

Fig. 6: At the center of this trichoscopic image, a yellowish pustule is visible. A tendency of tufting of hairs is seen at the periphery.

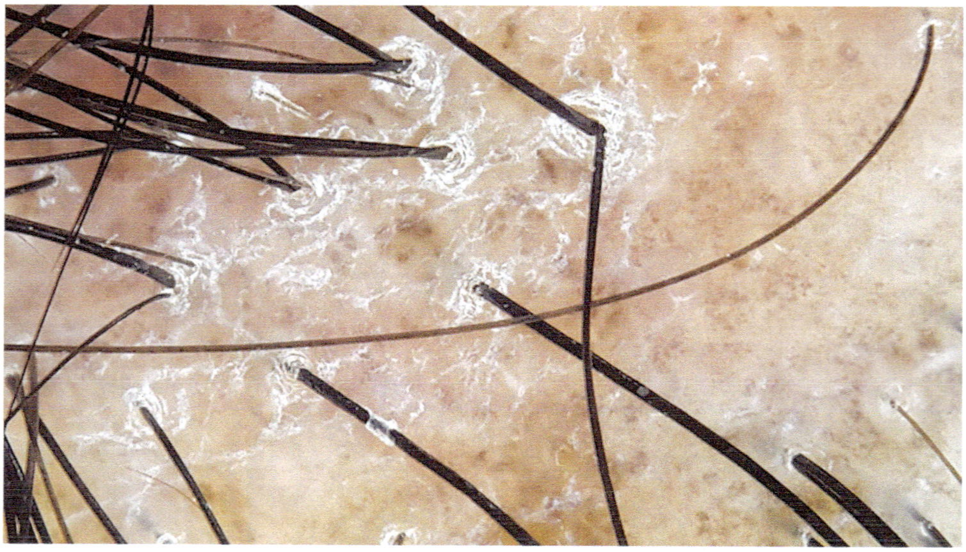

Fig. 7: Epidermal hyperplasia with incomplete formation of starburst pattern is seen in a case of folliculitis decalvans (FD). Marked perifollicular hyperkeratosis and scaling is commonly observed in FD.

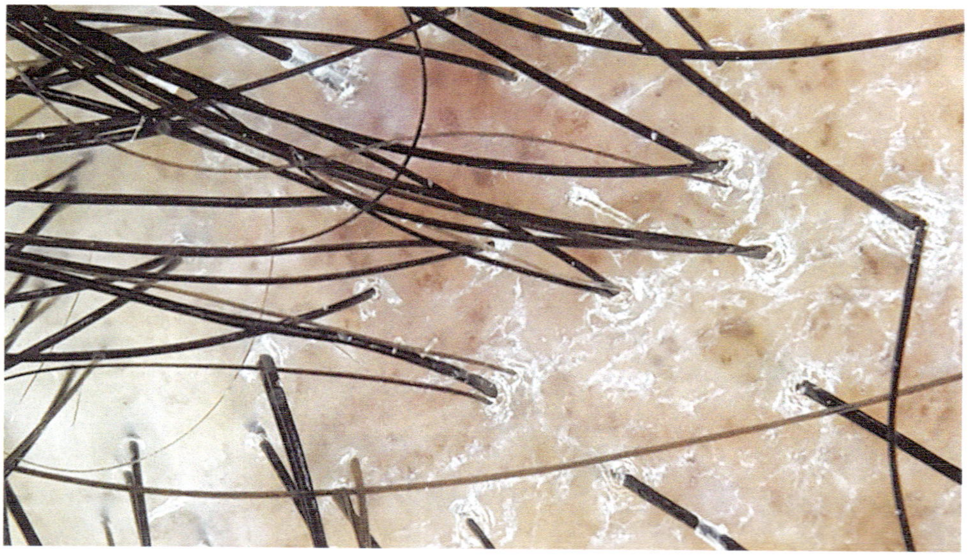

Fig. 8: Epidermal hyperplasia found on histopathology of folliculitis decalvans (FD) correspond to starburst pattern surrounding the hair shaft at its emergence.

REFERENCES

1. Otberg N, Kang H, Alzolibani AA, Shapiro J. Folliculitis Decalvans. Dermatol Ther. 2008:21:238-44.
2. Tosti A. Primary scarring alopecias. In: Tosti A (Ed). Dermoscopy of the Hair and Nails, 2nd edition. Philadelphia: Springer; 2016. pp. 61.
3. Rakaowska A, Slowinska M, Kowalska-Oledzka E, Warszawik O, Czuwara J, Olszewska M, et al. Trichoscopy in cicatricial alopecia. J Drugs Dermatol. 2012;11:753-8.

CHAPTER 22

Dissecting Cellulitis

Subrata Malakar

INTRODUCTION

- The disease begins with the follicular occlusion of vertex and occiput. In the due course, perifollicular pustules, nodules, abscesses, and sinus tracts develop.[1] It is a part of "follicular occlusion triad".[2]
- Though bacterial culture of the pustular discharge is sterile, secondary bacterial infection may occur. The course of the disease is chronic, relapsing, and progressive.[1]
- Alopecia is reversible in the early stage but in longstanding cases, scarring alopecia develops. Keloid formation is typical.

KEY TRICHOSCOPIC FEATURES

- Accentuated plugged follicular openings
- Black dots
- Broken hairs

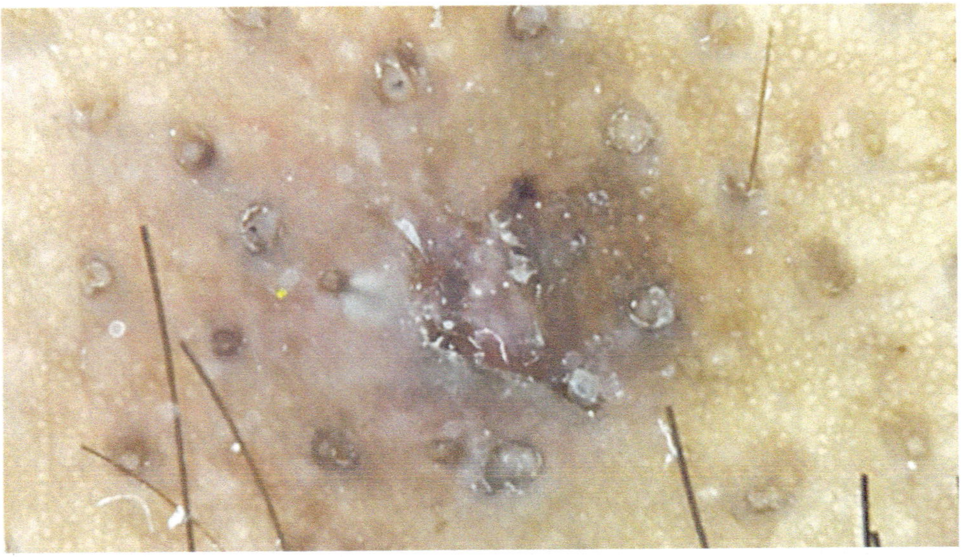

Fig.1: Trichoscopic image of dissecting cellulitis showing accentuated plugged follicular openings, broken hair and pin-point white dots.

REFERENCES

1. Mihic LL, Tomas D, Situm M, Krolo I, Sebetić K, Sjerobabski-Masnec I, et al. Perifolliculitis capitis abscedens et suffodiens in a caucasian: Diagnostic and therapeutic challenge. Acta Dermatovenerol Croat. 2011;19(2):98-102.
2. Thein M, Hogarth MB, Acland K. Seronegative arthritis associated with the follicular occlusion triad. Clin Exp Dermatol. 2004;29(5):550-2.

CHAPTER

23

Pseudopelade of Brocq

Subrata Malakar

INTRODUCTION

- It is a lymphocytic primary scarring alopecia and typically affects middle-aged women.[1]
- Clinically characterized by asymptomatic, noninflamed, white or porcelain-white, usually reticulate patches in the central scalp.[1,2]
- Small patches may coalesce to form larger patches. The course is slowly progressive. Characteristically, no inflammatory lesions are noticed throughout the course of disease.
- This is a distinct entity and should not be described as an end-stage scarring alopecia resulting from other inflammatory disease of the scalp.[2-4]

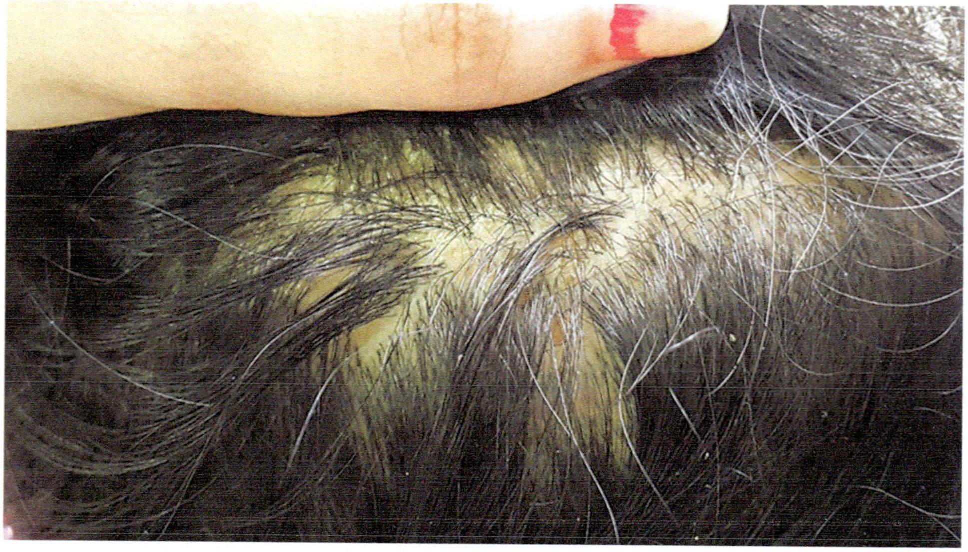

Fig. 1: Reticular irregular patches of scarring alopecia in pseudopelade of Brocq. Clinically, there is no sign of inflammation.

KEY TRICHOSCOPIC FEATURES

- Loss of follicular openings
- Lone dystrophic hairs at the margin of the lesion
- Smooth white areas
- Absence of features characteristic for other scarring alopecias
- The background has various shades of white such as porcelain-white, gray, beige (light yellow tan), and erythematous.

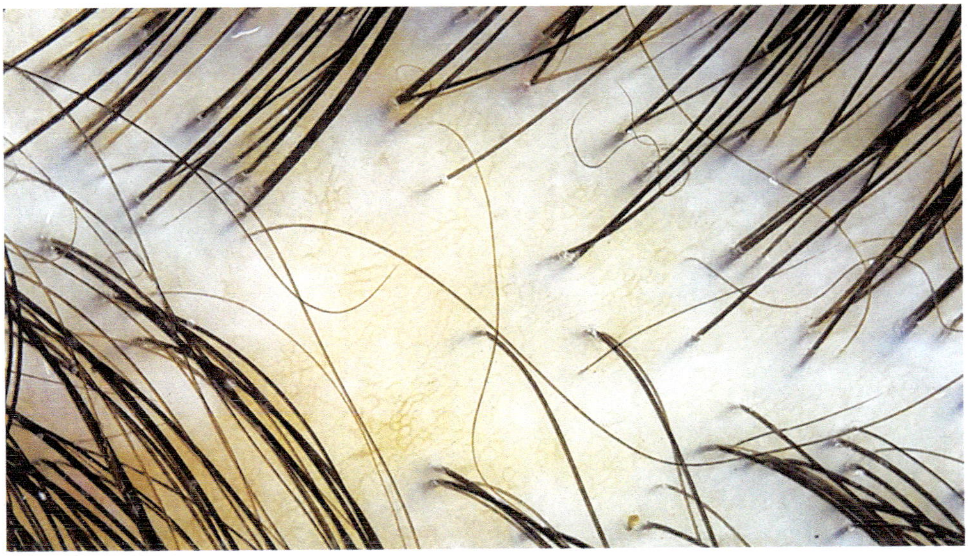

Fig. 2: Smooth scalp surface lacking follicular openings and presence of lone dystrophic hairs.

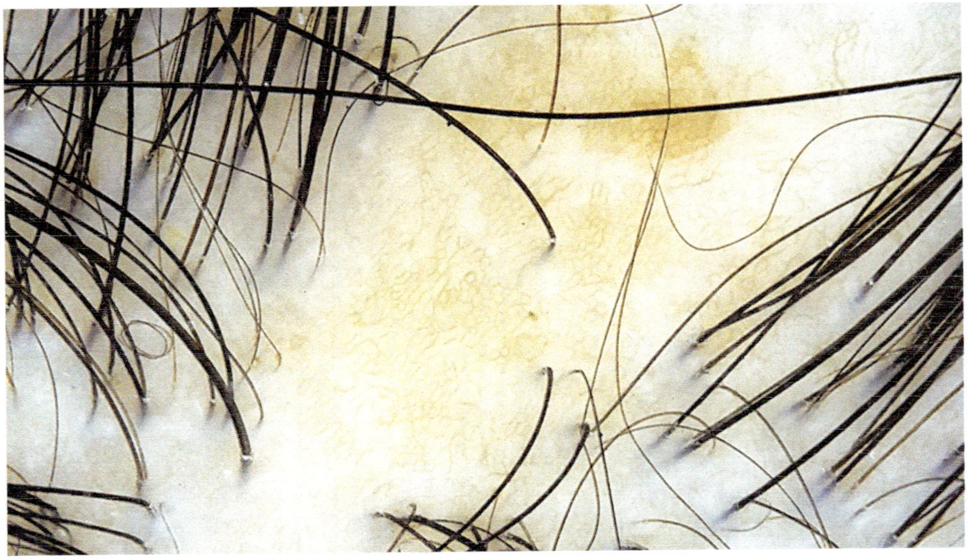

Fig. 3: Loss of follicular openings and presence of lone dystrophic hairs at the periphery of the patch. Note the background that has light yellow tan with subtle pigment network.

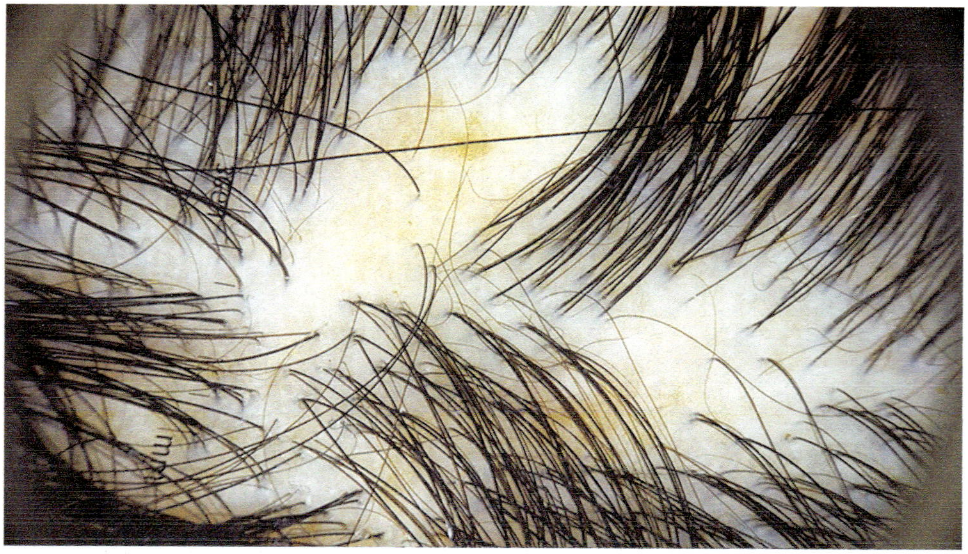

Fig. 4: Pseudopelade of Brocq: Scarring alopecic patches showing porcelain-white and beige background.

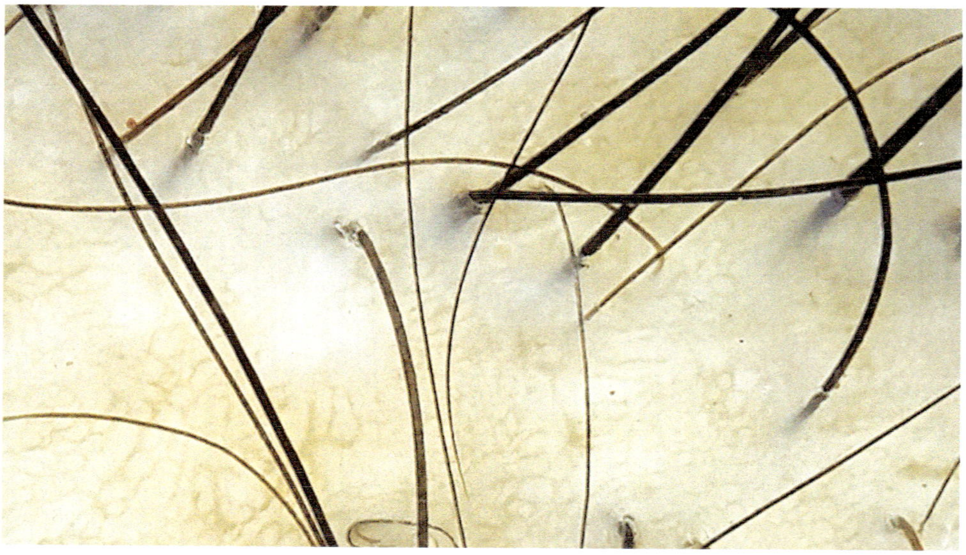

Fig. 5: Small smooth hairless area, loss of follicular openings, and absence of features indicating other scarring alopecias should raise the suspicion of pseudopelade of Brocq.

REFERENCES

1. Alzolibani AA, Kang H, Otberg N, Shapiro J. Pseudopelade of Brocq. Dermatol Ther. 2008;21(4):257-63.
2. Price V, Mirmirani P. Cicatricial Alopecia: An Approach to Diagnosis and Management. New York: Springer; 2011.
3. Trueb RM. Systematic approach to hair loss in women. J Dtsch Dermatol Ges. 2010;8(4):284-98.
4. Yu M, Bell RH, Ross EK, Lo BK, Isaac-Renton M, Martinka M, et al. Lichen planopilaris and Pseudopelade of Brocq involve distinct disease associated gene expression patterns by microarray. J Dermatol Sci. 2010;57(1):27-36.

ASSESSMENT IMAGES-BASED QUESTIONS

1. This is a trichoscopic image of a scarring alopecia with a background of beige tan color. What is the condition?

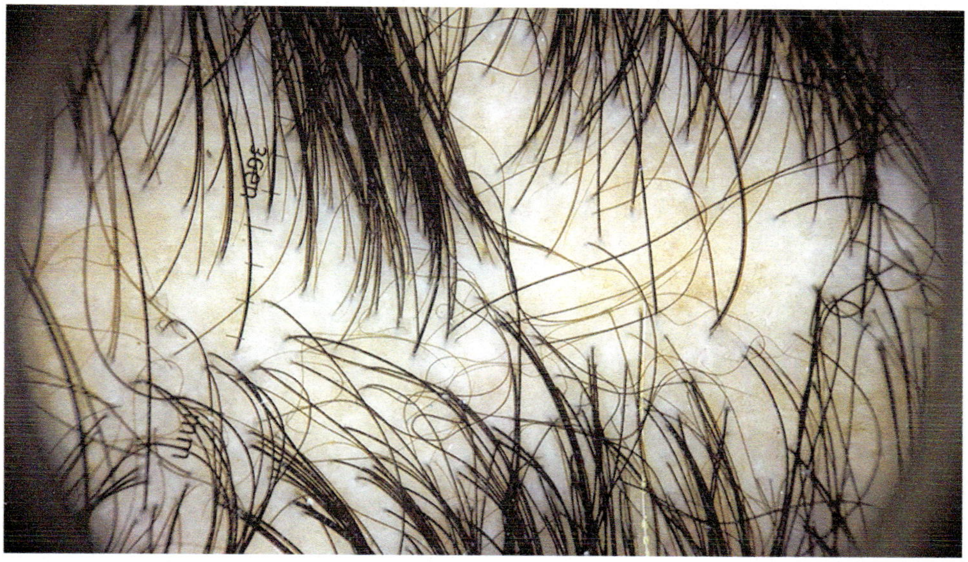

2. This trichoscopic image shows loss of follicular openings, decreased hair density and peripilar casts around single and two to three hair follicular units. What is your diagnosis?

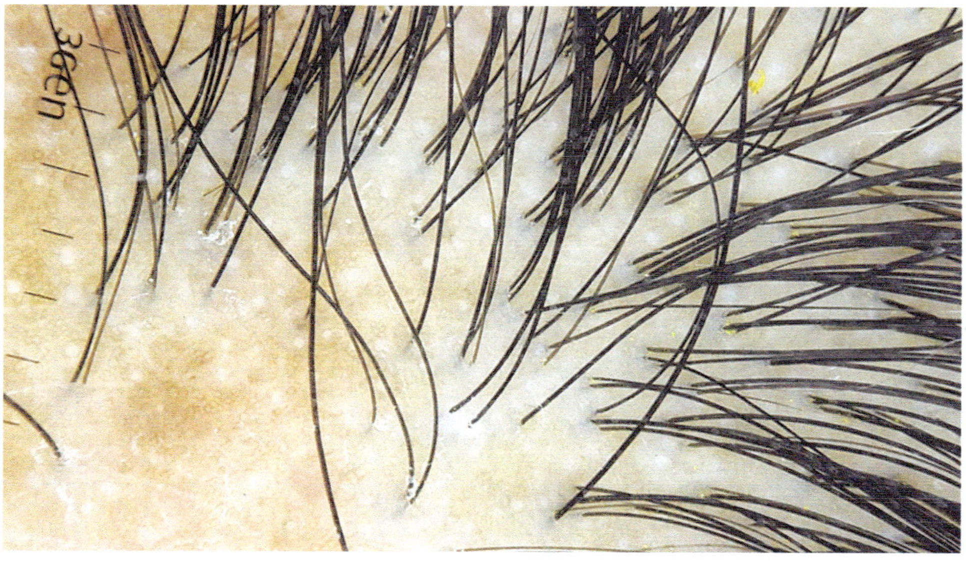

3. This is a trichoscopic image of discoid lupus erythematosus. Name its three trichoscopic features visible in this image.

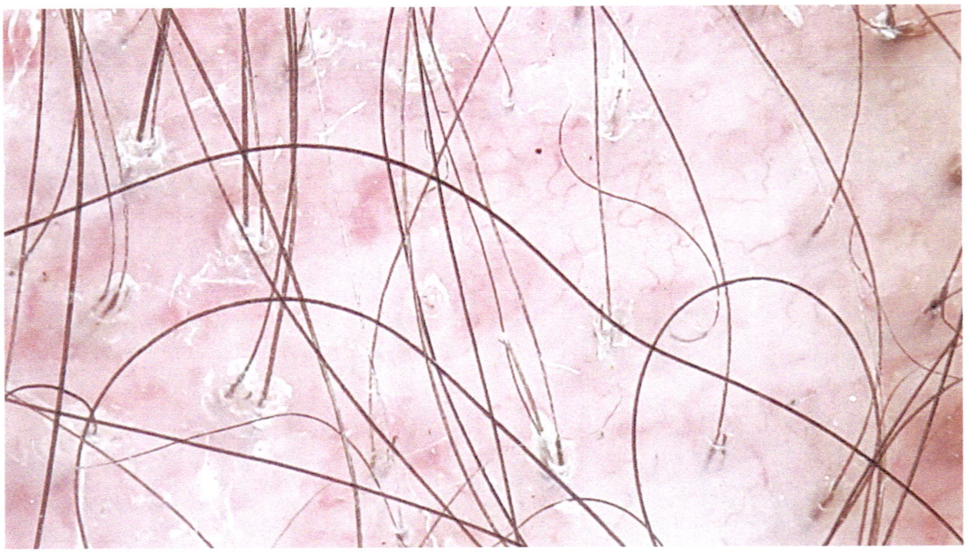

4. Blue-gray dots in a targetoid pattern are visible in this image. Name the scarring alopecia.

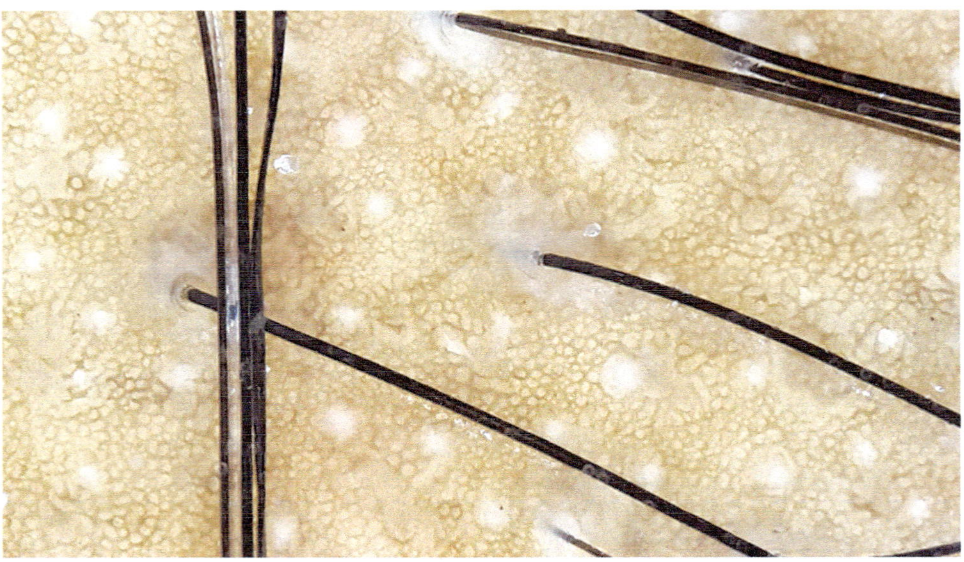

5. This patient had papulonodules over the nape of the neck. Trichoscopy shows tufting of hairs. Identify the scarring alopecia.

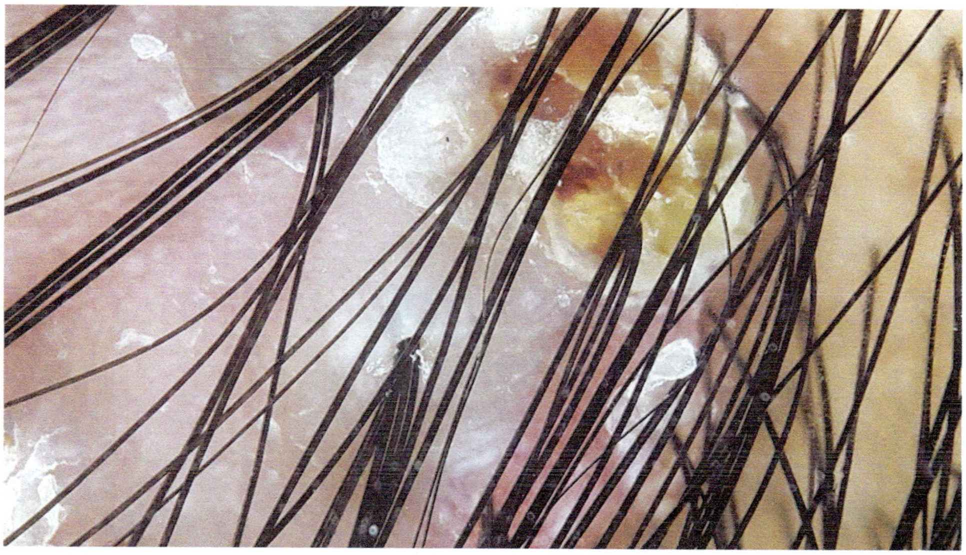

6. This is a case of lichen planopilaris. Name its three trichoscopic features seen in this image.

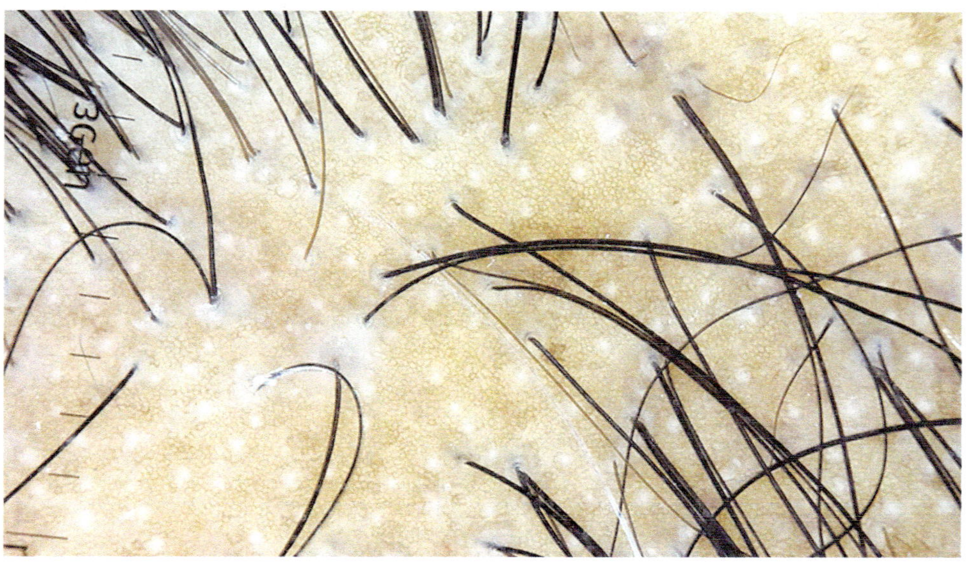

7. Tufting of hairs is strikingly present in this trichoscopic image. Name four scarring alopecias wherein tufting of hairs are found.

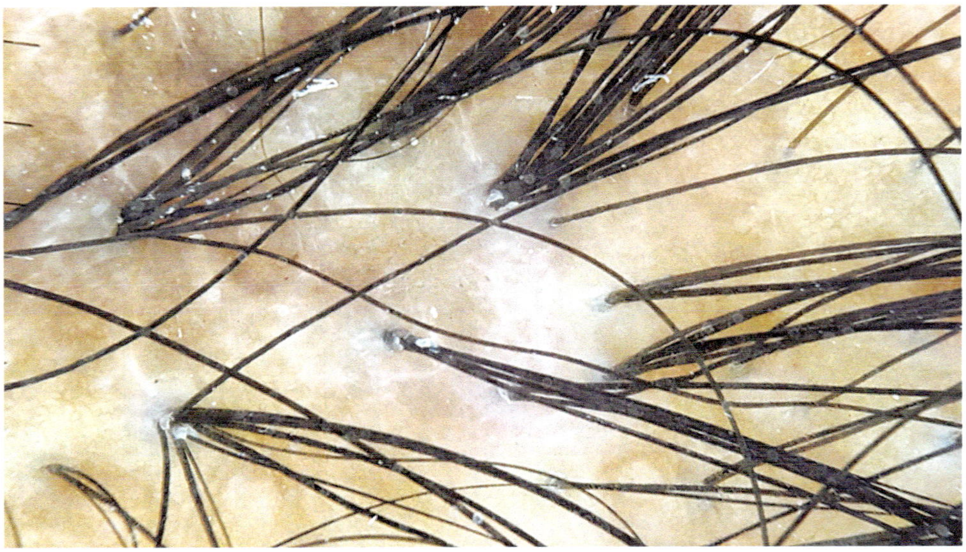

8. Peripilar casts mainly around two to three hair follicular units, blue-gray dots around hair follicles and in the interfollicular scalp are visible in the image. What is your diagnosis?

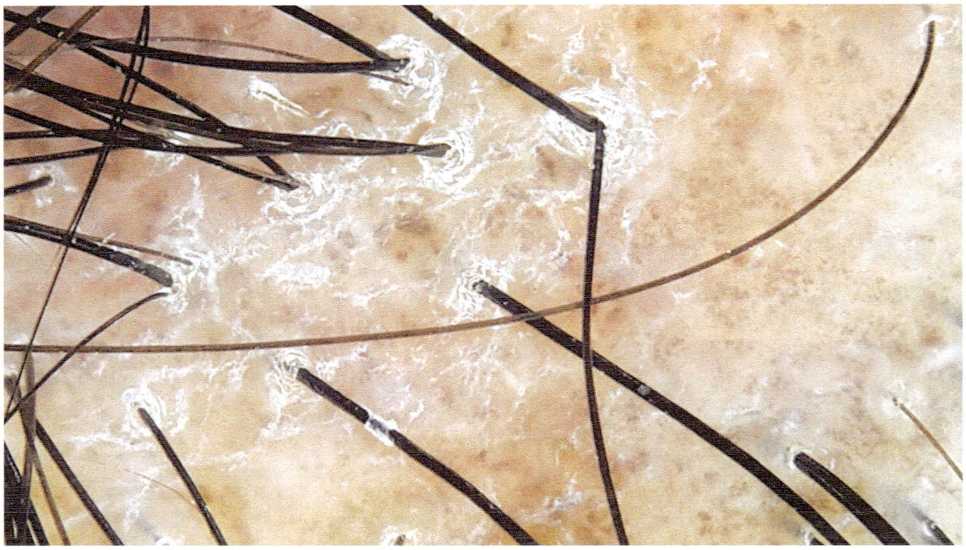

ANSWERS

1. Lichen planopilaris
2. Keratotic plugging, white areas, and giant irregular vessels
3. Lichen planus pigmentosus
4. Acne keloidalis nuchae
5. Peripilar casts around two to three hair follicular units, blue-gray dots in a targetoid pattern, and loss of follicular openings
6. Folliculitis decalvans, acne keloidalis nuchae, lichen planopilaris, and dissecting cellulitis of scalp
7. Lichen planopilaris

8

SECTION

Hair Weathering

CHAPTER

24 Trichoscopy of Damaged Hair

Samipa S Mukherjee, Subrata Malakar

INTRODUCTION

- Hair weathering is defined as the deterioration of the hair shaft from root to shoot resulting due to external factors.
- Cosmetic practices such as combing, brushing, braiding, weaving, hair extensions, straightening, waving, perming, repeated traction combing and dyeing, as well as environmental factors such as exposure to ultraviolet (UV) light, can induce structural damage to the hair fiber.
- The cuticle becomes raised and porous, exposing the cortex to further damage.
- A decrease in hair shine, elasticity, and strength is observed, with increase in dryness, frizziness ultimately leading to hair breakage.

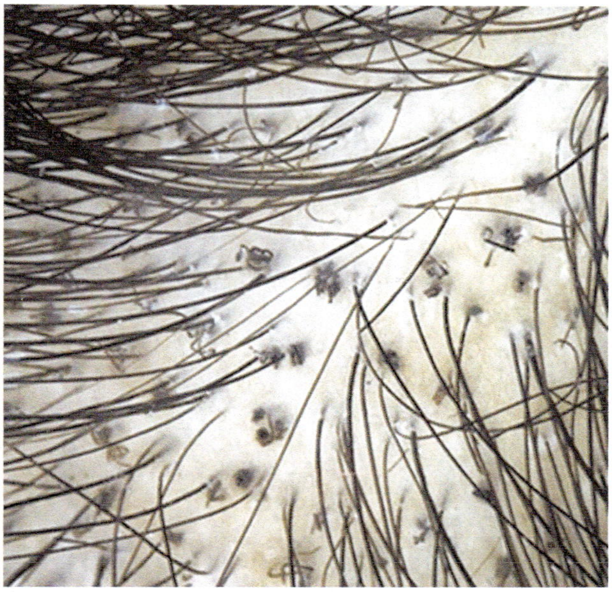

Fig. 1: Dystrophic hair due to singeing from usage of hot iron comb.

TRICHOPTILOSIS

INTRODUCTION

- Trichoptilosis literally is derived from the Greek word "tricho" meaning hair and "ptilos" meaning feather and commonly refers to the fraying of the distal hair shafts known as split ends.
- The split is longitudinal and may be divided into two or several divisions.

- Pathologically the frayed end is devoid of cuticle.
- This condition results due to external factors such as harsh combing, environmental factors, and heat.
- *Associations*: Trichorrhexis nodosa and trichonodosis[1]

KEY TRICHOSCOPIC FEATURES

- The distal end of the hair shaft is the examination field in cases of trichoptilosis.
- It reveals splitting of the hair shaft longitudinally in two or multiple divisions.
- At times, the split may be noted even proximal to the distal end.
- Sometimes, the split may be accentuated giving rise to a broom appearance.
- This can, however, be differentiated from trichorrhexis nodosa in being located at the distal end of the hair shaft rather than in the length of the hair shaft with just one end appearing like a broom stick.

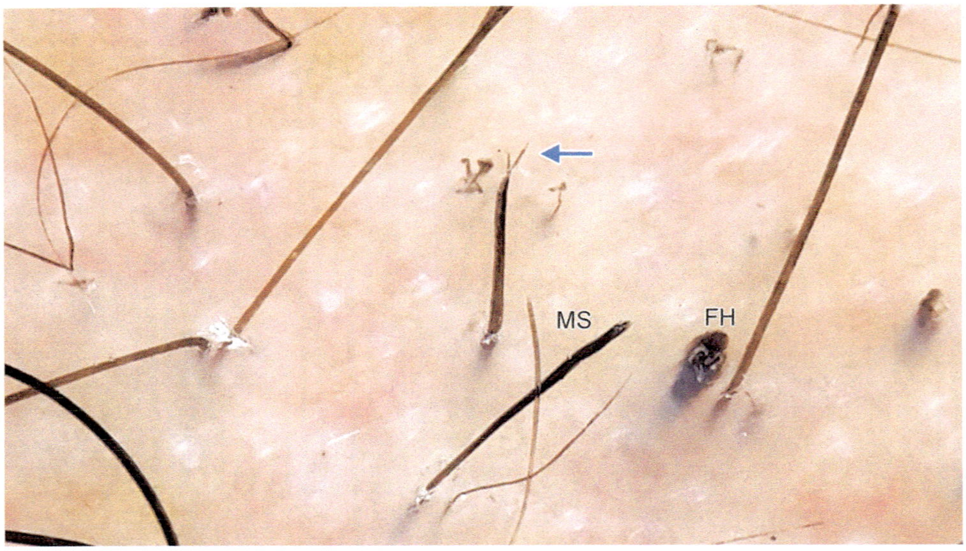

Fig. 2: Trichoptilosis showing longitudinal splitting of the distal end of hair shaft (blue arrow). Note also "mace sign" (MS) and flame hair (FH).

ACQUIRED TRICHORRHEXIS NODOSA

INTRODUCTION

- Trichorrhexis nodosa is defined as a fracture of the hair shaft affecting the distal ends of long hair resulting in easy fragility and occurs most commonly due to mechanical forces on the hair.
- Usage of heat for perming, curling, and styling of hair has also been associated in its causation along with chemical treatments of hair.
- Severe form results in matting of the hair in part or in toto at times.

KEY TRICHOSCOPIC FEATURES

- Gross dermatoscopy of the affected hair reveals multiple gray white areas corresponding to areas of swelling and fracture.
- On higher magnification the affected areas appear like two ends of a paint brush or broom aligned in opposition.

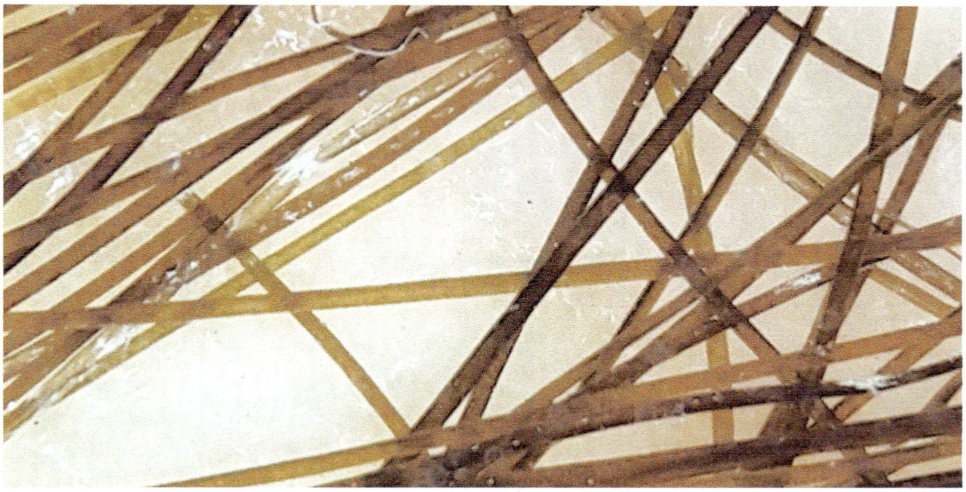

Fig. 3: Trichorrhexis nodosa resulting from traction combing. Brush-like hair fracturing are observed in multiple hairs.

TRICHONODOSIS

INTRODUCTION

- Trichonodosis is defined as knotting of hair on the distal portion of the hair shaft which could be spontaneous or secondary to exogenous trauma, chemical treatment, and mechanical forces.
- The knots are usually located on the outer third of the hair shaft. Rarely, more than one knot is found on a single hair and most were a simple half hitch knot.[2]
- Mechanical factors such as scratching, combing, washing, or friction may produce tangling and knotting of hairs.
- Most commonly this condition is found in curly hair predominant in the African population.
- This may further lead to tangling and matting of hair.
- Dermatoscopy is useful in differentiating this condition from other conditions such as knits on hair or particulate matter deposited post hair dyeing and chemical treatments.

KEY TRICHOSCOPIC FEATURES

- Evaluation of the distal third of the hair shaft reveals knotting of the hair shaft into a single, double, or multiple knots.
- Associated trichoptilosis and trichorrhexis nodosa may be observed.

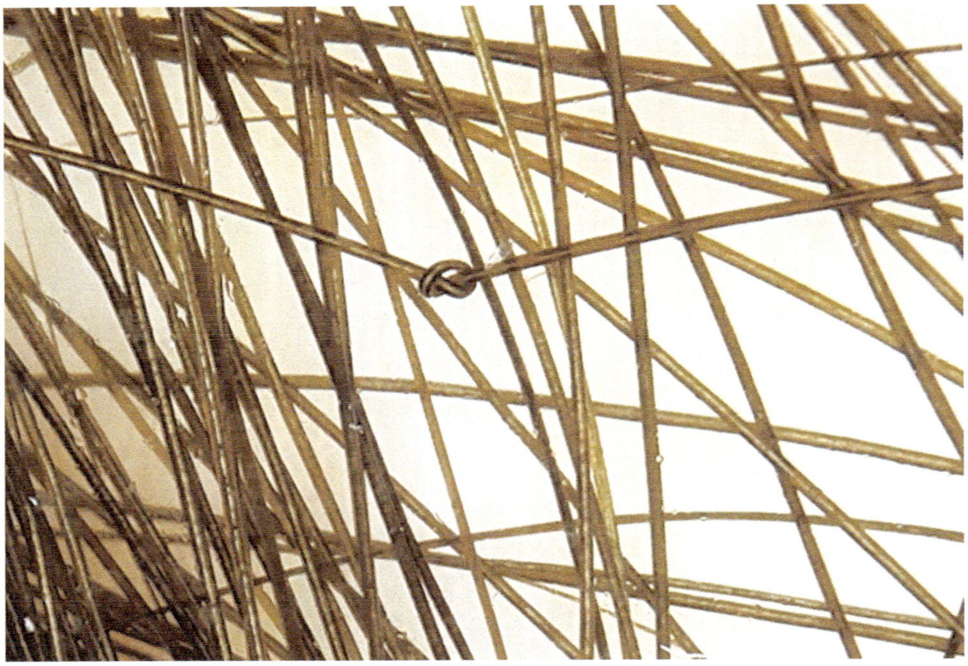

Fig. 4: Trichonodosis.

BUBBLE HAIR

INTRODUCTION

- Bubble hair is classically defined as an acquired hair shaft deformity characterized by bubble like areas in the hair shaft seen with light microscopy and corresponding cavitary defects with scanning electron microscopy.[3]
- It occurs due to exposure of wet hair to very high temperatures from blow dryers, curlers, or straighteners.
- The pathomechanism involves formation of steam filled cavities in the hair shaft due to sudden evaporation of water within the hair shaft.

KEY TRICHOSCOPIC FEATURES

- It reveals a spongy appearance of the hair shaft due to the presence of air bubbles within the hair shaft.
- Sometimes, it may be seen affecting the proximal end of the hair shaft as well.
- The appearance has been described as honeycomb or Swiss cheese appearance.[1]
- Dysmorphia of distal hair shaft was observed in bubble hair. In large hair samples, dermatoscopy can be used to highlight hair that warranted closer examination under light microscopy.[4]

CAMOUFLAGE PRODUCTS

INTRODUCTION

- There are in all five categories of camouflaging products available to reduce the appearance of hair loss—hair fibers, powder cakes, scalp lotions, scalp sprays, and hair crayons.[5]
- Most of them form a residue on the scalp and are thereby easily seen on dermatoscopy.
- Recently micropigmentation of the scalp is also being practiced widely as a method of camouflage.

KEY TRICHOSCOPIC FEATURES

- Most commonly used hair fibers are seen as small vertical, horizontal, or diagonally aligned pigmented fragments on the scalp surface differing in length present on the scalp and the hair shaft.
- Powder or crayon residue may appear like pigmented dots or give rise to a dirty scalp appearance.
- Micropigmentation on dermatoscopy not only gives an idea about the depth of pigmentation, color of the ink but also helps in establishing the pattern used for inducing pigmentation.

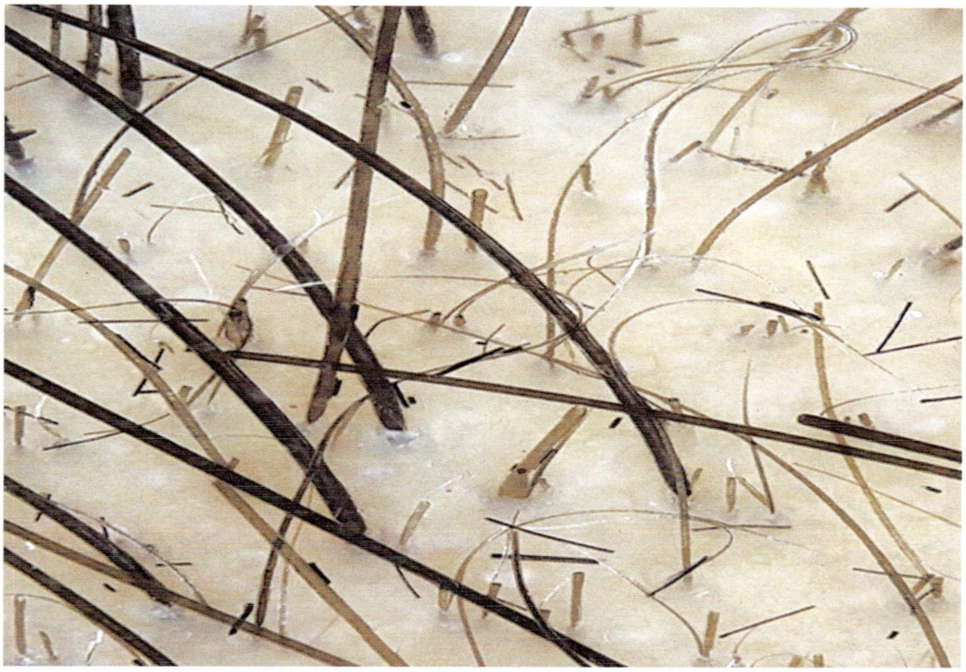

Fig. 5: Camouflage product in the form of hair fiber. The cosmetic hair fibers are strikingly thinner than the normal hair shafts and appear as short hair fragments.

HAIR COSMETICS

INTRODUCTION

- Hair cosmetics are routinely used for improving texture, imparting color, improving luster, thickness, and quality of hair.
- These particulate matter coat the hair shaft and form residues on the shaft which may be distributed regularly or in segments across the shafts.
- These products form concretions on the hair shaft which may be the presenting symptom of a few patients in the hair clinic.
- They need to be differentiated from other mimickers such as scale, nits, hair casts, and infective conditions such as trichomycosis.
- The products may form a residue on the scalp as well as the hair shaft.

KEY TRICHOSCOPIC FEATURES

- Dermatoscopy reveals micaceous white to refractile substances sticking to the hair shaft or encircling it completely.
- Similar deposition may also appear on the scalp.
- The color of concretions varies from white to black to brown depending on the product.
- Scalp erythema may be noted in case of allergic reaction to the cosmetics used.
- Other signs of weathering in the form of trichorrhexis nodosa, trichoptilosis may also be found.

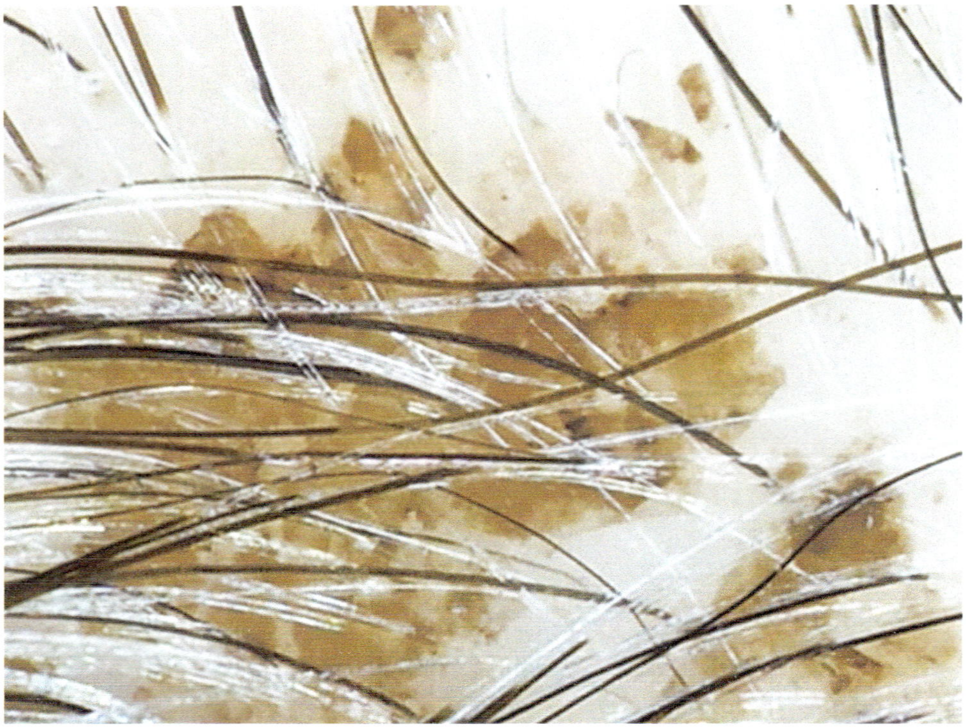

Fig. 6: Deposition of hair dye residue on the scalp.

EXTENSIONS

INTRODUCTION

Usage of extensions predisposes an individual to matting as telogen hairs that remain attached to the glued extensions easily tangle with the surrounding hair.

KEY TRICHOSCOPIC FEATURE

It is essential for revealing the trapped telogen hair in the glue causing damage.

REFERENCES

1. Tosti A. Dermoscopy of the Hair and Nails. New York: CRC Press; 2016.
2. English DT, Jones HE. Trichonodosis. Arch Dermatol. 1973;107:779.
3. Detwiler SP, Carson JL, Woosley JT, Gambling TM, Briggaman RA. Bubble hair: A case caused by an overheating hair dryer and reproducibility in normal hair with heat. J Am Acad Dermatol. 1994;30:5460.
4. Wallace MP, de Berker DA. Hair diagnoses and signs: The use of dermatoscopy. Clin Exp Dermatol. 2010;35:416.
5. Donovan JC, Shapiro Ran L, Shapiro P, Zupan M, Pierre-Louis M, Hordinsky MK. A review of scalp camouflaging agents and prostheses for individuals with hair loss. Dermatol Online J. 2012;18(8):1.

9

SECTION

Infection and Infestation

CHAPTER

25

Tinea Capitis

Subrata Malakar

INTRODUCTION

- Tinea capitis is a fungal infection affecting the hair and scalp and is most commonly seen in pediatric age group.[1]
- Tinea capitis is classified as—noninflammatory, inflammatory, and favus.[2,3]
- Tinea capitis in children is most commonly caused by *Microsporum* and *Trichophyton* species.[1]
- *Microsporum canis* causes ectothrix tinea capitis. Herein, fungal hyphae, and arthroconidia invade the outer part of hair shaft and may damage hair cuticle.[2,3]
- Trichophyton causes endothrix tinea capitis. Fungal hyphae and arthroconidia in endothrix occupy the hair shaft from within and the whole hair shaft may be weakened.[2,3]
- *Trichophyton schoenleinii* is associated with formation of air spaces within the shaft.[2,3]
- Diagnosis is based on direct microscopic exam of infected hair and mycological cultures.
- Scalp scaling and patchy alopecia are the frequent clinical presentations.
- Pustular lesions are seen in inflammatory tinea capitis.
- Cervical lymph nodes are commonly enlarged in tinea capitis.

KEY TRICHOSCOPIC FEATURES

- *Comma hairs*[4]: They are the dermoscopic markers of tinea capitis that appear as the punctuation mark "comma". The fungal elements infecting the hair shaft cause the hair to bend.
- *Corkscrew hairs*[5]: They are short hairs which are spiral in shape.
- *Broken hairs*[5,6]: Broken and dystrophic hairs are common but nonspecific findings.
- Black dots
- Hair casts
- Morse code (transverse white bands) hairs[7,8]
- i-hairs[9]
- Block hairs[9]

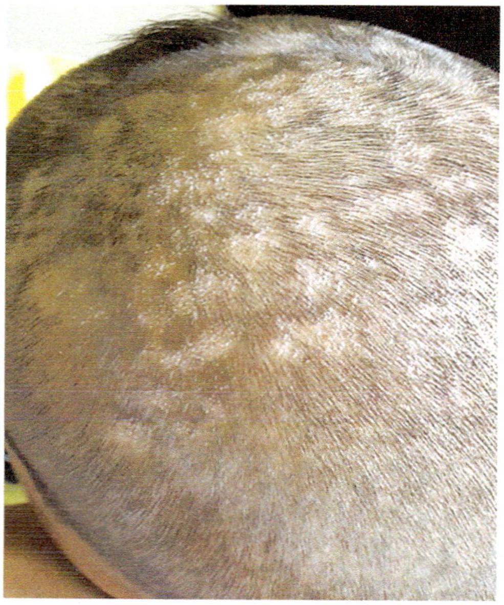

Fig. 1: Patches of alopecia is a characteristic feature of tinea capitis. Hairs may be broken at the scalp level due to endothrix fungus infection whereas in ectothrix invasion the shafts are broken 1–3 mm away from scalp level. In all types of tinea capitis, scalp scaling is a common occurrence.

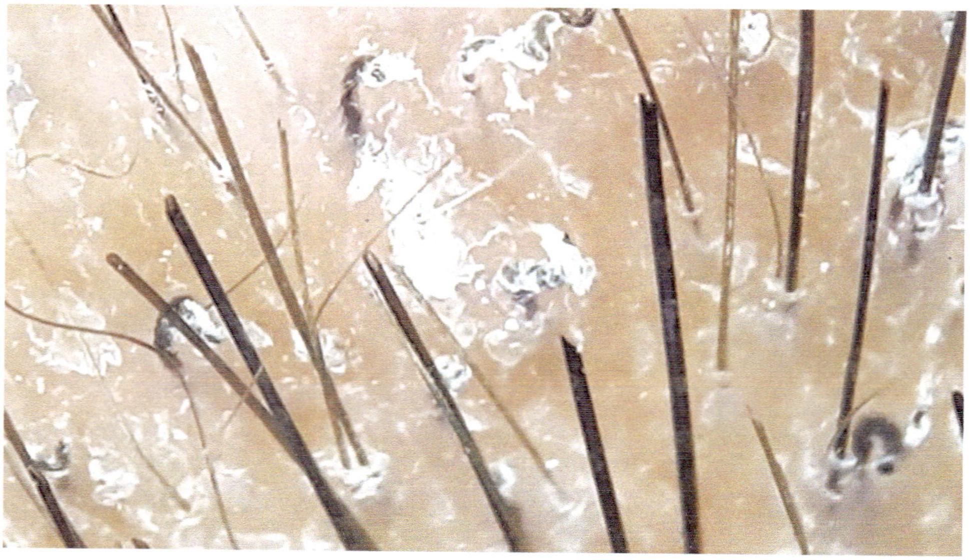

Fig. 2: Patchy alopecia with multiple comma hairs are evident. Bending of the short hairs (comma hairs) is due to partial damage to hair shafts by ectothrix parasitation. Comma hairs retain their normal thickness and color.

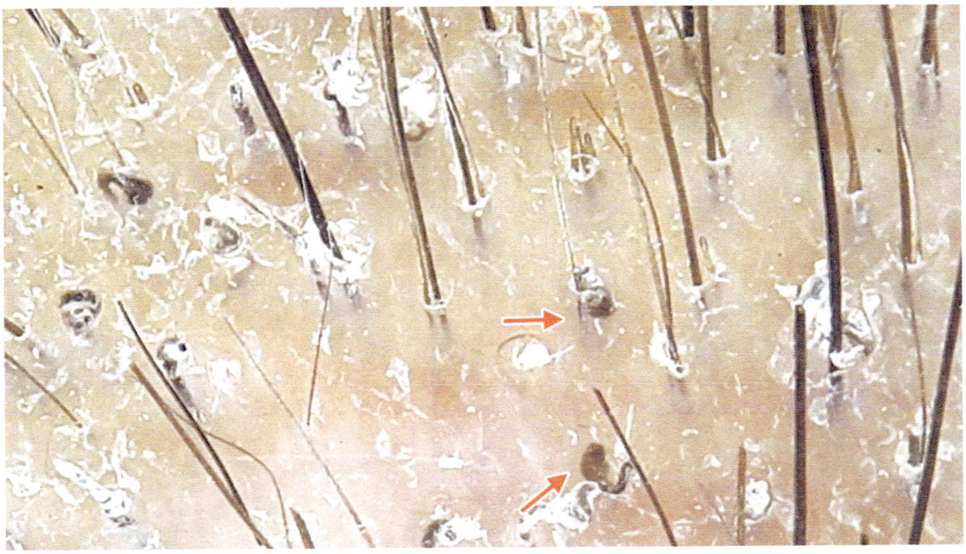

Fig. 3: Corkscrew hairs (arrows): They are short hairs which appear spiral on trichoscopy. They can be distinguished from comma hairs by their multiple twists.

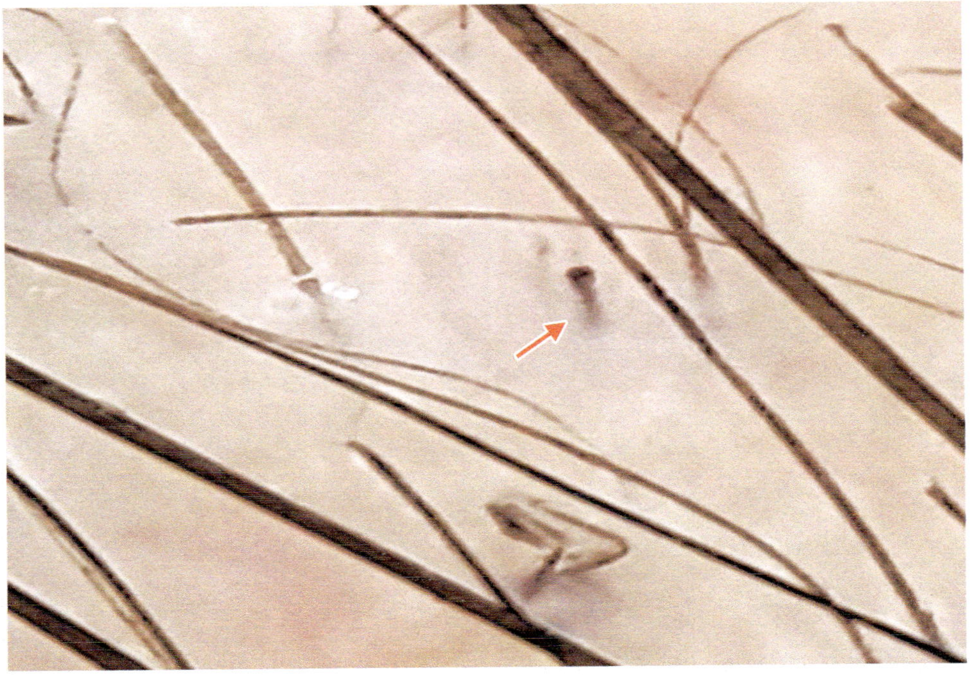

Fig. 4: "i-hair" (arrow) in tinea capitis: i-hair is a short broken hair that looks like the alphabet "I".[9] A corkscrew hair is also present in the field.

MORSE CODE HAIRS[7,8]

- They are a specific trichoscopic feature of fungal infection of scalp and eyebrow.
- *Polarized trichoscopy*: Horizontal white bands **(Fig. 5)**
- *Ultraviolet dermoscopy*: Fluorescence disappearing at the bands
- *Microscopy*: Numerous spores at the thinner fragment
- *Mechanism of formation of morse code hairs*: Horizontal bands correspond to localized areas of fungal infection, which result in hair perforation.

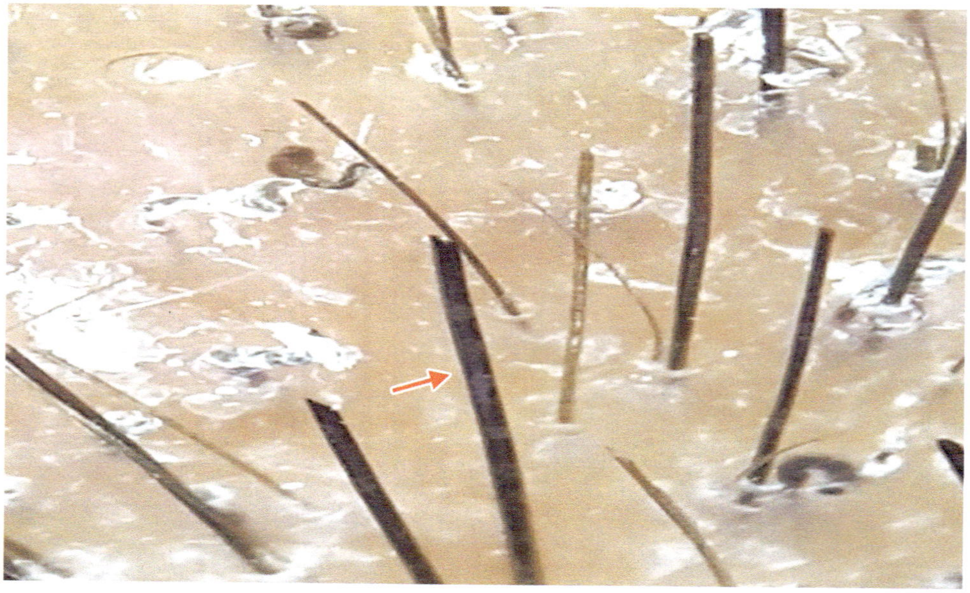

Fig. 5: "Morse code" hairs (arrow): Horizontal white bands present in a regular distribution along the hair shaft.

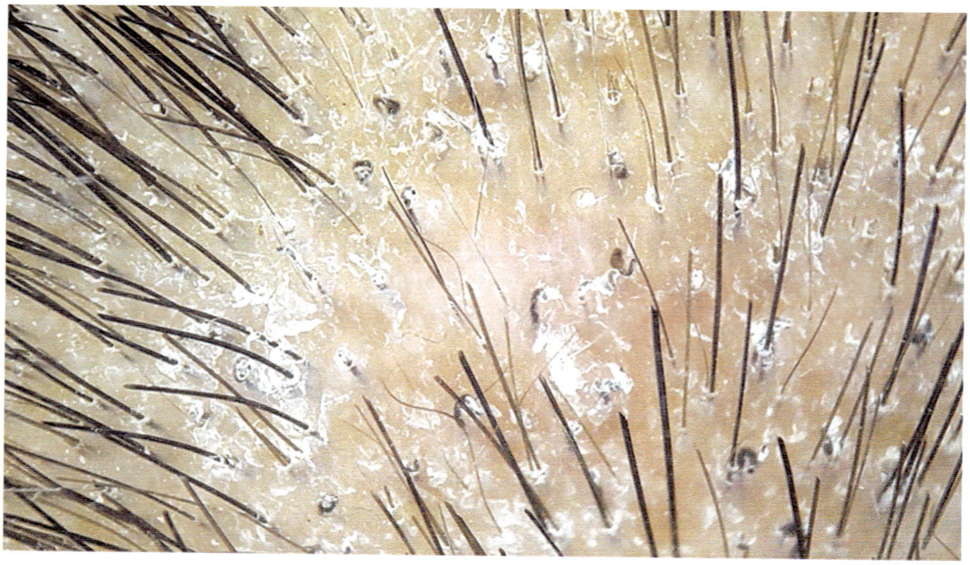

Fig. 6: Tinea capitis showing multiple comma and corkscrew hairs.

REFERENCES

1. Grimalt R. A practical guide to scalp disorders. J Investig Dermatol Symp Proc. 2007;12(2):10-4.
2. Mebazaa A, Oumari KE, Ghariani N, Mili AF, Belajouza C, Nouira R, et al. Tinea capitis in adults in Tunisia. Int J Dermatol. 2010;49(5):513-6.
3. Ilkit M. Favus of the scalp: an overview and update. Mycopathologia. 2010;170(3):143-54.
4. Tangjaturonrusamee C, Piraccini BM, Vincenzi C, Starace M, Tosti A. Tinea capitis mimicking folliculitis decalvans. Mycoses. 2011;54:87-8.
5. Hughes R, Chiaverini C, Bahadoran P, Lacour JP. Corkscrew hair: A new dermoscopic sign for diagnosis of tinea capitis in black children. Arch Dermatol. 2011;147:355-6.
6. Slowinska M, Rudnicka L, Schwartz RA, Kowalska-Oledzka E, Rakowska A, Sicinska J, et al. Comma hairs: a dermoscopic marker for tinea capitis; A rapid diagnostic method. J Am Acad Dermatol. 2008;59(suppl):S77-9.
7. Lin YT, Li YC. The dermoscopic comma, zigzag, and bar code-like hairs: markers of fungal infection of the hair follicles. Dermatologica Sinica. 2014;32(3):160-3.
8. Wang HH, Lin YT. Bar code-like hair: dermoscopic marker of tinea capitis and tinea of the eyebrow. J Am Acad Dermatol. 2015;72(1):S41-S42.
9. Rudnicka L, Szepietowski JC, Slowinska M. Tinea capitis. In: Rudnicka L, Olszewska M, Rakowska A (eds). Atlas of trichoscopy. London: Springer; 2012. pp. 367.

ASSESSMENT QUESTIONS

1. Mention two common trichoscopic features of tinea capitis.
2. Morse code hairs are specific trichoscopic features of fungal infection of scalp. What is its mechanism of formation?

ANSWERS

1. Comma hair and corkscrew hair.
2. Horizontal white bands of morse code hairs correspond to the areas of fungal infection, which result in hair perforation.

CHAPTER

26

Pediculosis Capitis

Subrata Malakar

INTRODUCTION

- Infestation of *Pediculus capitis* (*Pediculus humanus* var *capitis*) is common and can easily be diagnosed clinically upon close examination.
- Diagnostic signs of head lice infestation are lice and/or nits. Nonetheless, it may be time consuming and nits may be confused with pseudonits (scales of different origin).[1]
- Trichoscopy allows straightforward identification of head lice and nits and also can differentiate nit (louse egg) and nit cast (empty egg).
- As trichoscopy can assess the viability of the contents of the nits, it can be used to monitor the treatment efficacy.

KEY TRICHOSCOPIC FEATURES

- *Nit*: Louse egg attached to hair shaft.
- *Nit cast*: Empty egg appearing as a translucent structure fixed to a hair shaft.
- Head louse

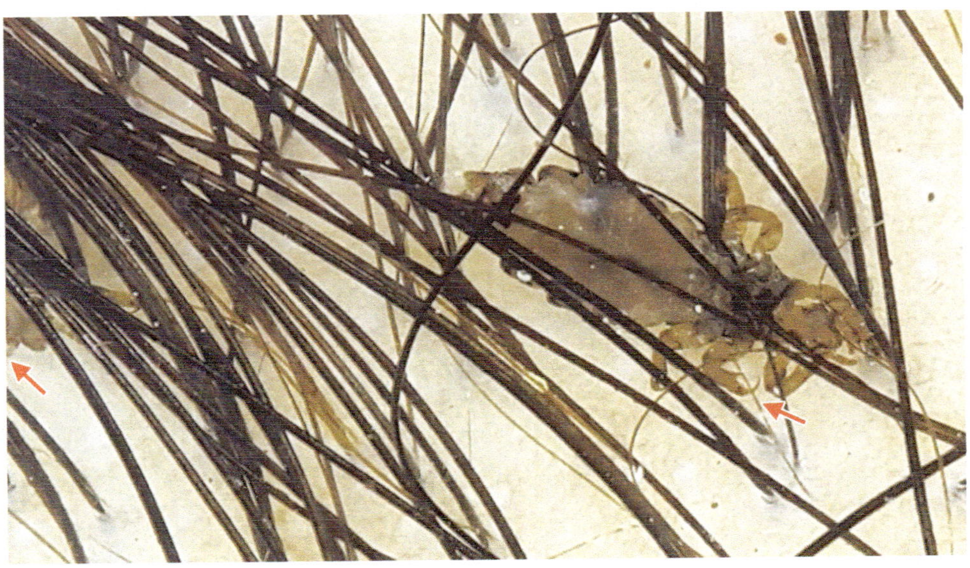

Fig. 1: Adult head lice are dorsoventrally flattened and wingless. One pair of antennae protrude from the insects' head; Segments of the antenna are clearly visible (arrow). Six legs project from the thorax. These legs terminate with a single claw and opposing thumb. Between its claw and the thumb, the louse grasps the hair of the host (arrow).

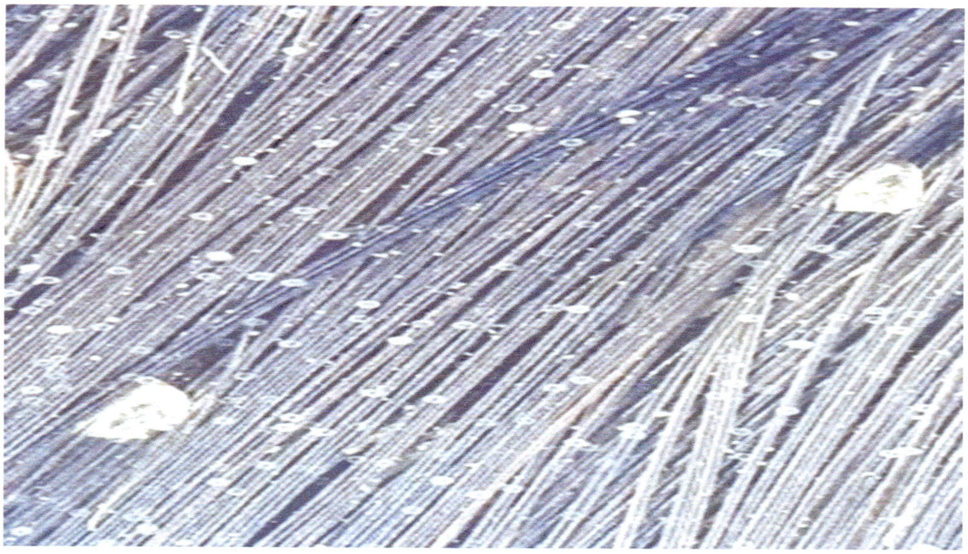

Fig. 2: Nit cast: Empty egg appearing as a translucent structure fixed to a hair shaft.[2]

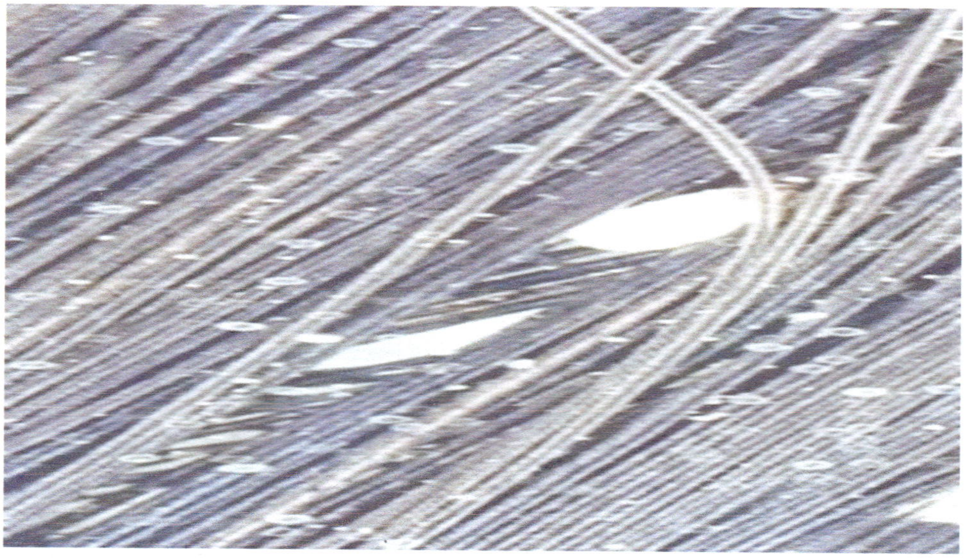

Fig. 3: Nit: Louse egg attached to hair shaft.[2]

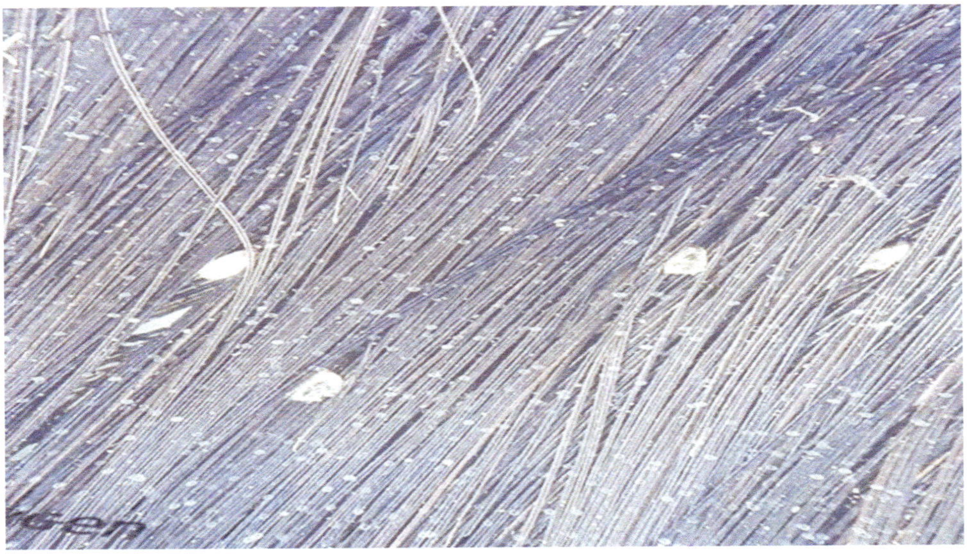

Fig. 4: In this trichoscopic field, both nits and nit casts are seen attached to hair shafts.

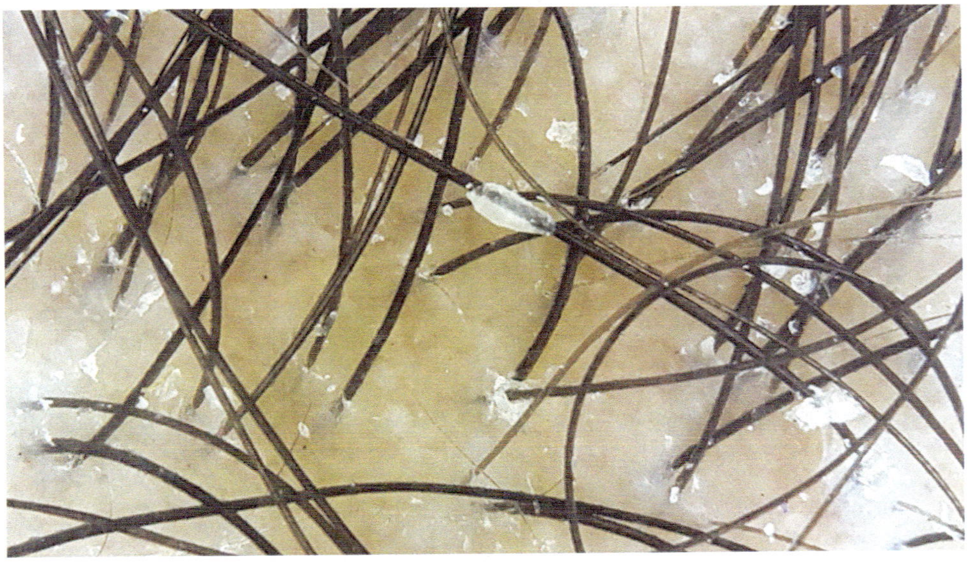

Fig. 5: Pseudonits: They are scales of different origins. At the center is a pseudonit which encircles the hair shaft, whereas a nit does not encircle the shaft but is attached to one side of the shaft.[3] Single scales and yellowish background are clues to diagnosis of seborrhoeic capitis.

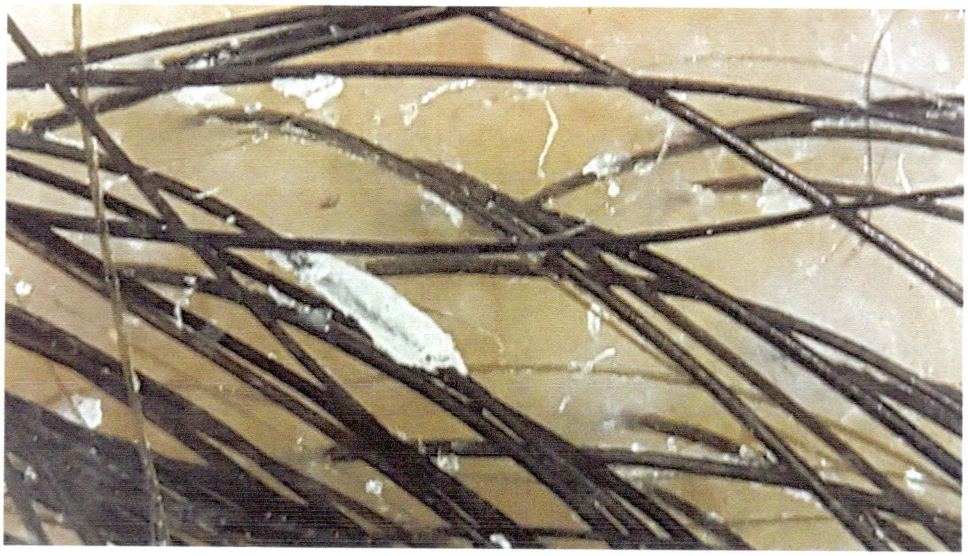

Fig. 6: Pseudonit: Close-up view.

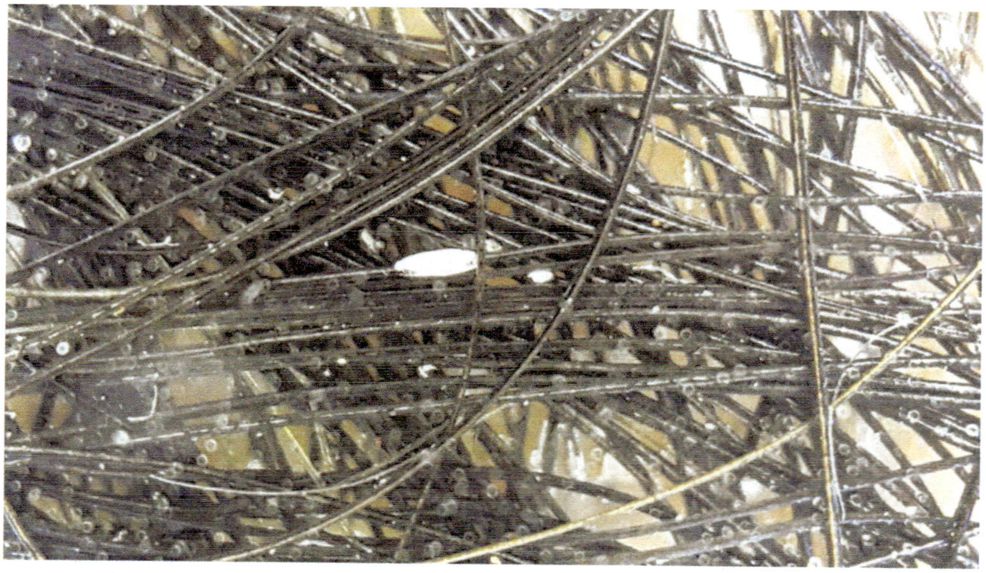

Fig. 7: A nit is attached to one side of hair shaft which differentiates it from a pseudonit shown in this image.

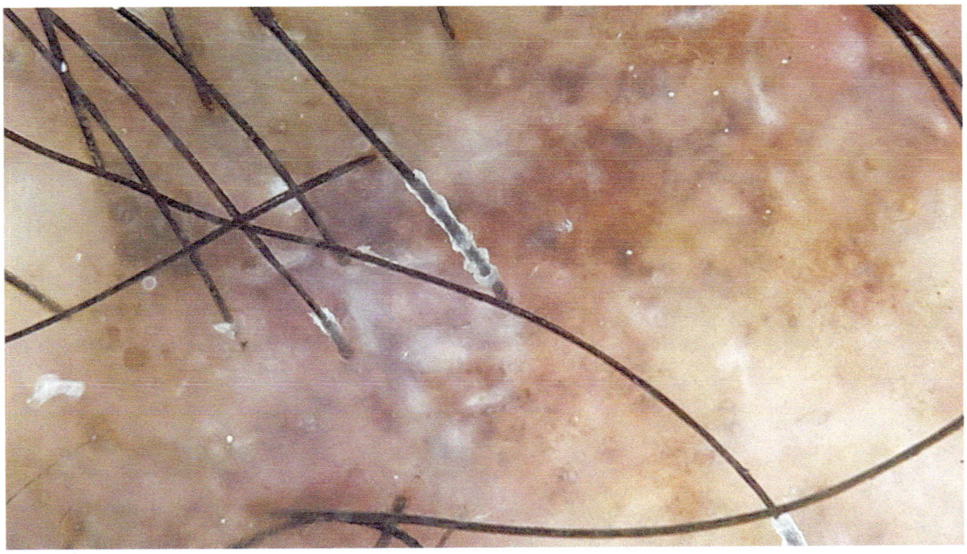

Fig. 8: Nits should also be differentiated from hair casts. Hair casts may be an important feature of scarring alopecia and they surround hair shafts. Other features of scarring alopecia are present in this image.

REFERENCES

1. Micali G, Lacarrubba F, Massimino D, Schwartz RA. Dermatoscopy: Alternative uses in daily clinical practice. J Am Acad Dermatol. 2011;64:1135-46.
2. Bowling J. General dermatology. In: Bowling J, (Ed). Diagnostic Dermoscopy. Oxford: Wiley; 2012. pp. 123.
3. Lacarrubba F, Dinotta F, Micali G. Parasitic scalp infections. In: Rudnicka L, Olszewska M, Rakowska A (Eds). Atlas of Trichoscopy. London: Springer; 2012. pp. 357.

ASSESSMENT IMAGE-BASED QUESTIONS

1. Name the insect and mention the trichoscopic diagnostic clue of these infestations.

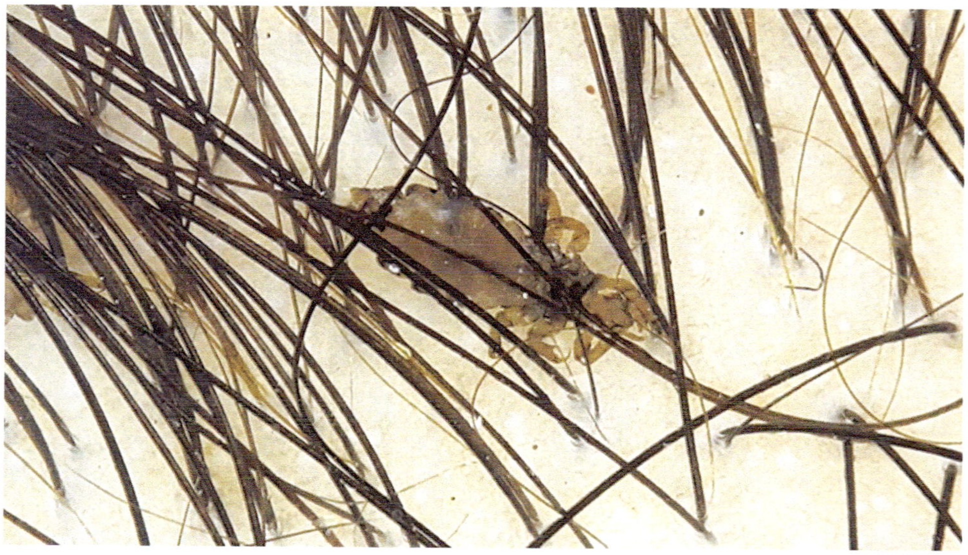

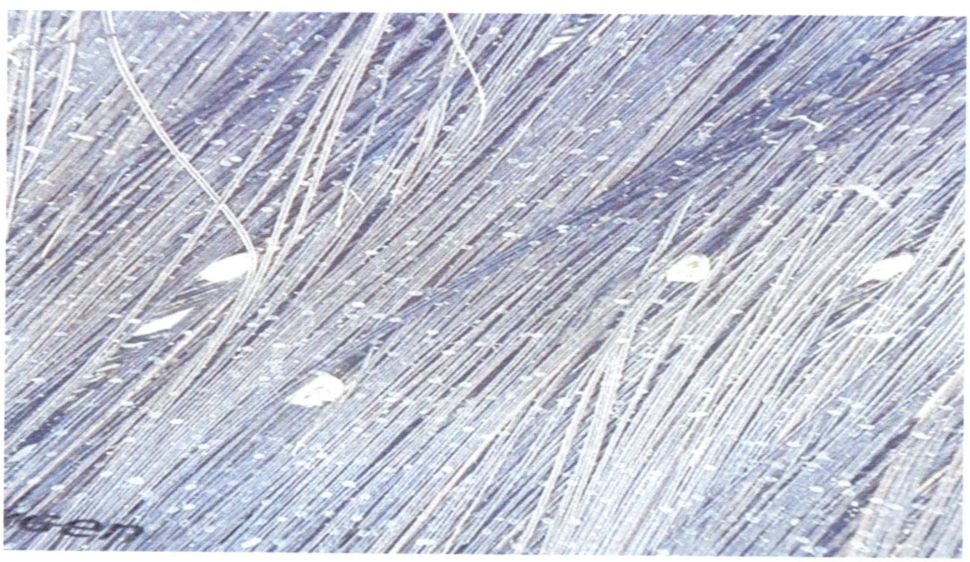

2. Nits are visible in this image. What is the main trichoscopic differential diagnosis of the nits?

ANSWERS

1. Head louse (*Pediculus humanus capitis*). Diagnostic clues are lice or nits or both.
2. Pseudonits or scales of different origins.

CHAPTER 27

Scalp Psoriasis, Seborrheic Dermatitis, and Sebopsoriasis

Subrata Malakar

SCALP PSORIASIS, SEBORRHEIC CAPITIS, AND SEBOPSORIASIS

INTRODUCTION

- Psoriasis is a chronic, multifactorial inflammatory disease associated with other disorders that fall under the term "metabolic syndrome".
- Scalp psoriasis causes scaling and itching with a clinical picture that closely mimics seborrheic dermatitis.
- Scalp can often be the only site of involvement in psoriasis.
- The lesions frequently spread over the anterior hair line onto the forehead.
- The diagnosis of scalp psoriasis is usually clinical. Rarely, histopathology is required for diagnosis.
- In patients with scalp psoriasis, seborrheic dermatitis commonly coexists. An overlap between them is known as sebopsoriasis.[1]
- Seborrheic capitis is characterized by scaling and poorly defined erythematous patches. Young adult men are affected more often than women.
- One hypothesis about its etiopathogenesis is that, it develops as an altered cutaneous response to *Malassezia* species or their toxins, or to the free fatty acids produced by the *Malassezia* species.[2]

KEY TRICHOSCOPIC FEATURES

- Psoriasis is a chronic, multifactorial inflammatory disease associated with other disorders that fall under the term "metabolic syndrome".
- Scalp psoriasis causes scaling and itching with a clinical picture that closely mimics seborrheic dermatitis.
- Scalp can often be the only site of involvement in psoriasis.
- The lesions frequently spread over the anterior hair line onto the forehead.
- The diagnosis of scalp psoriasis is usually clinical. Rarely, histopathology is required for diagnosis.
- In patients with scalp psoriasis, seborrheic dermatitis commonly coexists. An overlap between them is known as sebopsoriasis.[1]
- Seborrheic capitis is characterized by scaling and poorly defined erythematous patches. Young adult men are affected more often than women.
- One hypothesis about its etiopathogenesis is that, it develops as an altered cutaneous response to *Malassezia* species or their toxins, or to the free fatty acids produced by the *Malassezia* species.[2]
- Trichoscopy can differentiate scalp psoriasis from scalp seborrheic dermatitis depending on the vascular patterns.[3]
- *Scalp psoriasis*: Red dots and globules, twisted red loops, and glomerular vessels. Dots appear as twisted red loops on higher magnification.[2]
- *Seborrheic capitis*: Arborizing vessels and atypical red vessels in the absence of red dots and globules.[4]
- *Scales of scalp psoriasis*: Thick and silvery
- *Scales of seborrheic dermatitis*: Yellow and greasy

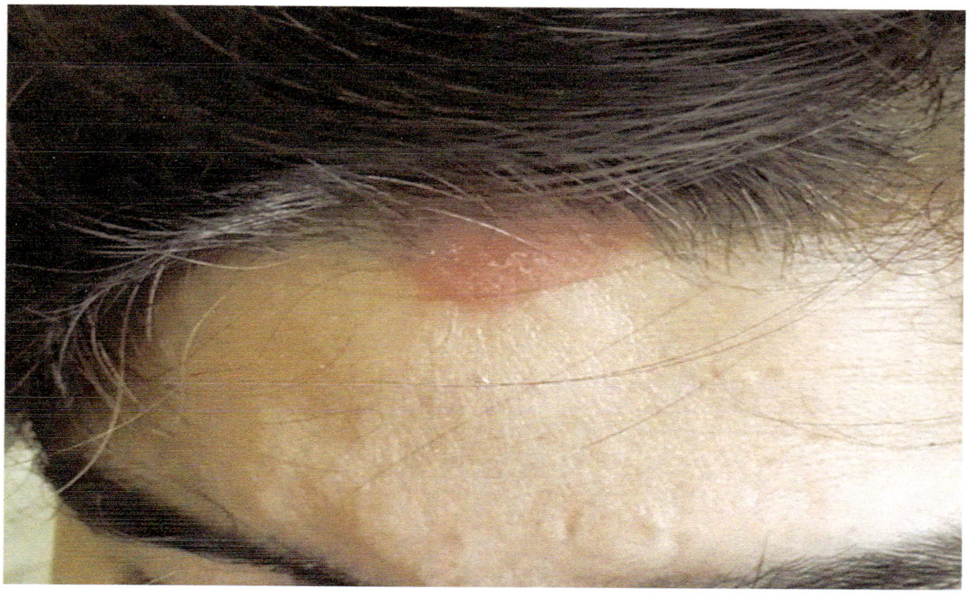

Fig. 1: Sharply bordered erythematous lesion covered by silvery-white scales is characteristic of psoriasis. The lesions spread frequently onto the forehead. Pruritus may be moderate to severe.

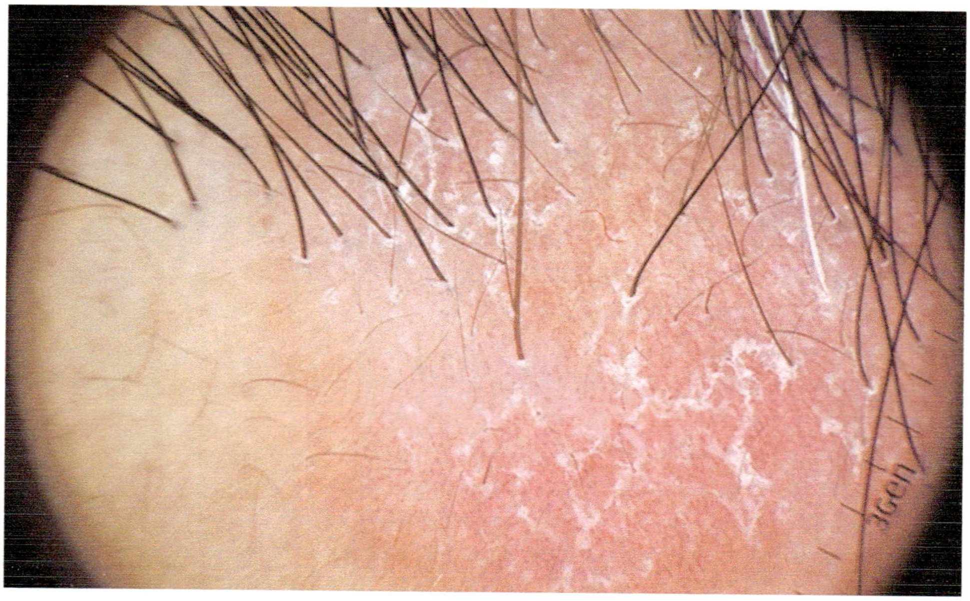

Fig. 2: On trichoscopy, regular red dots and globules are observed at low magnification in psoriasis.

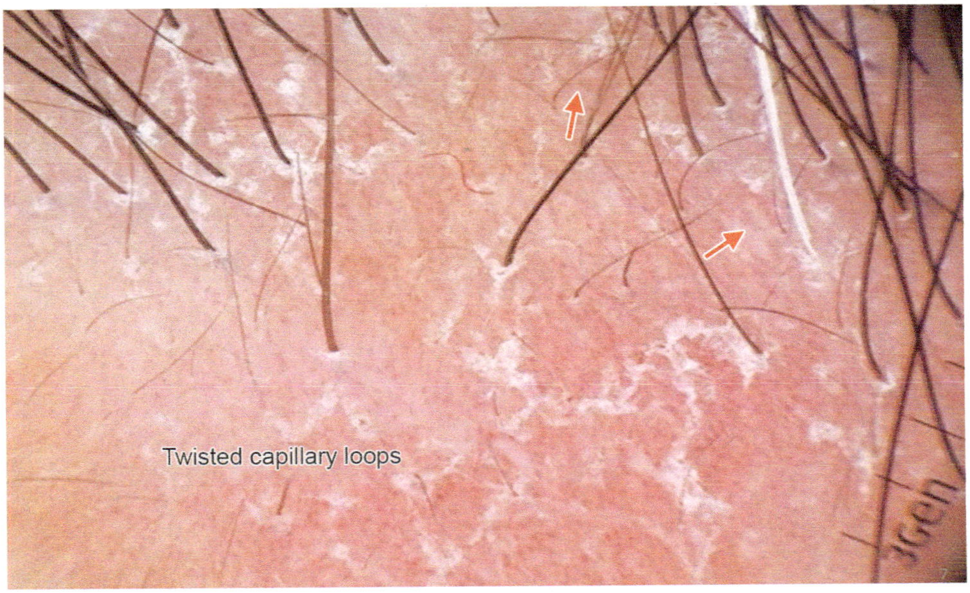

Fig. 3: After zooming or on higher magnification, red dots and globules appear as twisted capillary loops (arrow).

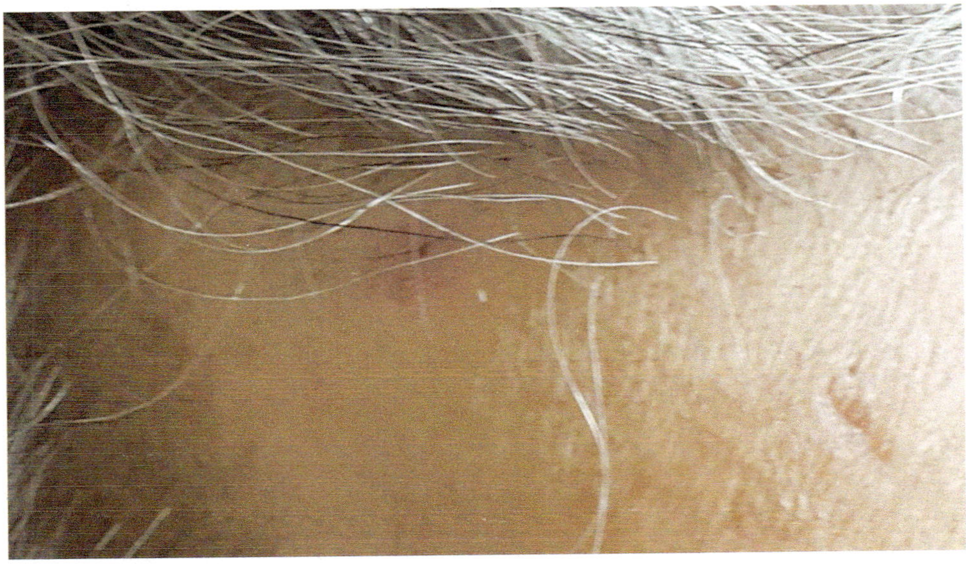

Fig. 4: A small plaque of scalp psoriasis.

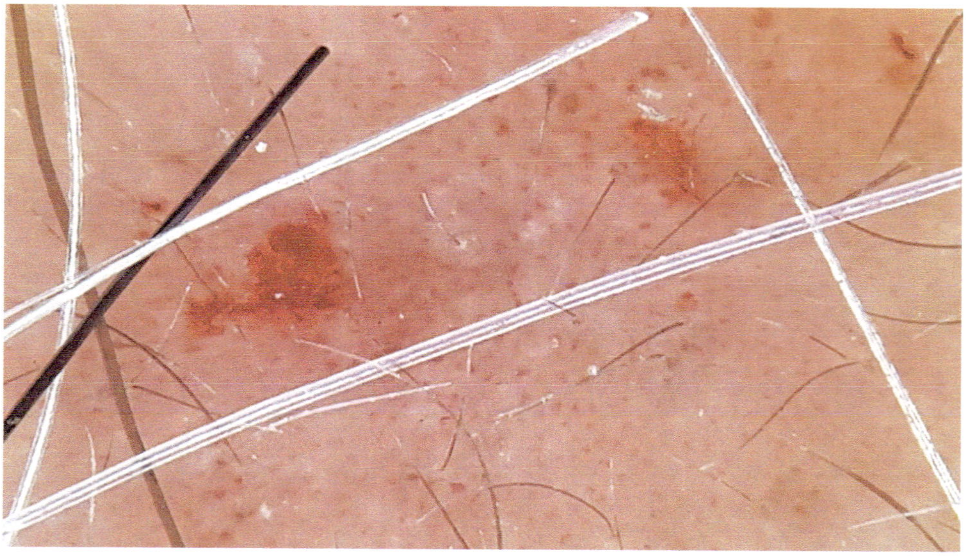

Fig. 5: Trichoscopy of the previous patient: Regularly distributed twisted capillary loops are seen. The vascular patterns such as red dots and globules, and twisted capillary loops differentiate psoriasis from seborrheic capitis where arborizing vessels and atypical vessels are seen. Extravasation of blood, a feature of psoriasis, is also present in this trichoscopic field.

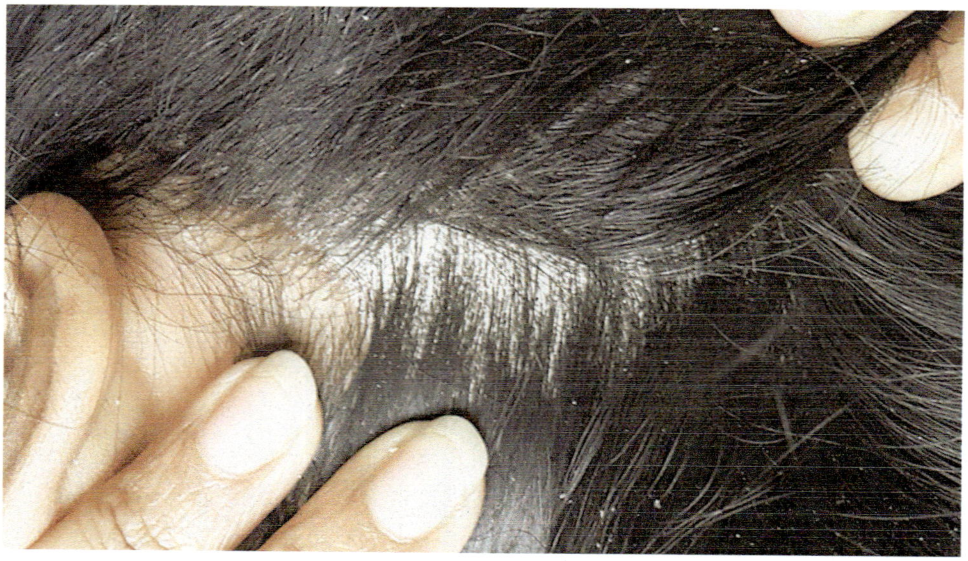

Fig. 6: Sometimes clinical differentiation between psoriasis and seborrheic capitis may be difficult.

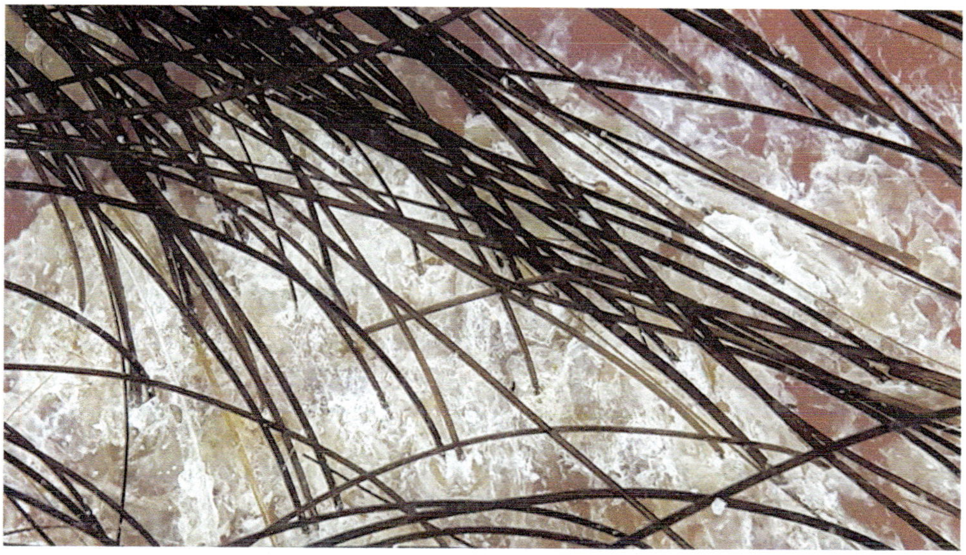

Fig. 7: Diffuse white, feathery scaling is a characteristic though not a specific finding of scalp psoriasis.

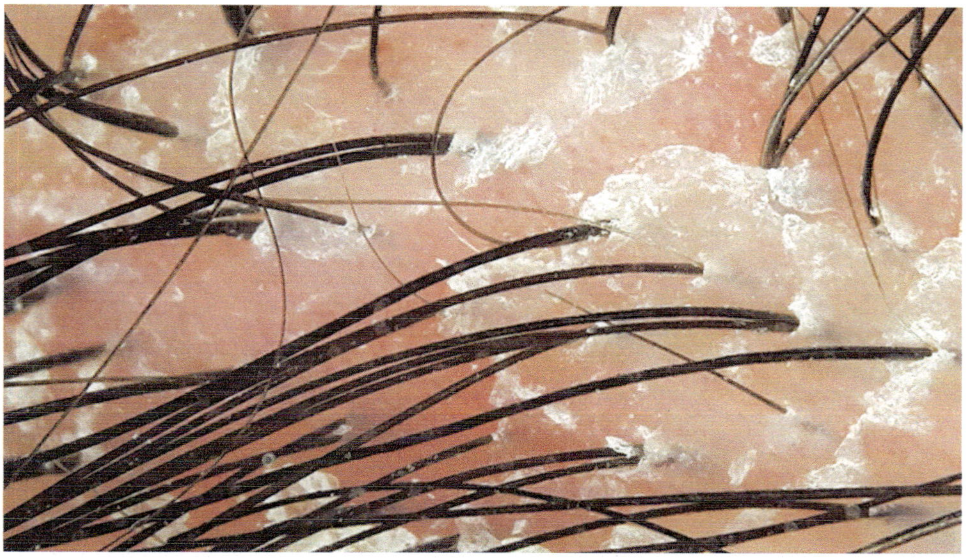

Fig. 8: Large sheets of white silvery scales, extravasation of blood, and twisted capillaries are seen. After removal of sheets of scales, more vascular patterns will be visible. The scales can be removed after approximately 2 weeks of treatment with keratolytics (such as salicylic acid) along with topical corticosteroids.

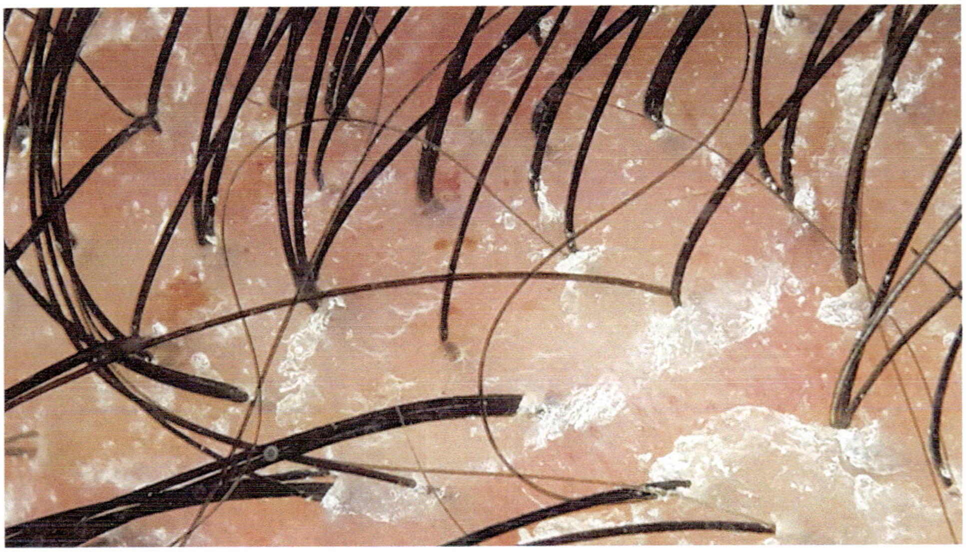

Fig. 9: In psoriasis, extravasation of blood is usually circular or oval in shape[5] that differentiates it from post-traumatic extravasation. Note the presence of silvery-white scales.

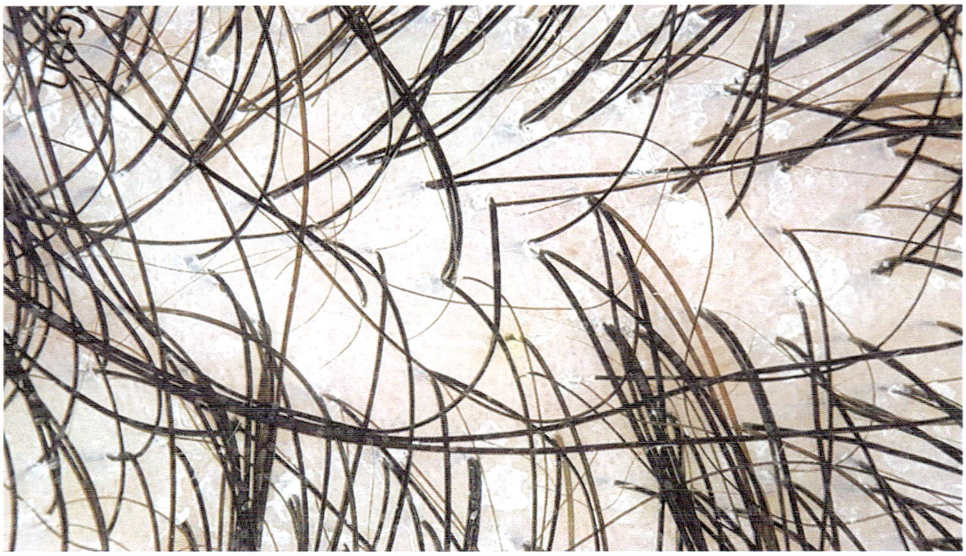

Fig. 10: Extensive interfollicular silvery-white scales in psoriasis. Red dots and globules are arranged regularly. Perifollicular scales and hair casts are rarely seen. Unlike seborrheic capitis, discrimination of single scale is not always possible.

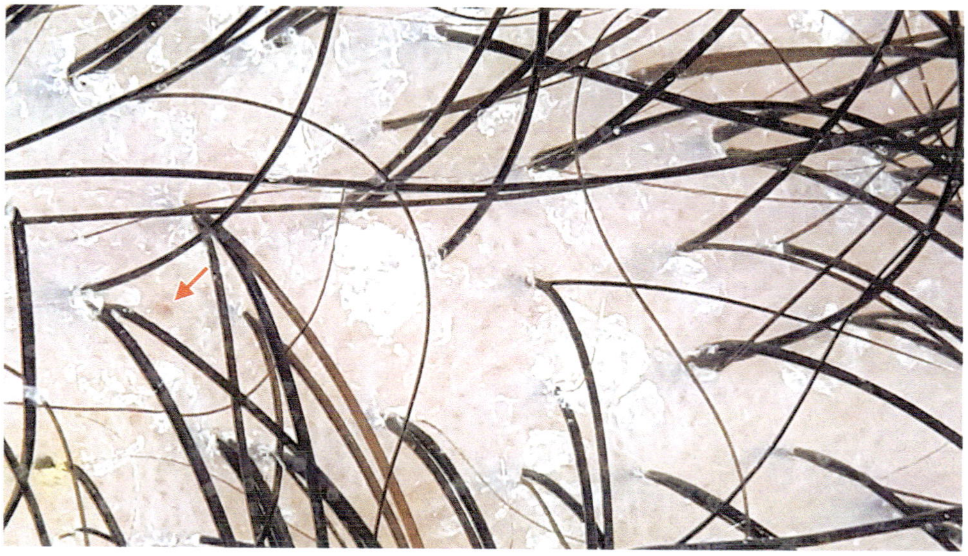

Fig. 11: White silvery scales distinguish psoriasis from seborrheic capitis. Scaling is extensive and interfollicular. In active psoriasis, often there is extravasation of blood (arrow). Twisted capillaries are seen in nonscaly areas.

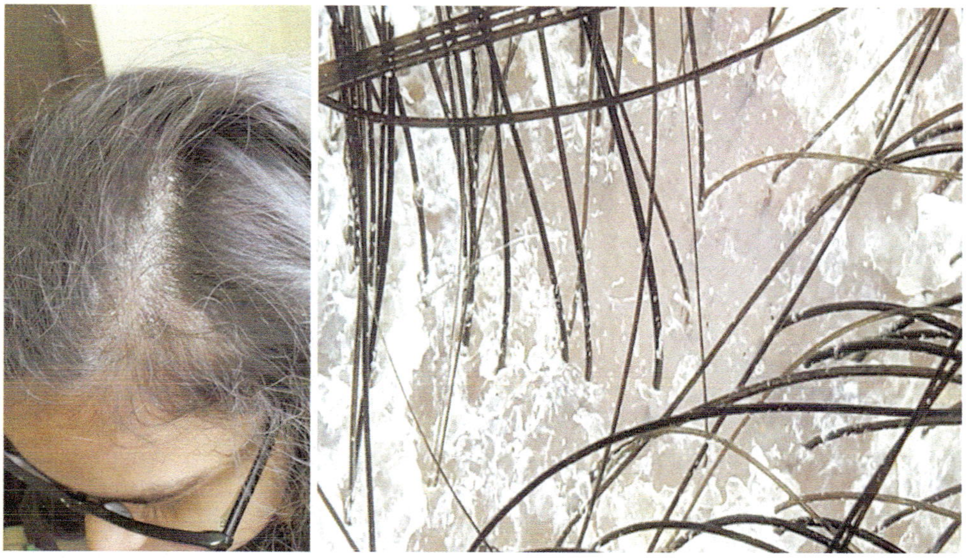

Fig. 12: Erythematous, moderate-to-severe scaly patch with an ill-defined margin is the characteristic clinical picture of seborrheic capitis. Scales in some areas appear slightly yellow trichoscopically.

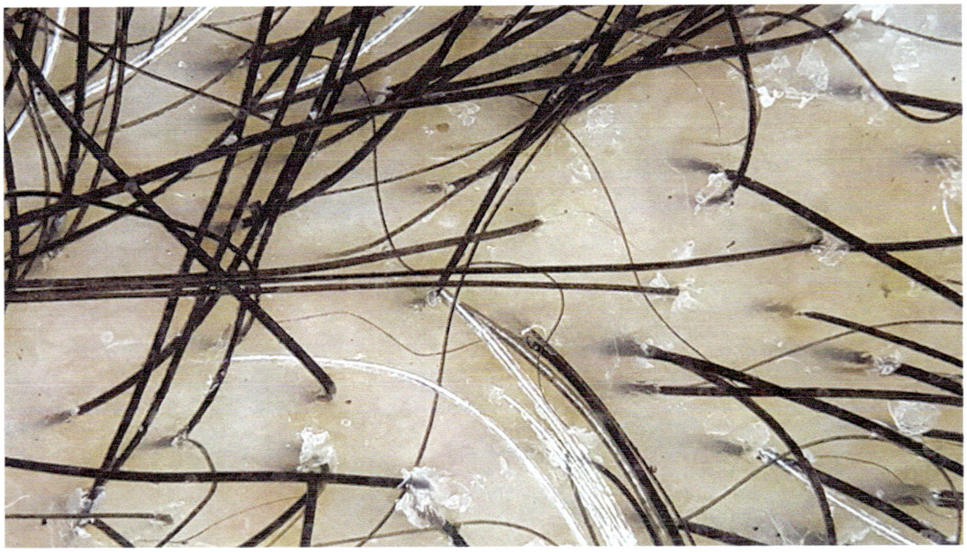

Fig. 13: Yellowish background in seborrheic capitis. Mostly single scales are present.

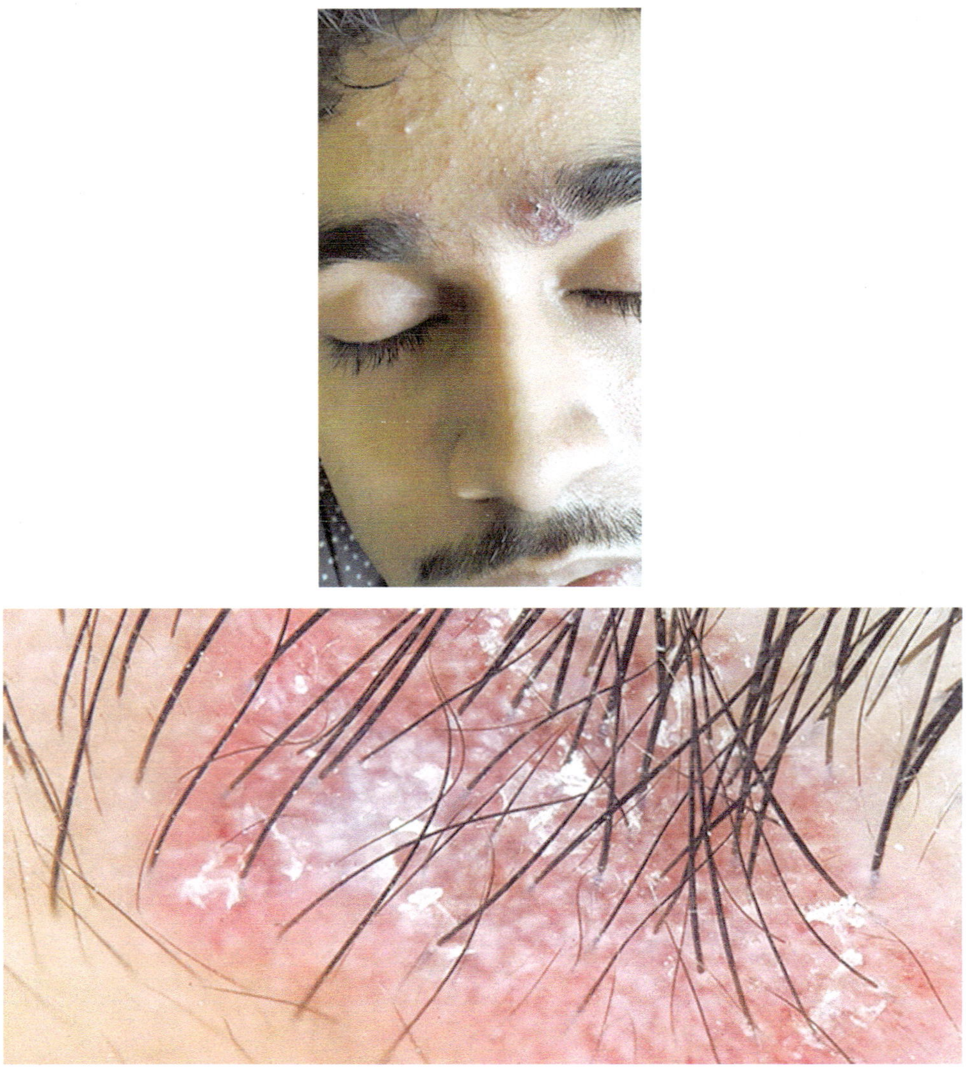

Fig. 14: Seborrheic dermatitis of eyelid: Perifollicular and interfollicular scales with erythema at the background.

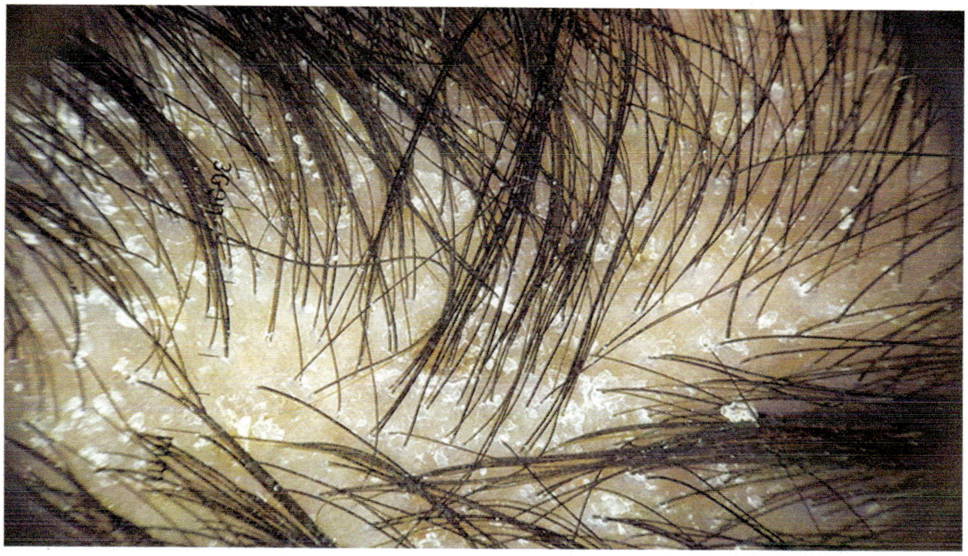

Fig. 15: Yellowish scales in diffuse distribution in a case of seborrheic capitis. Single scales and clusters of scales are present.

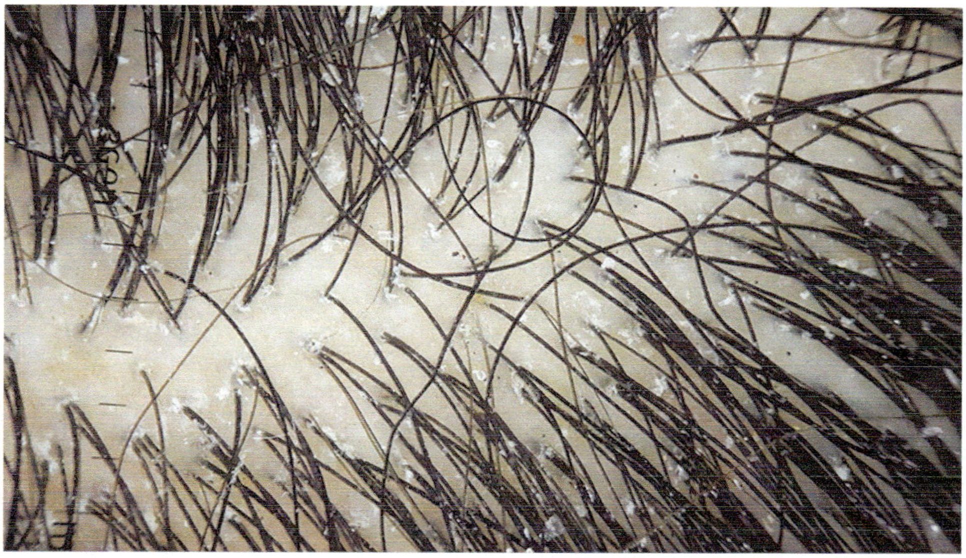

Fig. 16: Mostly single scales are visible on a slightly yellowish background. Scales are also visible over the hair shafts.

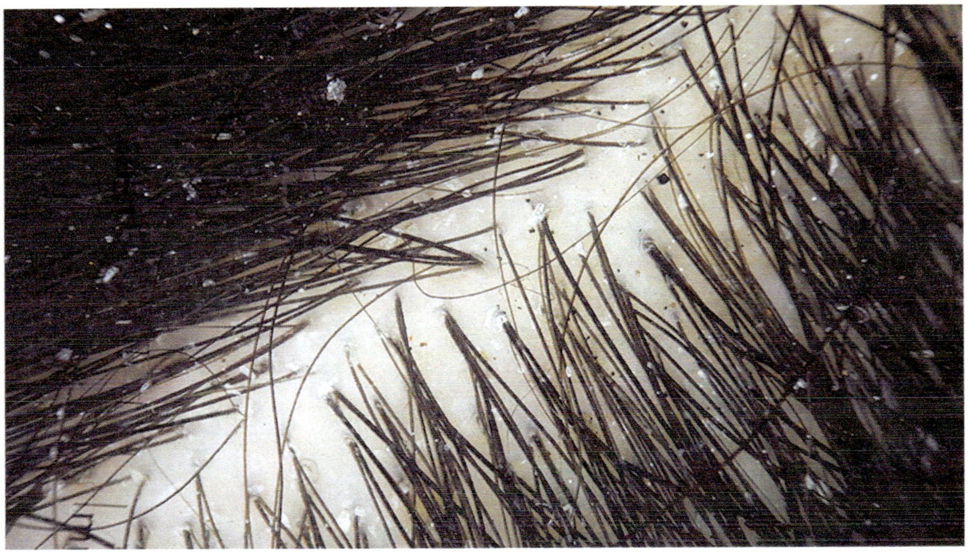

Fig. 17: Moderate scaling mostly seen over hair shafts as well as in the interfollicular areas in a case of seborrheic capitis. Note the presence of dirty dots which are environmental particles.

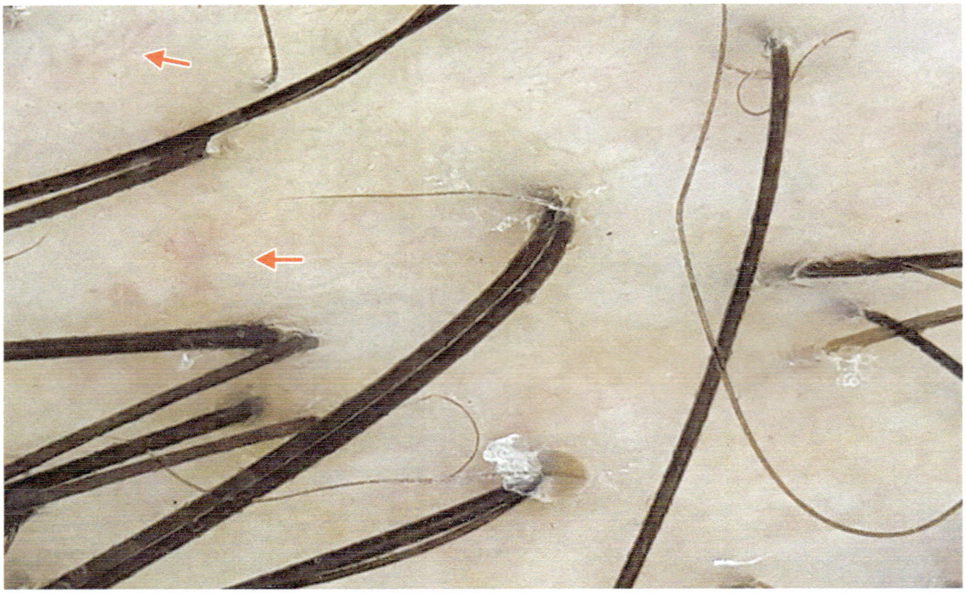

Fig. 18: Scaling in seborrheic capitis may be very mild. Note the presence of thin arborizing vessels and slightly yellowish background.

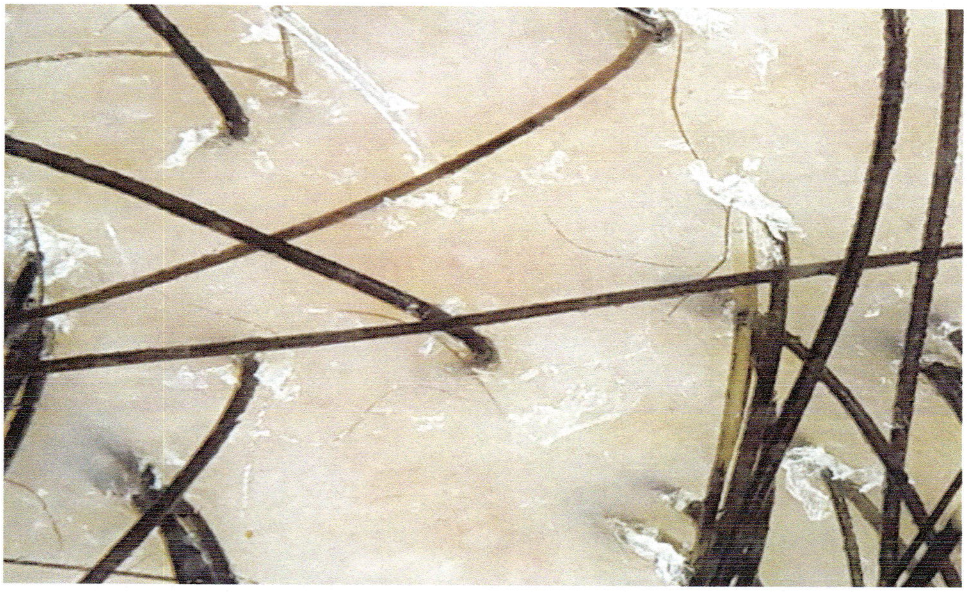

Fig. 19: Multiple dotted, comma, very small arborizing and linear vessels are seen in this image. This multicomponent vascular pattern.[6] is highly characteristic of seborrheic capitis. This differs from psoriasis where a regular, homogeneous vascular pattern is observed.

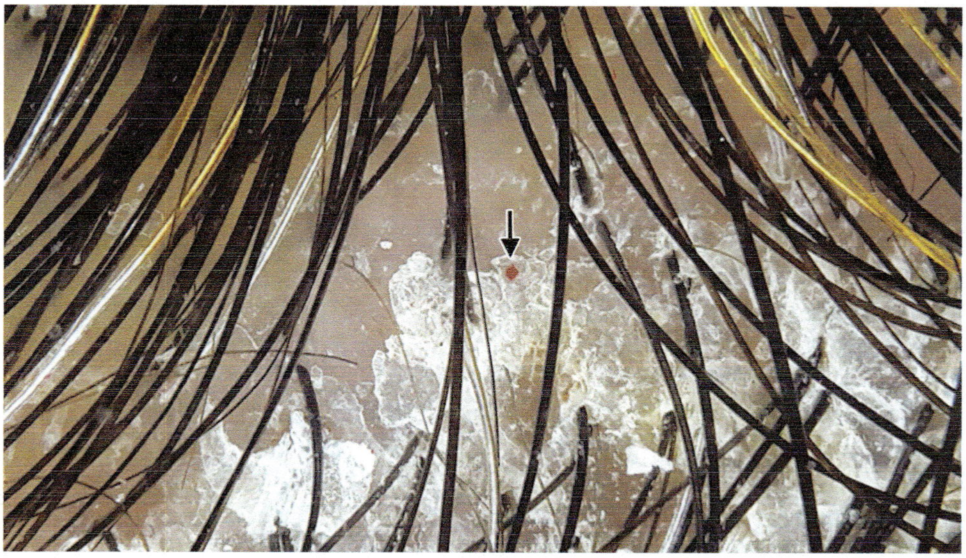

Fig. 20: In sebopsoriasis, yellow greasy scales as well as silvery white scales are present. Extravasation of blood is also seen. In psoriasis, extravasation of blood is usually circular or oval in shape[5] which differentiates it from post-traumatic extravasation.

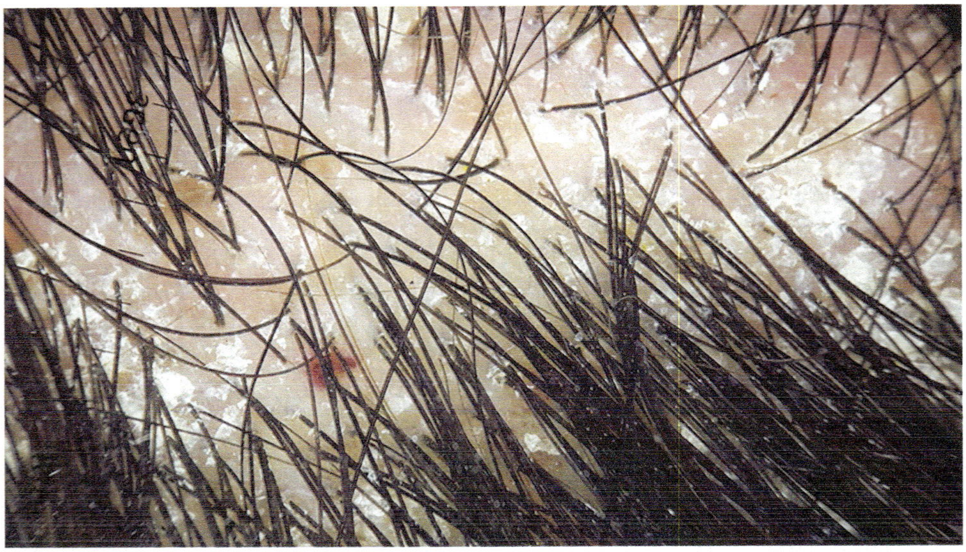

Fig. 21: In this case of sebopsoriasis, both silvery white scales and yellow scales are present.[7] Extravasation of blood which is circular in shape is seen indicating a psoriatic component.

REFERENCES

1. Wozel G, Klein E, Mrowietz U, Reich K, Sebastian M, Streit V. Scalp psoriasis. J Dtsch Dematol Ges. 2011;9(1):70-4.
2. Kim GK. Seborrhoeic dermatitis and Malassezia species: How are they related? J Clin Aesthet Dermatol. 2009;2(11):14-7.
3. Ross EK, Vincenzi C, Tosti A. Videodermatoscopy in the evaluation of hair and scalp disorders. J Am Acad Dermatol. 2006;55:799-806.
4. Kim GW, Jung HJ, Ko HC, Kim MB, Lee WJ, Lee SJ, et al. Dermatoscopy can be useful in differntiating scalp psoriasis from seborrhoeic dermatitis. Br J Dermatol. 2011;164:652-6.
5. Rudnicka L, Rakowska A, Olszewska M, Sicinska J, Maj M, Majsterek M, et al. Psoriasis. In : Rudnicka L, Olszewska M, Rakowska A (Eds). Atlas of Trichoscopy. London: Springer; 2012. pp. 386.
6. Rudnicka L, Sicinska J, Rakowska A, Warszawik-Hendzel O. Seborrheic dermatitis. In: Rudnicka L, Olszewska M, Rakowska A (Eds). Atlas of Trichoscopy. London: Springer; 2012. pp. 376.
7. Vincenzi C, Tosti A. Inflammatory Scalp Disorders. In: Tosti A (Ed). Dermoscopy of the Hair and Nails. Boca Raton: CRC Press; 2016. pp. 114.

ASSESSMENT IMAGE-BASED QUESTIONS

1. What is your trichoscopic diagnosis? What are the points in favor of your diagnosis?

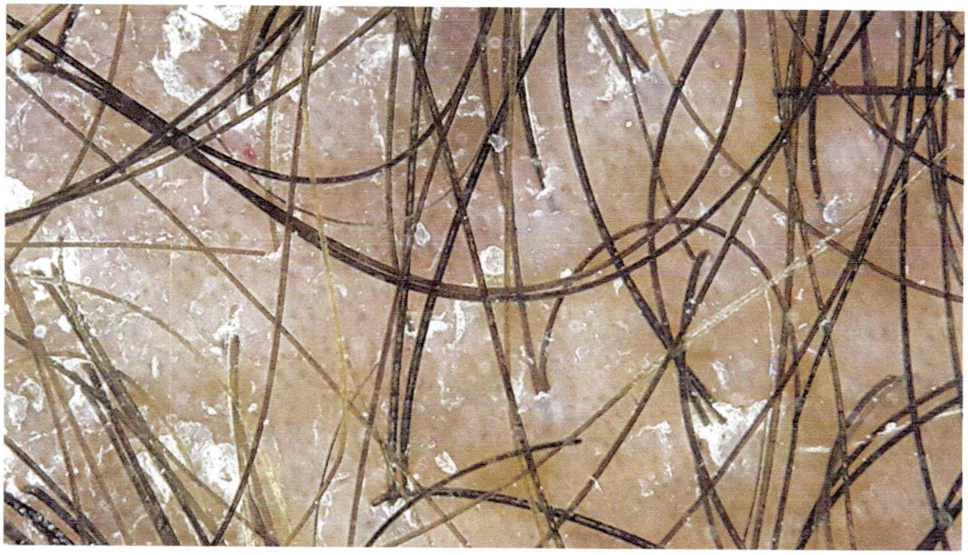

2. Trichoscopic diagnosis of sebopsoriasis is made on the basis of extravasation of blood, presence of silvery white scales and yellowish scales. What is the difference between psoriatic extravasation and traumatic extravasation of blood?

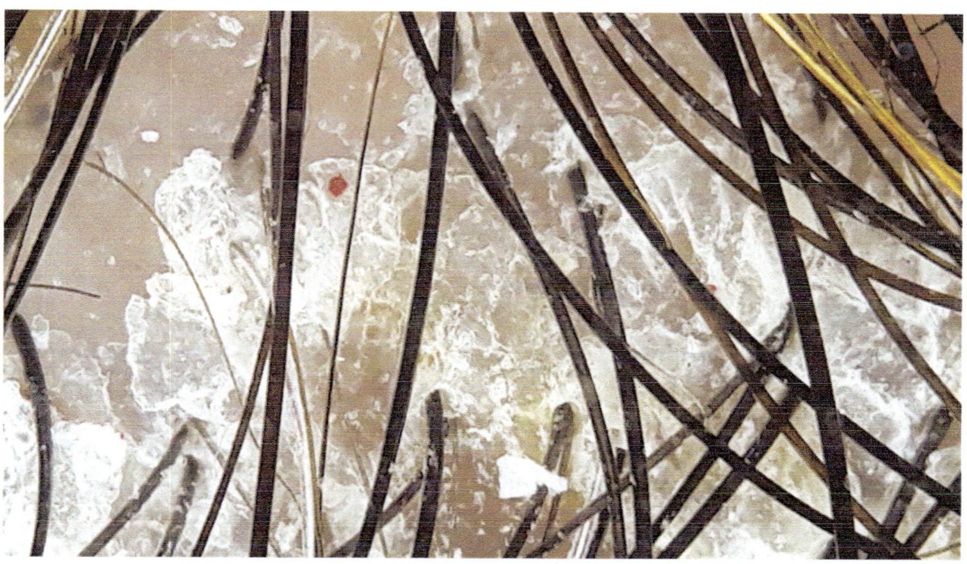

3. Some vascular patterns are seen in this image. In which scaly condition of the scalp this vascular pattern is found?

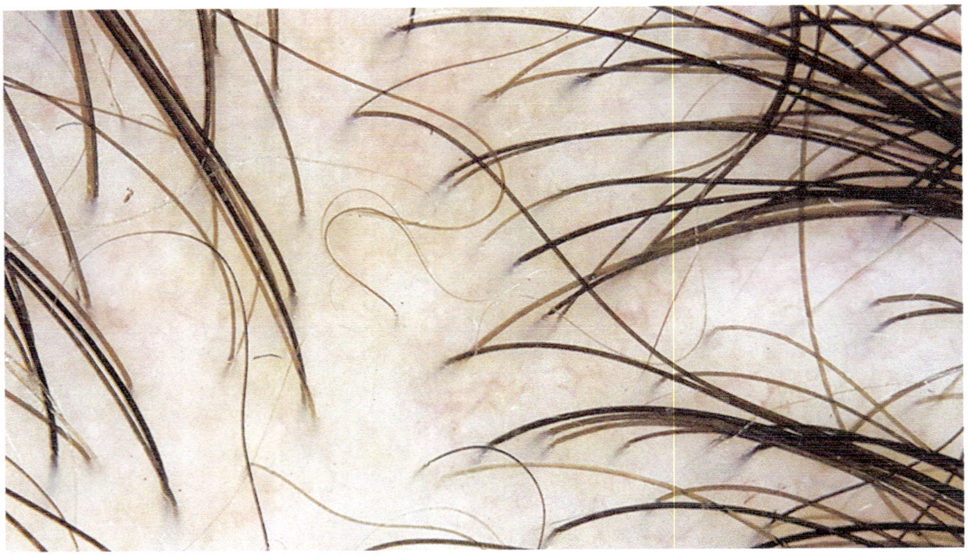

4. Single scales against a yellowish background are found in a particular inflammatory scalp disease. Name that condition.

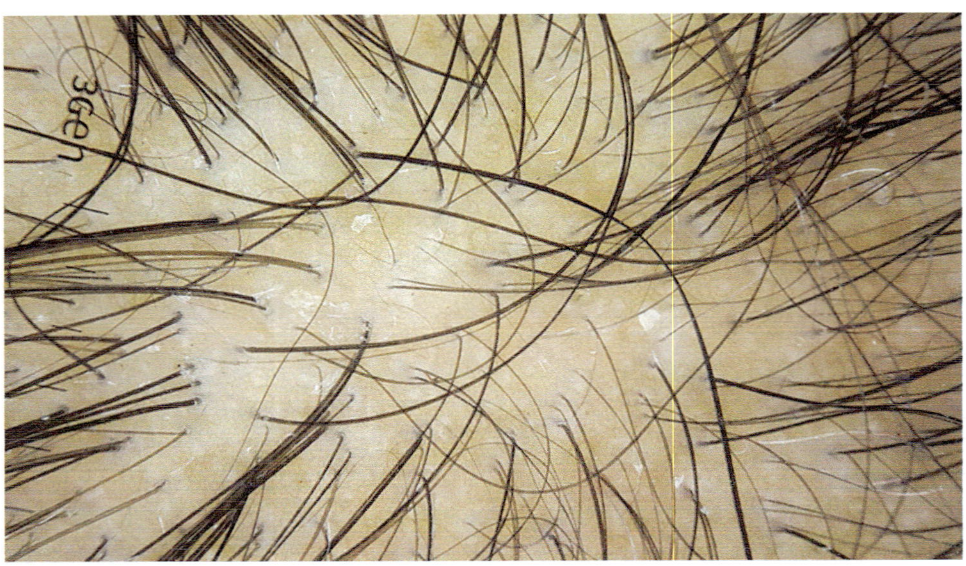

5. Large sheets of silvery white scales, single scales and yellowish scales on an erythematous background are visible. Name the condition.

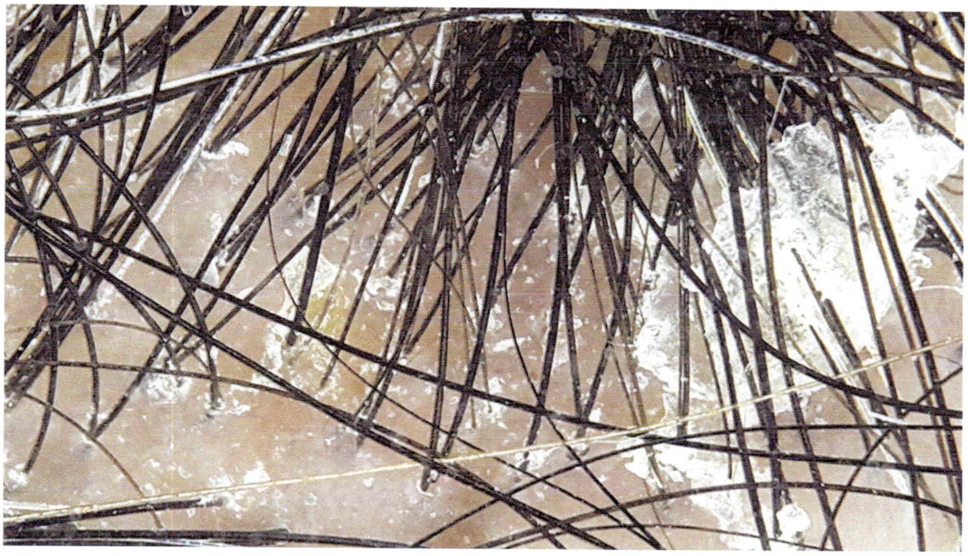

6. Silvery white scales and regularly distributed dots and globules are seen in this image. Identify the scalp condition.

ANSWERS

1. Psoriasis. Red dots, globules, and silvery white scales
2. Extravasation in psoriasis is circular or oval in shape whereas in mechanical trauma the shape is irregular.
3. This is seborrheic capitis where thin arborizing vessels are seen.
4. Seborrheic capitis
5. Sebopsoriasis
6. Psoriasis

CHAPTER 28

Trichoscopy in Autoimmune Bullous Disorders

Souvik Sardar, Subrata Malakar

INTRODUCTION

- This group of diseases clinically manifests with formation of spontaneous vesicles or bulla as the primary lesion in the skin and mucous membrane due to production of autoantibodies.
- Scalp may be involved in some of the variants but literatures on trichoscopic findings are very limited.
- It must be mentioned here that none of the trichoscopic features are pathognomonic for the diseases hence, patients presenting solely with scalp lesions are a diagnostic challenge.
- The common trichoscopic findings in some of the autoimmune bullous diseases with scalp manifestations have been discussed here.

PEMPHIGUS VULGARIS

Key Trichoscopic Features

- Polygonal hemorrhagic patches with sharp demarcation (recent lesions) correspond to the areas of erosion. This is the most consistent feature of pemphigus but not a specific one.[1]
- Large yellow dots with whitish halo correspond to blocked sebaceous gland openings by the detached epidermis giving a "fried-egg" appearance.[1]
- White lamellar structures correspond to areas of detached epidermis.[1]
- Vessels—dotted vessels with whitish halo, elongated serpentine vessels,[1] linear helical vessels, glomerular vessels, and lace-like vessels[2] may be found.
- Yellow hemorrhagic crusts, if found, is an indication for antibiotic therapy.[2]
- Hair casts—hair shafts encircled by hair casts may be seen in immediate perilesional areas due to acantholysis of the outer root sheath (ORS) keratinocytes drawn outside the follicular ostia containing Dsg3. It denotes subclinical involvement.[3] Some have described it as the Nikolsky's sign of hair.[4]
- But in one study hair casts has also been found in cases of pemphigus foliaceus which they have explained to be a sign of diffuse scaling rather than acantholysis.[2]

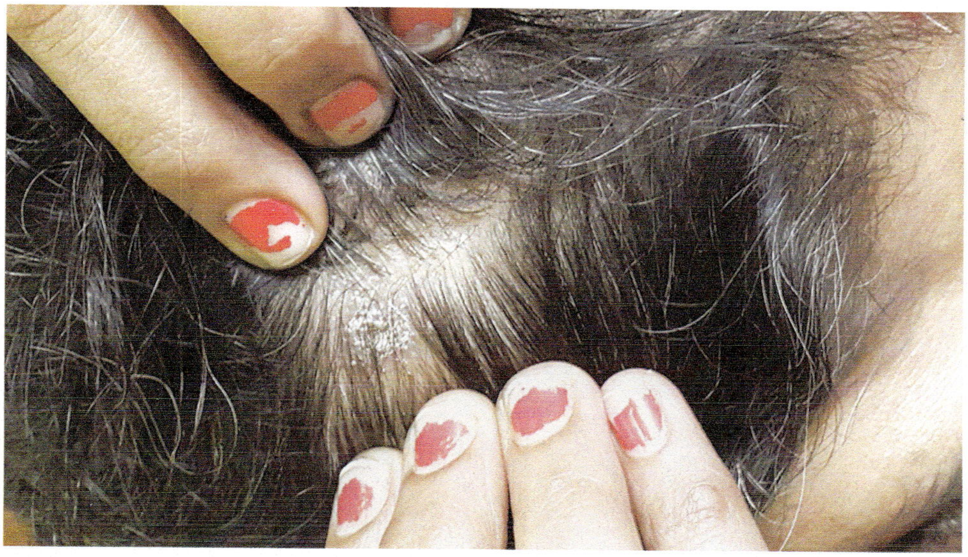

Fig. 1: Clinical picture showing a lesion of pemphigus vulgaris (in healing phase) over the scalp.

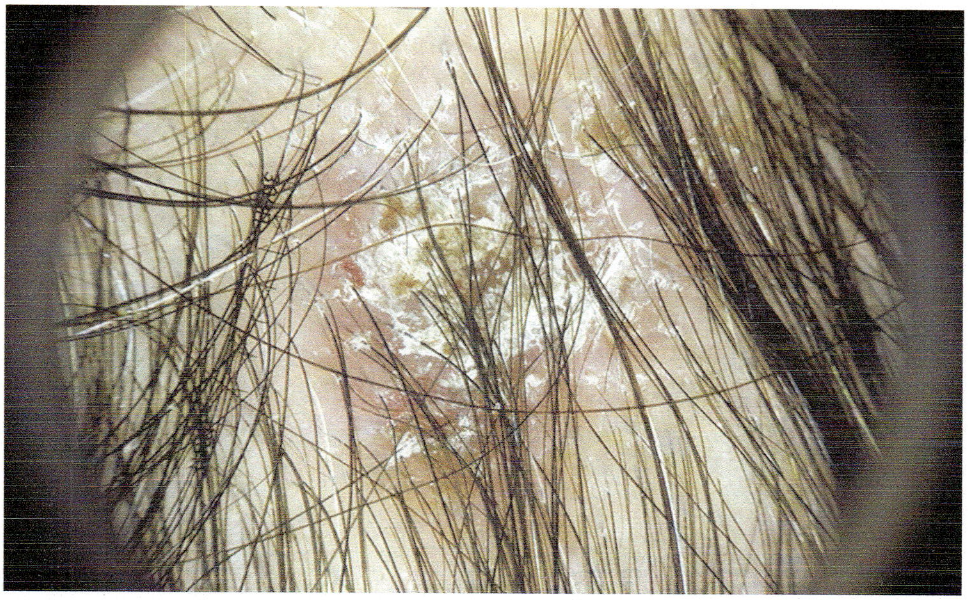

Fig. 2: Trichoscopic image of the same patient showing areas of hemorrhage, white scales, and yellowish crusts.

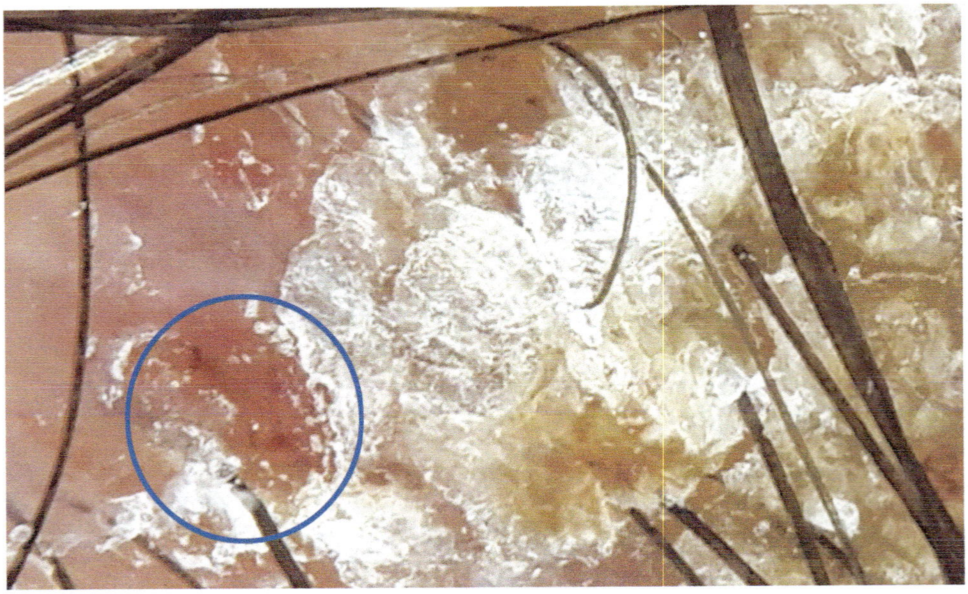

Fig. 3: Image (zoomed 2×) showing hemorrhagic area (blue circle), white scales, and yellowish crusts.

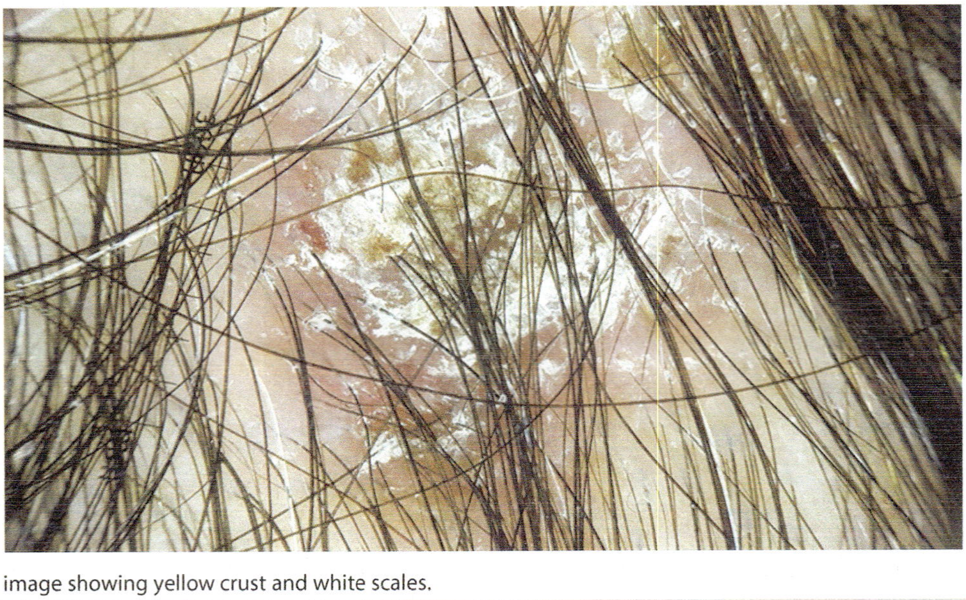

Fig. 4: Trichoscopic image showing yellow crust and white scales.

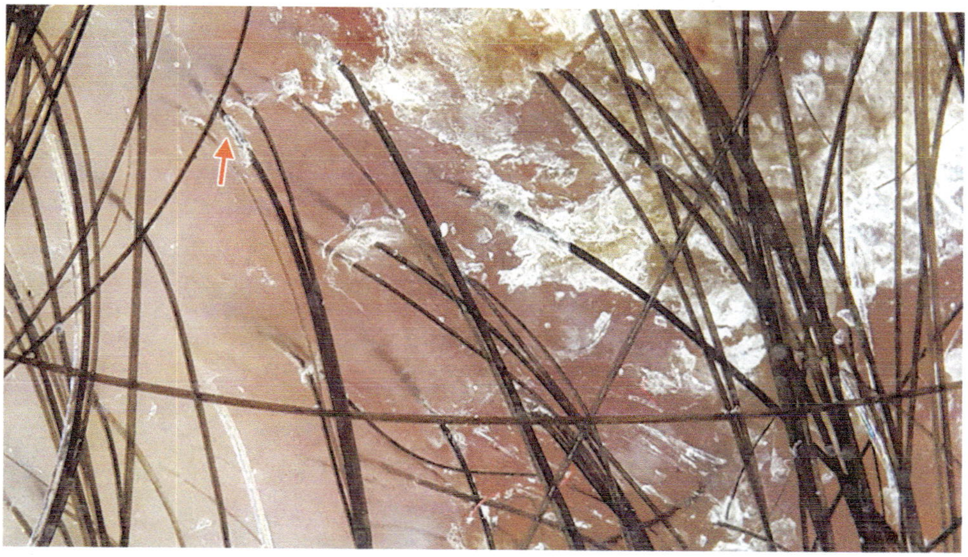

Fig. 5: Nikolsky's sign of the hair: It is the trichoscopic image of acantholytic hair cast (red arrow).

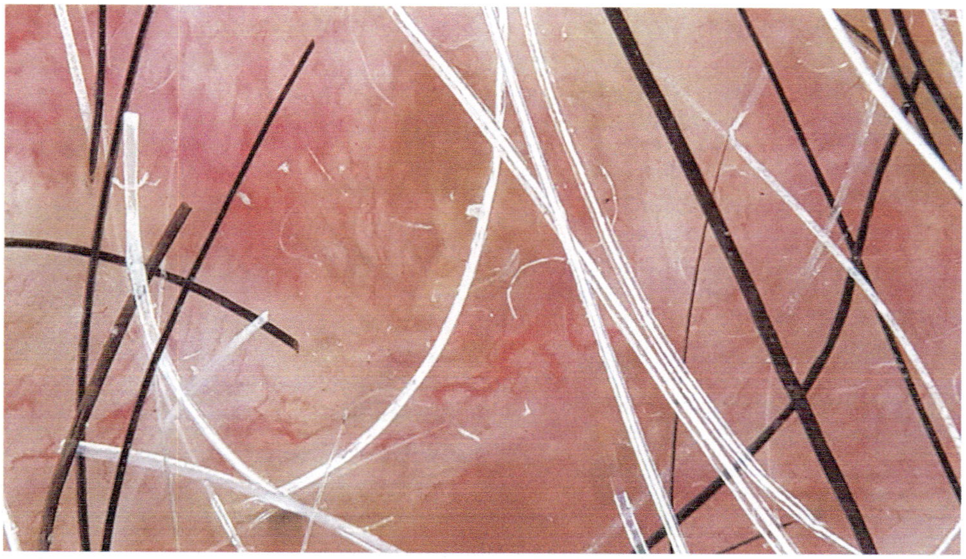

Fig. 6: Trichoscopic image of scalp in another case of pemphigus vulgaris showing elongated serpentine blood vessels.

PEMPHIGUS FOLIACEOUS

Key Trichoscopic Features

- Thick white polygonal lamellar crust,[5] white and yellow diffuse scaling.[2] Feature of scaling is more consistent with pemphigus foliaceus than pemphigus vulgaris.
- Hair casts—well-defined yellowish or whitish hair casts[2]
- Vessels—linear serpentine, linear helical, and glomerular vessels may be observed but less common than pemphigus vulgaris.[2]
- Hemorrhagic patches[2]

DERMATITIS HERPETIFORMIS

Key Trichoscopic Features

Regularly distributed polymorphic vessels (linear, dotted, or comma shaped) in linear or circular arrangements giving impression of psoriasis.[5]

BULLOUS PEMPHIGOID

Key Trichoscopic Features

- White circular or oval transparent structures with sharp demarcation—corresponding with bulla.[1]
- Decreased number of follicular openings[1]
- Yellow dots with whitish halo[1]—sebum underlying the follicular openings which are blocked by detached epidermis shows yellow dots, whereas the perifollicular area is white due to absence of sebaceous glands. This feature is also found in pemphigus.

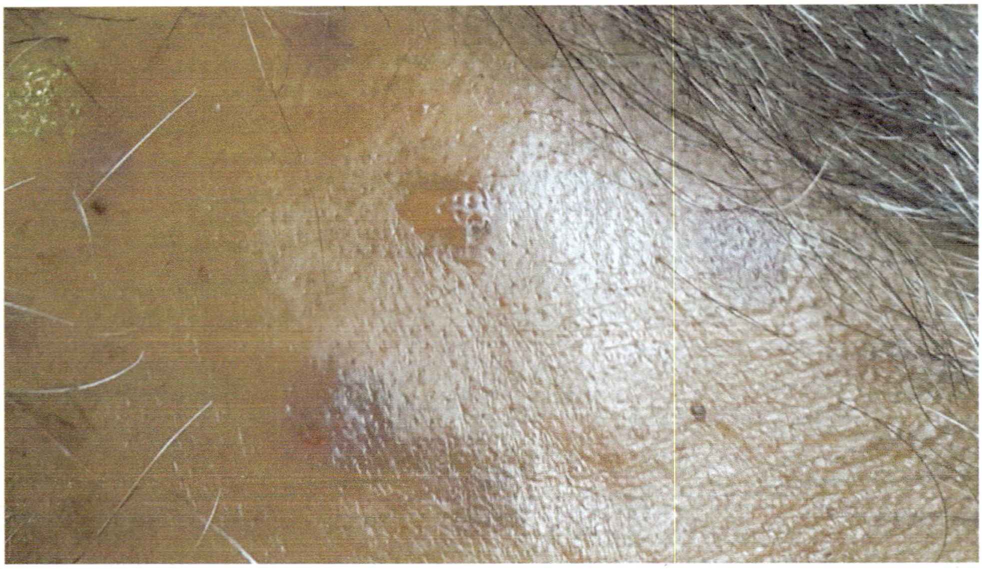

Fig. 7: Clinical photograph of an intact bulla over forehead in a patient of Bullous pemphigoid. A recently ruptured bulla is present in the lower forehead.

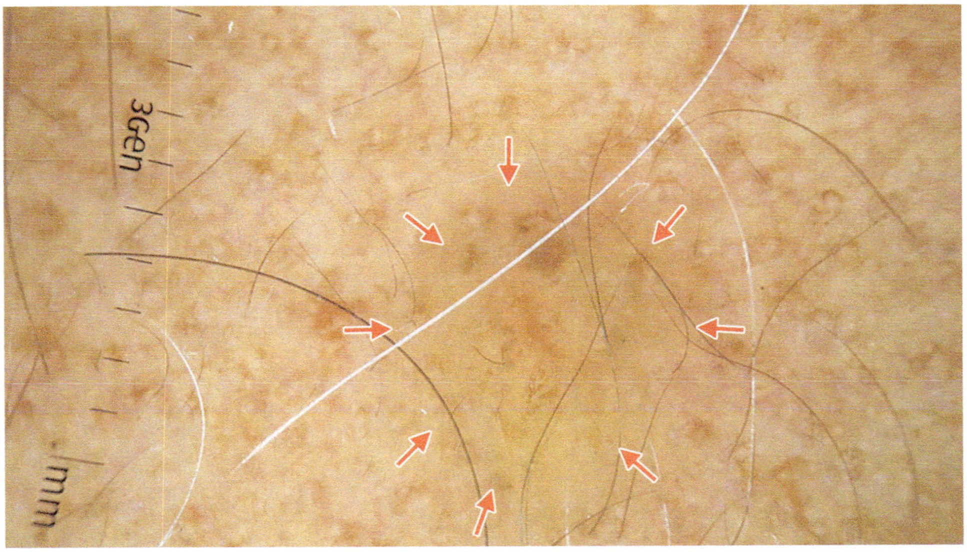

Fig. 8: Trichoscopic image of the previous patient showing a transparent membrane of the intact bulla whose border has been delineated with red arrows. Note clear fluid in the bulla.

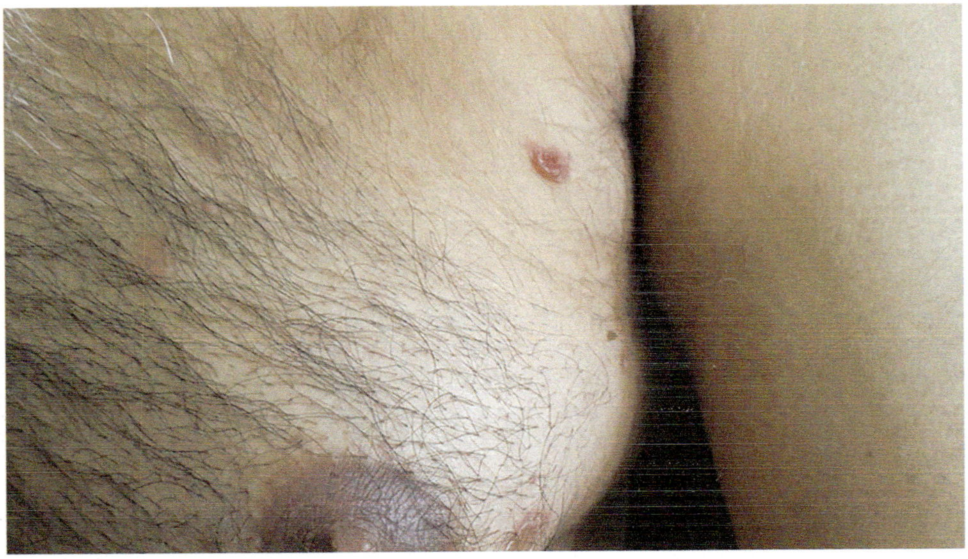

Fig. 9: Clinical picture of the same patient with bullous pemphigoid showing ruptured bulla over chest.

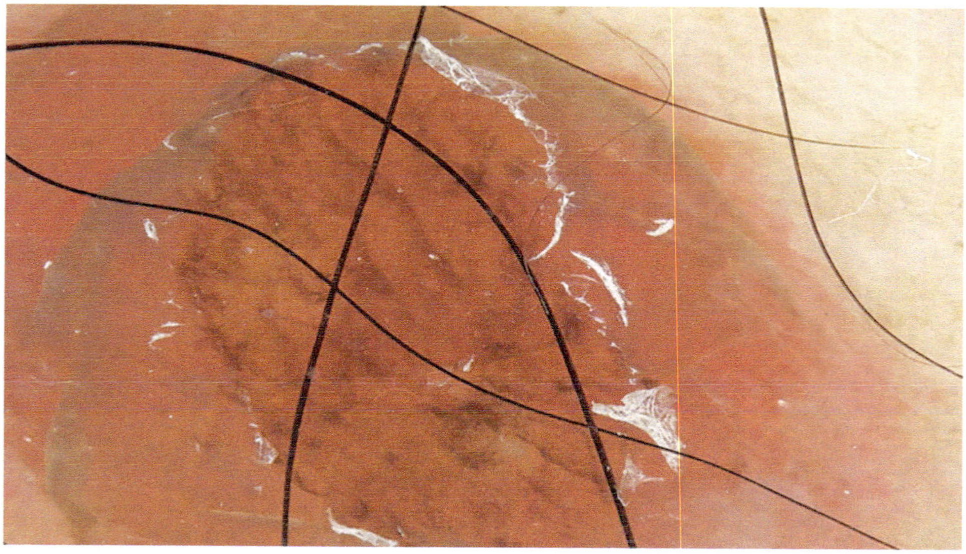

Fig. 10: Trichoscopic image of the chest bulla showing a transparent ruptured membrane (white lamellar scales indicating the ruptured margin) and areas of hemorrhage.

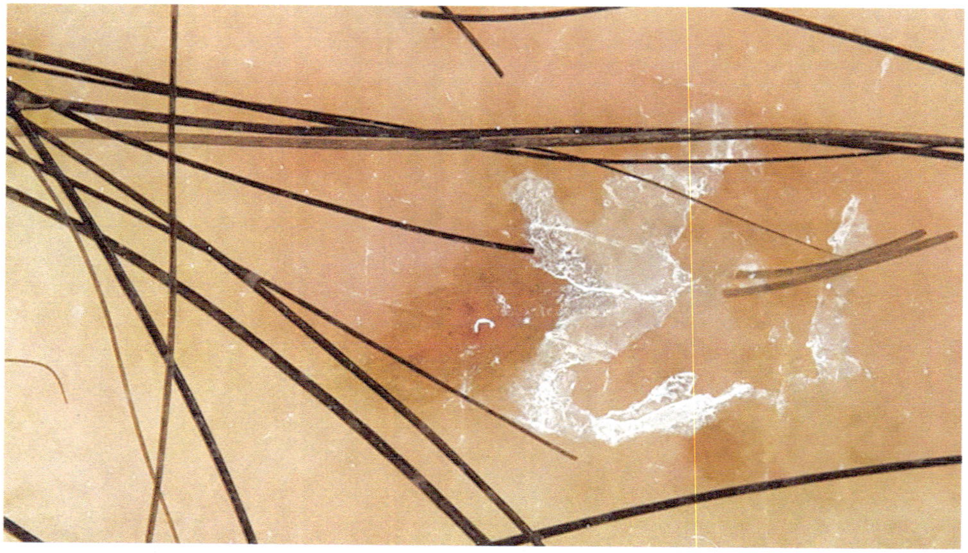

Fig. 11: Trichoscopic image showing detached lamellar white scales from a lesion of bullous pemphigoid over scalp.

REFERENCES

1. Kurzeja M, Rakowska A, Olszewska M, Rudnicka L. Trichoscopy (dermoscopy of the scalp) in autoimmune bullous skin diseases. Abstract CD. Prague: 21st Congress of the European Academy of Dermatology and Venereology; 2012.
2. Sar-Pomian M, Kurzeja M, Rudnicka L, Olszewska M. The value of trichoscopy in the differential diagnosis of scalp lesions in pemphigus vulgaris and pemphigus foliaceus. An Bras Dermatol. 2014;89(6):1007-12.
3. Pirmez R. Acantholytic hair casts: A dermoscopic sign of pemphigus vulgaris of the scalp. Int J Trichol. 2012;4:172-3.
4. Delmonte S, Semino MT, Parodi A, Rebora A. Normal anagen effluvium: a sign of pemphigus vulgaris. Br J Dermatol. 2000;142(6):1244-5.
5. Kurzeja M. Application of reflectance confocal microscopy in diagnosing pemphigus vulgaris and pemphigus foliaceus. PhD Thesis. Warsaw: Medical University of Warsaw; 2013.

CHAPTER 29

Trichoscopy in Autoimmune Connective Tissue Diseases

Souvik Sardar, Subrata Malakar

INTRODUCTION

- Autoimmune connective tissue diseases (AI-CTD) are a group of diseases characterized by unregulated immune activation against self-antigens leading to inflammation of the connective tissues.
- Different types of circulatory autoantibodies are found which can be detected by serological tests.
- AI-CTD has a strong female predilection.
- The disease manifests with either cutaneous or systemic features or both.
- Scalp involvement is quite common and mostly manifests as alopecia.
- Some of the important trichoscopic features in common AI-CTD have been described in this chapter.

SYSTEMIC LUPUS ERYTHEMATOSUS

Key Trichoscopic Features[1,2]

- Diffuse nonscarring alopecia shows trichoscopic features of acute telogen effluvium.
- Patchy nonscarring alopecia shows:
  - Vessels:
    - Interfollicular arborizing vessels: Most common finding in the hair loss area.
    - Perifollicular vessels (red dots)
    - Pan follicular vessels—both in follicular units and around follicles
  - Vellus hairs: First thing to appear with treatment
  - Hair shaft hypopigmentation: First sign to disappear after treatment
  - Hair shaft thinning
  - Peripilar sign
  - Honeycomb pigment patterns
- Patchy scarring alopecia shows trichoscopic features of discoid lupus erythematosus (DLE) (mostly), lupus profundus.

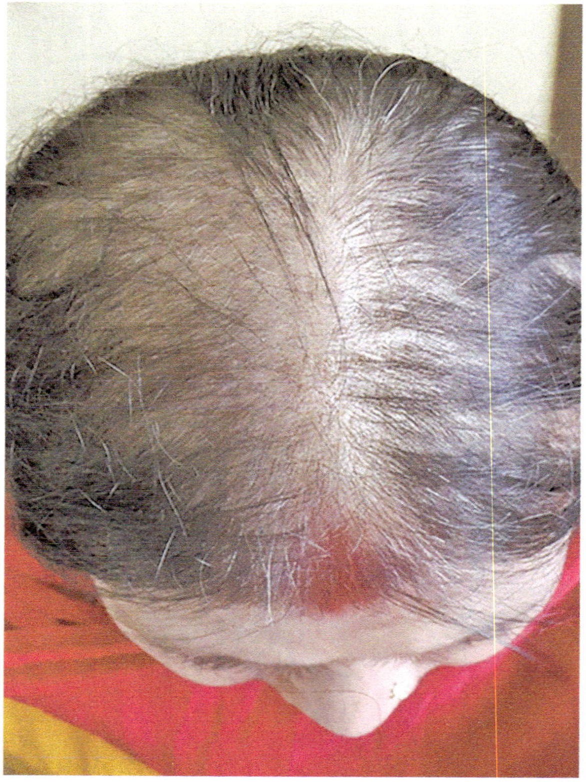

Fig. 1: Pretreatment clinical picture of a patient of systemic lupus erythematosus (SLE) showing diffuse non-scarring alopecia over scalp.

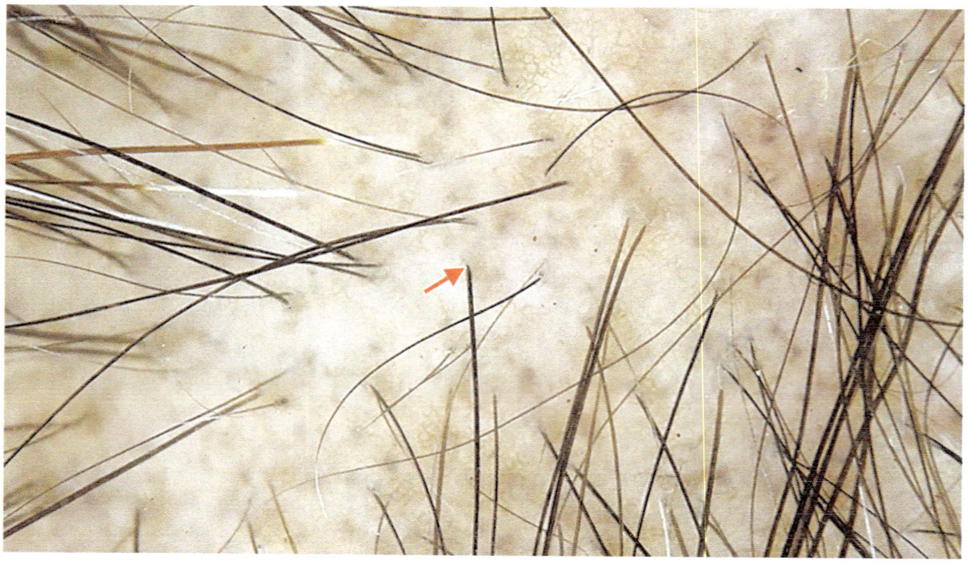

Fig. 2: Trichoscopic image of the previous patient showing predominance of single-unit hair follicles (arrow), reduced hair follicle density. Also note upright re-growing hairs which indicates telogen effluvium.

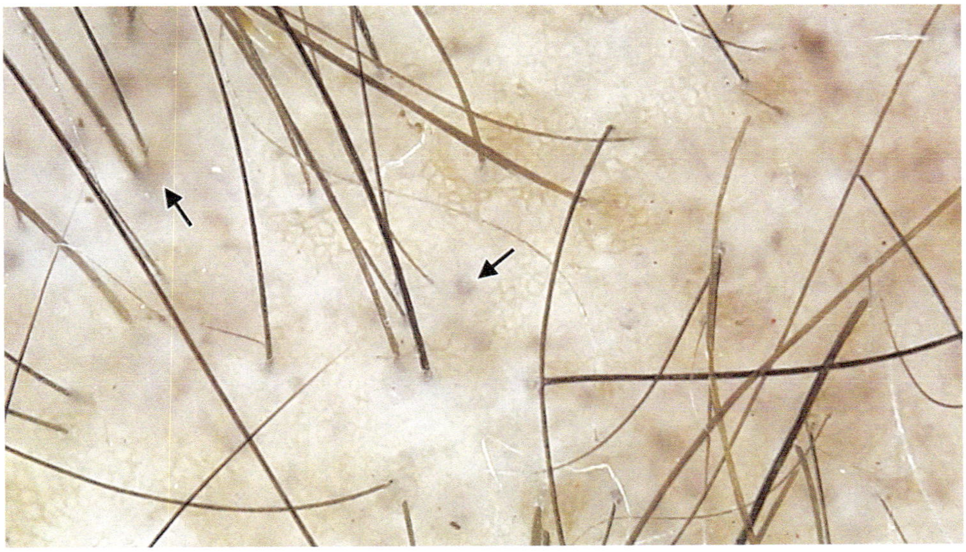

Fig. 3: Trichoscopic image of the same patient showing prominent blue-gray dots (arrows) corresponding to areas of interface dermatitis and pigmentary incontinence.

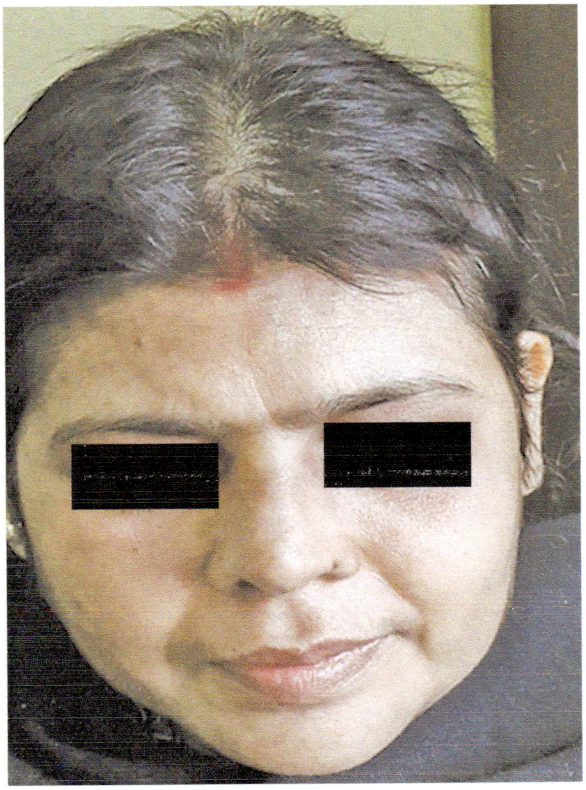

Fig. 4: After 4 months of treatment mainly with systemic steroid, the same patient showing remarkable improvement in the diffuse alopecia. Note also the slight development of moon facies.

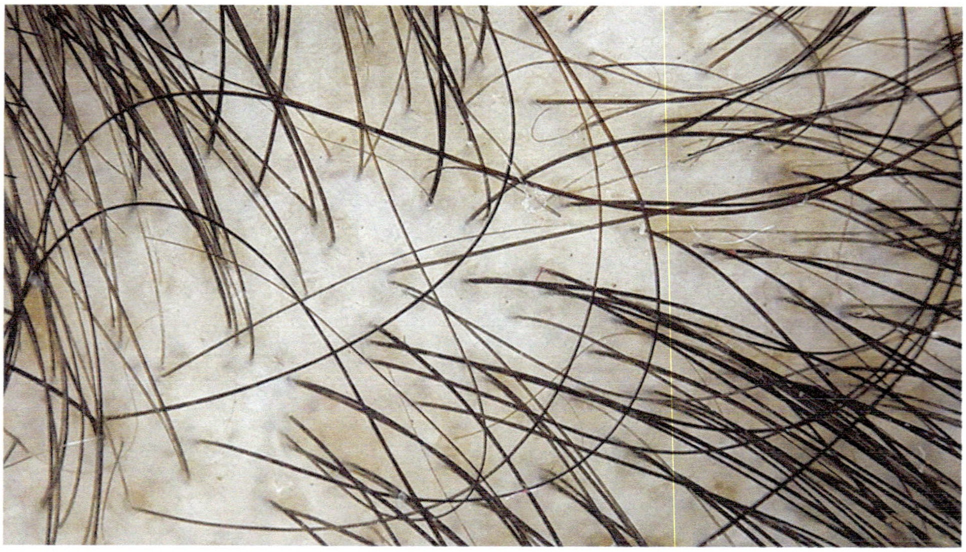

Fig. 5: Trichoscopic image of the same patient (post-treatment) showing increased hair density. Please note the increased number of 2- and 3-unit hair follicles as well as remarkable reduction of blue-gray dots.

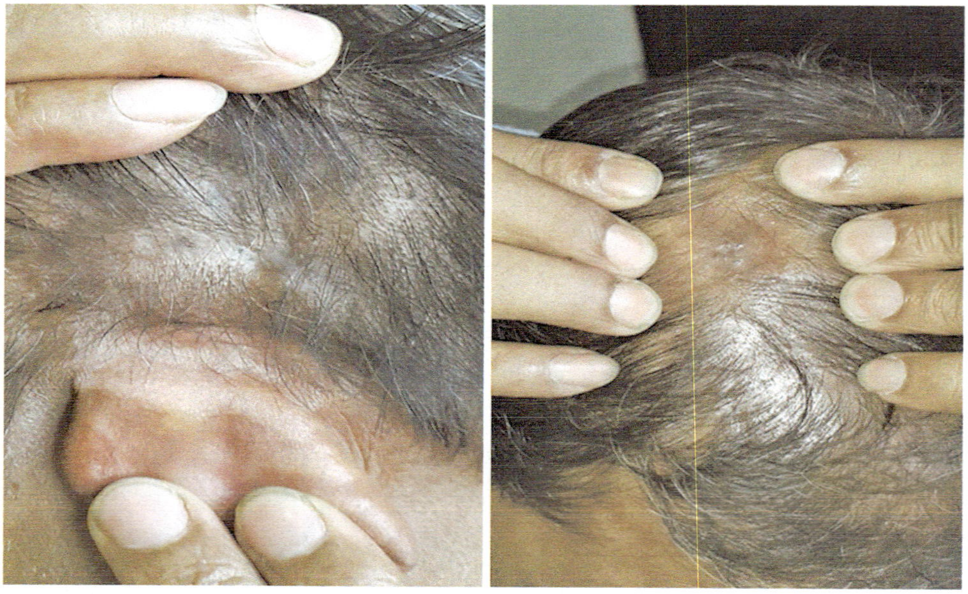

Fig. 6: Clinical picture showing patchy scarring alopecia with areas of nodularity along with depressed scars corresponding with lupus profundus over scalp in another patient of systemic lupus erythematosus (SLE).

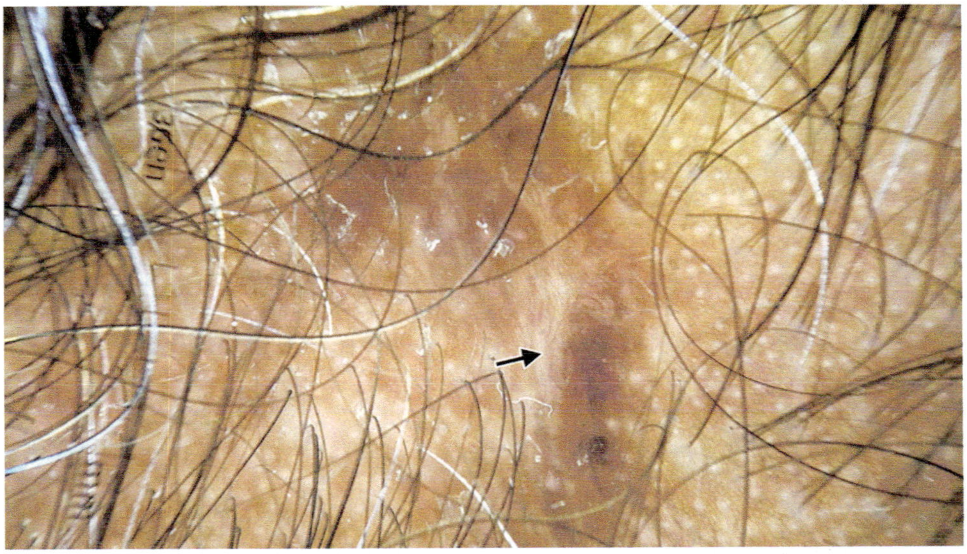

Fig. 7: Trichoscopy of the previous patient with lupus profundus showing peripheral scales with blotchy grayish brown homogeneous pigmentation and white structureless areas of scarring (arrow) in-between.

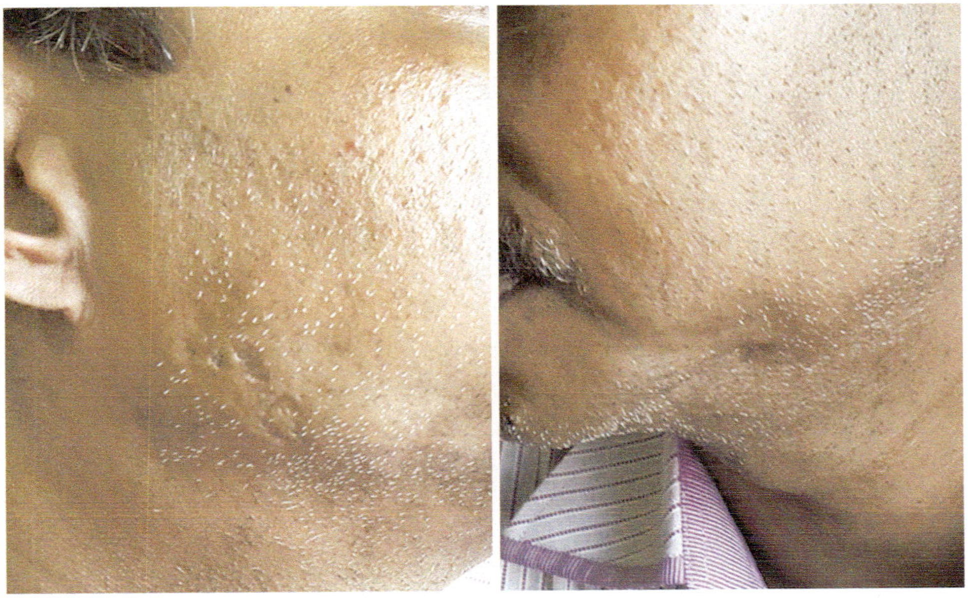

Fig. 8: The same patient who showed lesions of lupus profundus over the scalp had more lesions elsewhere in the body. These clinical images show the healed phase of lupus profundus over the beard region.

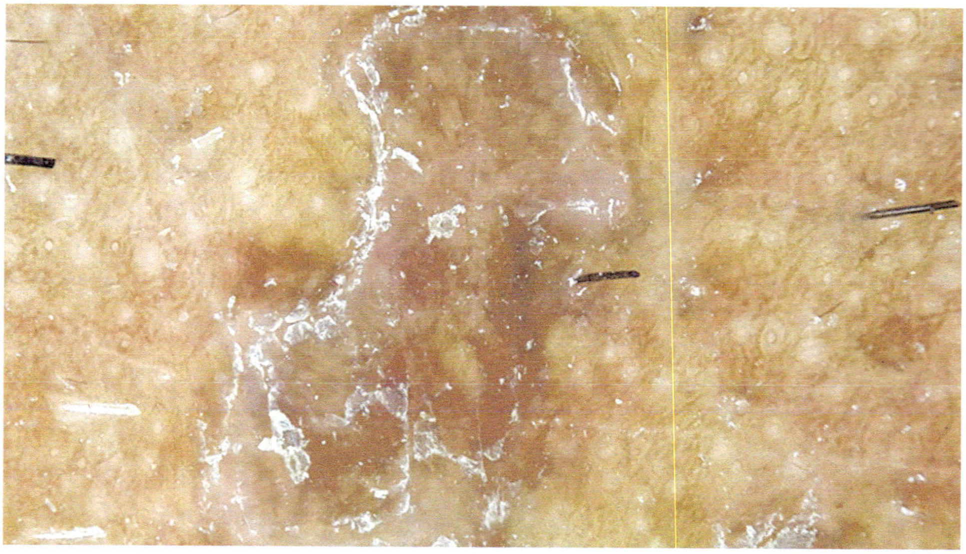

Fig. 9: Trichoscopy from the beard area of the previous patient with lupus profundus showing peripheral white scaling with blotchy grayish-brown pigmentation and white structureless areas.

DERMATOMYOSITIS

Key Trichoscopic Features[2]

- Features of acute telogen effluvium may be seen.
- Nonscarring diffuse alopecia may show polymorphous interfollicular vessels.
- Gray dots and patches (authors' observation)

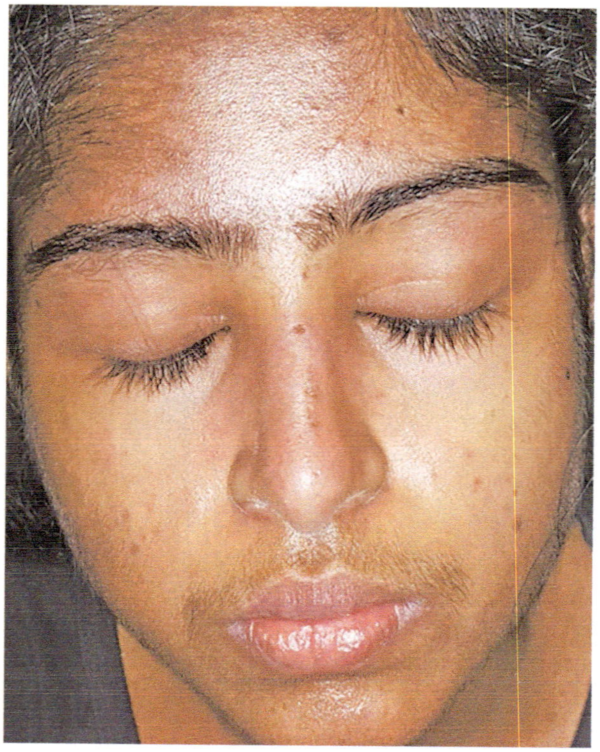

Fig. 10: Heliotrope rash in a woman with dermatomyositis (DM). Note periorbital edema. Heliotrope rash is highly suggestive of DM.

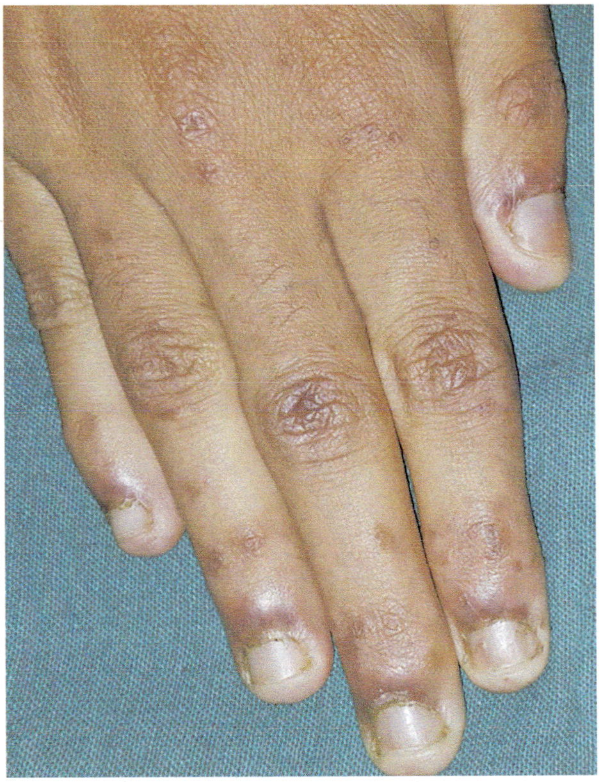

Fig. 11: Gottron papules: Flat topped, erythematous to violaceus papules and plaques found over bony prominences, particularly the metacarpophalangeal and interphalangeal joints. They may mimic the lesions of lupus erythematosus or lichen planus.

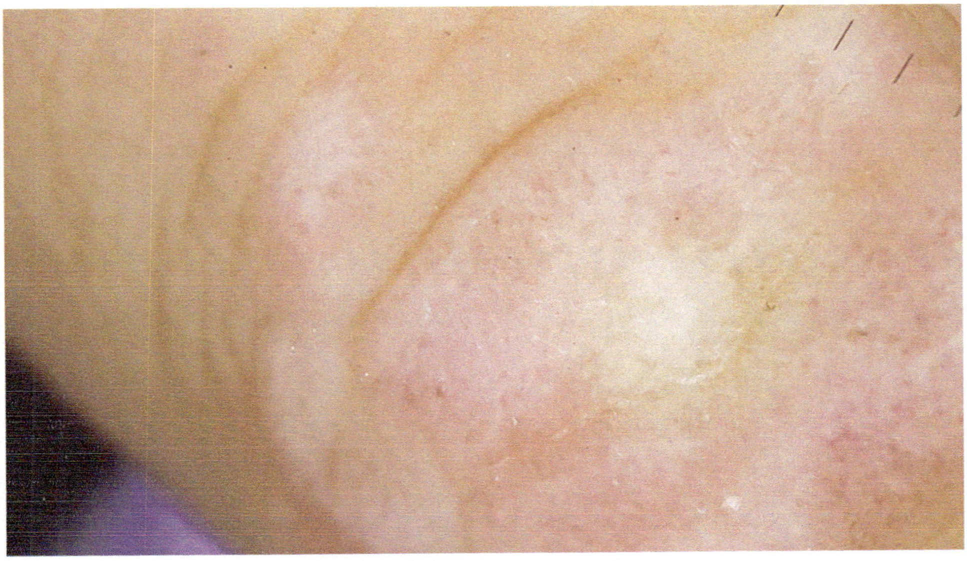

Fig. 12: Dermoscopy of Gottron papules: Polymorphic vessels (authors' observation).

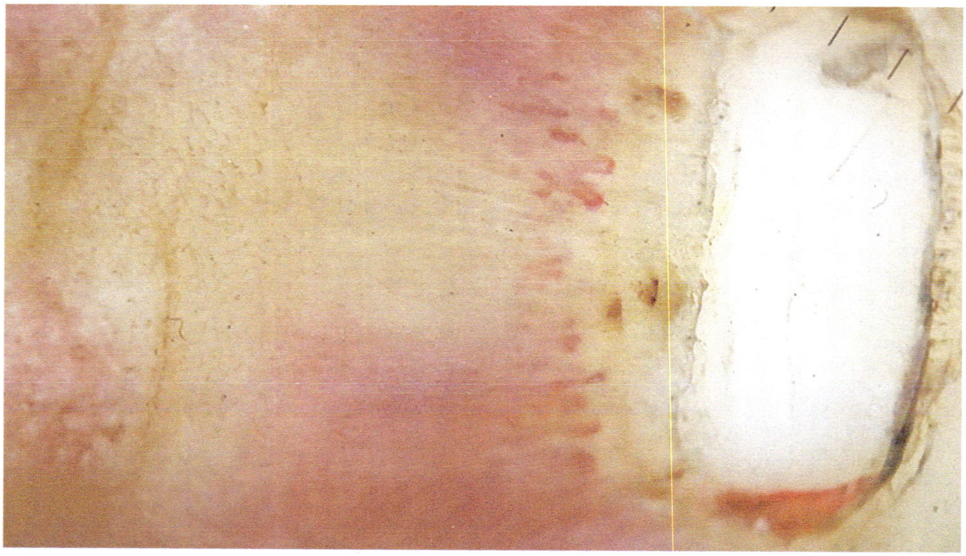

Fig. 13: Dermoscopy of the proximal nail-fold showing irregular capillary loop enlargement and cuticle hemorrhage.

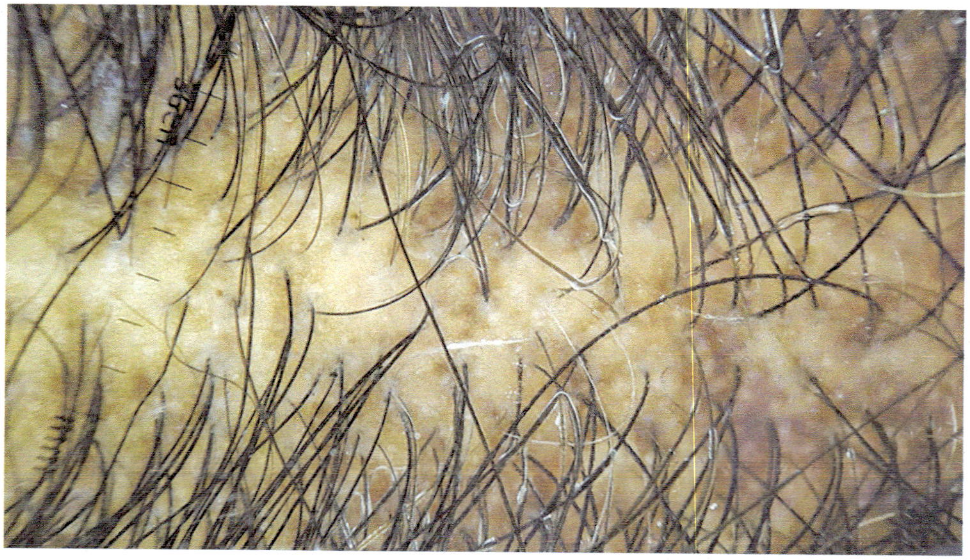

Fig. 14: Trichoscopy of the same patient **(Fig. 10)** showing blue gray dots and patches corresponding to areas of pigmentary incontinence which is a consequence of interface dermatitis.

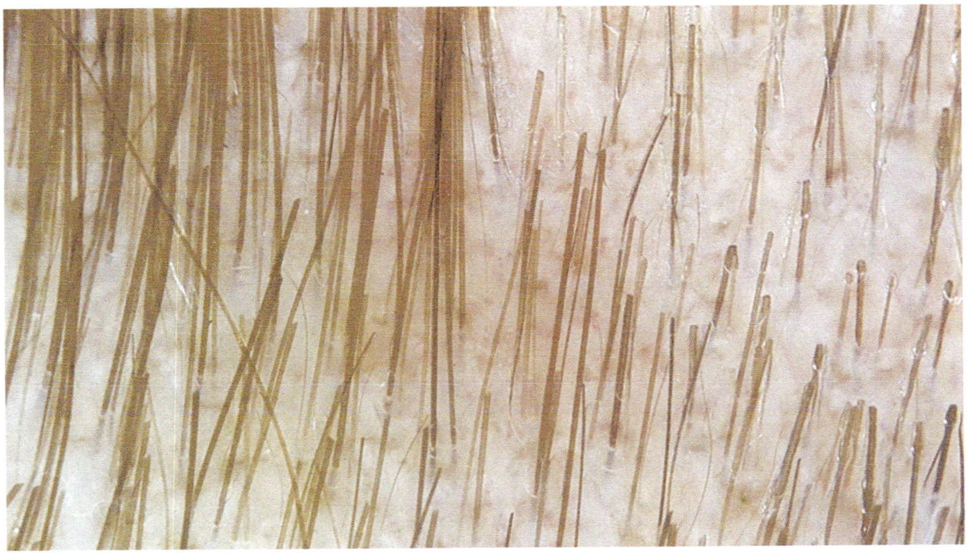

Fig. 15: Trichoscopy of another patient of DM showing polymorphic vessels. Note blue-gray dots.

SYSTEMIC SCLEROSIS

Key Trichoscopic Features[3]

- Polymorphous (thick arborizing, capillary loops, or spider) vessels in the frontal area
- Telangiectasia (dilated and deformed capillary, may have microhemorrhage)
- Avascular areas interspersed between vascular areas may be noted.
- Perifollicular salt and pepper pigmentation
- Hair shaft thinning

REFERENCES

1. Ye Y, Zhao Y, Gong Y, Zhang X, Caulloo S, Zhang B, et al. Non-scarring patchy alopecia in patients with systemic lupus erythematosus differs from that of alopecia areata. Lupus. 2013;22(14):1439-45.
2. Tosti A. Systemic diseases. In: Toshi A (Ed). Dermoscopy of the Hair and Nails, 2nd edition. Boca Raton: CRC Press. 2016;111.
3. Kwiatkowska M, Rakowska A, Walecka I, Rudnicka L. The diagnostic value of trichoscopy in systemic sclerosis. J Dermatol Case Rep. 2016;10(2):21-5.

CHAPTER

30

Pediatric Hair Disorders

Samipa S Mukherjee, Subrata Malakar

INTRODUCTION

- Dermoscopy of the hair and scalp (trichoscopy) facilitates the differential diagnosis of hair diseases in children, including alopecia areata, trichotillomania, and tinea capitis.
- It can also assist in the diagnosis of multiple genetic hair shaft disorders, such as monilethrix, trichorrhexis invaginata, trichorrhexis nodosa (TN), pili torti, and pili annulati.
- The noninvasive nature of the diagnostic tool makes it a favorite which can be used not only to diagnose and assess the progress of treatment but also for the ease of convincing the parents.

LOOSE ANAGEN HAIR SYNDROME

INTRODUCTION

- Loose anagen syndrome (LAS) is a benign, self-limiting condition where anagen hairs are easily and painlessly extracted leading to a positive hair pull test and is mainly reported in childhood; with a variable adulthood onset as well.
- Dermatoscopy of the scalp is not specific. It may, however, be used for the evaluation of the plucked hair which shows an anagen hair devoid of a sheath.
- The confirmation of the diagnosis can only be done by light microscopy showing a floppy sock appearance and a trichogram.

KEY TRICHOSCOPIC FEATURES

- Scalp features are nonspecific.
- Predominance of single hair follicular units
- Marked reduction of terminal hair (authors' observation)
- Empty follicles
- The evaluation of the plucked hair which shows an anagen hair devoid of a sheath.

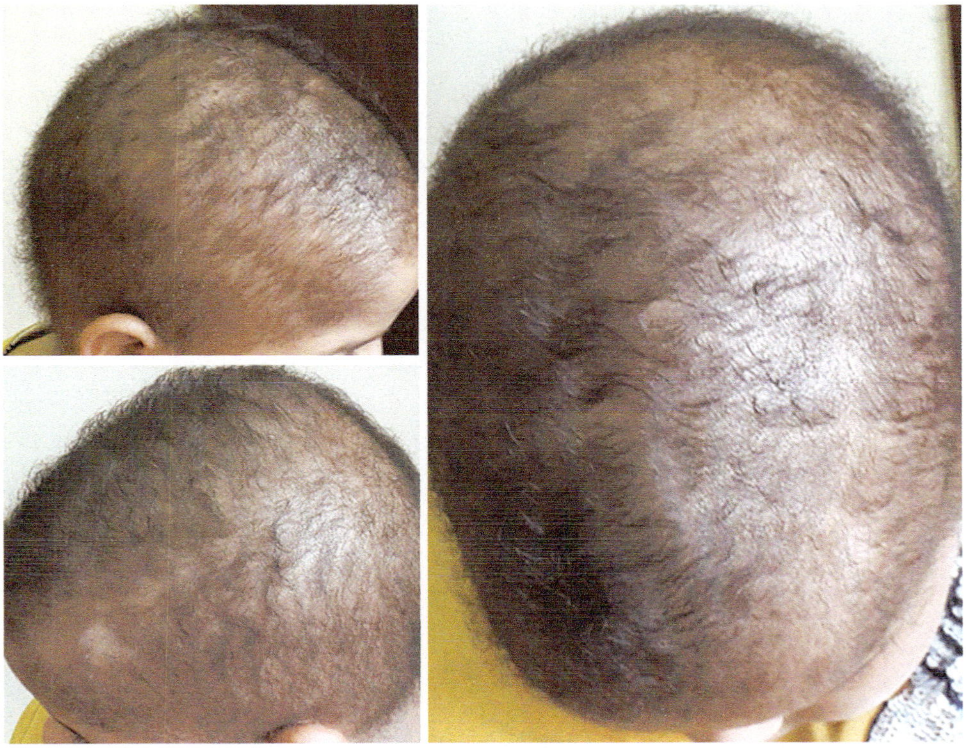

Fig. 1: Sparse, short, wiry hair present all over the scalp since birth without any systemic involvement. Clinical differentials include isolated wooly hair and loose anagen hair syndrome.

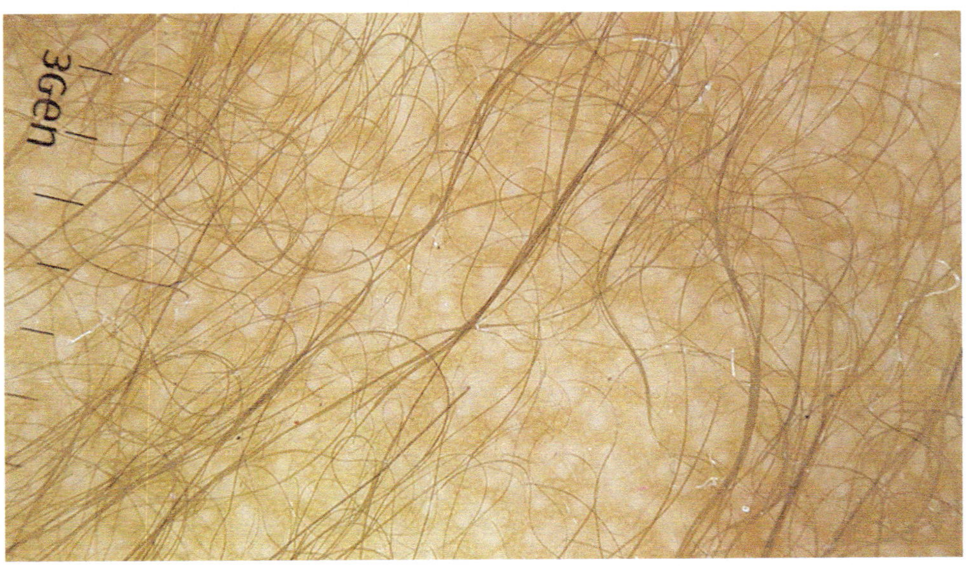

Fig. 2: On trichoscopy of the above patient: (1) Predominance of single hair follicular units; (2) Reduced number of terminal hair; (3) Empty follicles.

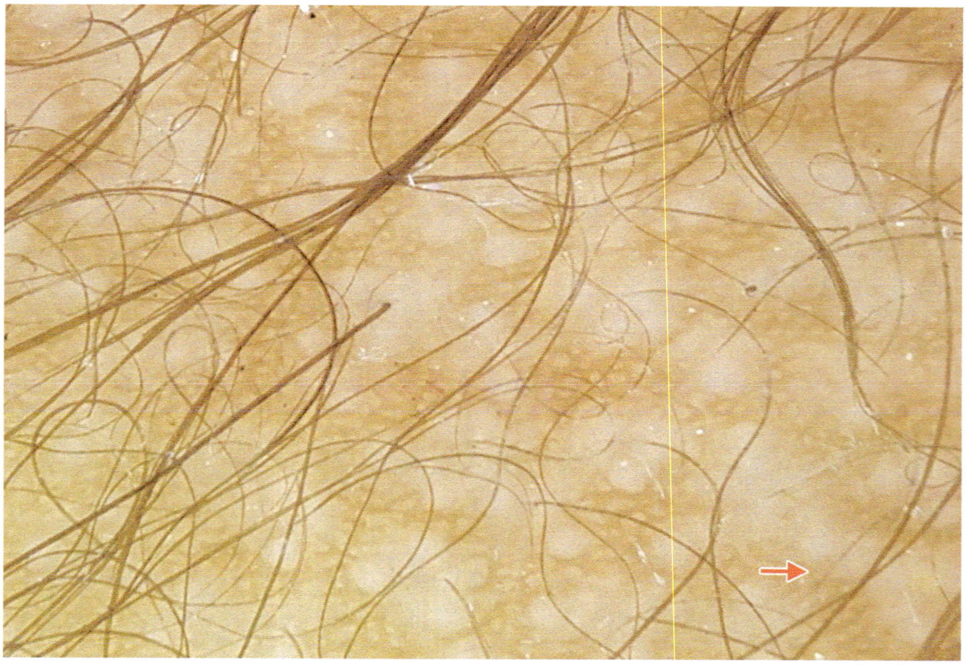

Fig. 3: Marked reduction of terminal hairs. Note also the empty follicles.

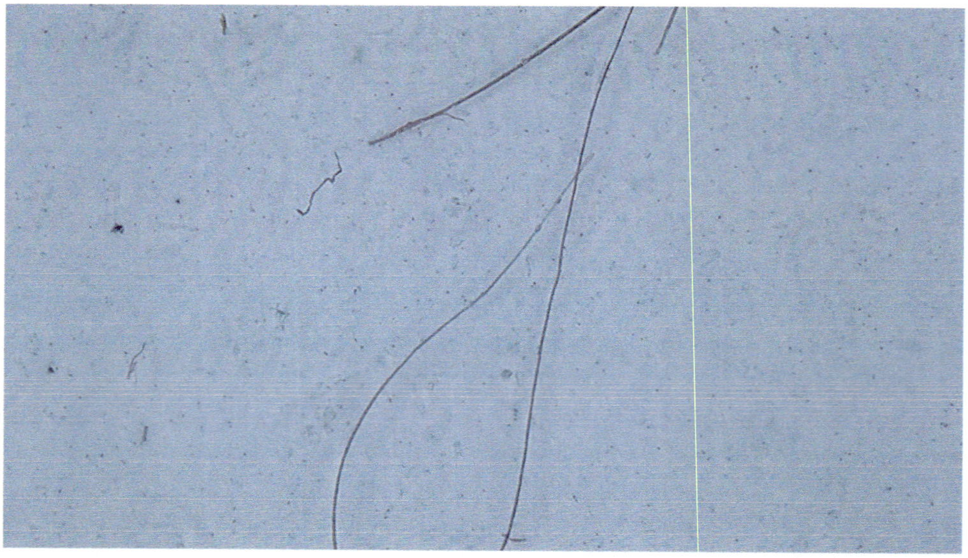

Fig. 4: Dermoscopy of the root shows anagen hair devoid of outer root sheath making it easier to choose the hair for light microscopy showing floppy sock appearance.

CONGENITAL TRIANGULAR ALOPECIA

INTRODUCTION

- Congenital triangular alopecia (CTA) also known as temporal triangular alopecia is a benign noncicatricial pattern of hair loss presenting at birth or may develop later in life.
- It presents with a patchy hair loss which on closer inspection reveals lack of terminal hair but presence of vellus hair.

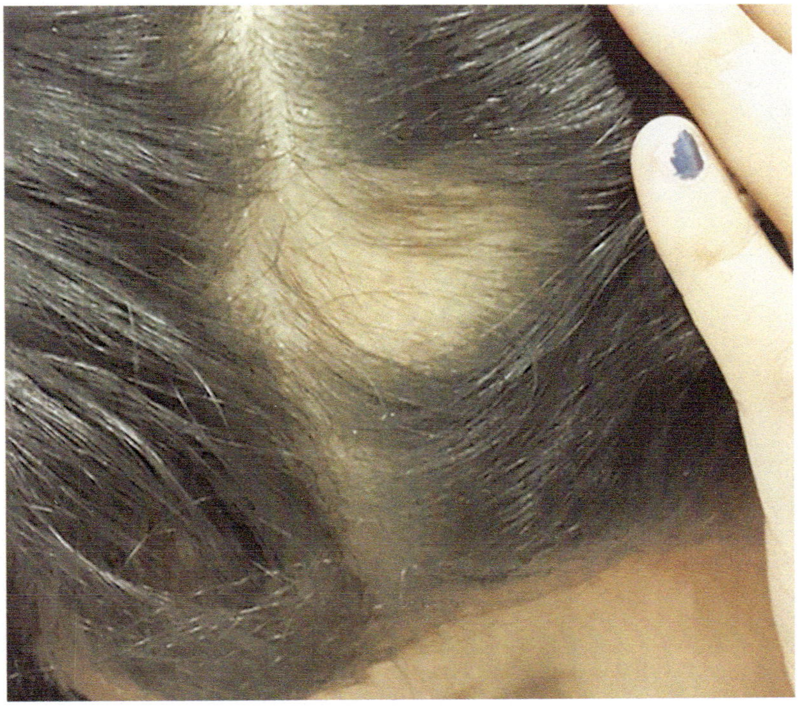

Fig. 5: Congenital triangular alopecia is not rare and is usually diagnosed between 2 and 9 years of age. A triangular or oval patch is observed in the temporal region but may be present in any area of scalp.

KEY TRICHOSCOPIC FEATURES

- Follicular features of CTA include short vellus hairs with varying hair length diversity, as well as white hairs in the absence of diagnostic features for other types of localized alopecia.[1]
- The presence of epidermal scaling, as well as interfollicular features such as arborizing red lines and a honeycomb pigment pattern, may also be useful clues.
- Vellus hairs are a highly sensitive but not specific marker for CTA.
- Shim et al. demonstrated clustered short vellus hairs without other specific findings.[2]

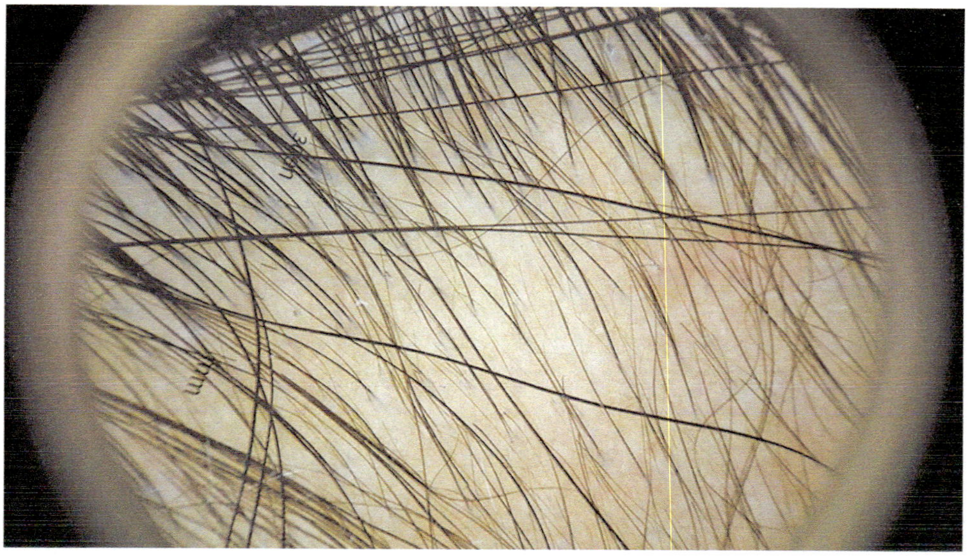

Fig. 6: (1) Short vellus hairs with varying hair length diversity, as well as white hairs in the absence of diagnostic features for other types of localized alopecia.[1] (2) Vellus hairs are a highly sensitive but not specific marker for congenital triangular alopecia (CTA).

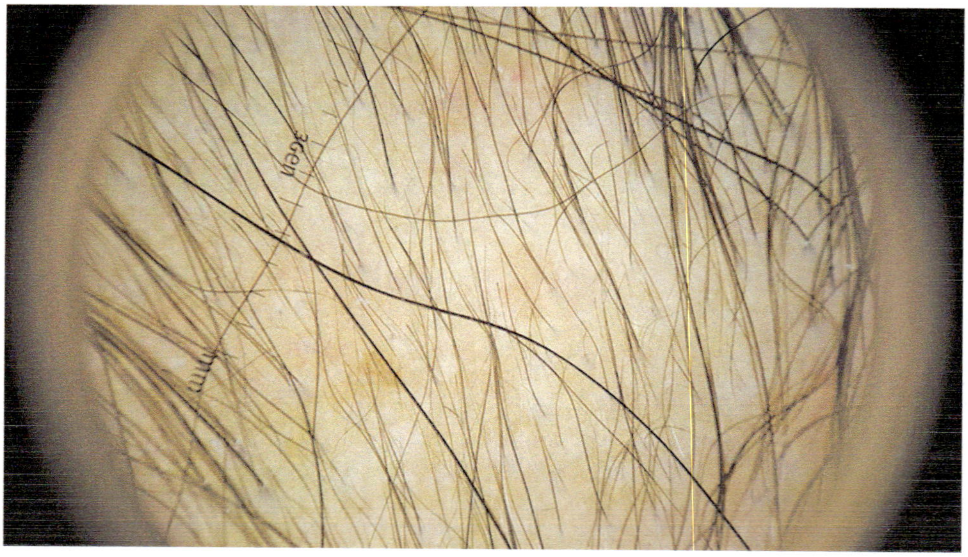

Fig. 7: Clustered short vellus hairs.[2]

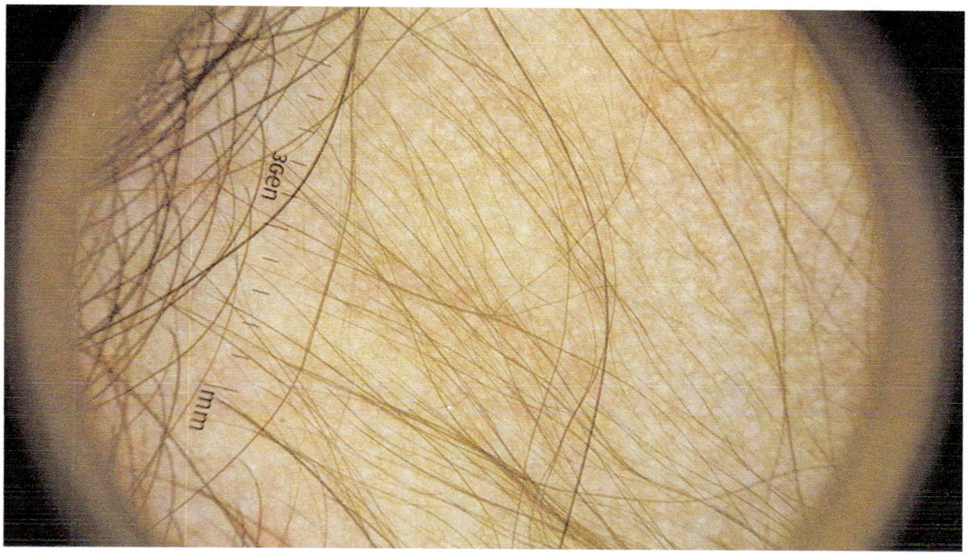

Fig. 8: Note the carpet of vellus hair with clustering of short vellus hair.

TRICHORRHEXIS NODOSA

INTRODUCTION

- Trichorrhexis nodosa, one of the most common hair shaft disorders, appears as minute grayish nodes along the hair shaft.
- It may be acquired or inherited.
- These nodes represent loss of cuticle along with frayed cortical fibers.
- On light microscopy, these changes appear like two paint brushes thrust into one another.

KEY TRICHOSCOPIC FEATURES

- The scalp in TN is unremarkable.
- The nodes appear gray-white areas on lower magnification.
- The hair shaft reveals the classical thrust paint brush appearance which are seen as gray-white nodes.[3]
- In addition to scalp hair, eyebrow hair also reveals similar changes in affected individuals.

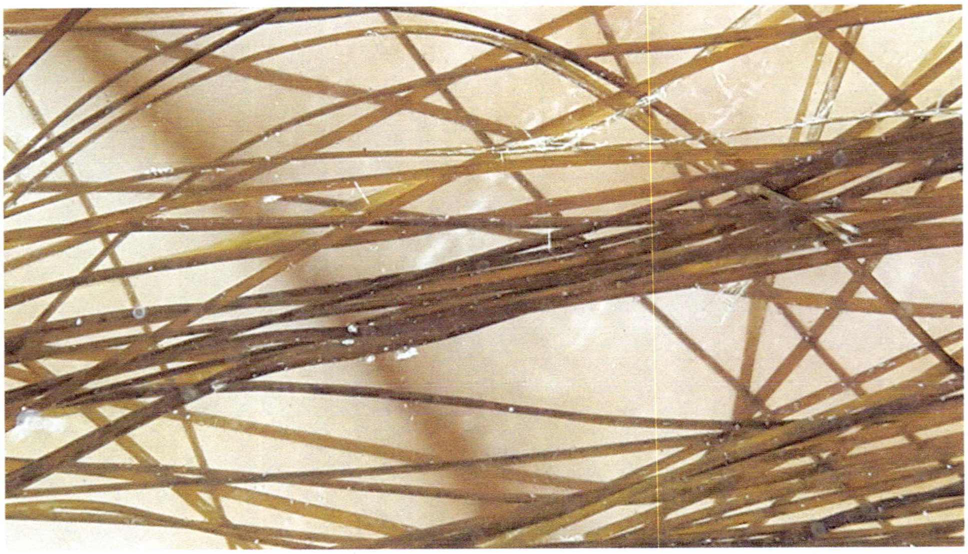

Fig. 9: Trichorrhexis nodosa. Note brush-like hair shafts and broken fragments.

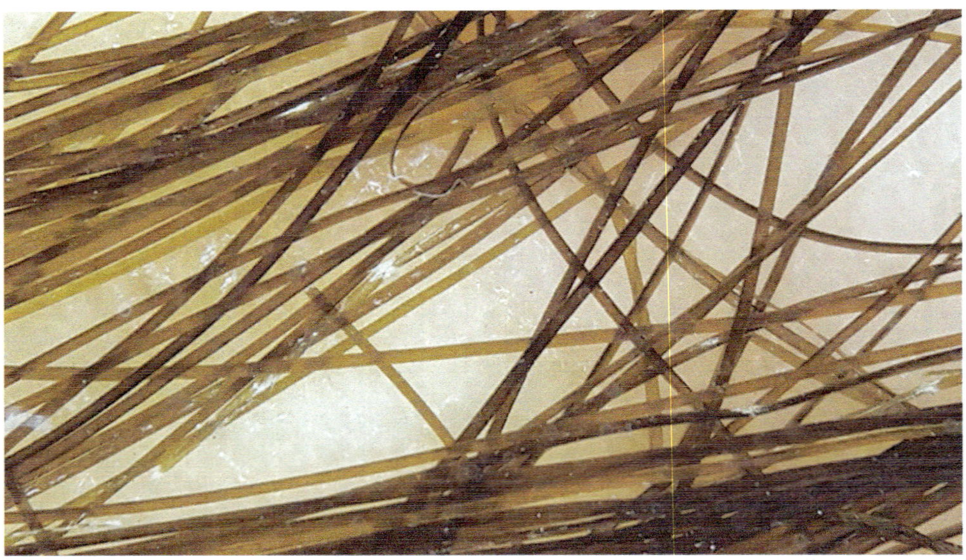

Fig. 10: Trichoscopy of trichorrhexis nodosa (TN) shows a hair splits into multiple fibers producing the appearance of two brushes aligned together.

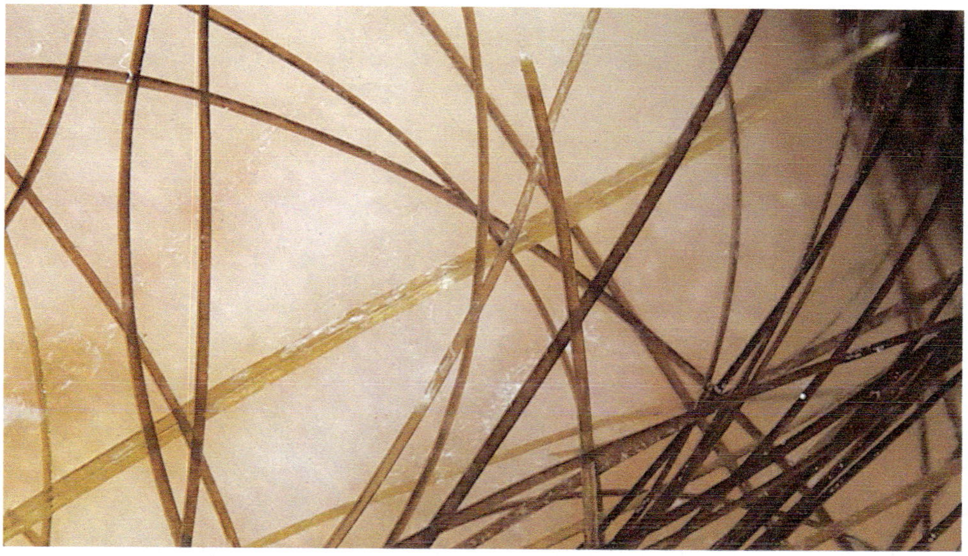

Fig. 11: Location of the nodules in trichorrhexis nodosa (TN). In acquired TN they are usually located at the distal end whereas in congenital TN nodules are observed proximally in the hair shafts.

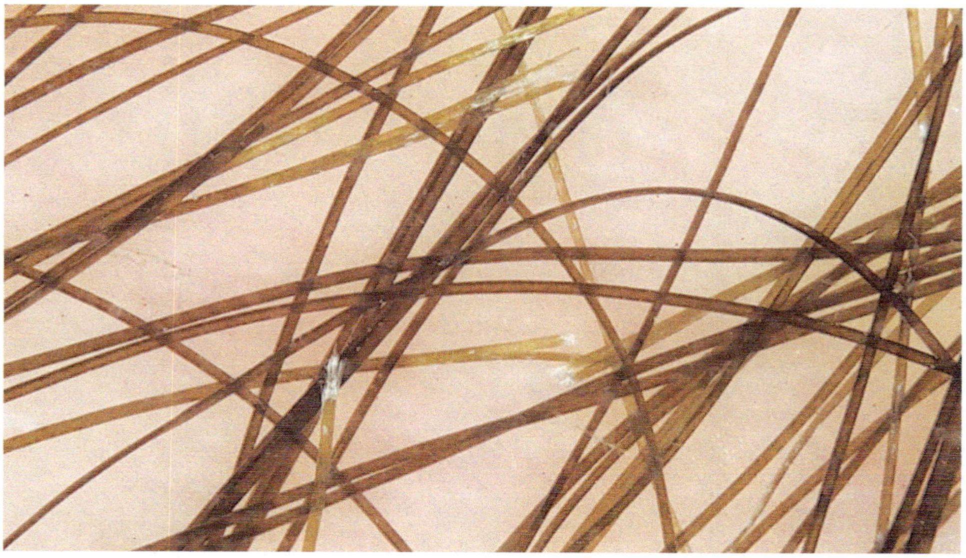

Fig. 12: Paint brush appearance of the broken ends of the hair.

CONGENITAL ATRICHIA WITH PAPULAR ERUPTION

INTRODUCTION

- *Atrichia congenita* with *papular* lesions represents a complex and heterogeneous group of genodermatoses characterized by irreversible complete hair loss soon after birth, and associated with the development of keratin-filled cysts over the body.
- Diagnosis of this particular genotrichoses is important for planning and counseling the patient.

KEY TRICHOSCOPIC FEATURES

- The dermoscopic feature of this particular entity has not been described in literature so far.
- According to the authors the feature noted consistently in these patients is a cluster of star appearance which may be defined aggregates of pinpoint white dots on the scalp in clusters of 8–10 arranged in a regular pattern all over the scalp.
- In the view of the authors, this appearance may be the result of the stranded hair bulbs and dermal papilla in the dermis which probably undergo fibrosis in due course of time and appear as white dots.

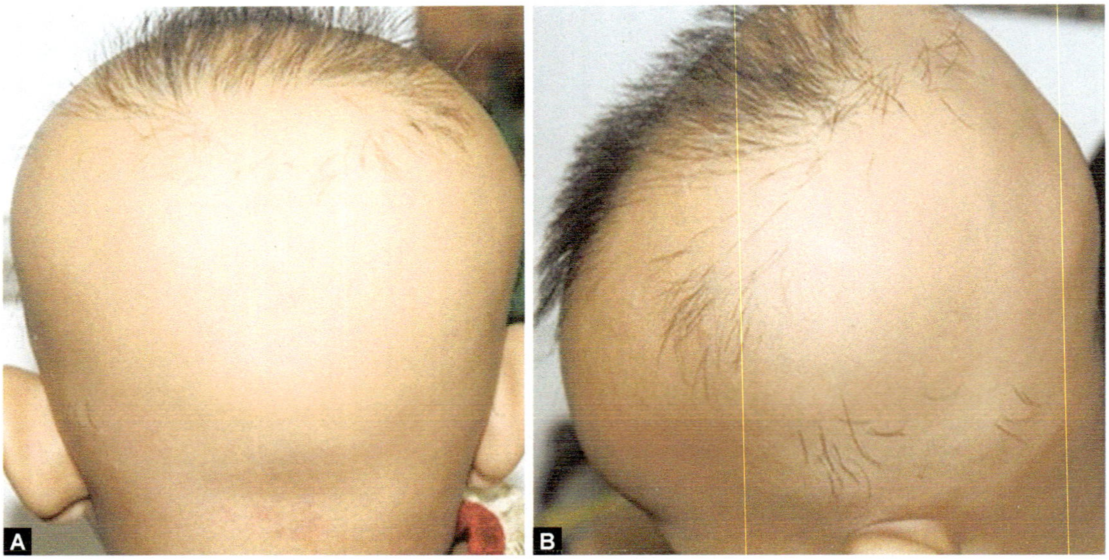

Figs. 13A and B: Congenital atrichia with papular eruption.

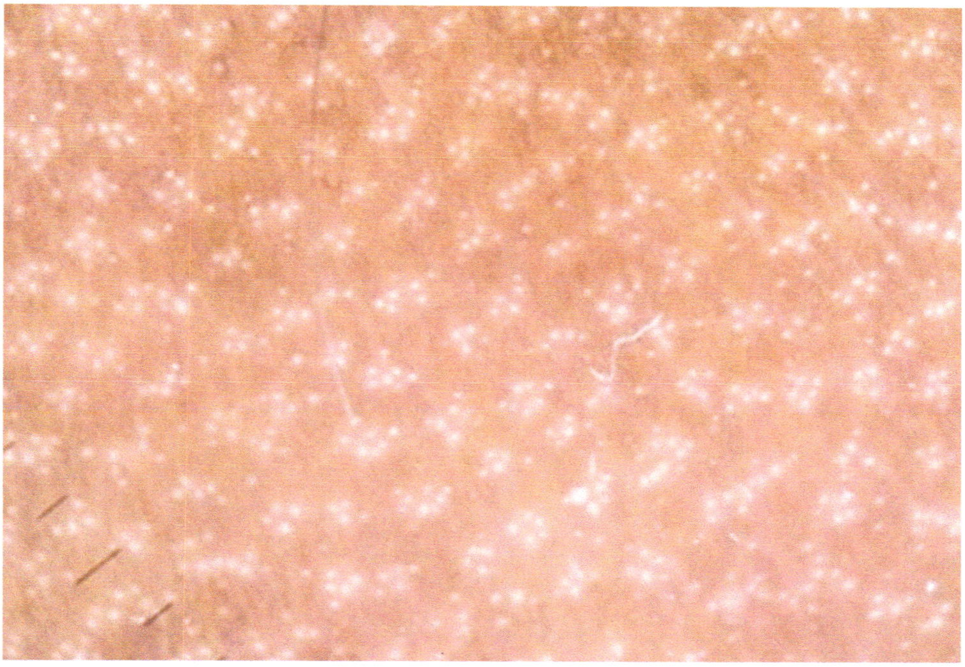

Fig. 14: Cluster of star appearance which may be defined aggregates of pin-point white dots on the scalp in clusters of 8–10 arranged in a regular pattern all over the scalp.

MONILETHRIX

INTRODUCTION

- It is defined as a hair shaft disorder characterized by easy fragility of the hair shafts leading to hair loss.
- The hair is normal at birth; however, in a few months the patient develops keratotic papules, alopecia and brittle hair.
- Light microscopy aided in demonstrating the regular beaded appearance which clinched the diagnosis.

KEY TRICHOSCOPIC FEATURES

- The scalp in monilethrix is unremarkable with a normal vasculature, follicular, and interfollicular patterns.
- Hair of varying lengths with many broken hair.
- Examination of the hair reveals multiple beaded hair with equidistant nodes and internodes.[4]
- Dermoscopy of body hair and of the eyebrows may also reveal regular beading of the hair which may not be apparent clinically.

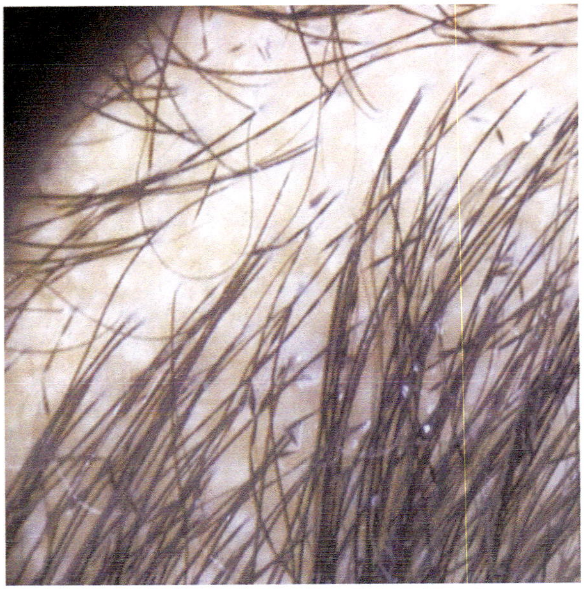

Fig. 15: Trichoscopic examination of the hair reveals multiple beaded hair with equidistant nodes and internodes.[4]

REFERENCES

1. Karadag Köse O, Güleç AT. Temporal triangular alopecia: Significance of trichoscopy in differential diagnosis. J Eur Acad Dermatol Venereol. 2015;29(8):1621-5.
2. Shim WH, Jwa SW, Song M, Kim HS, Ko HC, Kim BS, et al. Dermoscopic approach to a small round to oval hairless patch on the scalp. Ann Dermatol. 2014;26:214-20.
3. Kharkar V, Gutte R, Thakkar V, Khopkar U. Trichorrhexis Nodosa with Nail Dystrophy: Diagnosis by Dermoscopy. Int J Trichol. 2011;3(2):105-6.
4. Sharma VK, Chiramel MJ, Rao A. Dermoscopy: A rapid bedside tool to assess monilethrix. Indian J Dermatol Venereol Leprol. 2016;82:73-4.

ASSESSMENT IMAGE-BASED QUESTIONS

A case of patchy hair loss present since childhood over the right temporal area not responding to treatment.

1. What are the clinical differential diagnosis?

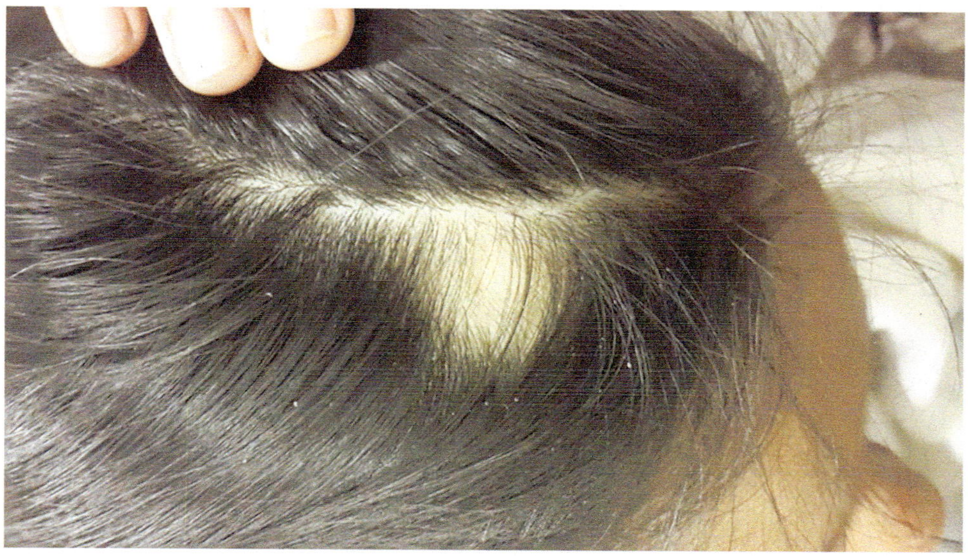

Trichoscopic findings of the above patient shows vellus hairs as the prominent feature.

2. What is the final diagnosis?

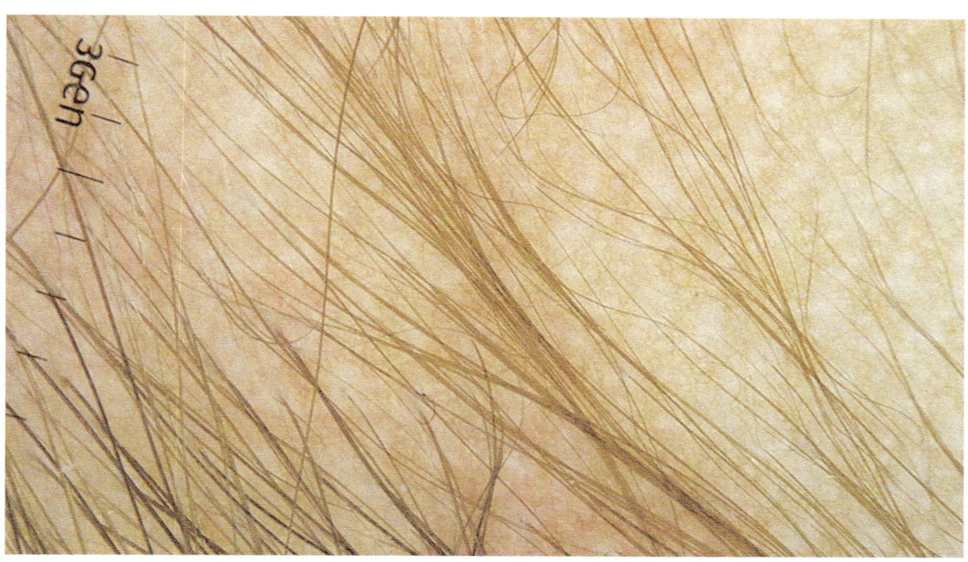

ANSWERS

1. Alopecia areata and congenital triangular alopecia
2. Congenital triangular alopecia because of the presence of carpet of vellus hairs and no other signs suggestive of alopecia areata

CHAPTER 31

Body Hair

Subrata Malakar

INTRODUCTION

- Along with the diagnosis of scalp hair disorders, trichoscopy can also help diagnosing body hair disorders including keratosis pilaris, trichostasis spinulosa, etc.
- Trichoscopy can quickly scan the whole body hairs.
- Trichoscopy reduces the necessity of other painful diagnostic procedures such as biopsy and hair plucking.

KEY FEATURES

- Circle hairs
- Rolled hairs
- Ingrown hairs
- Trichostasis spinulosa
- Keratosis pilaris
- Pili multigemini
- Eruptive vellus hair cyst (EVHC)
- Body hairs in other dermatoses
- *Demodex* at the emergence of facial hairs

Circle Hairs

- It represents a body hair growth disorder and is characterized by asymptomatic presence of circular or spiral hairs.[1]
- Usually seen on the trunk and upper legs of overweight patients.[1]
- It can occasionally be detected on the scalp.[2]
- Several theories are there about its pathogenesis. According to the latest one, these hairs are genetically determined disorders that correspond to vestigial of the mammalian undercoat.[3]
- *Histopathology*: Presence of "riverbed" dilated follicle infundibulum with entrapped hair shafts.[1]
- *Trichoscopy*: Hairs may protrude from the skin or may be seen under thin skin layer (subcorneal hair coiling).[1]
- Clinical significance is unknown.

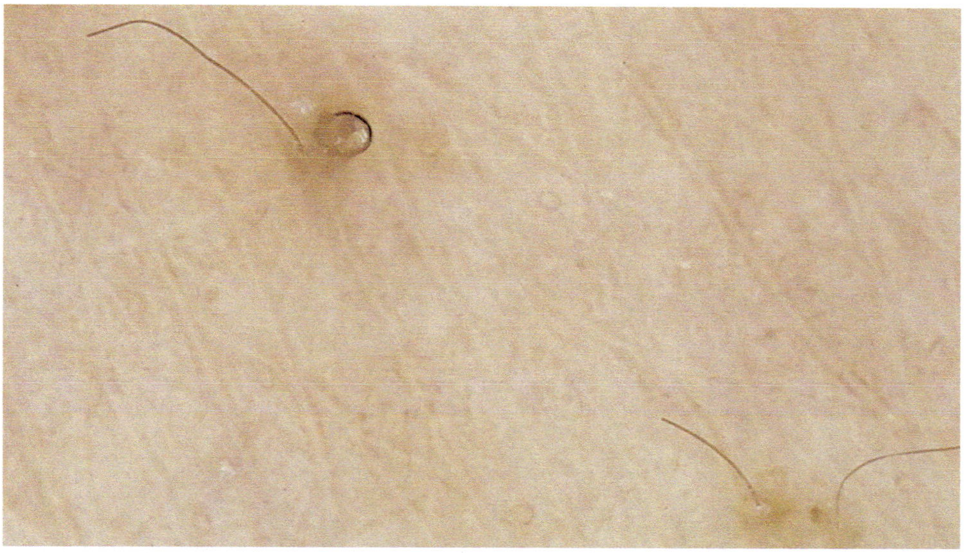

Fig. 1: Circle hair presents as dark hair circle which is located under a thin layer of stratum corneum.

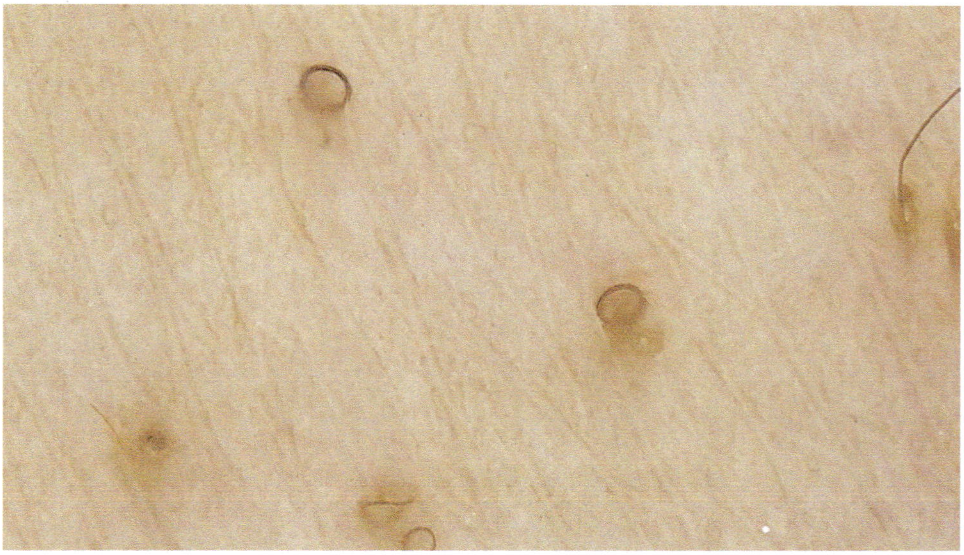

Fig. 2: Subcorneal circle hairs. There is no evidence of follicular obstruction or perifollicular inflammation.

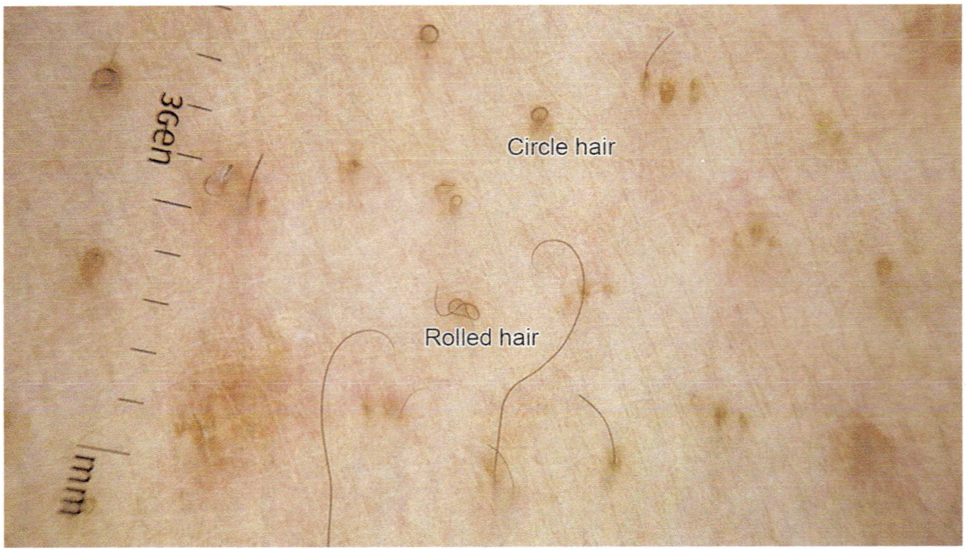

Fig. 3: Circle hairs are present among normal hairs. One rolled hair is also visible in this field.

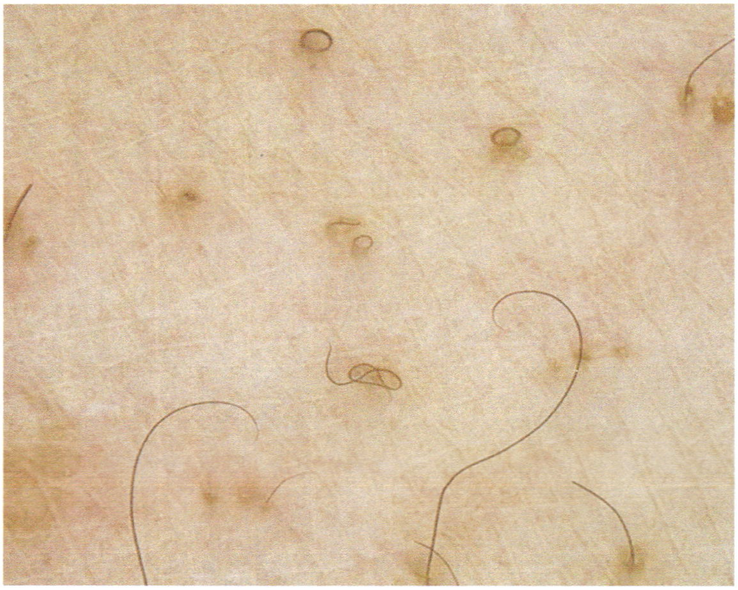

Fig. 4: Circle hairs and rolled hairs among normal body hairs. Under microscopy they show dystrophic bulb in anagen phase and there is absence of inner root sheath.

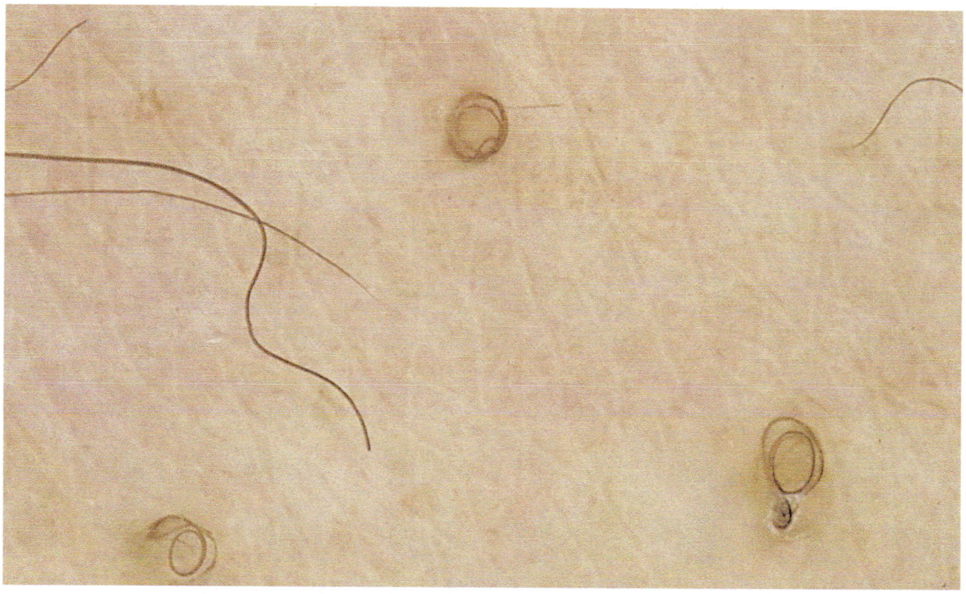

Fig. 5: Circle hairs may be found in overweight patients and in those who perform frequent waxing procedures.

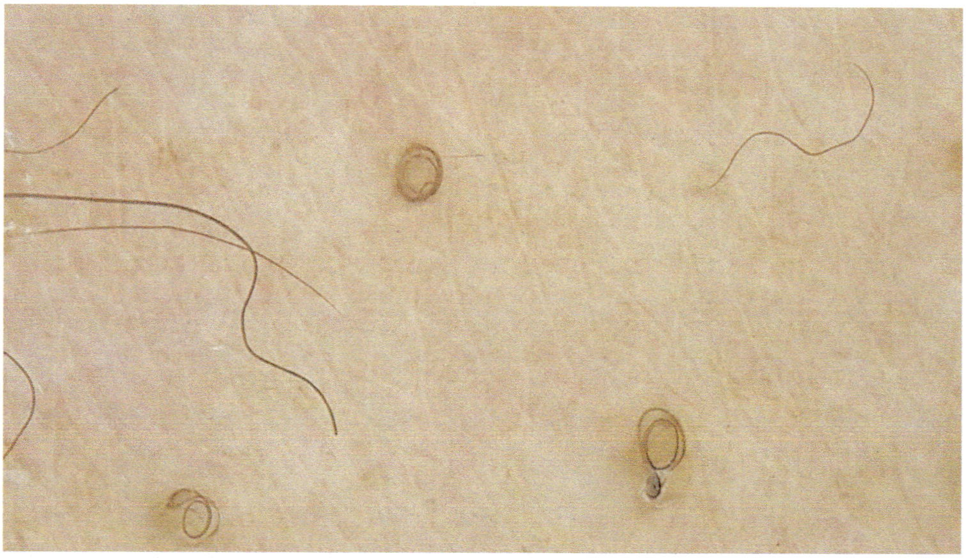

Fig. 6: Dark hairs forming circles are observed among normal hairs. There is controversy about its pathogenesis. However, recently circle hair is hypothesized as a genetic disorder corresponding to remnants of the mammal undercoat.

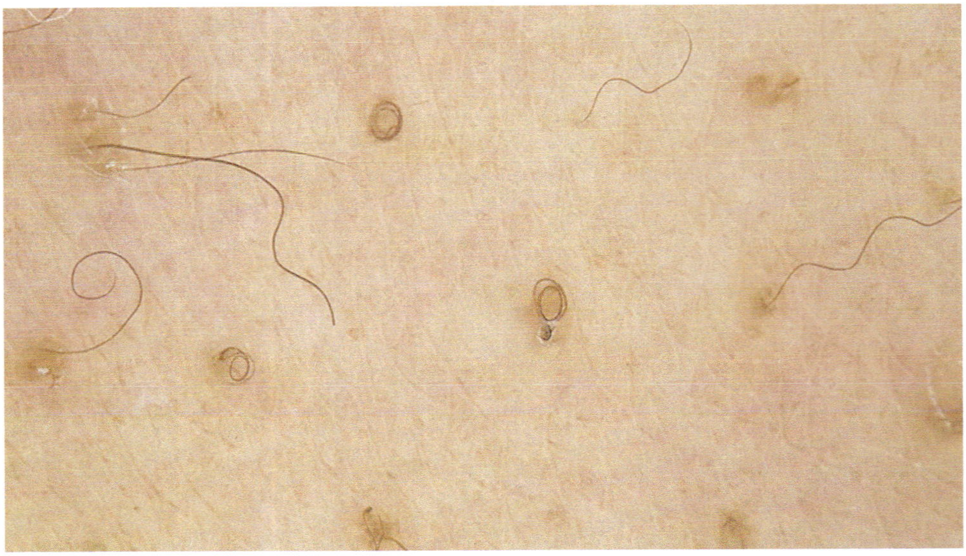

Fig. 7: Circle hairs are found incidentally on different regions of the body including extremities and abdomen where they are surrounded by normal hairs.

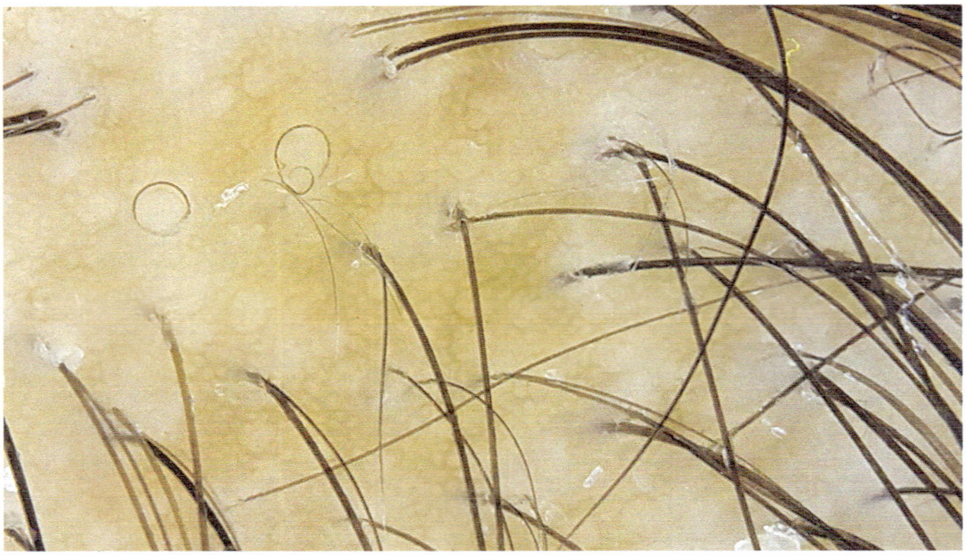

Fig. 8: Circle hairs can also be observed occasionally over the scalp. Clinical significance is unknown.

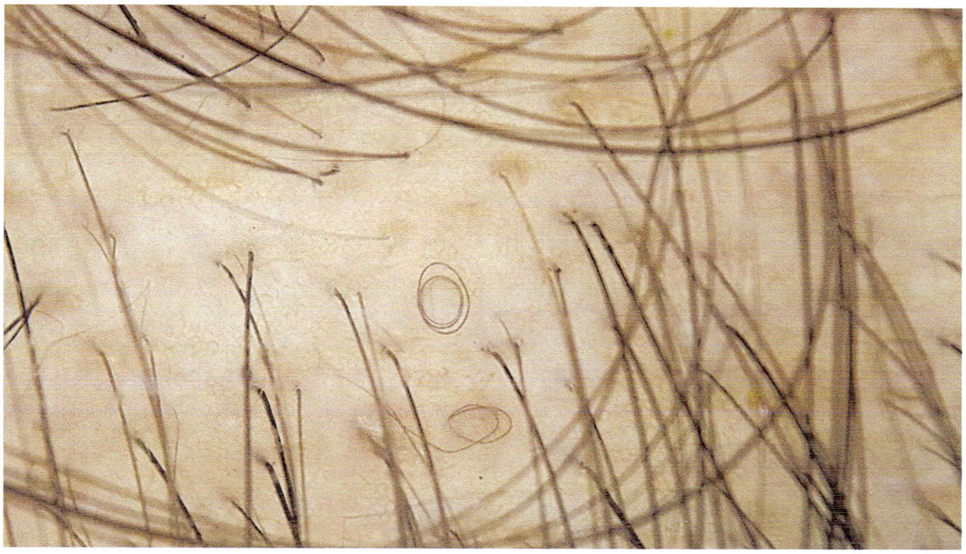

Fig. 9: Not uncommonly circle hairs may be present in healthy individual.

Rolled Hairs

- Present as keratotic inflammatory follicular papules with twisted hairs.[4]
- Probably caused by trauma due to vigorous rubbing.[2]
- More common than circle hairs
- Association has been reported with treatment with cyclosporin and corticosteroid, keratosis pilaris, xerosis, ichthyosis, etc.[5-8]
- Present over extensor of extremities, back, buttocks, and shoulder.[5-8]
- It is postulated that rolled hair is the result of inability of the hair follicle to emerge through the infundibulum.
- *Histopathology*: Follicular hyperkeratosis
- *Trichoscopy*: Twisted hairs and peripilar casts

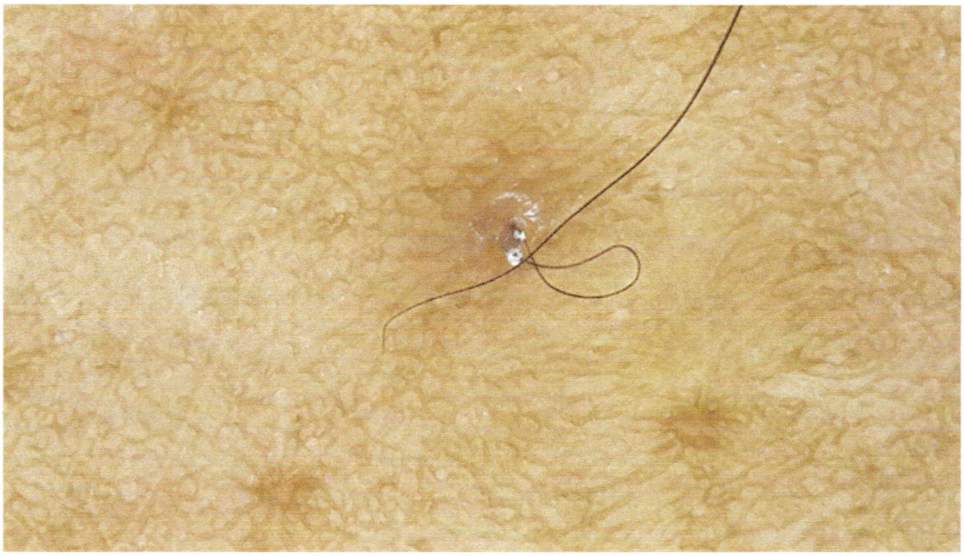

Fig. 10: Rolled hair on trichoscopy shows twisted hair with peripilar cast.

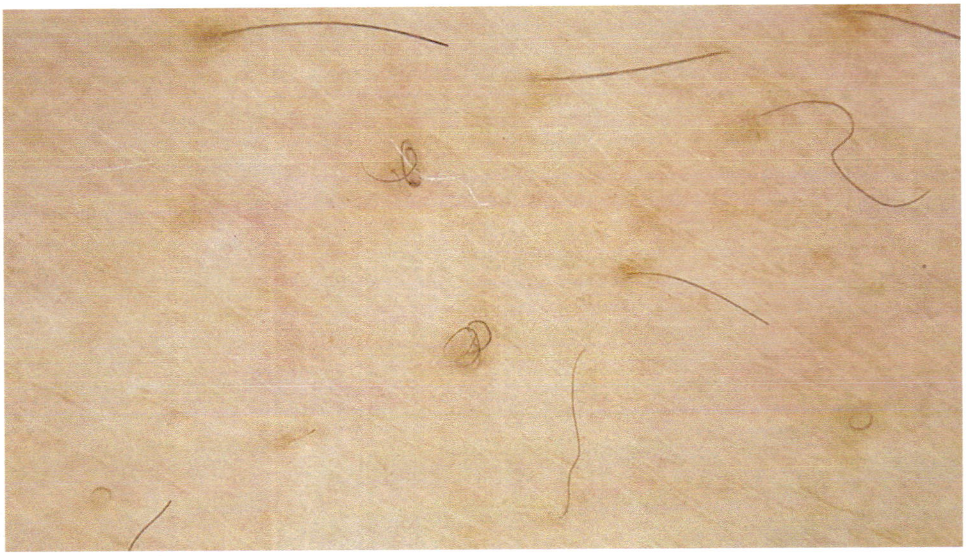

Fig. 11: Rolled hair—subcorneal spiral hairs interspersed with normal hairs.

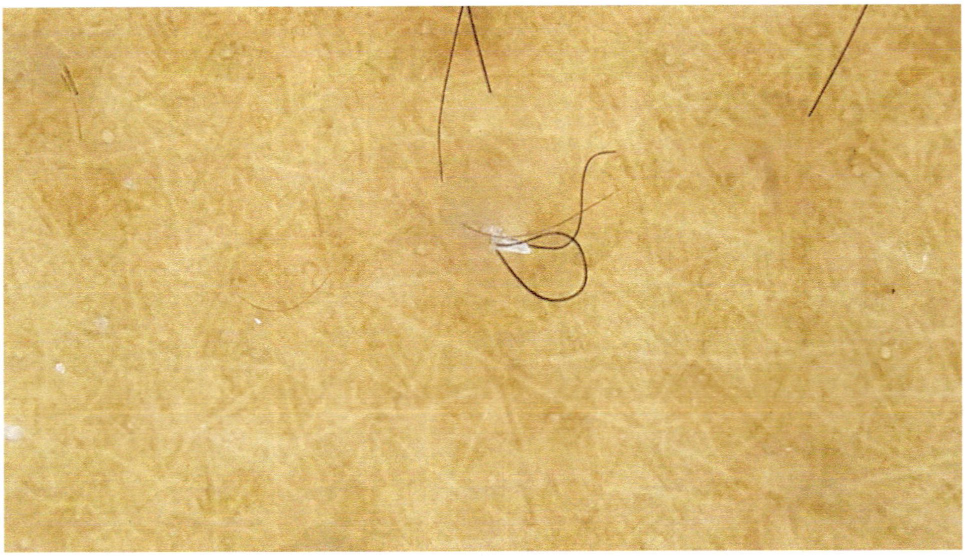

Fig. 12: On trichoscopy, rolled hair appear as irregularly twisted hair into a hyperkeratotic papule.

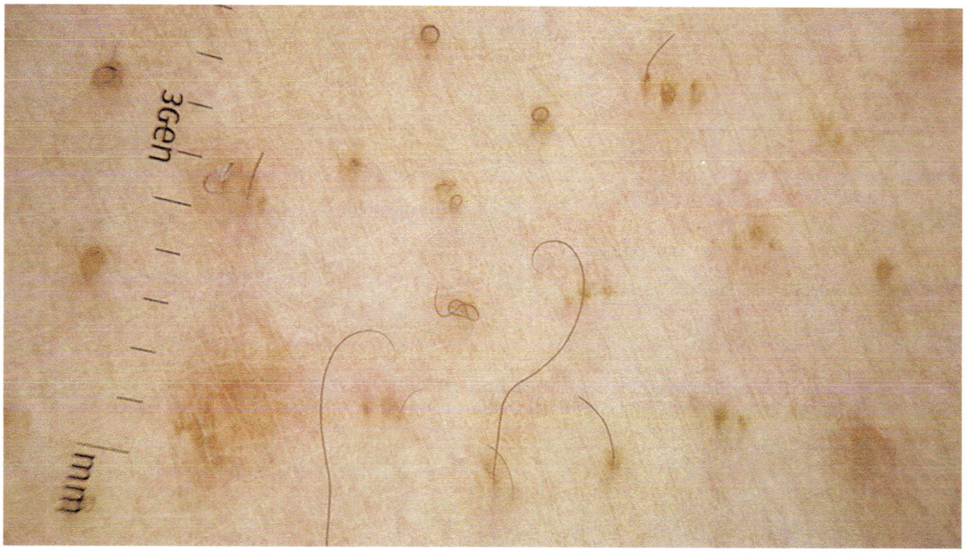

Fig. 13: Irregularly twisted subcorneal hairs with peripilar cast.

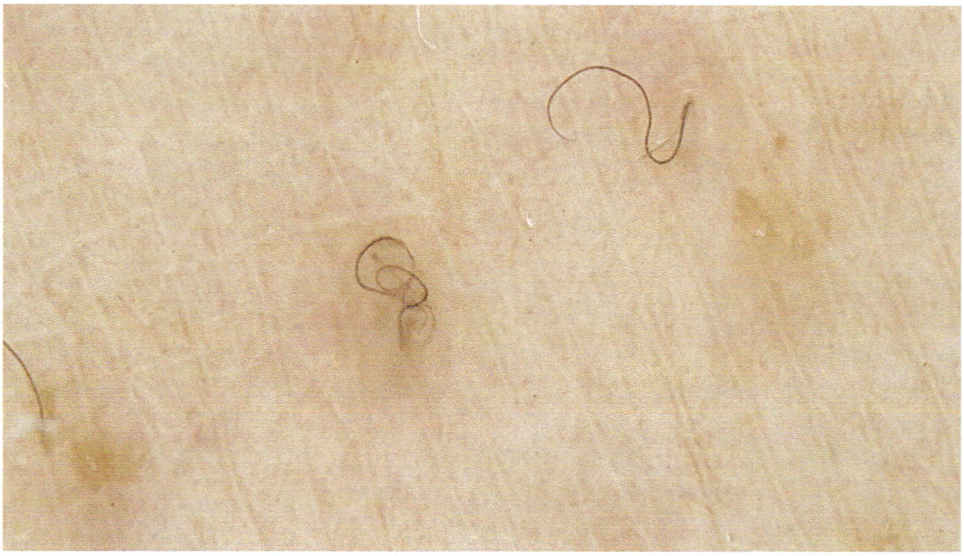

Fig. 14: Irregularly twisted subcorneal hairs. (magnified image).

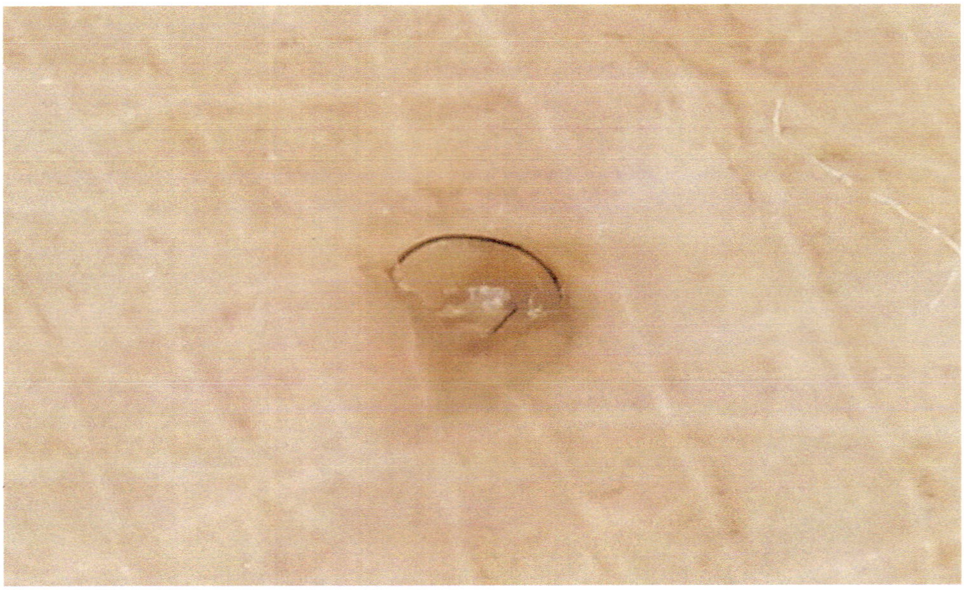

Fig. 15: Rolled hair—keratotic inflammatory follicular papule with twisted hair.

Ingrown Hairs

- Other names are pseudofolliculitis barbae, pseudofolliculitis of beard.[2]
- Usually occurs over beard area, nape of neck, axillae, legs and pubic area.
- Frequently is precipitated by shaving or plucking.
- Two types of ingrowing hairs occur—(1) transfollicular and (2) extrafollicular when sharp hair re-enters the skin 1–2 mm away from its emergence.[9]
- Papulopustular lesions are the main presentation of ingrown hairs in men located commonly in the beard and submental areas. Neck also may be involved.
- Whereas in women they are usually seen on the chin and inguinal area. It may be accompanied by itch, pain, or secondary infection. Hypertrophic scar and keloid, as a consequence may be produced.[10,11]
- Trichoscopy is very useful to educate the patient who can observe and appreciate the condition. So it may serve to monitor the patient compliance to treatment.
- *Chin and inguinal areas*: Dermoscopy shows "U"-shaped ingrowing hairs under a papular lesion which correlate with transfollicular penetration.
- *Histopathology*: Foreign body reaction, giant cells, and fibrosis
- Extrafollicular penetration is commonly observed over beard area and neck.

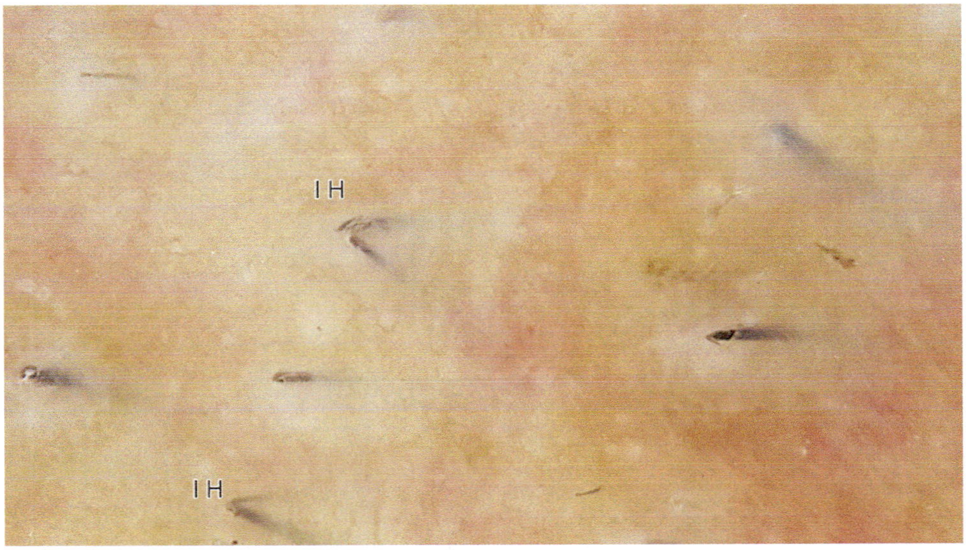

Fig. 16: "U"-shaped ingrown hairs (IH) over neck.

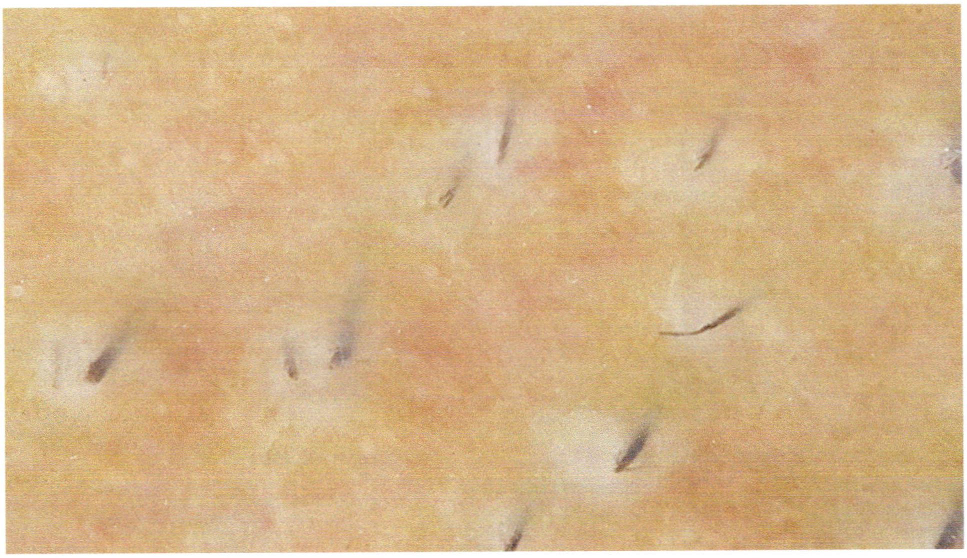

Fig. 17: Hair shaft embedding with foreign body reaction and inflammation.

Trichostasis Spinulosa

- Hyperkeratosis of a dilated follicle with retention of multiple telogen vellus hairs.[2]
- Open comedo-like lesions or horny spinous plugs are seen primarily on the tip of the nose, alae nasi, and cheeks.[2]
- It can also present as itchy papules on the trunk and upper extremities in young adults.[2]
- In chronic renal failure, diffuse trichostasis spinulosa has been reported.[2]
- *Histology*: Dilated follicular infundibulum with numerous pigmented vellus hairs of up to 50 hairs and keratinous material.[2]
- Many diagnostic procedures are there including microscopic examination and biopsy.
- Dermoscopy provides fast and easy diagnosis. On dermoscopy, there are tufts of multiple vellus hairs emerging from the dilated follicles. Other follicular openings are occluded by keratotic plugs.[2]

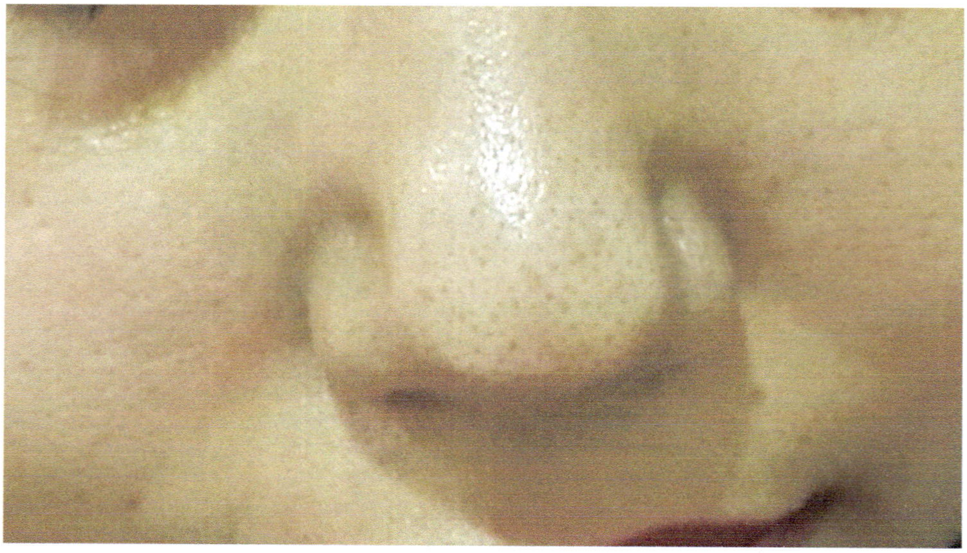

Fig. 18: Clinical photography of trichostasis spinulosa over nose, alae nasi, and adjacent cheeks.

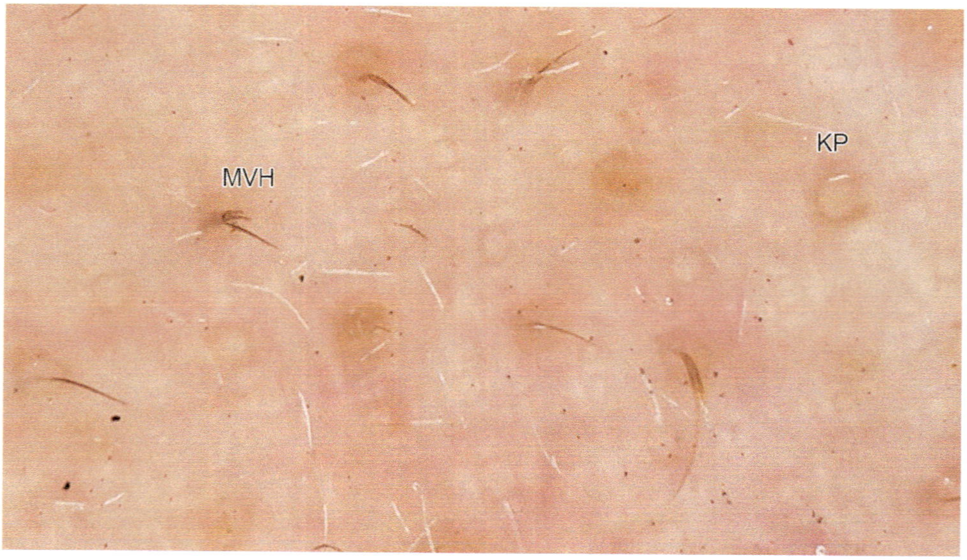

Fig. 19: Trichoscopy of trichostasis spinulosa shows tufts of multiple vellus hairs (MVH) and keratotic plugs (KP).

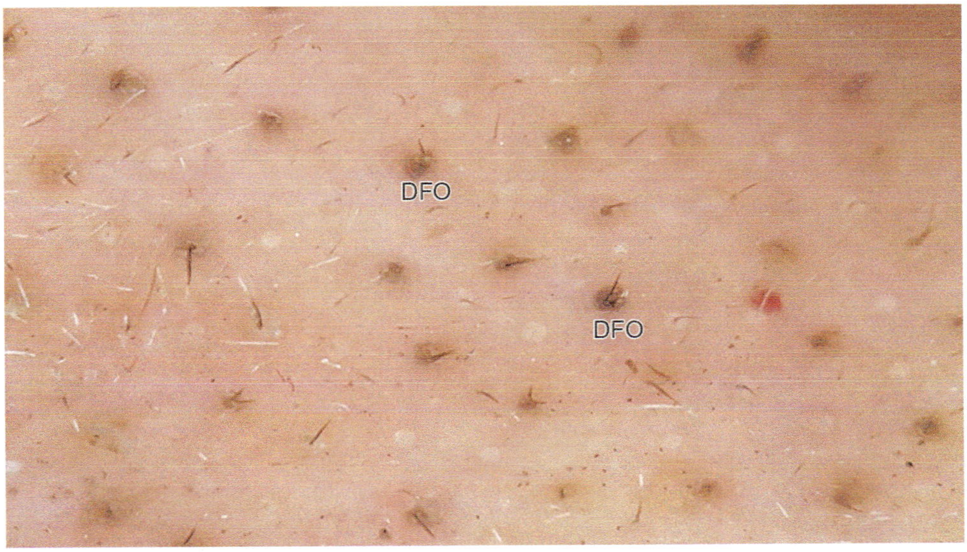

Fig. 20: Tufts of vellus hairs emerging from dilated infundibular openings (DFO).

Keratosis Pilaris

- It is a common autosomal dominant disorder characterized by keratinous plugs in the follicular infundibulum with varying degrees of perifollicular erythema.
- The most accepted theory regarding its pathogenesis is defective keratinization of the follicular epithelium resulting in a keratotic infundibular plug.[12]
- Asymptomatic or pruritic keratotic papules over upper arm, thigh, face, and buttock.[13,14]
- *Dermoscopy*: Vellus hair surrounded by peripilar casts. Vellus hairs may be twisted or coiled. In severe cases, vellus hairs are coiled and embedded in the horny layer. Perifollicular erythema and hyperpigmentation is frequently seen.[2]

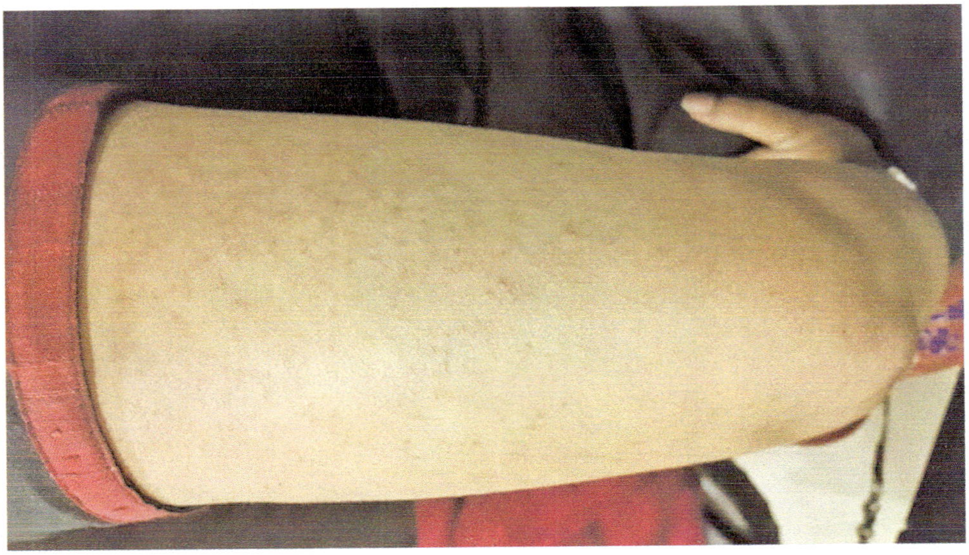

Fig. 21: Clinical picture of keratosis pilaris.

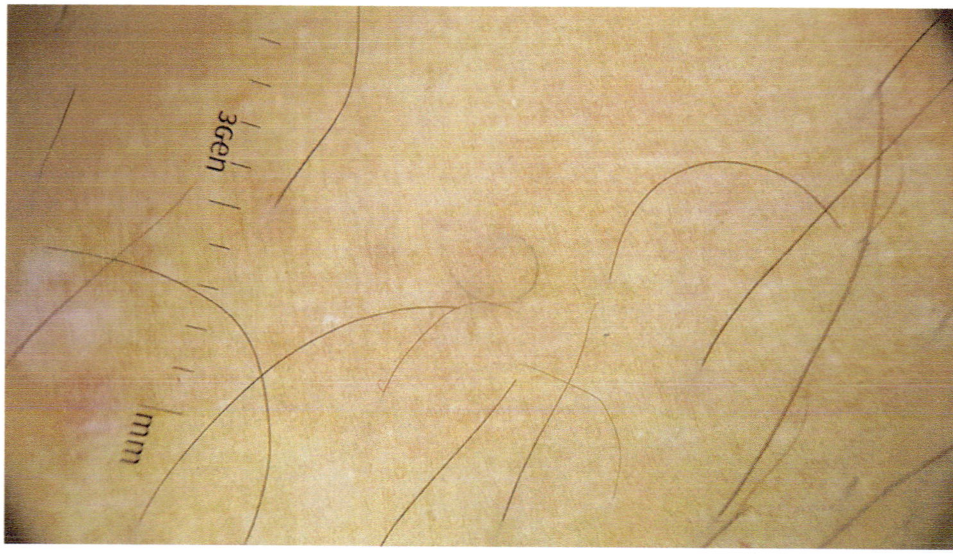

Fig. 22: Trichoscopy of keratosis pilaris—coiled vellus hair embedded in the subcorneal layer.

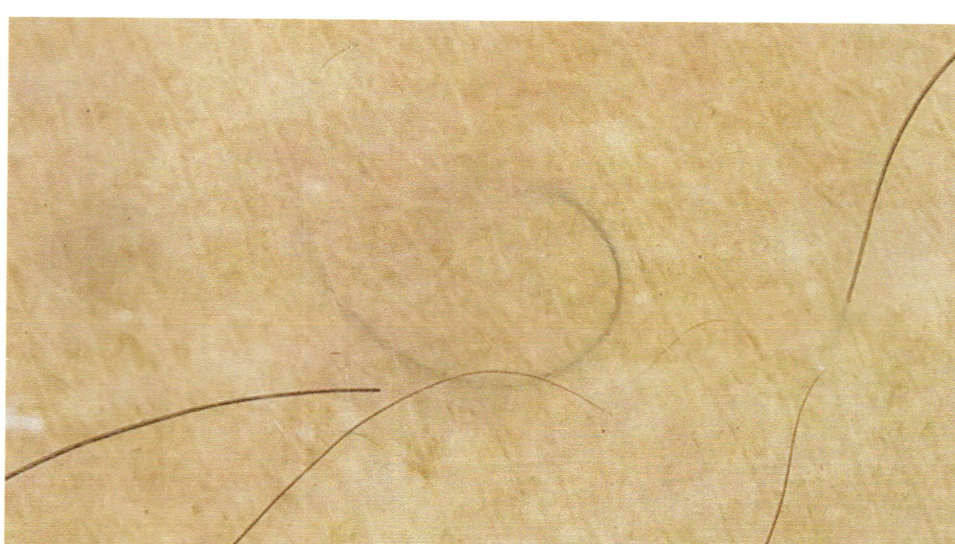

Fig. 23: Zooming of previous image—coiled vellus hair is clearly seen under thin stratum corneum.

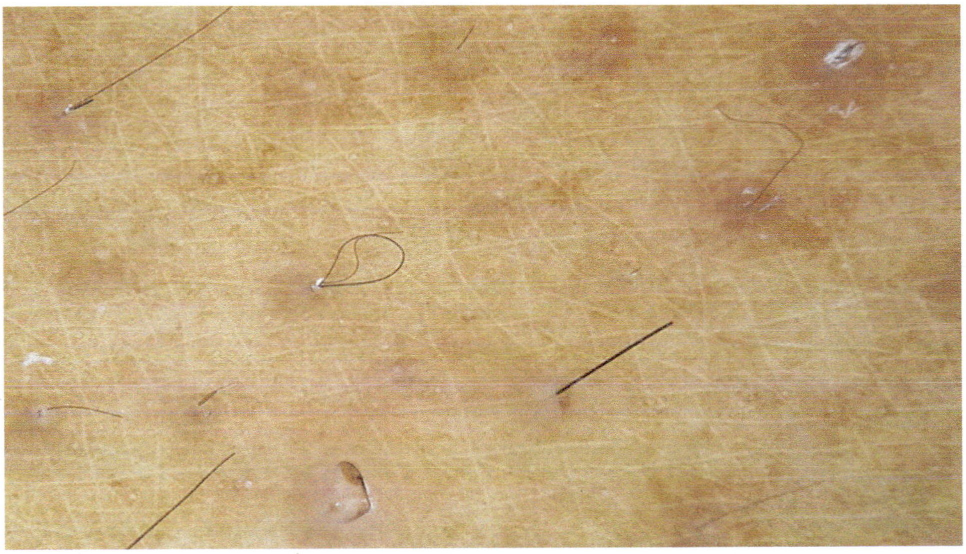

Fig. 24: Irregularly coiled vellus hairs embedded into horny layer. Perifollicular erythema with hyperpigmentation is also seen.

Pili Multigemini

- It is a developmental defect of hair follicles where multiple hair shafts emerge from a single follicle. Hair shafts are separated from each other by IRS but enclosed in a common ORS.[15]
- The common age group affected are childhood to adolescent.
- It should be suspected in males showing remarkably thick hair. Recurrent inflammatory papules leaving atrophic or hypertrophic scars are the common presentation. Multigeminate follicles occur mainly along the jaw lines.[16]
- *Histology*: Multiple separated hair shafts enclosed in a common ORS but separated from each other by IRS.
- *Dermoscopy*: Bundles of multiple pigmented hairs of similar thickness emerging from each hair follicle. Each tuft has a peripilar cast.[2]
- *Treatment*: Q-switched ruby laser

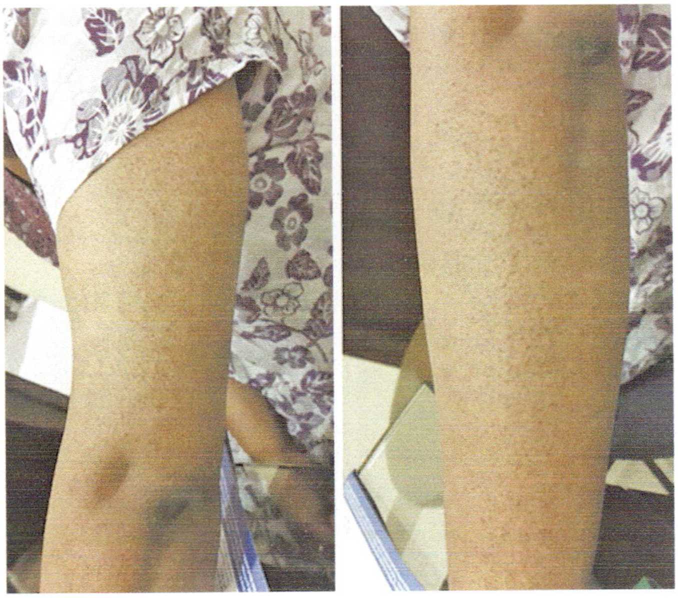

Fig. 25: Clinical picture of keratosis pilaris.

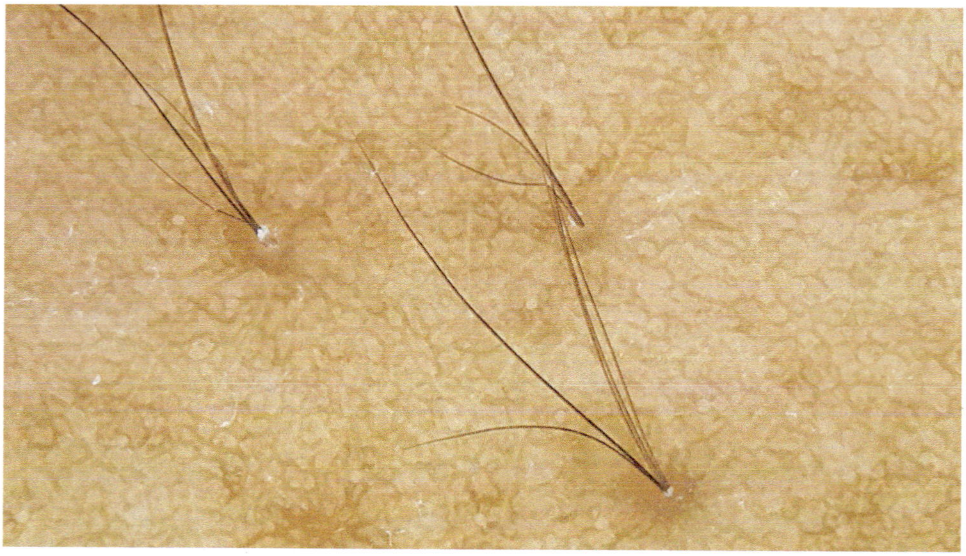

Fig. 26: Pili multigemini: Each hair tuft has a peripilar cast.

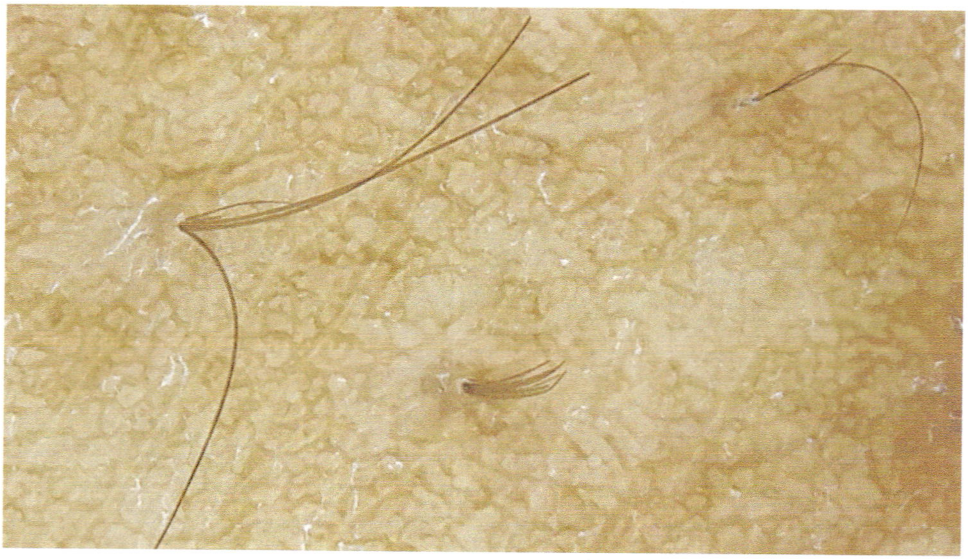

Fig. 27: Bundles of pigmented hairs emerging from the same follicular opening. Note the equal thickness of all the hairs. The hair tufts are surrounded by peripilar casts.

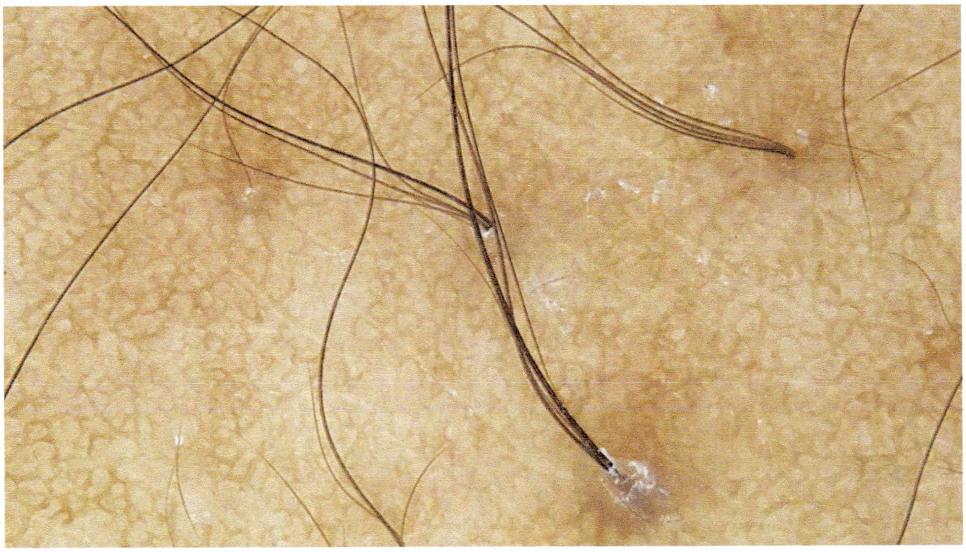

Fig. 28: Hair tufts surrounded by peripilar cast. The patients showing strikingly thick hairs may have pili multigemini trichoscopically.

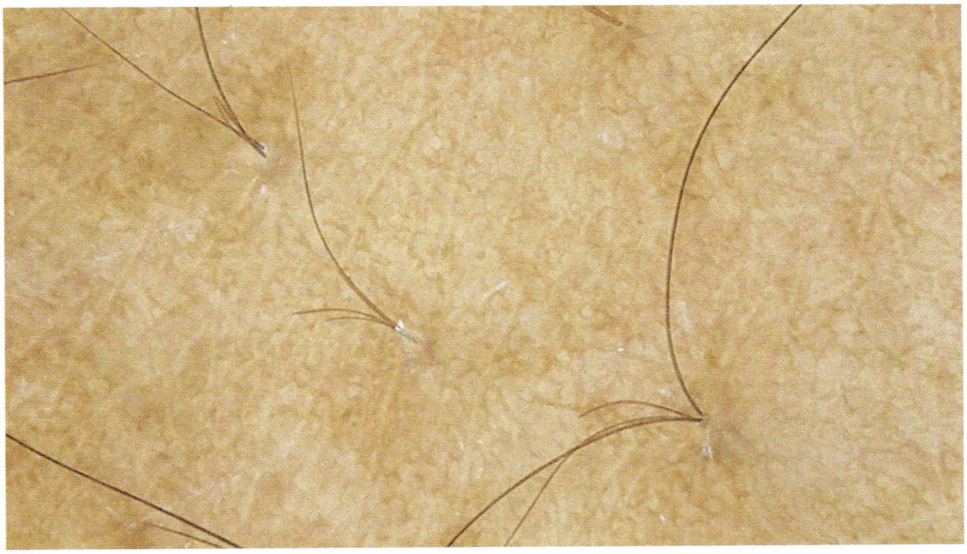

Fig. 29: Pili multigemini: Nearly 2% of patients presenting with other dermatological conditions have this disorder.

Eruptive Vellus Hair Cysts

- Present as multiple, asymptomatic papules over chest and abdomen with a smooth or centrally umbilicated surface. Affects children in their second decade of life. There is occlusion and dilatation of vellus hair follicles.[17-19]
- Inheritance—sporadic/autosomal dominant
- Coexistence of EVHC and steatocystoma multiplex is common.[2]
- *Histopathology*: Small epidermoid cyst containing multiple vellus hairs (overlapping feature of steatocystoma and EVHC)
- *Dermoscopy*: Well-defined whitish circular structures[2]
- *Treatment*: Topical retinoid, CO_2 laser

Body Hairs in Other Dermatoses

Body hairs can be affected in dermatoses involving both the scalp hairs and body hairs, like lichen planopilaris.

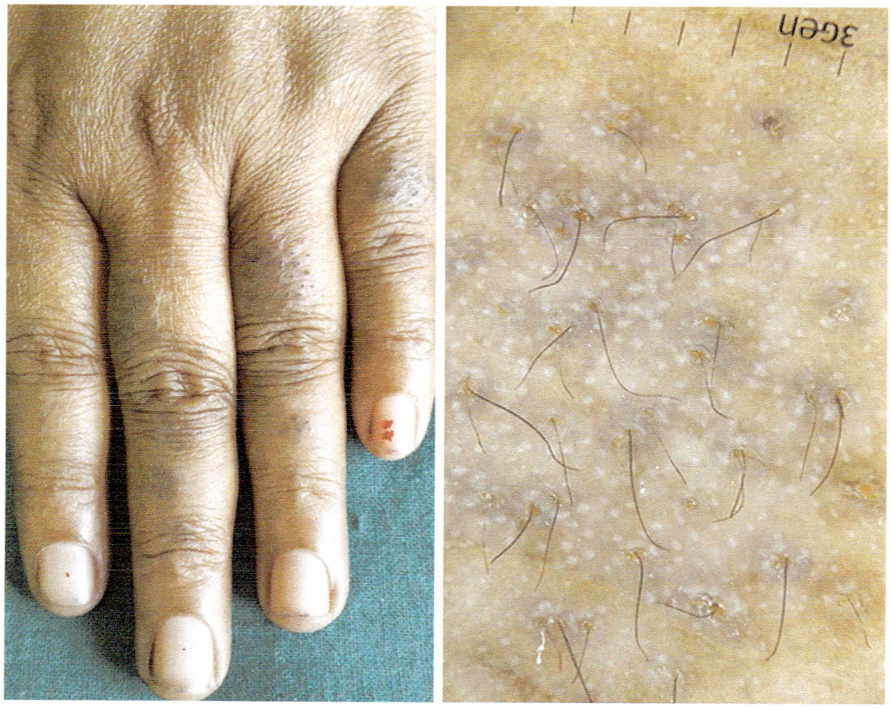

Fig. 30: Blue-gray dots in target pattern involving body hairs in a case of lichen planopilaris.

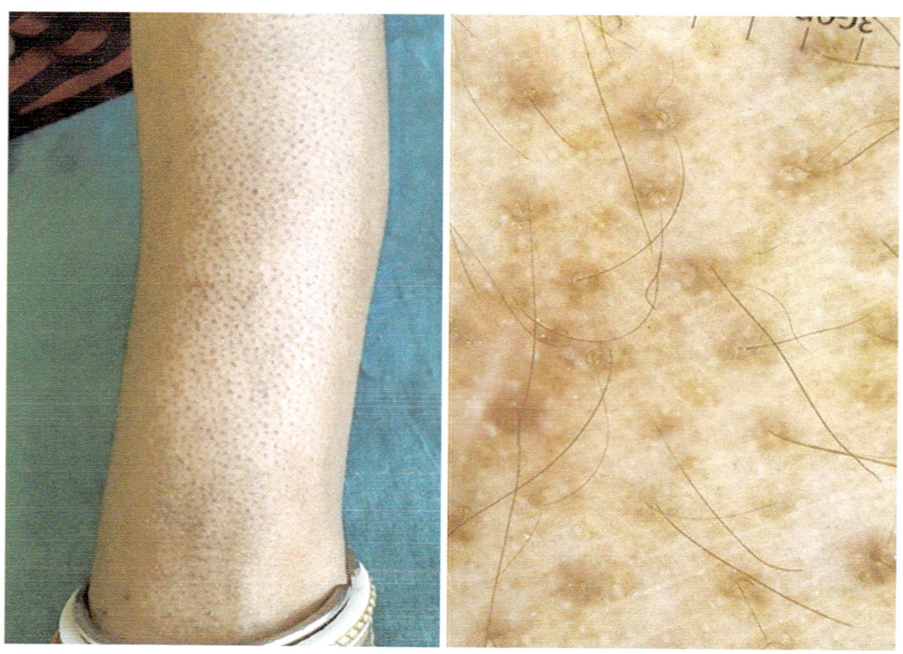

Fig. 31: Blue-gray target pattern around forearm hairs in a case of lichen planopilaris.

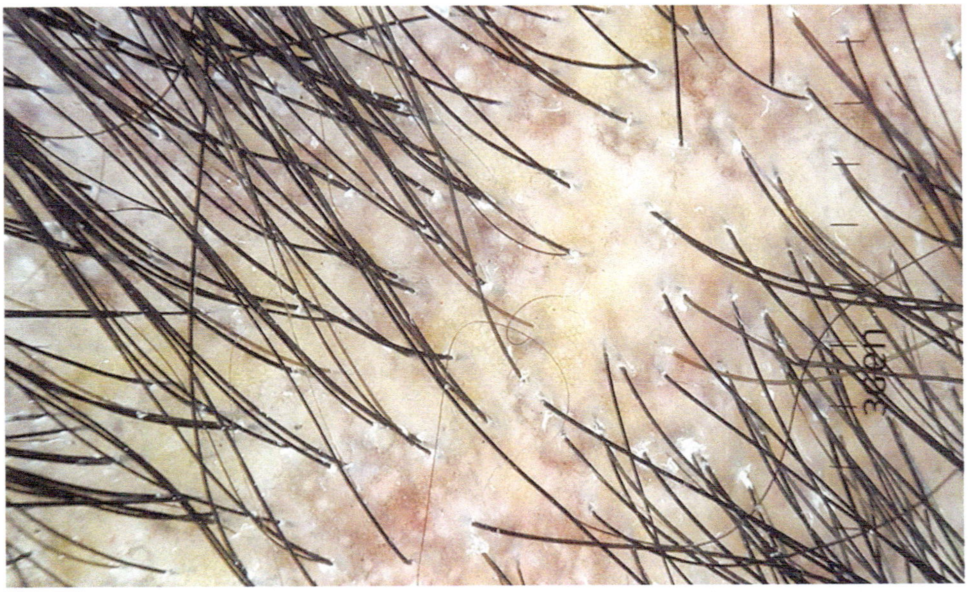

Fig. 32: Same patient as Figures 30 and 31. The patient presents with severe scalp itching and on routine trichoscopy blue-gray dots, peripilar scales and erythema were found. Histopathology confirmed it as a case of lichen planopilaris. Target pattern is due to melanin incontinence surrounding only the perifollicular area and sparing interfollicular region.

Demodicosis

- It results from infestation with the *Demodex* mite, an obligate human parasite having two species, *Demodex folliculorum* and *Demodex brevis*. *Demodex* can only live in the human hair follicle.[20]
- *Demodex* is an ectoparasite of pilosebaceous follicle and sebaceous gland, typically found on the face including cheeks, nose, chin, forehead, temples, eyelashes, brows, and also on the balding scalp, neck, and ears.
- Clinically, it may present as erythema, burning, and stinging sensation or a nonspecific rash over the face.
- Demodicosis is diagnosed when there is high density of *Demodex* mites (>5/sq cm)
- *Dermoscopy*: White spicules protruding from the follicular openings. White spicules represent mite tails.[21]

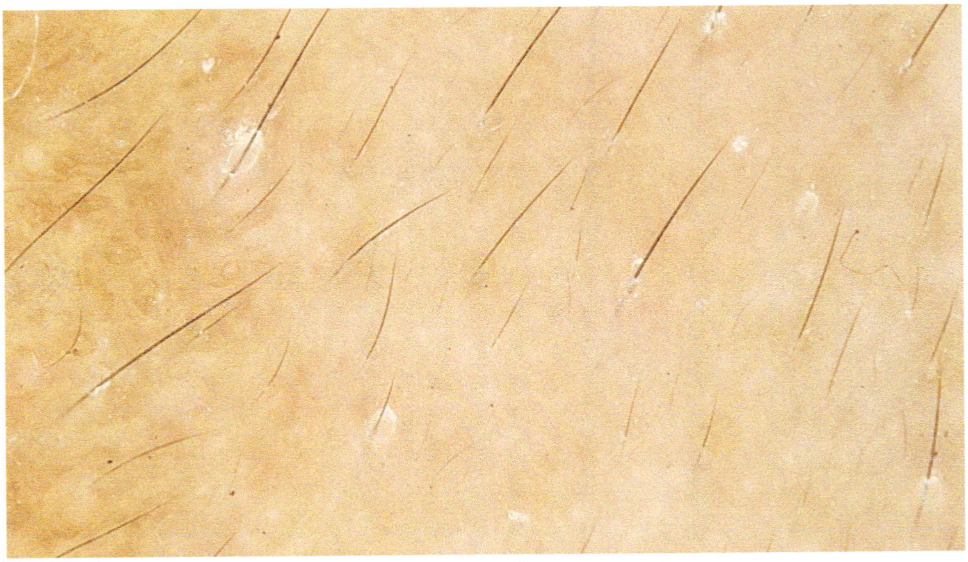

Fig. 33: *Demodex* at the emergence of facial hairs. It presents as white spicules from the follicular openings representing the mite tail.

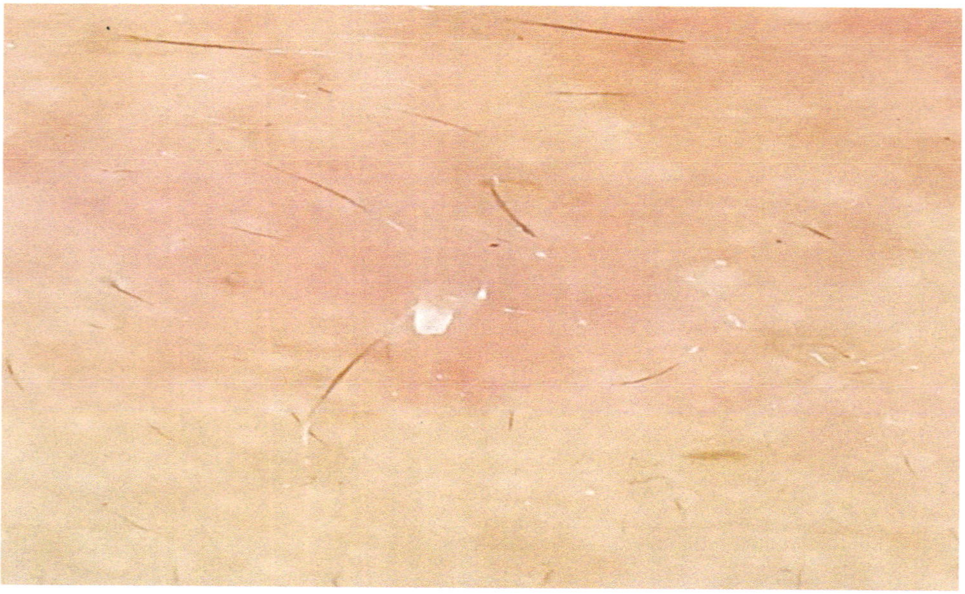

Fig. 34: *Demodex* at the follicular opening of face. Note the white spicule representing the tail of *Demodex* and some erythematous rash. The patient also had mild burning sensation which all favors the diagnosis of demodicosis.

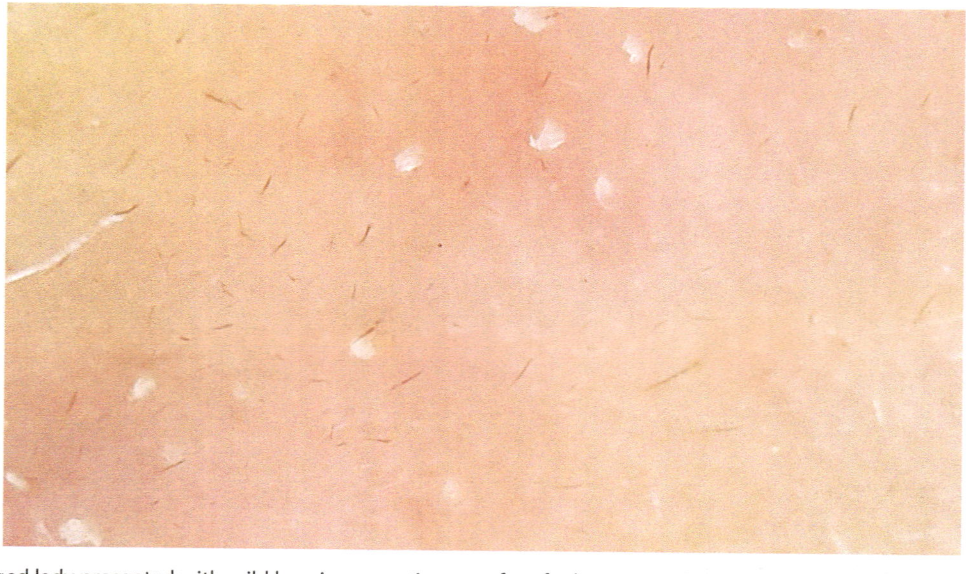

Fig. 35: A middle-aged lady presented with mild burning sensation over face for last 1 year. On examination, there is erythematous rash and on trichoscopy, the field is studed with white spicules. Thus, trichoscopy is very fast and definitive to diagnose demodicosis.

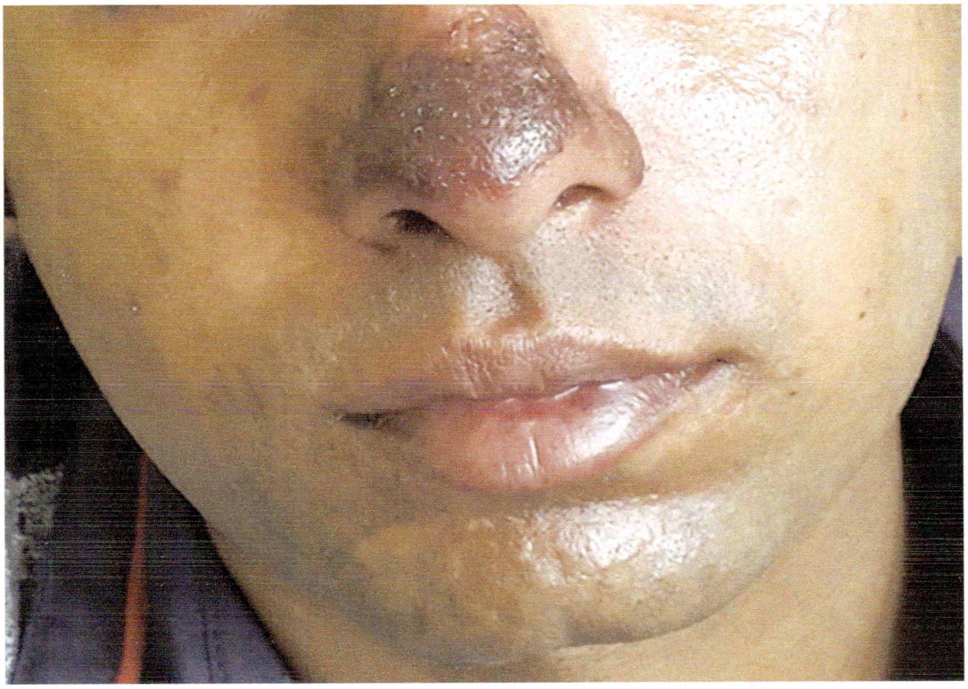

Fig. 36: Asymptomatic dull erythematous rash over nose for last 1 year.

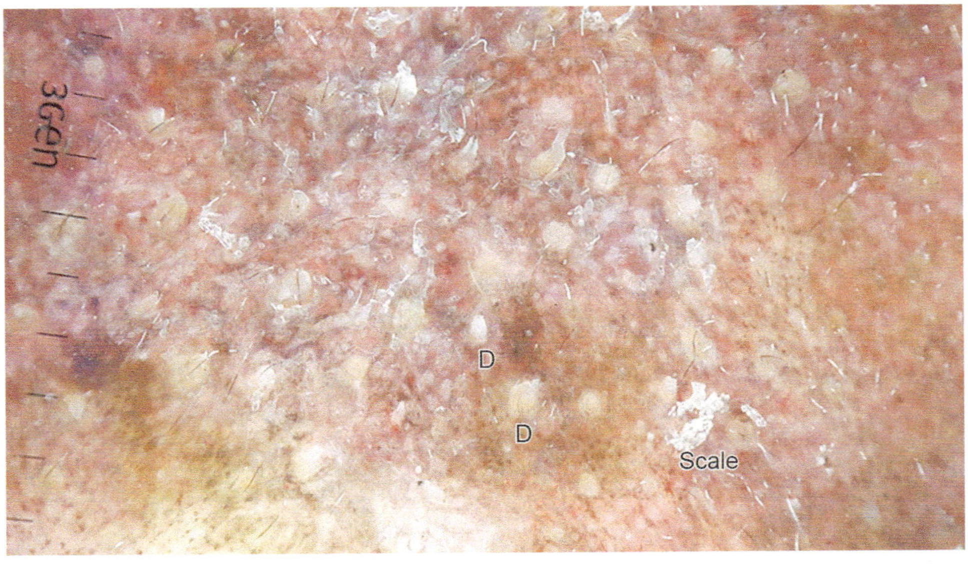

Fig. 37: On trichoscopy of previous image, the field is full of white spicules of *Demodex* (D) on an erythematous background. Some scales are also present. Histopathology showed the presence of *Demodex* infundibulum.

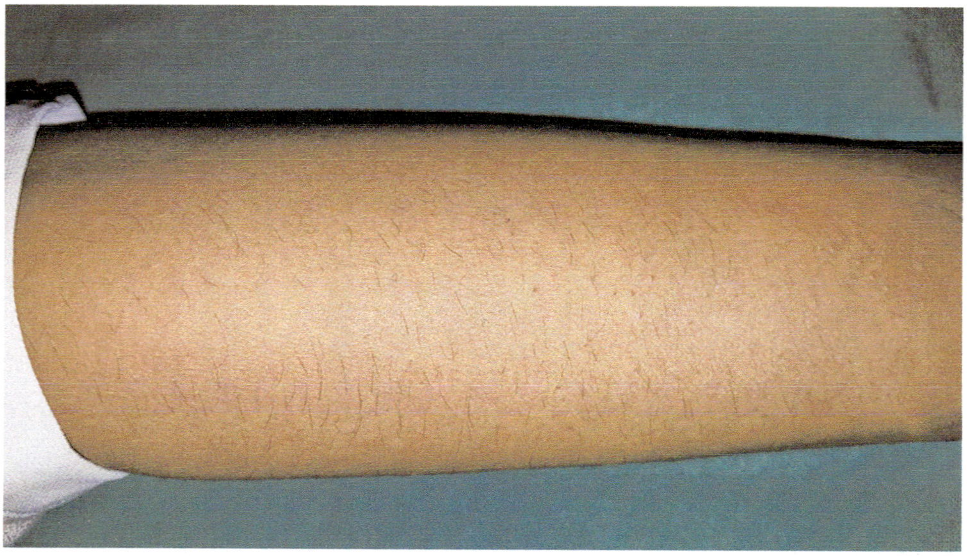

Fig. 38: A 23-year-old girl presented with minute papular eruptions and mild irritation over forearms and legs. There is a history of regular waxing is present.

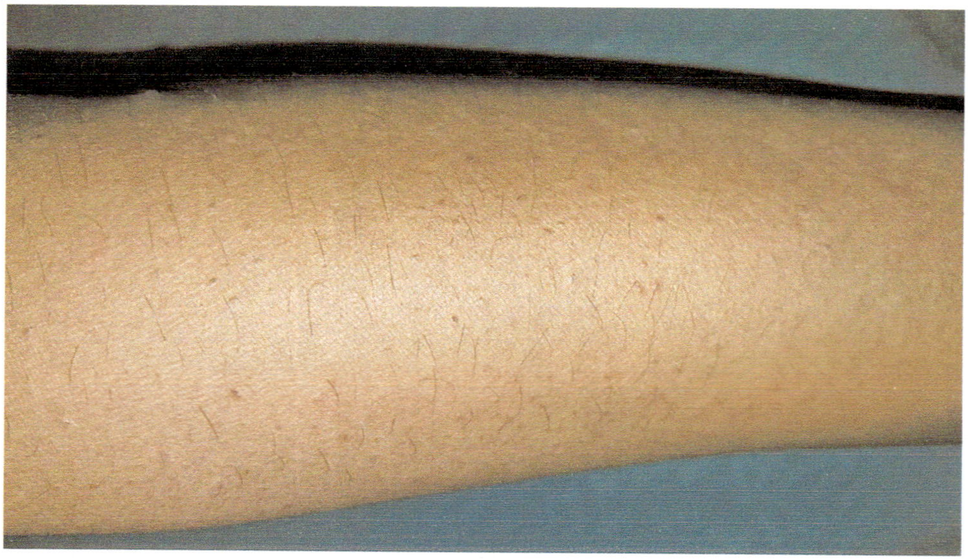

Fig. 39: Same patient with minute papular eruption over leg.

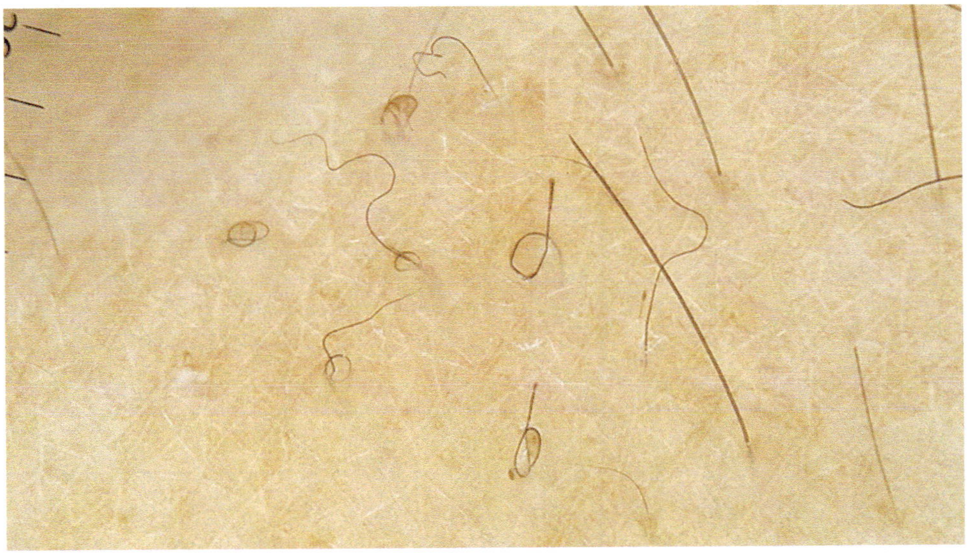

Fig. 40: On trichoscopy of previous patient, multiple trichoscopic derformities of body hairs are seen namely rolled, subcorneal and ingrown hairs. This is a result of mechanical force applied in different directions while performing waxing.

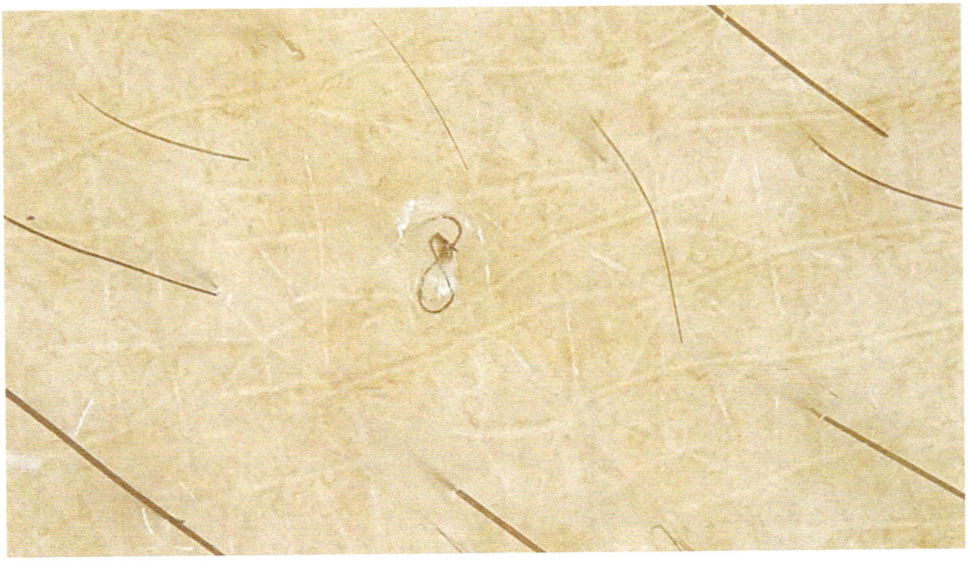

Fig. 41: Rolled hair in the same patient.

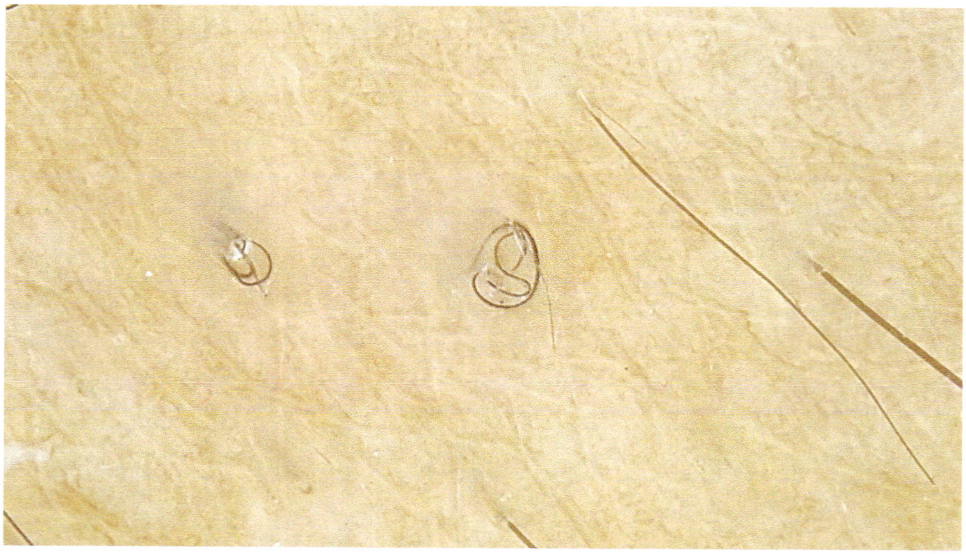

Fig. 42: Twisted and ingrown hair in the same patient.

REFERENCES

1. Lacarrubba F, Misciali C, Gibilisco R, Micali G. Circle hairs: Clinical, trichoscopic and histopathologic findings. Int J Trichol. 2013;5:211-3.
2. Panchaprateep R, Tanus A, Tosti A. Clinical, dermoscopic, and histopathologic features of body and hair disorders. J Am Acad Dermatol. 2015;72:890-900.
3. Contreras-Ruiz J, Duran-McKinster C, Tamayo-Sanchez L, Orozco-Covarrubias L, Ruiz-Maldonado R. Circle hairs: a clinical curiosity. J Eur Acad Dermatol Venerol. 2000;14:495-7.
4. A Tosti. Body hair disorders. In: Tosti A. Dermoscopy of the Hair and Nails, 2nd ed. Boca Raton: CRC press. 2016. pp. 126-32.
5. Fergusson AG, Derblay PR. Rolled hairs: A possible complication of corticosteroid therapy. Arch Dermatol. 1963;87:311-4.
6. Seckin D, Gulec TO, Haberal M. Higher incidence of rolled hairs in renal transplant recipients: A possible complication of corticosteroid and cyclosporine therapy. Acta Derm Venereol. 1998;78:384.
7. Ortonne JP, Juhlin L, el Baze P, Pautrat G. Familial rolled and spiral hairs with palmoplantar keratoderma. Acta Derm Venereol. 1985;65:250-54.
8. Itin PH, Bircher AJ, Lautenschlager S, Zuberbuhler E, Guggenheim R. A new clinical disorder of twisted and rolled body hairs with multiple, large knots. J Am Acad Dermatol. 1994;30:31-5.
9. Kelly AP. Pseudofolliculitis barbae and acne keloidalis nuchae. Dermatol Clin. 2003;21:645-53.
10. Kundu RV, Patterson S. Dermatologic conditions in skin of color, part II: disorders occurring predominately in skin of color. Am Fam Physician. 2013;87:859-65.
11. Edlich RF, Haines PC, Nichter LS, Silloway KA, Morgan RF. Pseudofolliculitis barbae with keloids. J Emerg Med. 1986;4:283-6.
12. Hwang S, Schwartz RA. Keratosis pilaris: A common follicular hyperkeratosis. Cutis. 2008;82:177-80.
13. Lalit G, Anubhav G, Kumar KA, Asit M. Familial erythromelanosis follicularis faciei et colli with extensive keratosis pilaris. Int J Dermatol. 2011;50:1400-1.
14. Otberg N, Shapiro J. Tufted folliculitis. In: Bolognia J, Jorizzo J, Schaffer JV (eds). Dermatology. Philadelphia: Elsevier Saunders; 2012. pp. 1109.
15. Pinkus H. Multiple hairs (Flemming-Giovannini; report of two cases of pili multigemini and discussion of some other anomalies of the pilary complex. J Invest Dermatol. 1951;17(5):291-301.
16. Cambiaghi S, Barbareschi M, Cambiaghi G, Caputo R. Scanning electron microscopy in the diagnosis of pili multigemini. Acta Derm Venereol. 1995;75:170-1.
17. Piepkorn MW, Clark L, Lombardi DL. A kindred with congenital vellus hair cysts. J Am Acad Dermatol. 1981;5:661-5.
18. Lee S, Kim JG, Kang JS. Eruptive vellus hair cysts. Arch Dermatol. 1984;120:1191-5.
19. Oiso N, Matsuda H, Kawada A. Eruptive vellus hair cysts of the labia majora: detection of openings of the cysts to the epidermis by dermoscopy. Eur J Dermatol. 2013;23:417-8.
20. Forton F, Germaux MA, Brasseur T, De Liever A, De Liever A, Laporte M, Mathys C, et al. Democidosis and rosacea: Epidemiology and significance in daily dermatologic practice. J Am Acad Dermatol. 2005;52(1):74-87.
21. Mangold A, Swanson DL. Dermoscopy in general dermatology. In: Johr RH, Stolz W. Dermoscopy, 2nd edition. New York: McGraw-Hill; 2015. pp. 505-28.

ASSESSMENT IMAGE-BASED QUESTIONS

1. What is your diagnosis?

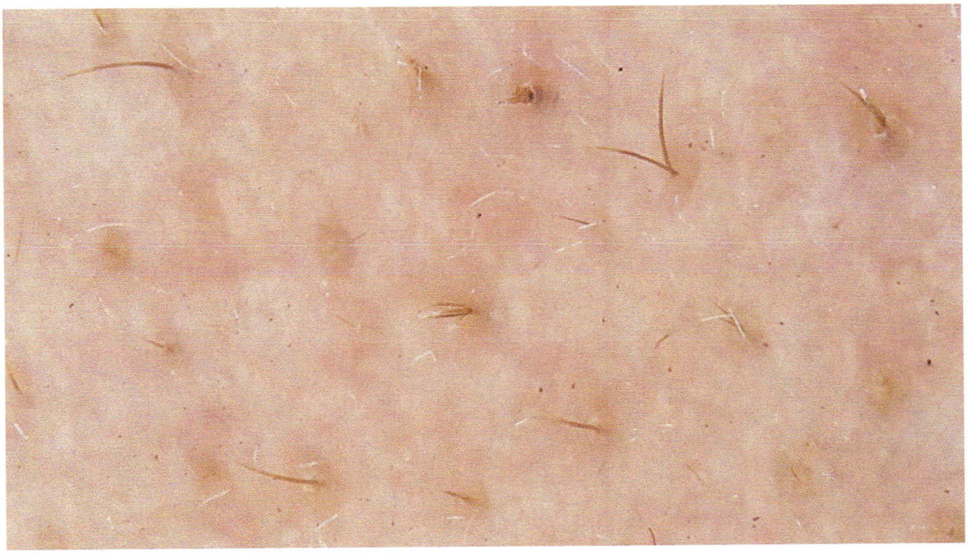

2. Arrow A and B indicate which trichoscopic features?

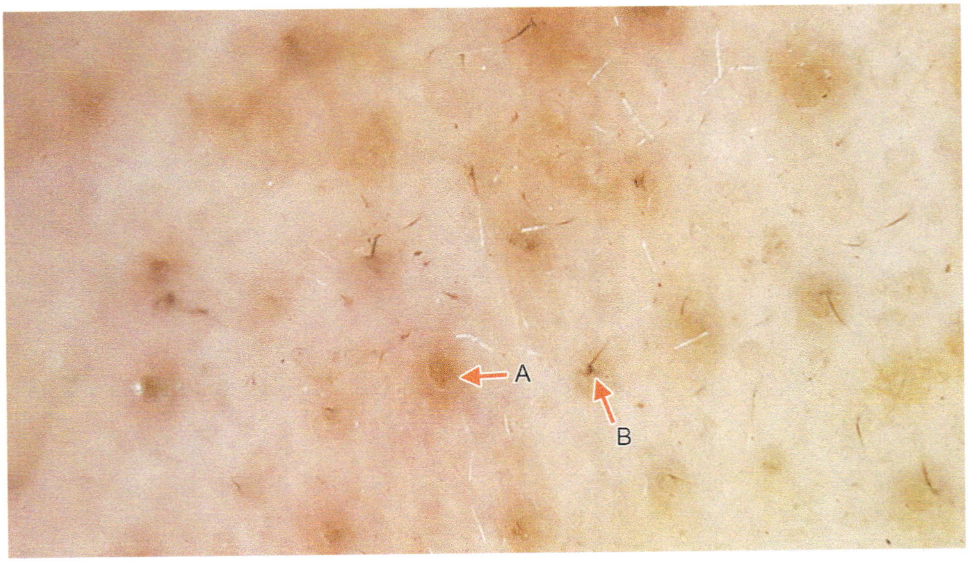

3. It is a developmental defect of hair follicles where multiple hair shafts emerge from a single follicle. What is your diagnosis?

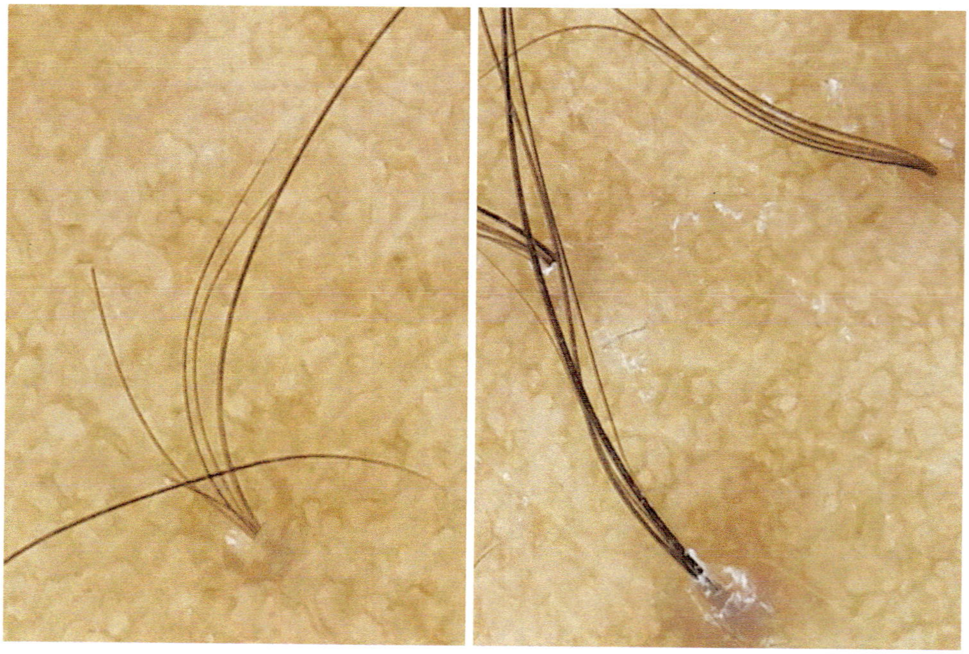

4. This is the trichoscopic feature of a condition where the patient presents with erythema, burning and stinging of face. Diagnose the condition.

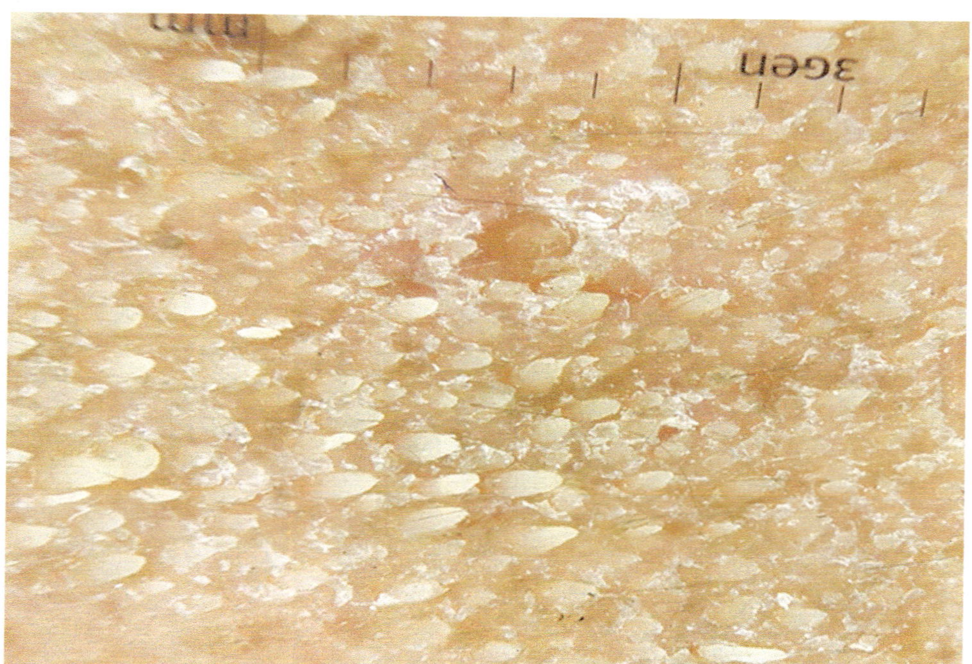

5. Name the body hair abnormality.

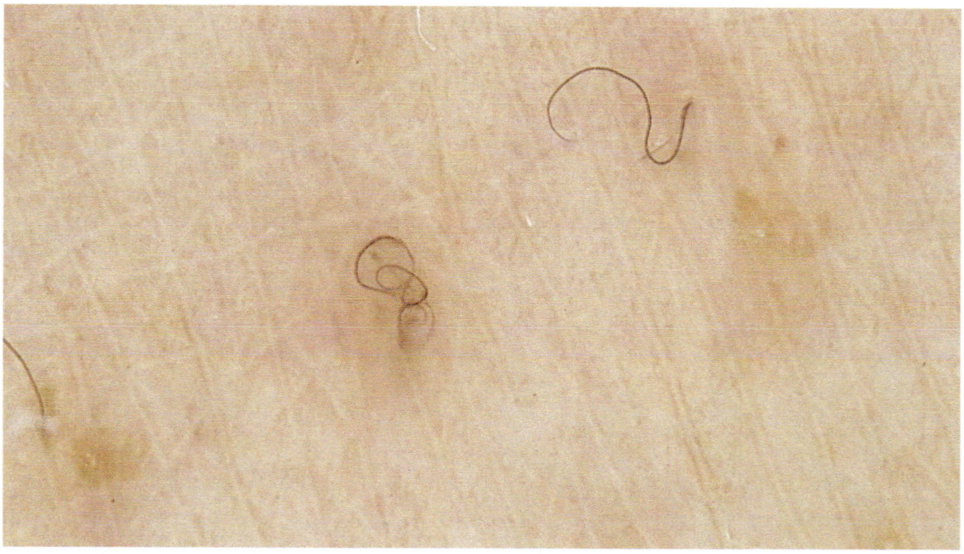

6. Which types of body hair abnormalities are seen?

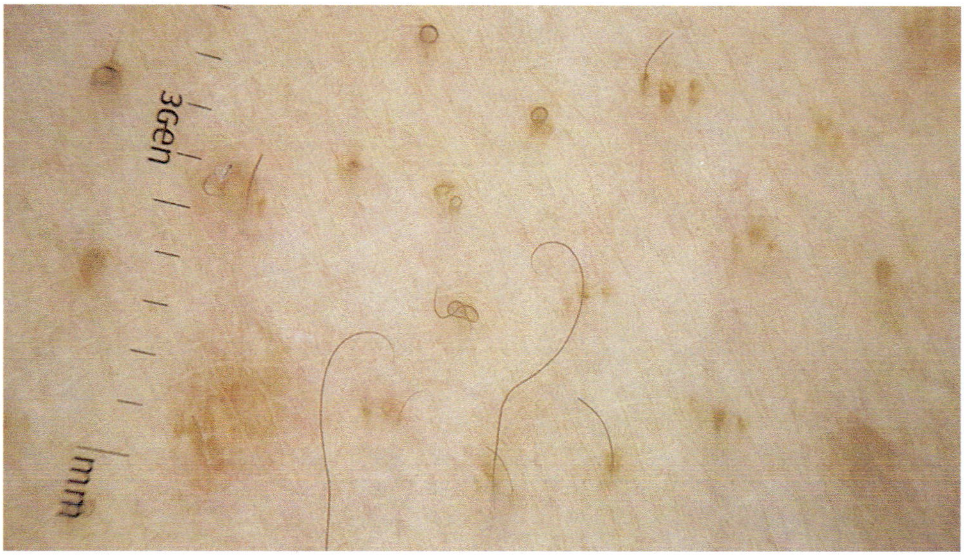

7. Name the trichoscopic feature.

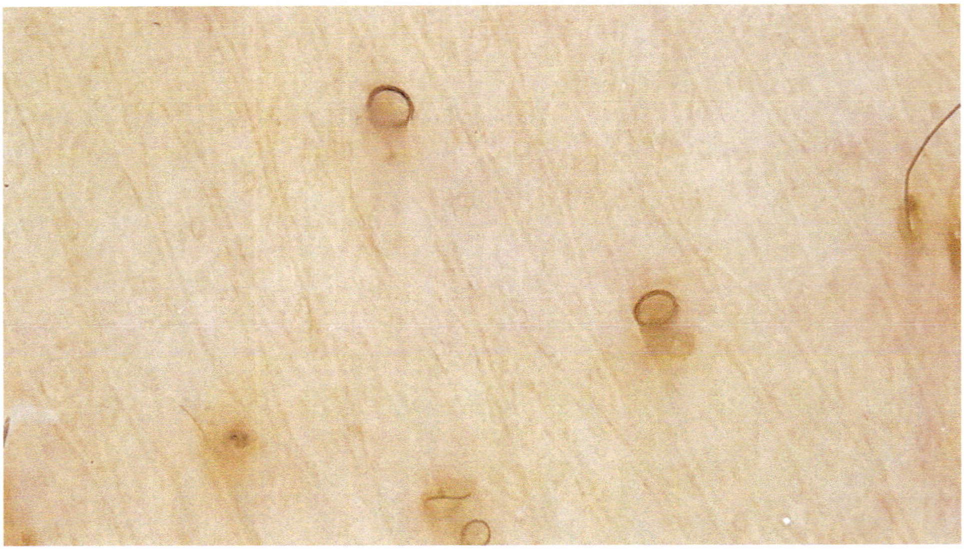

8. Name the type of body hair abnormality.

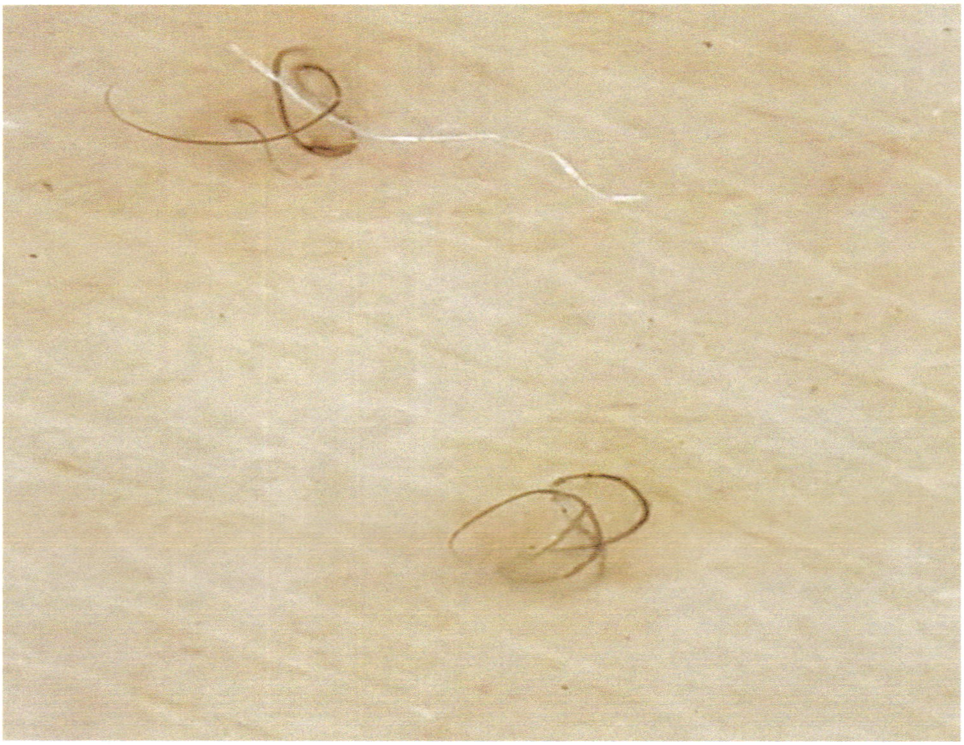

ANSWERS

1. Trichostasis spinulosa
2. A. Keratotic plug; B. Dilated infundibular opening
3. Pili multigemini
4. Demodecosis
5. Rolled hair
6. Circle hair, rolled hair
7. Circle hair
8. Rolled hair

CHAPTER 32

Trichoscopy in Hair Transplantation

Madura C, BS Chandrashekar

INTRODUCTION

Trichoscopy is a technique used to facilitate the diagnosis of hair and scalp disorders.[1] It is performed with handheld dermascope of 10× magnification or video dermascope with lenses ranging from ×20 to ×1,000.[2,3] The trichoscopic digital imaging (FotoFinder 10× to 160×) is a versatile, reliable digital imaging system with epiluminescence microscopy with video documentation. Both dermoscopy and hair transplantation are the growing fields in dermatology. The steps in hair transplantation involve assessment, harvest, and transfer of thousands of individual follicular units to the recipient site. This mandates usage of technology at all points. This chapter describes the application trichoscopy for scalp assessment in hair transplantation patient. It is a diagnostic tool, monitors treatment response, and also gives an insight on prognosis.

Hair transplantation is now performed by majority of dermatologists, who is the true trichologist. It involves transplantation of individual follicular units from safe donor zone to the recipient site by various techniques. The most successful hair transplant surgeon is the one who assesses the patient's needs, calculates the total donor harvest, selects proper technique accordingly, plans the present and future surgery and give good unnoticeable aesthetically pleasing hairline. The success of results depends on the patients' donor and recipient area hair characteristics.[4,5] Hence, proper assessment of donor zone is the important step. It is assessed in terms of scalp condition (rule out disease pathology), scalp elasticity, hair density, grouping, thickness, and texture of hair.

ROLE OF TRICHOSCOPE IN HAIR TRANSPLANTATION

For accurate diagnosis: The diagnosis of androgenic alopecia is straight forward with definitive clinical and dermoscopic picture. The common trichoscopic findings in AGA are hair shaft thickness heterogeneity (HSTH), brown peripilar sign (BPPS), white peripilar sign (WPPS), yellow dots, pinpoint white dots, scalp honeycomb pigmentation, focal atrichia, epidermal scaling, and arborizing red lines. HSTH is an essential criterion for diagnosing AGA. BPPS is more common in early AGA. However, WPPS, yellow dots, pinpoint white dots, focal atrichia, and scalp pigmentation are positively correlated with advanced AGA.[6-8] The trichoscopy can be important tool to differentiate classical case of AGA from DUPA (diffuse unpatterned androgenic alopecia), an under reported entity. It is a rapidly progressive androgenic alopecia that starts in early decades and progresses rapidly and there will be diffuse scalp involvement without sparing donor zone. DUPA poses challenge for hair transplant surgeon. It is seen in both men and women. It differs from MPHL by lacking the stable permanent zone. Diagnosing DUPA is very important because selecting them for hair transplantation can prove to be disaster **(Fig. 1)**.[9] On dermoscopy, the occipital region in classic androgenic alopecia and that of normal control do not show any difference in the area; however, in DUPA, features of HSTH of >10%, WPPS and focal atrichia are common findings in patients with diffuse scalp involvement in authors experience.[10-12]

The other diagnostic dilemma is diffuse alopecia areata and alopecia incognito. Diffuse alopecia areata is characterized by diffuse involvement of scalp including donor zone with uniform miniaturization of hair shafts without shaft diameter variation. Dermoscopically, we see vellus hair and yellow dots (seen in both AGA and AA, but more in latter). The presence of specific markers, black dots and broken and exclamation mark hairs are predictors of disease activity.[8,13,14] Alopecia incognita is characterized by androgenetic alopecia and telogen effluvium with occurrence of disperse and severe hair thinning in short time. There are numerous, diffuse yellow dots of different size and uniform colors within the follicular orifices of both empty and hair-bearing with a large number of re-growing of tapered terminal hairs in the entire scalp.[3]

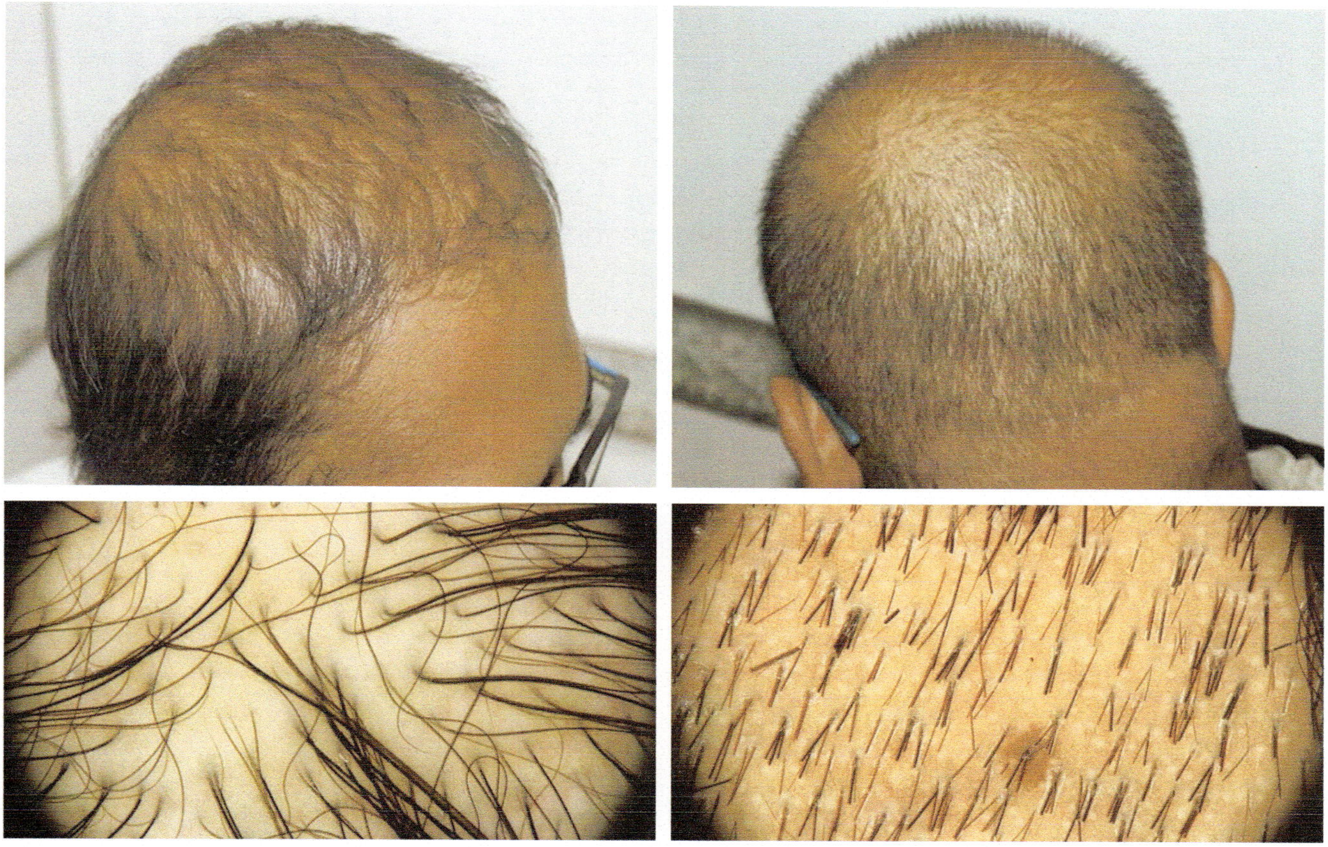

Fig. 1: Shows diffuse unpatterned androgenetic alopecia with transparent donor zone. Trichoscopy shows miniaturization of donor zone and features of AGA.

- *To assess the donor area*:
  - The trichoscope is a user-friendly tool to assess the donor zone. The safe donor zone is the horseshoe-shaped area of 5–7 cm width overlying the mid-occipital region. The occipital notch is the inferior limit and 5 cm above this line is safe zone. The lateral limit is marked by a vertical line drawn upwards along the preauricular area. However, the boundaries of safe zone should be individual to each patient. The trichoscopic evaluation is very valuable here.
  - *To calculate yield of donor area*: The trichoscopy helps in assessing the density, grouping so that number of sessions and graphs for a patient can be planned and documented. Trichoscopy of normal scalp shows follicular units containing 2–4 terminal hairs (>55 mm) and 1 or 2 vellus hairs (<0.03 mm in width).[15] A normal terminal hair is uniform in thickness and color. The devise assesses the demand of recipient area and at expanse of ongoing hair loss. A donor supply to recipient demand ratio is estimated that helps the physician determine the good/poor candidate for surgery.

- The folliscope is a handheld microscopic imaging device (1× to 300× magnification) attached to a computer and a monitor through a USB port. It can measure subtle differences in hair density, hair caliber, hair growth rates, terminal versus miniaturized (vellus) hair, or the amount of anagen versus telogen hair in an area that can be quantified and compared. These information help in finding patient's eligibility for surgery.
- The donor density can be quickly and accurately measured in multiple areas providing an estimate of donor supply. A decreased density or a greater percentage of miniaturized hair in the donor area would warn against the risk of poorer results. A patient with higher density and very few miniaturized hairs would be a better candidate **(Figs. 2 and 3)**. Visualizing increased miniaturization in the donor area may warrant DUPA and also to diagnose reverse AGA **(Fig. 1)**. The assessing density is needed to calculate length and breadth of strip and also to pick number of follicular unit excision (FUE) graphs/cm^2. It can be used to counsel and educate patient to set realistic expectations. The regular systematic analysis of the donor and recipient area parameters of all patients and maintaining records may create patient selection standard parameters.
- The device assesses the parafollicular area for any disease pathology (seborrhea, dermatitis, psoriasis, and healed folliculitis scar) **(Figs. 4 and 5)**. In patients with recurring folliculitis of scalp, the healed folliculitis scar can make extraction difficult because of fibrosis which requires deeper scoring with punch in FUE sessions. It can also affect the yield of graphs which can be explained to the patients in advance.
- The device not only assesses the density but also the emergence of hair and intracutaneous direction of follicle can be assessed. It can vary from center to lateral. In beard it is more acute angle with parallel intracutaneous course **(Figs. 6A and B)**. Additionally, the shaft texture and graying of hair can be noted.

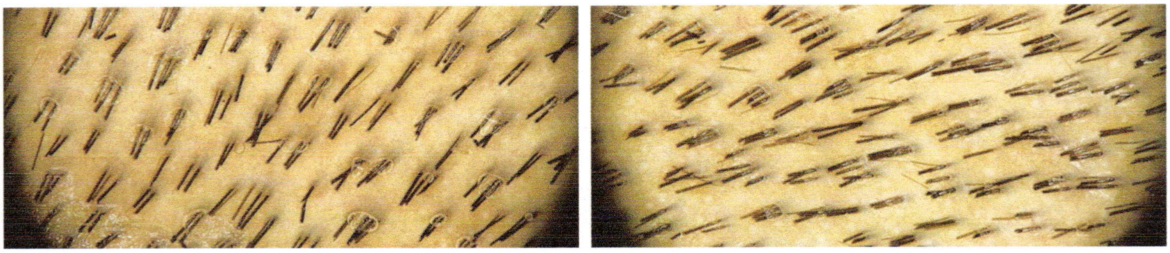

Fig. 2: Shows good density donor zones.

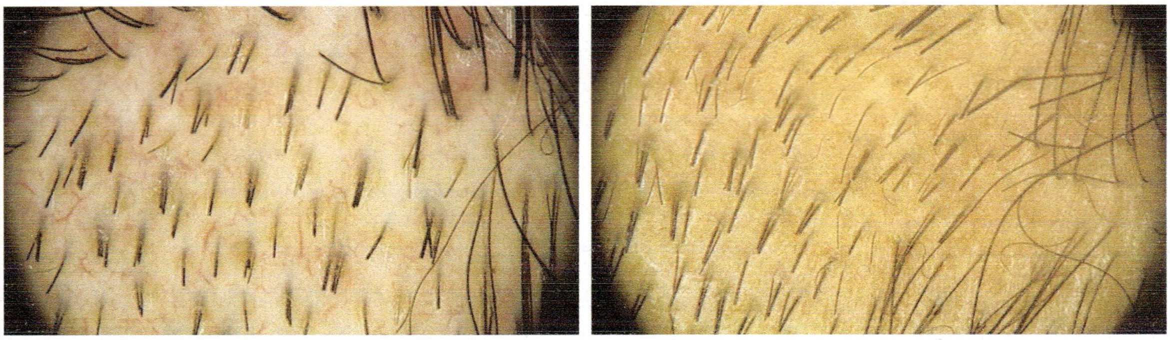

Fig. 3: Shows poor density donor zones.

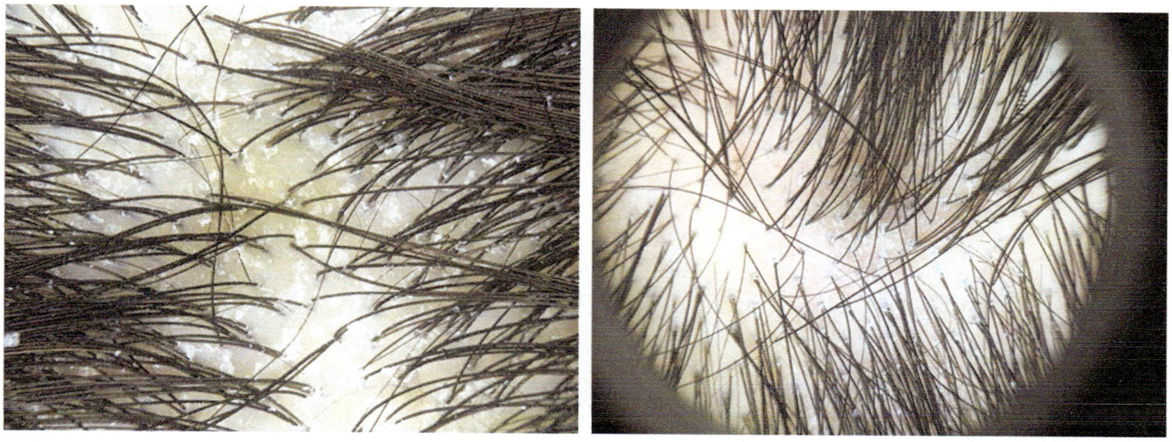

Fig. 4: Shows scalp surface changes (seborrhea and seborrheic dermatitis).

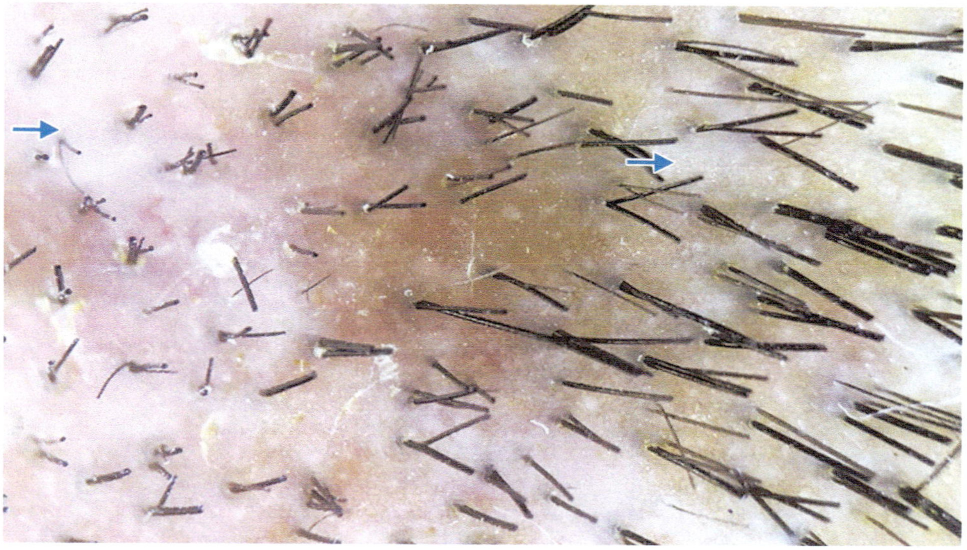

Fig. 5: Shows healing folliculitis and healed folliculitis, white flare is seen (arrows).

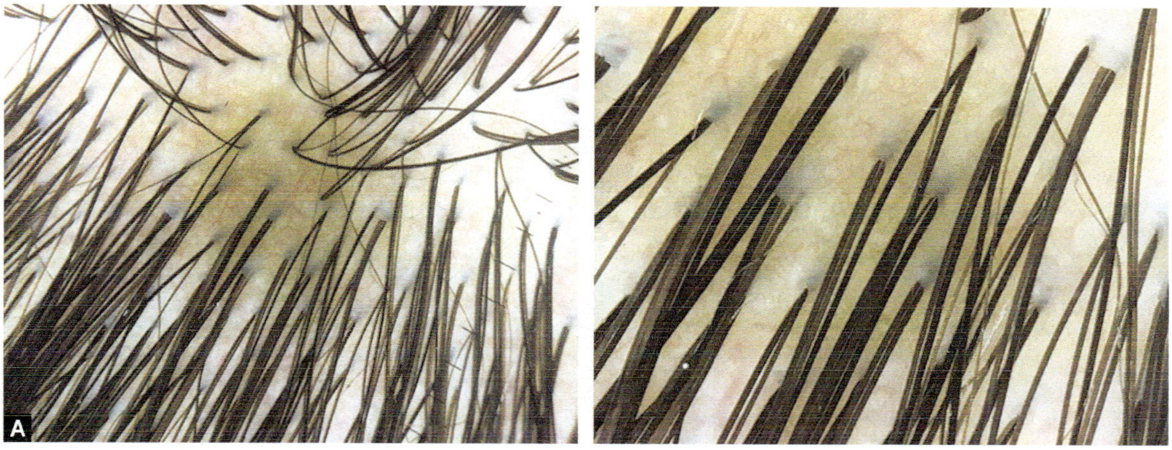

Continued

Continued

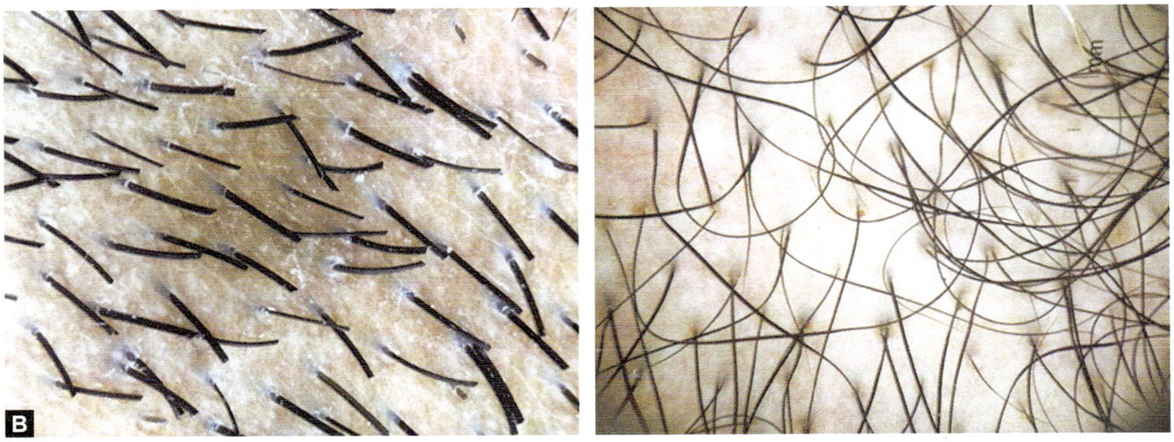

Figs. 6A and B: (A) Shows very good donor zone. Visualize the intracutaneous course of follicle in scalp and (B) Shows beard and chest hair, note they have got more parallel intracutaneous course.

- *Graft survival*: The transilluminating light source and magnifying optics of dermascope with both polarized and nonpolarized light gives complimentary information of transplanted grafts positioning by nonpolarized light at epidermal level. Whereas blood vessels and circumferential epithelial proliferation looking as red color and white streaks respectively indicates early development and survival of the grafts at dermal level with polarized light.
- *Assess the results after surgery*: The trichoscopy documents the hair growth and loss. The trichoscopic image of pretransplant area can be compared with image of post-transplant area of single point. This is more important in handling dissatisfied patients. Author recommends to take baseline trichoscopic image and repeat the image at 9th or 12th month to see the effectiveness of therapy. It easily differentiates the thicker transplanted hair growing in the midst of thinner vellus hair **(Fig. 7)**. This type of assurance is more important in patients undergoing hair transplantation in Ludwig's patterns and also FPHL. The device also assesses the other features of hair transplantation such as angle of hair **(Figs. 8A and B)** and aesthetic complications (pits and cobbling) **(Figs. 9A and B)**.
- *The trichoscan of donor area after hair transplantation [FUE/follicular unit transplantation (FUT)]*: Shows white flairs at the sight of FUE Graph harvest **(Fig. 10)**. The FUT scar which is closed by trichophytic method shows regrowth of hair from within the scar **(Fig. 11)**. These pictures can motivate the patients undergoing hair transplantation to accept the FUT technique who have scar phobia.

To conclude, trichoscopy is a convenient, noninvasive, and well-accepted method in evaluation of hair disorders. Hair transplant surgeons run a busy clinic and this user-friendly tool can aid patient assessment more scientifically to evaluate surgical candidacy. This can optimize the chances of achieving more consistent and aesthetic results by eliminating poor and borderline candidates.

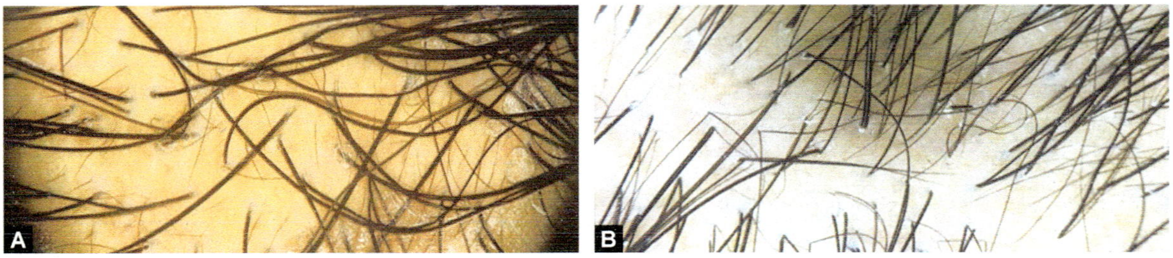

Fig. 7: Shows post-transplanted area after 18 months, thick transplanted hairs in between vellus hairs.

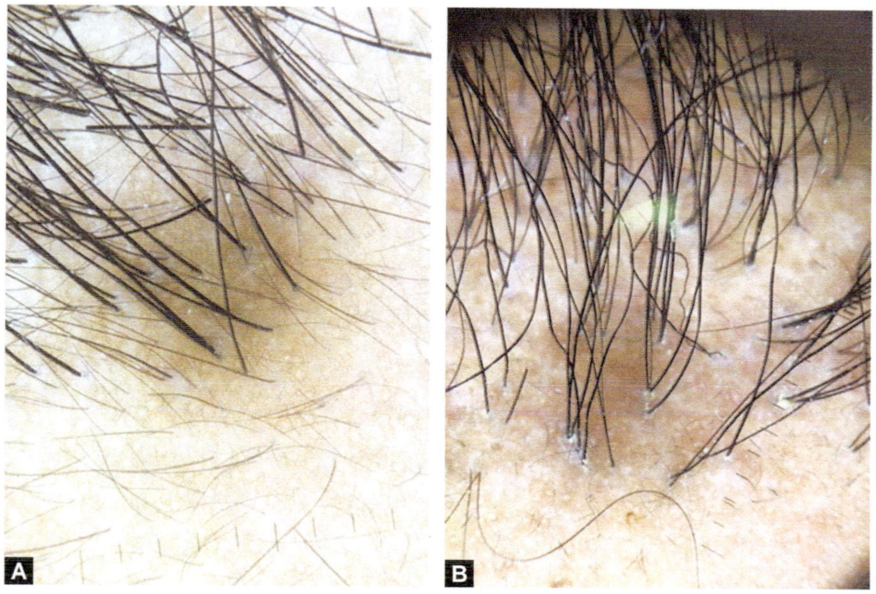

Figs. 8A and B: (A) Uncomplicated natural hair line; and (B) Hair line cobbling deformity and also wrong angle.

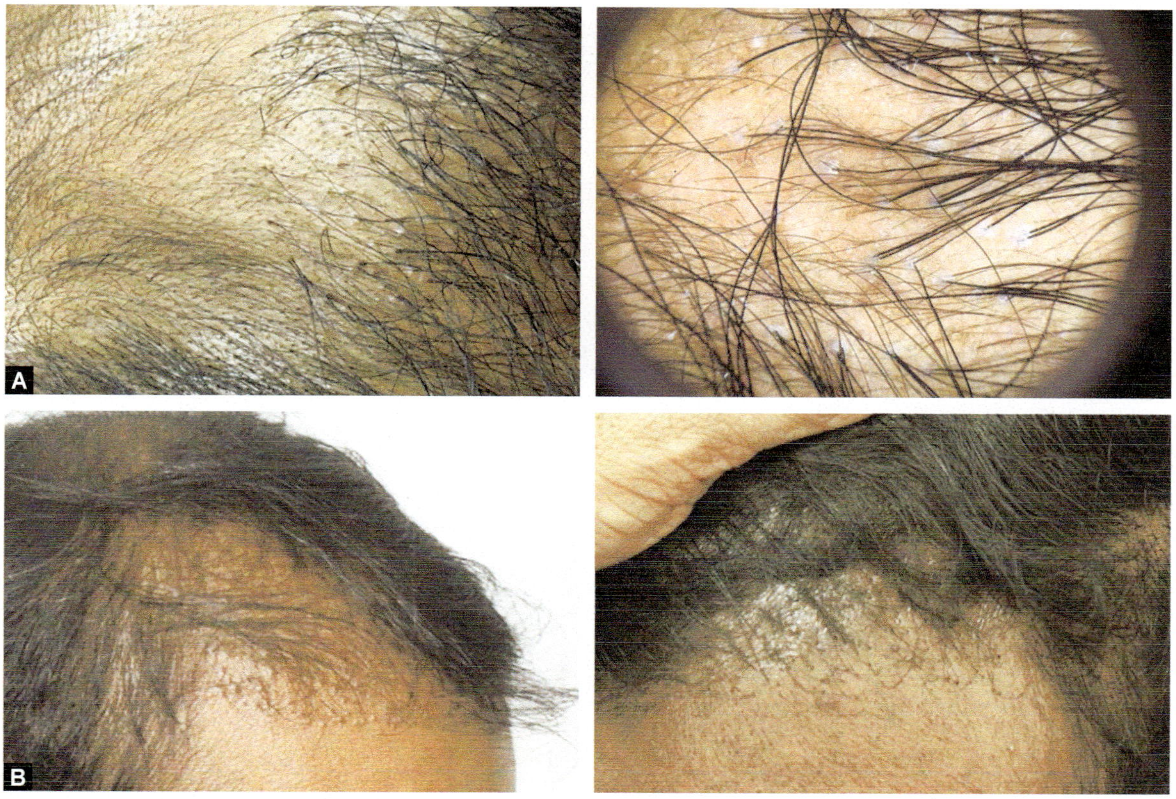

Figs. 9A and B: (A) Post-transplant cobble stoning/tenting with dermoscopic image and (B) Cobbling and pitting deformities.

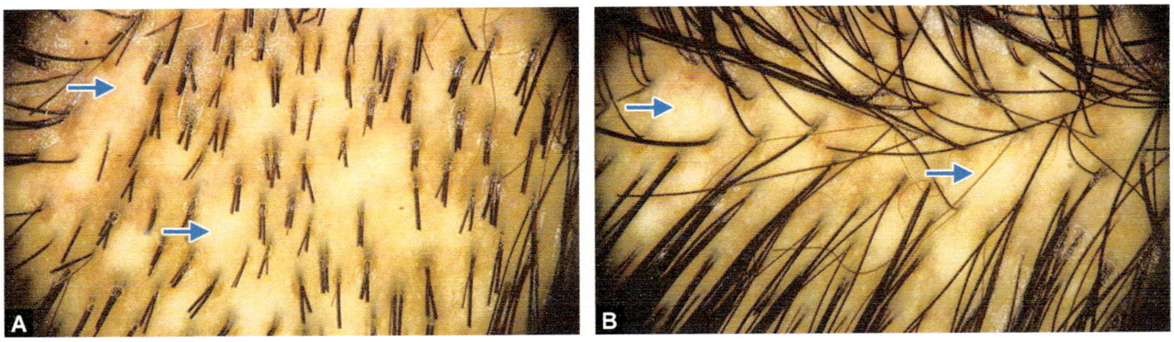

Figs. 10A and B: Shows post-follicular unit excision donor zone. White flares (arrows) are areas of fibrosis after follicular graft harvest.

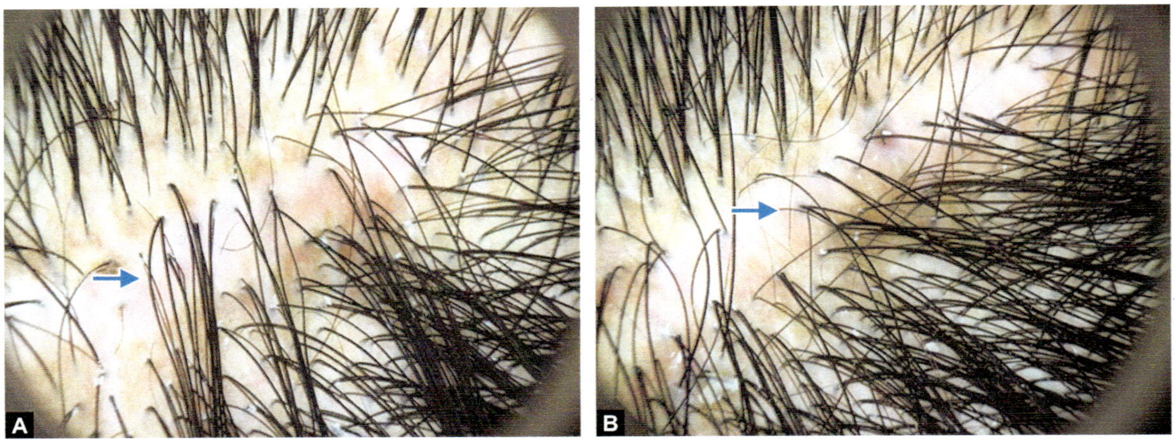

Figs. 11A and B: Shows post-trichophytic closure of follicular unit transplantation (FUT) scar. The hairs are growing within scar of FUT (arrows).

REFERENCES

1. Tosti A. Hair shaft disorders. In: Tosti A (ed). Dermoscopy of Hair and Scalp: Pathological and Clinical Correlation. Illustrated ed. USA: CRC Press; 2007. pp. 51-3.
2. Rudnicka L, Olszewska M, Rakowska A, Kowalska-Oledzka E, Slowinska M. Trichoscopy: A new method for diagnosing hair loss. J Drugs Dermatol. 2008;7:651-4.
3. Tosti A, Duque-Estrada B. Dermoscopy in hair disorders. J Egypt Womens Dermatol Soc. 2010;7:1-4.
4. Unger WP, Unger RH. Hair transplanting: an important but often forgotten treatment for female pattern hair loss. J Am Acad Dermatol. 2003;49(5):853-60.
5. Bernstein RM, Rassman WR. Follicular unit transplantation: 2005. Dermatol Clin. 2005;23(3):393-414.
6. Inui S, Nakajima T, Itami S. Scalp dermoscopy of androgenetic alopecia in Asian people. J Dermatol. 2009;36:82-5.
7. Miteva M, Tosti A. Hair and scalp dermatoscopy. J Am Acad Dermatol. 2012;67(5):1040-8.
8. Inui S. Trichoscopy for common hair loss diseases: Algorithmic method for diagnosis. J Dermatol. 2011;38(1):71-5.
9. Bernstien RM. Follicular unit hair transplantation. In: Robinson JK, Hanke CW, Siegel DM, Fratila A (eds). Surgery of Skin, 2nd edition. Mosby: Elsevier; 2010. pp. 485-512.
10. Hu R, Xu F, Han Y, Sheng Y, Qi S, Miao Y, et al. Trichoscopic findings of androgenetic alopecia and their association with disease severity. J Dermatol. 2015;42(6):602-7.
11. Rakowska A, Slowinska M, Kowalska-Oledzka E, Olszewska M, Rudnicka L. Dermoscopy in female androgenic alopecia: method standardization and diagnostic criteria. Int J Trichology. 2009;1(2):123-30.
12. Galliker NA, Trüeb RM. Value of trichoscopy versus trichogram for diagnosis of female androgenetic alopecia. Int J Trichology 2012;4(1):19-22.
13. Miteva M, Tosti A. Hair and scalp dermatoscopy. J Am Acad Dermatol. 2012;67(5):1040-8.
14. Inui S, Nakajima T, Itami S. Coudability hairs: A revisited sign of alopecia areata assessed by trichoscopy. Clin Exp Dermatol. 2010;35(4):361-5.
15. Elghblawi E. Trichoscopy simplified. Open Dermatol J. 2015;9:12-20.

CHAPTER 33

Algorithm

Samipa S Mukherjee

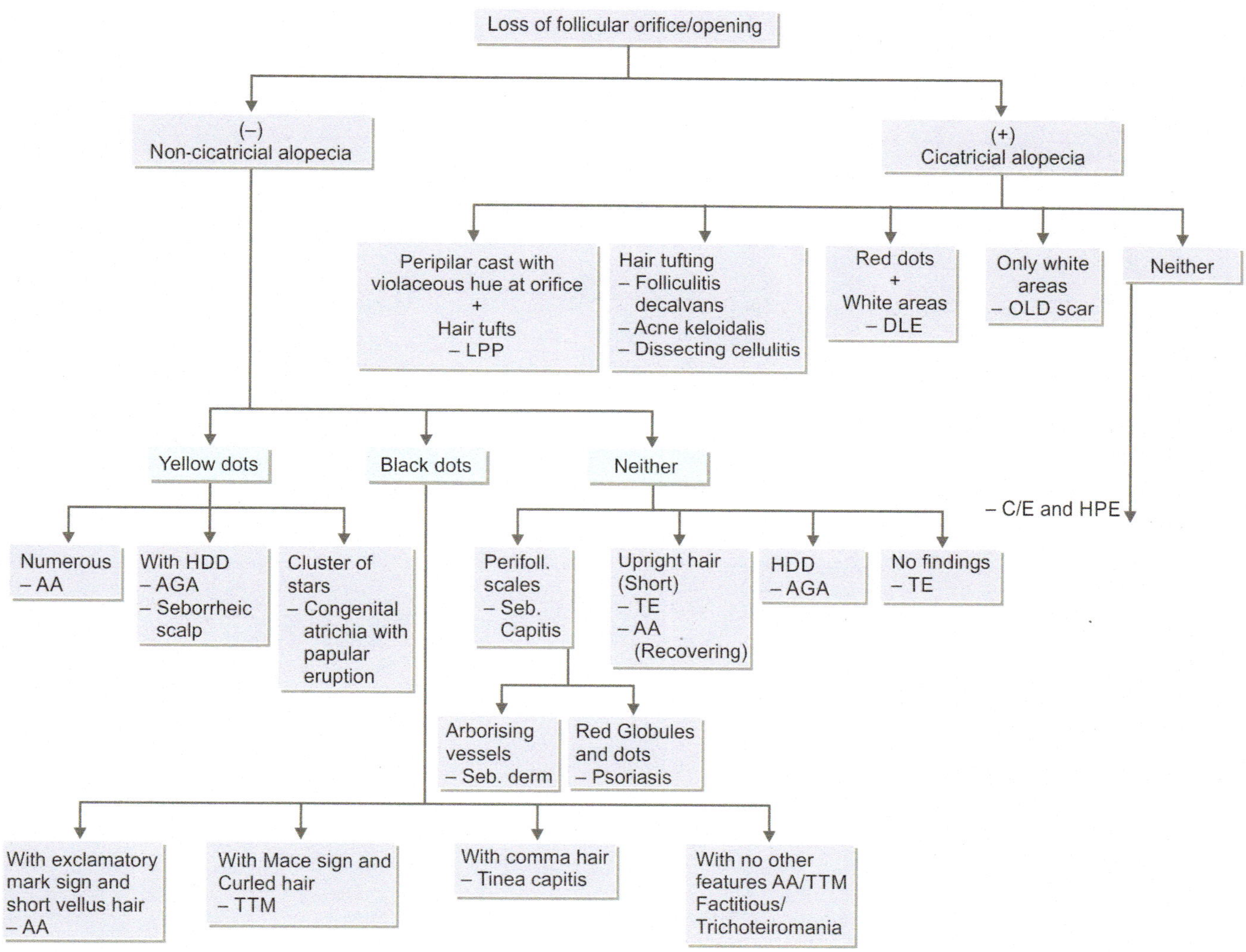

Flowchart 1: Loss of hair follicle openings.
(AA: alopecia areata; AGA: androgenetic alopecia; DLE: discoid lupus erythematosus; HDD: hair diameter diversity; LPP: lichen planopilaris; TTM: trichotillomania)

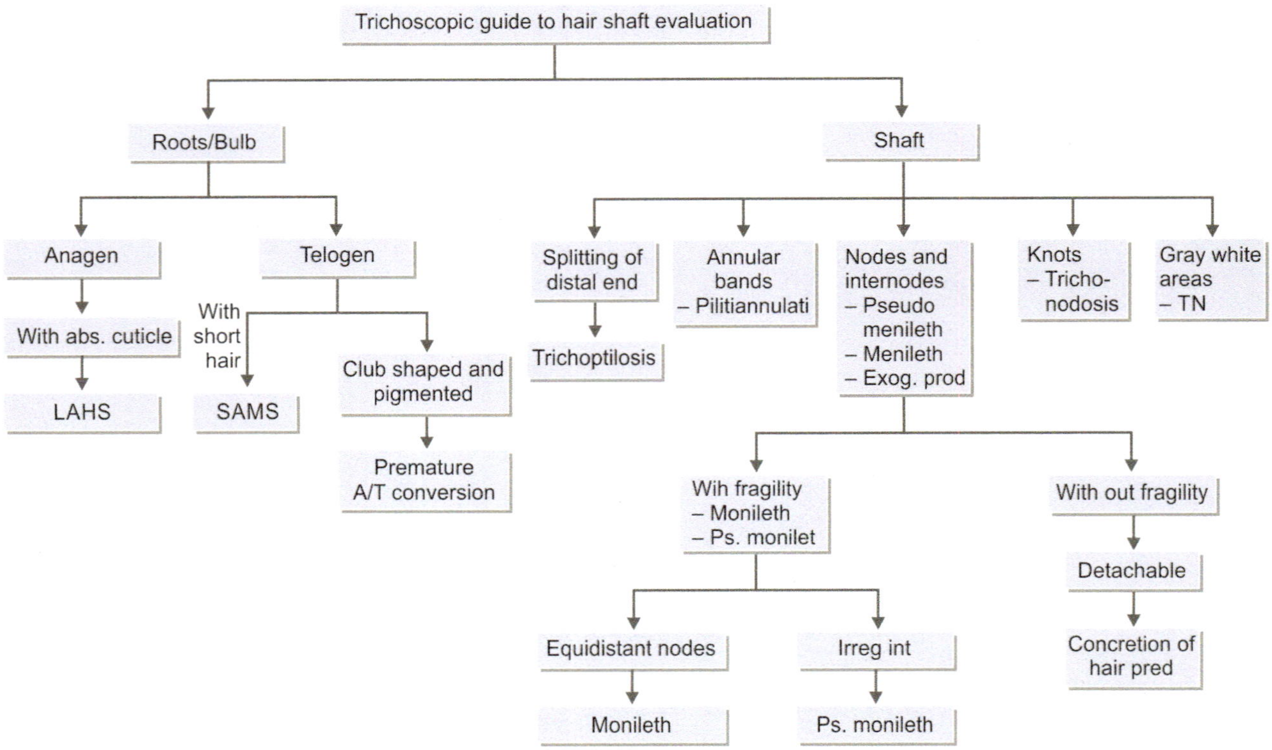

Flowchart 2: Hair shaft evaluation.
(LAHS: loose anagen hair syndrome)

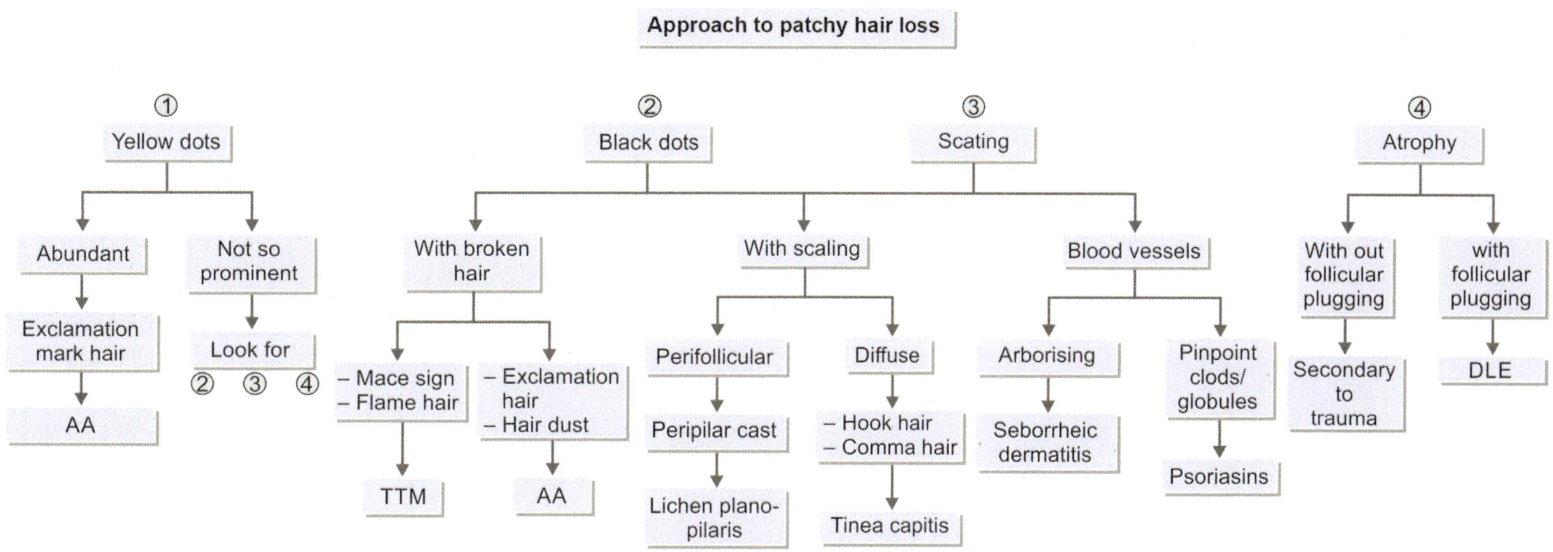

Flowchart 3: Patchy hair loss.
(AA: alopecia areata; DLE: discoid lupus erythematosus; TTM: trichotillomania)

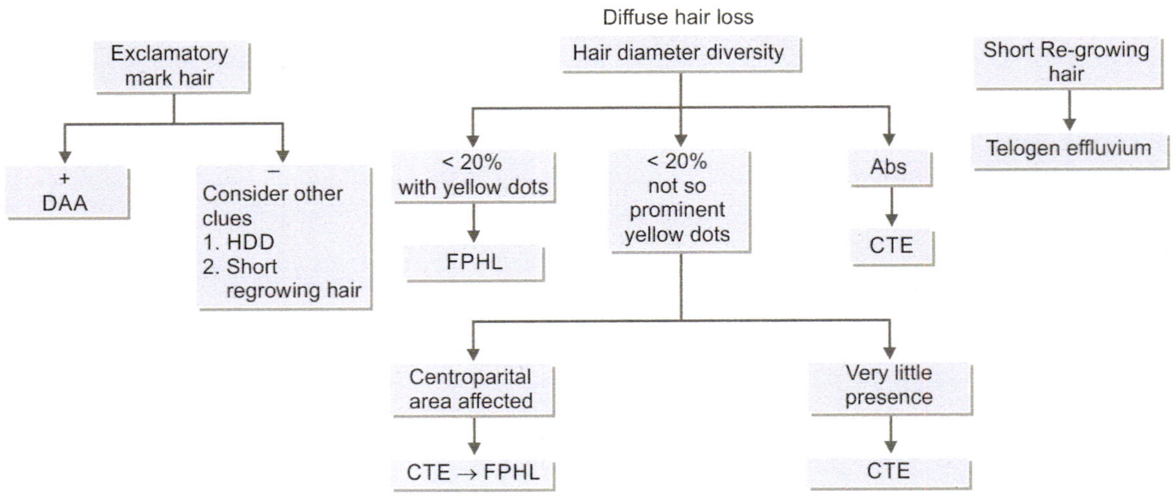

Flowchart 4: Diffuse hair loss.
(CTE: chronic telogen effluvium; DAA: diffuse alopecia areata; DLE: discoid lupus erythematosus; FPHL: Female pattern hair loss; HDD: hair diameter diversity)

CHAPTER 34

Trichoscopic Monitoring and Follow-up

Subrata Malakar

INTRODUCTION

- Besides diagnosis, trichoscopy helps in following up of diseases such as alopecia areata, trichotillomania, androgenetic alopecia, tinea capitis, and other scarring and nonscarring alopecias.
- Olszewska and Rudnica in 2005 first monitored treatment efficacy in female androgenetic alopecia.[1] They measured hair shaft thickness before and during therapy. Peripilar sign, yellow dots, and hair shafts per follicular units were the parameters they took for monitoring.[2]
- Monitoring the diseases may be complex but can be simplified by taking some easy parameters. For example in scalp psoriasis instead of looking for psoriasis severity index score, we can determine the success of scalp psoriasis therapy by looking for the disappearance of scaling and fading or disappearance of dotted vessels.
- In alopecia areata, inactivity or improvement of the disease process can be assessed by disappearance or reduction of exclamation mark hairs, black dots, etc., and presence of regrowing hairs.[3]
- In a similar manner, trichotillomania, telogen effluvium, tinea capitis, and pediculosis also can be monitored trichoscopically.
- Scarring alopecia shows disease-specific trichoscopic signs which also can be followed up for therapy maintenance, or reduction of the dose of the drugs.
- So trichoscopy is a highly effective investigative tool not only for the diagnosis of the disease but also for the monitoring and sequential follow-up of the treatment efficacy, and can well be utilized for several researches.

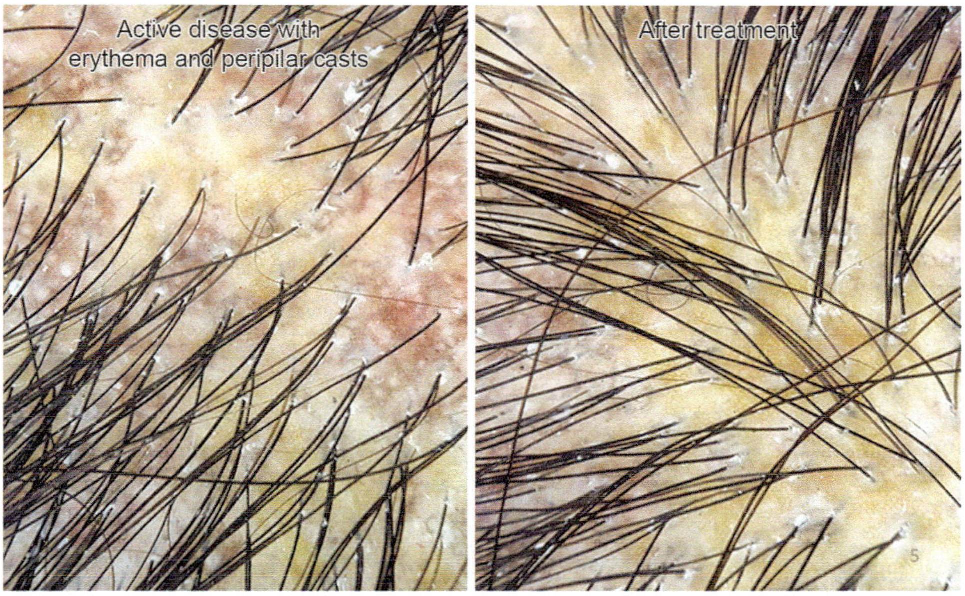

Fig. 1: Lichen planopilaris (LPP) case 1. Trichoscopy helps to follow-up the treatment response. Visible improvement of LPP after treatment can be appreciated by trichoscope.

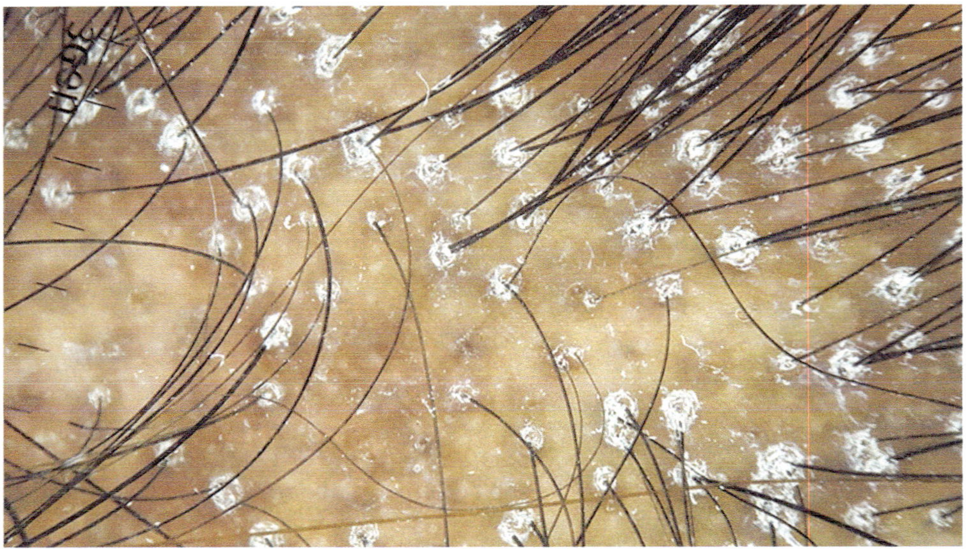

Fig. 2: Lichen planopilaris (LPP) case 2. A case of active LPP where the trichoscopic field is studded with peripilar casts and blue-gray dots and areas, and erythema.

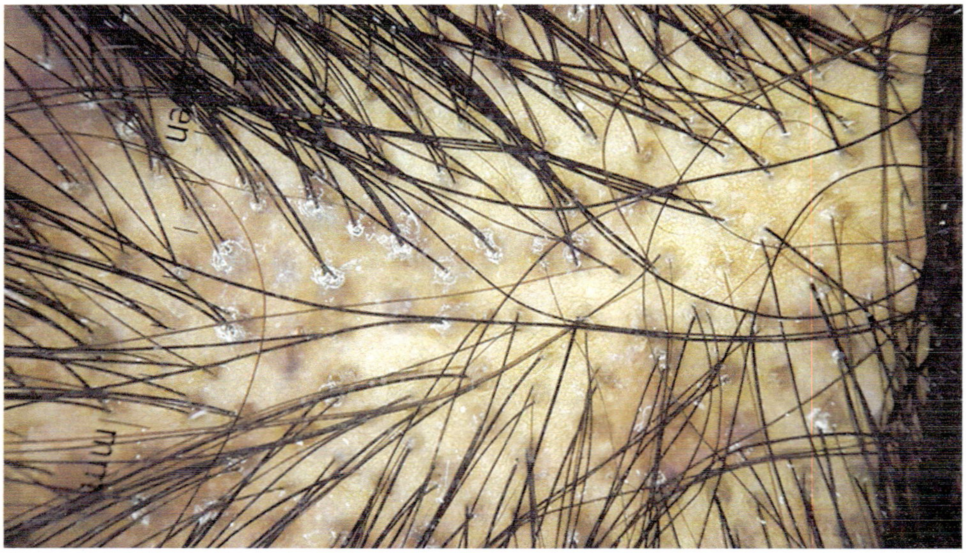

Fig. 3: Lichen planopilaris (LPP) case 2. Significant improvement after treating with oral steroid minipulse and hydroxychloroquine for two-and-half months. There is notable reduction of peripilar casts and erythema.

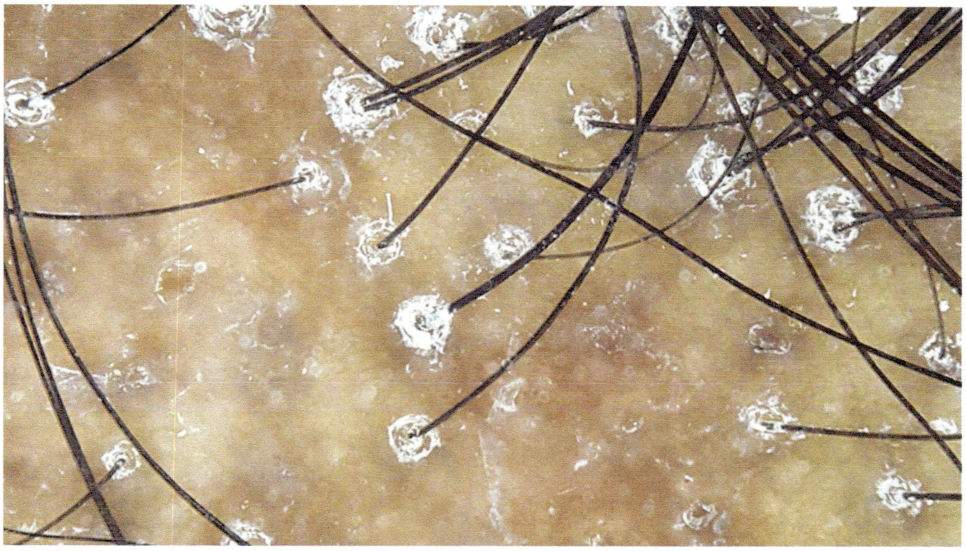

Fig. 4: Lichen planopilaris (LPP) case 3. Trichoscopy reveals prominent peripilar casts, blue-gray dots and mild erythema. Histopathology confirms the diagnosis of LPP.

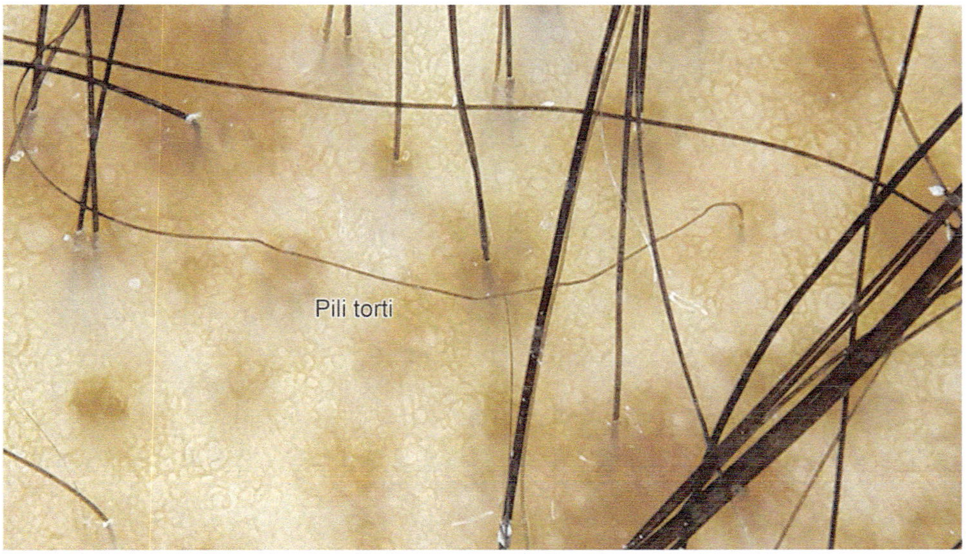

Fig. 5: Lichen planopilaris (LPP) case 3. Trichoscopic follow-up shows remarkable improvement after 3 months of treatment. Peripilar casts are not visible and blue-gray dots and patches are replaced by postinflammatory hyperpigmentation. Erythema is no more visible. Note the horizontally placed pili torti at the center of the image. In pili torti, the affected hair is flattened and twisted on its axis. It has several causes. In LPP, it results from hair follicular deformation due to perifollicular fibrosis.

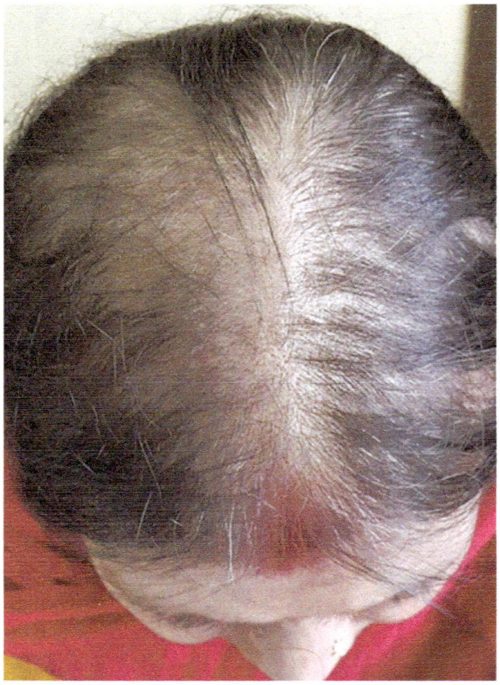

Fig. 6: Systemic lupus erythematosus (SLE) 1. A case of SLE with diffuse hair loss.

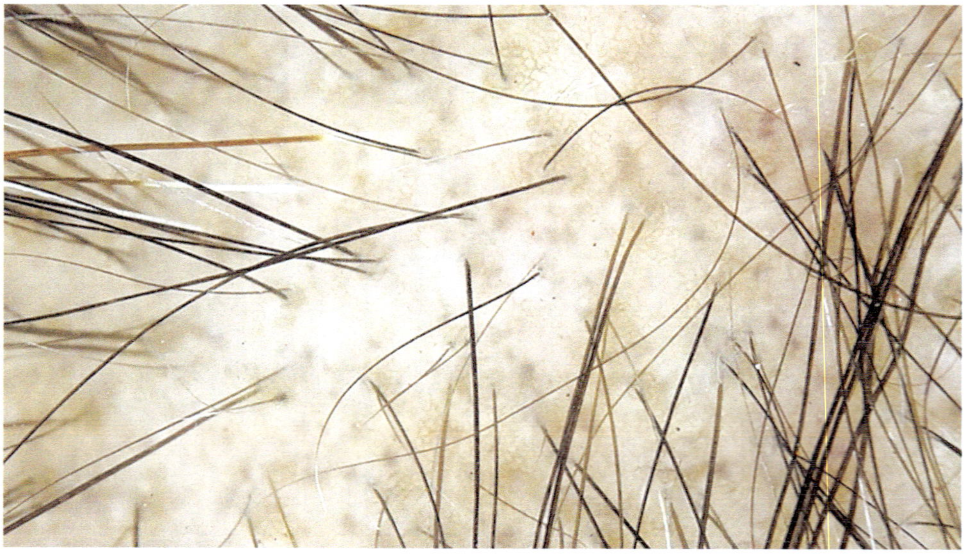

Fig. 7: Systemic lupus erythematosus (SLE) 2. Trichoscopy shows blue-gray dots in a speckled pattern. As there is interface dermatitis in SLE, melanin incontinence occur all throughout the dermis including perifollicular area. Lichen planopilaris (LPP) differs from SLE in that, there is only perifollicular incontinence of melanin in LPP, resulting in blue-gray target pattern whereas in SLE the process occurs all throughout dermis and as a consequence blue-gray dots are present as a speckled pattern.

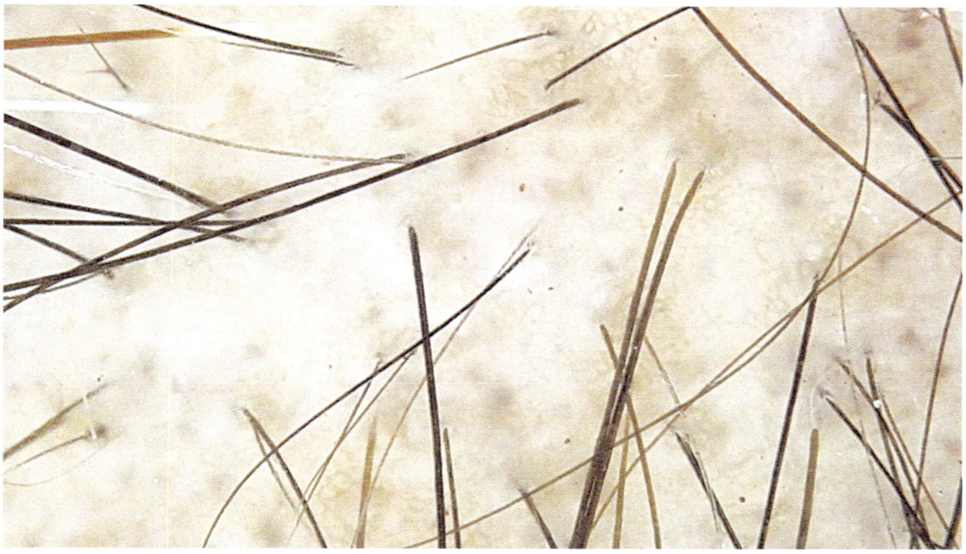

Fig. 8: Systemic lupus erythematosus (SLE) 3. Another field from same patient showing blue-gray dots in speckled pattern. Note there is loss of hair density.

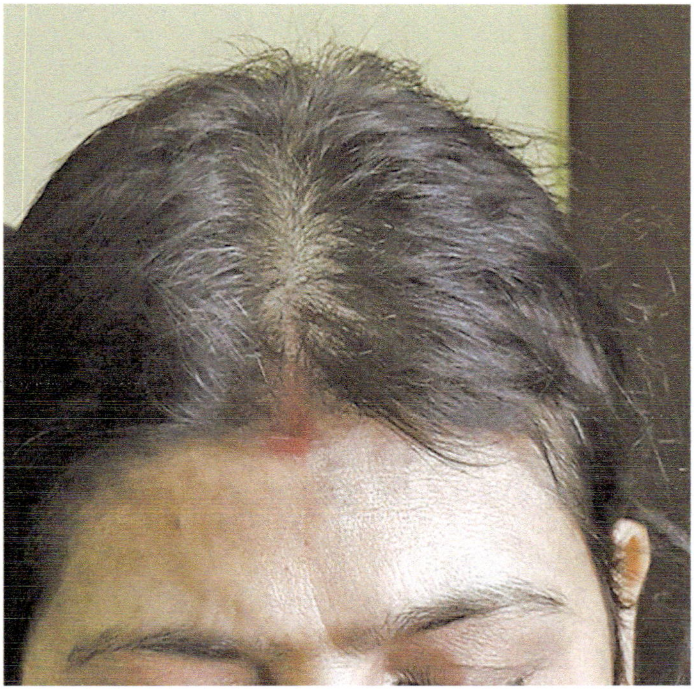

Fig. 9: Systemic lupus erythematosus (SLE) 4. Same patient after treatment for 3 months showing remarkable improvement of hair density along with improvement of other parameters of SLE. Regrowing hairs are not visible.

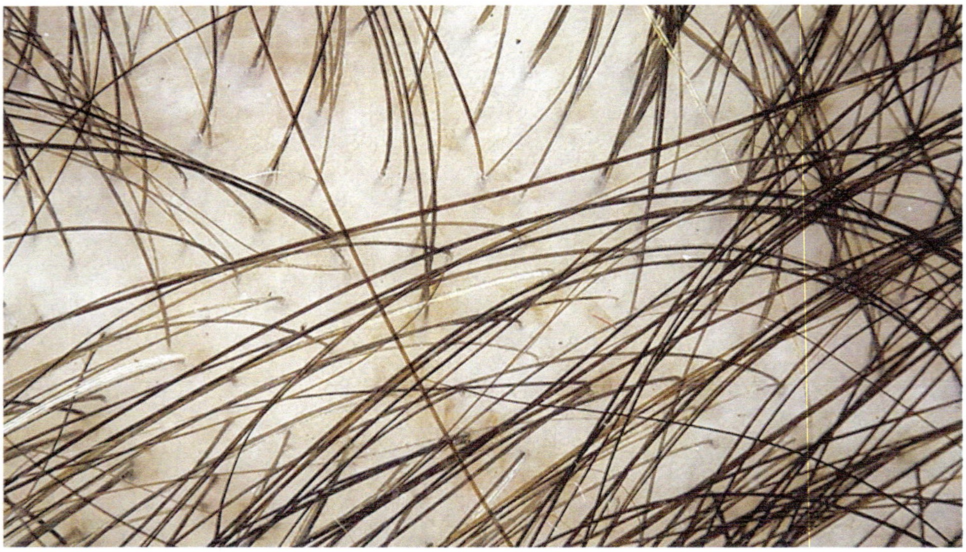

Fig. 10: Systemic lupus erythematosus (SLE) 5. This is the image of trichoscopic follow-up of the previous patient. Blue-gray dots in a speckled pattern are not observed after 3 months of treatment. Hairs have become dense.

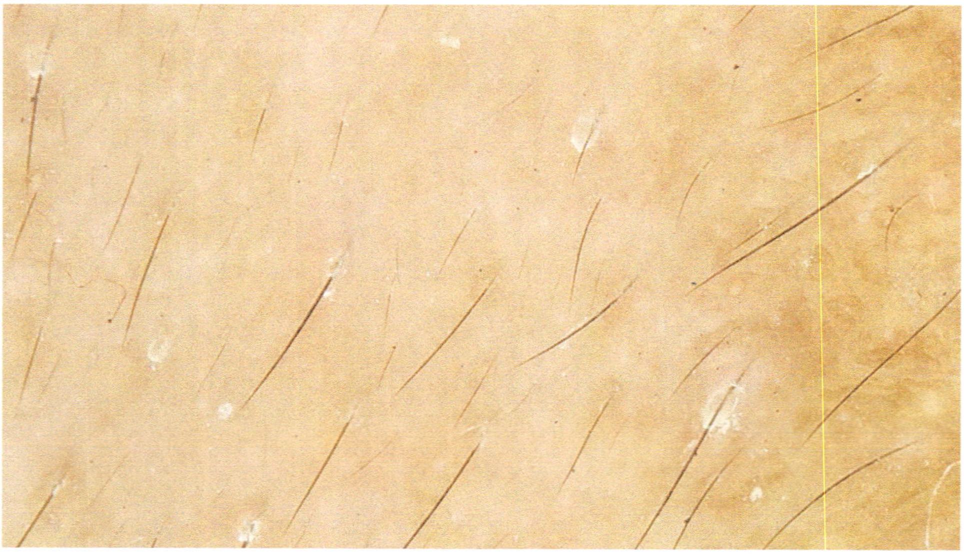

Fig. 11: Demodicosis 1. White spicules of *Demodex* in the infundibulum of the facial hairs. The protruded part of spicules are tails of *Demodex*.

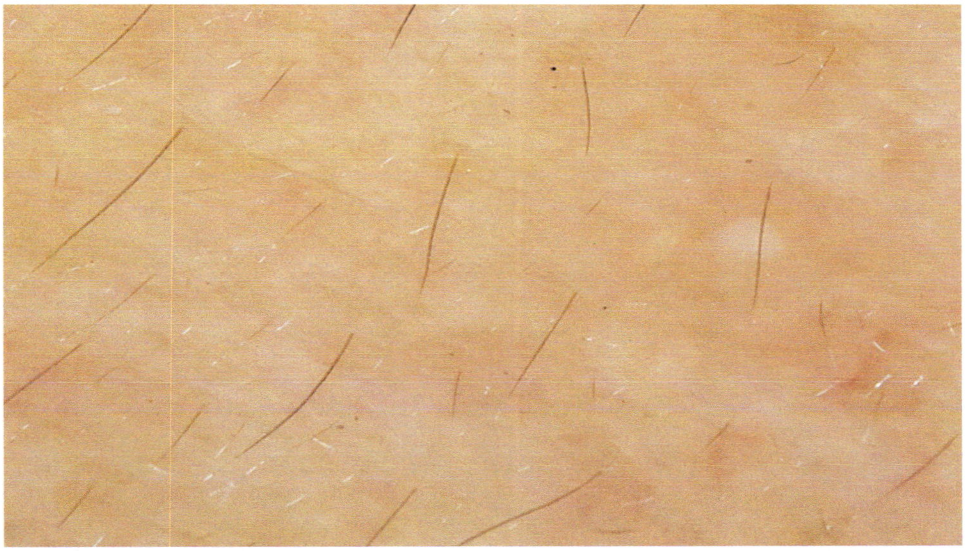

Fig. 12: Demodicosis 2. Trichoscopic follow-up after 2 weeks of treatment with oral and topical ivermectin. Improvement is highly significant with no trace of *Demodex*.

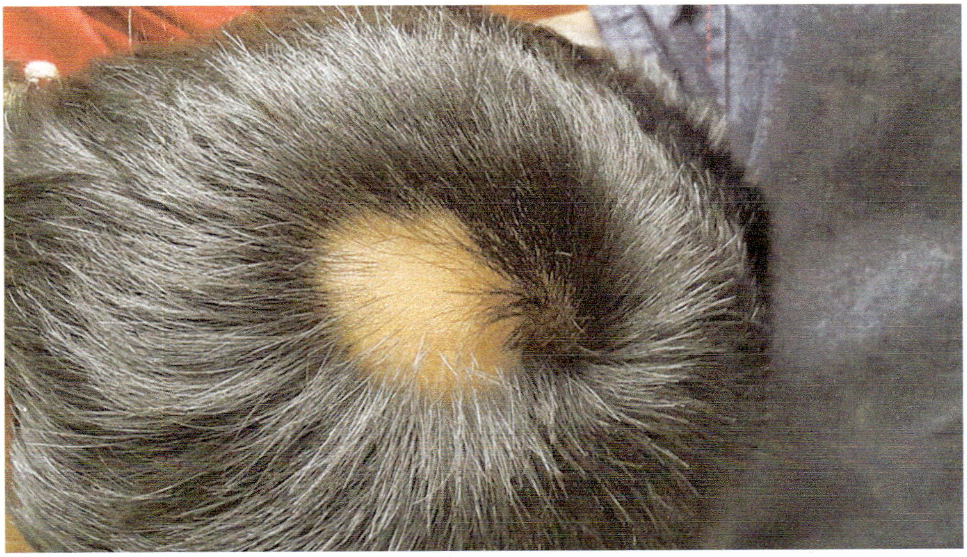

Fig. 13: Alopecia areata (AA) 1. A case of AA.

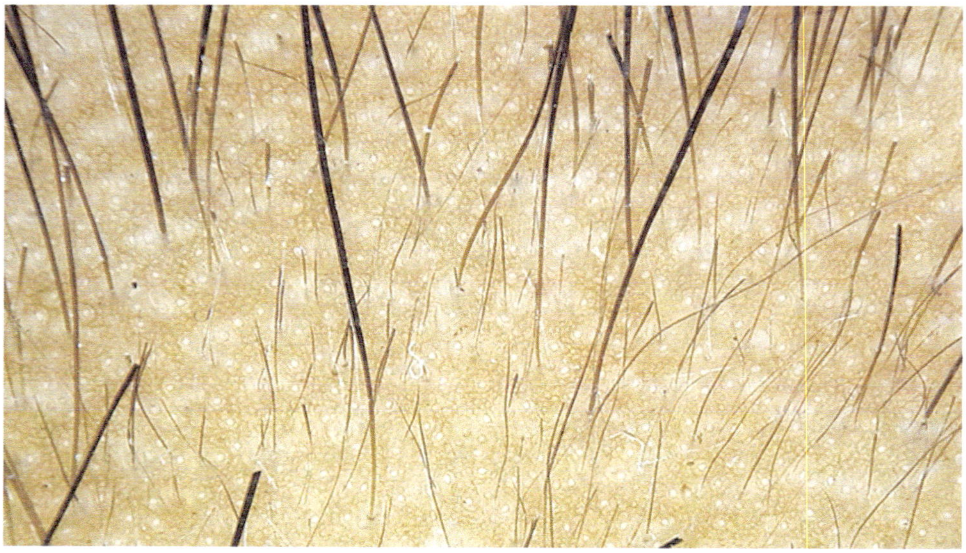

Fig. 14: Alopecia areata (AA) 2. Exclamation mark hairs and coudability hairs seen in this image are trichoscopic marker of AA.

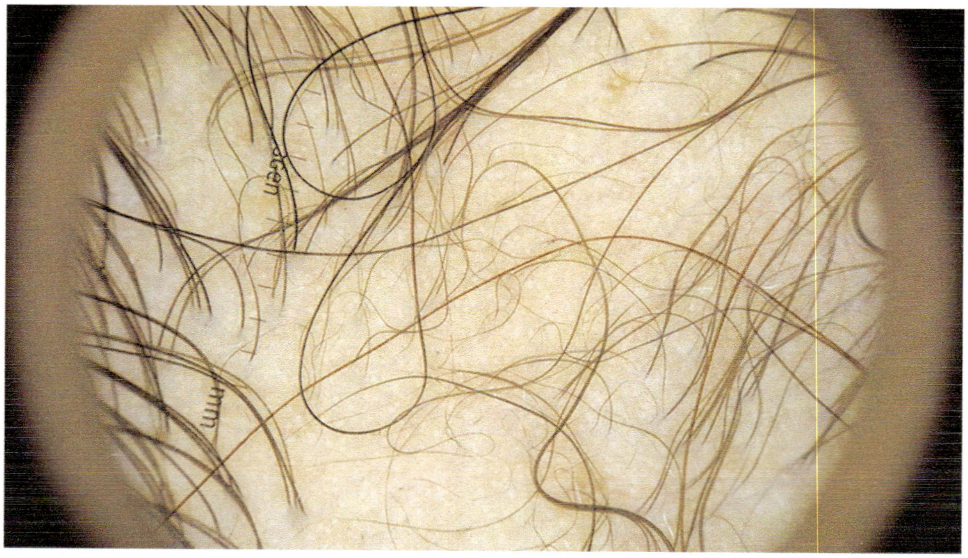

Fig. 15: Alopecia areata (AA) 3. Trichoscopic follow-up after one-and-half months of treatment showing appearance of vellus hairs.

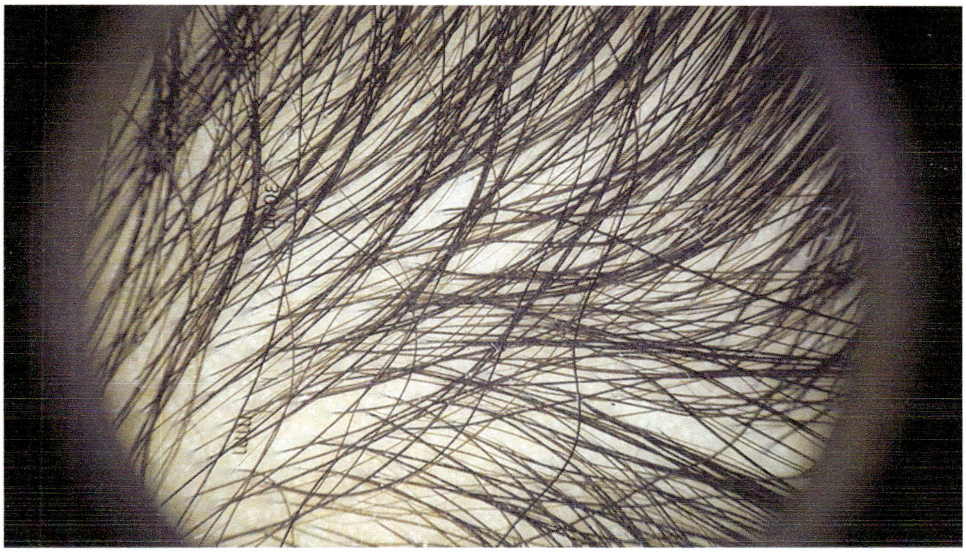

Fig. 16: Alopecia areata (AA) 4. Trichoscopic follow-up of the same patient after 6 months showing full recovery.

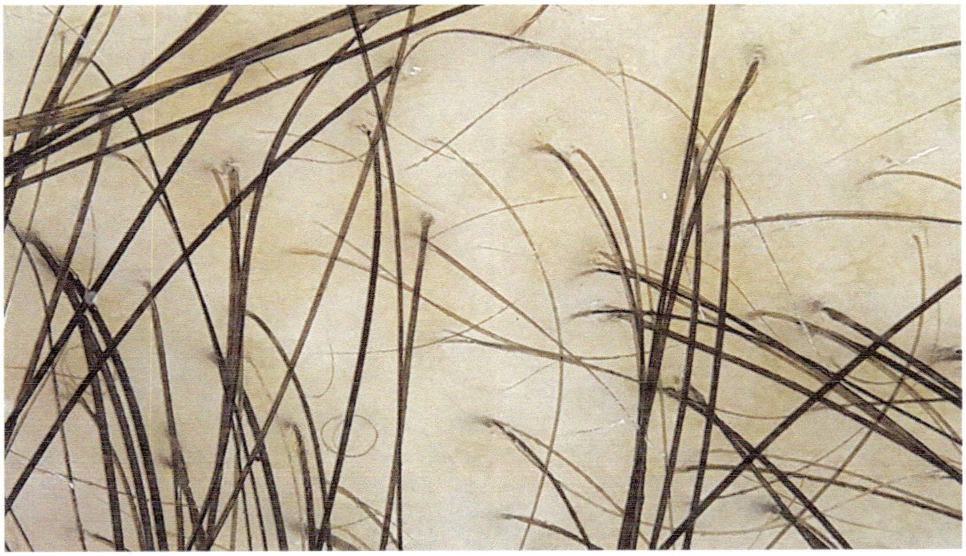

Fig. 17: Telogen effluvium (TE) 1. Regrowing hairs in a case of TE.

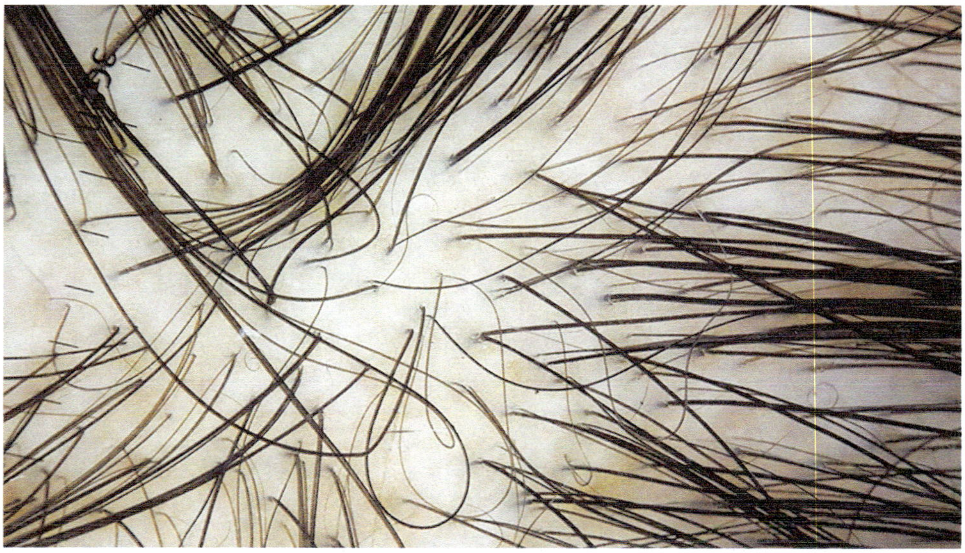

Fig. 18: Telogen effluvium (TE) 2. After 4 months of trichoscopic follow-up of the same patient.

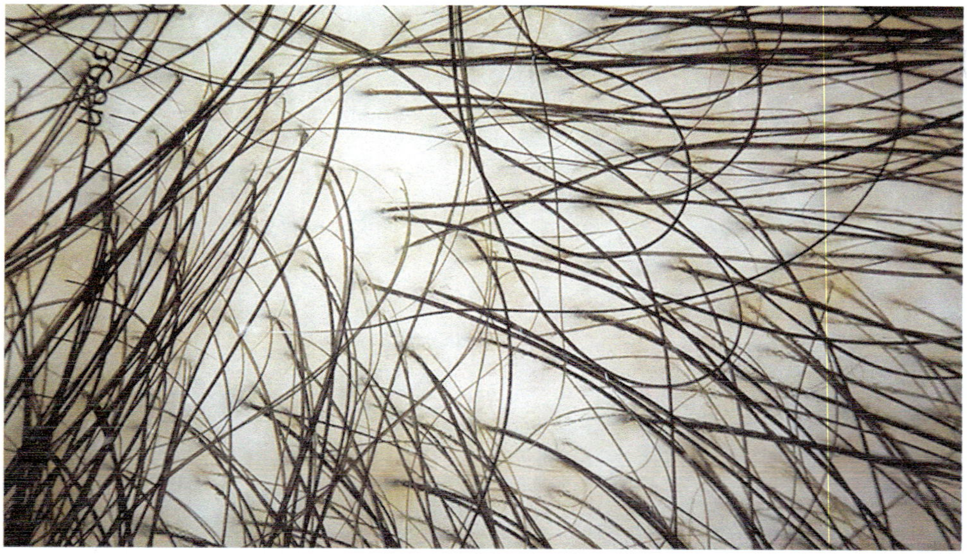

Fig. 19: Telogen effluvium (TE) 3. Full recovery after 6 months. Regrowing hairs are not visible.

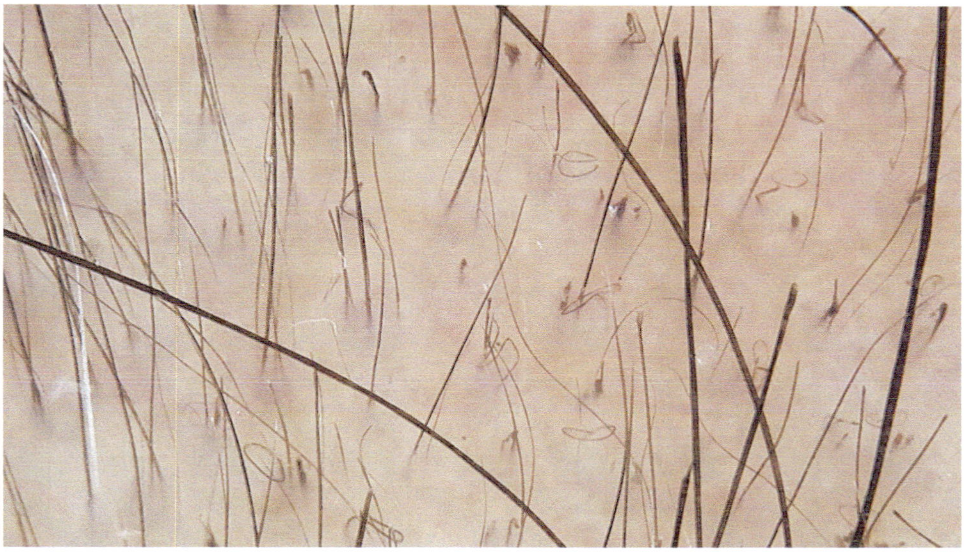

Fig. 20: Trichotillomania (TTM) 1. This is a case of TTM showing coiled hair, flame hair, "Mace" sign, broken hairs, and question mark hair.

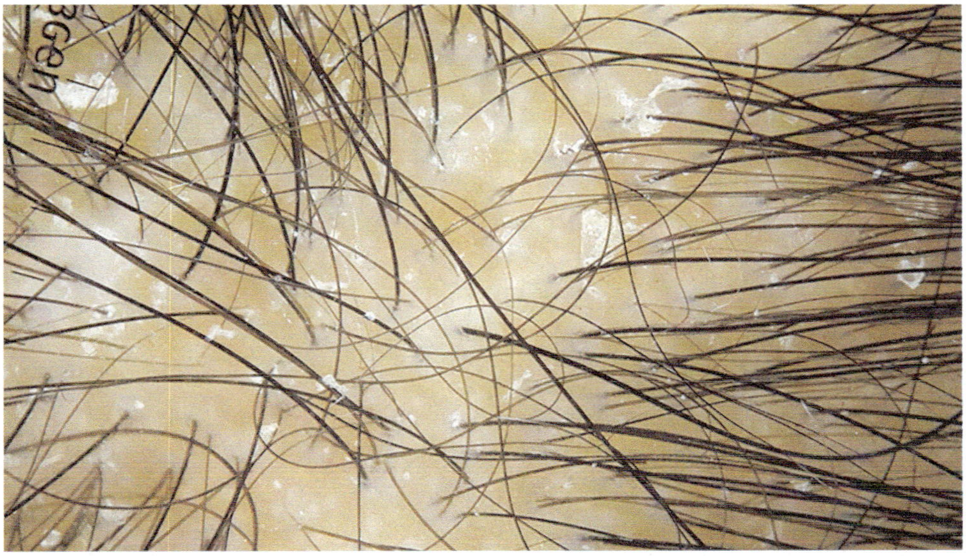

Fig. 21: Trichotillomania (TTM) 2. after counseling and treatment the patient left the habit of pulling the hairs and showed marked improvement after 4 months.

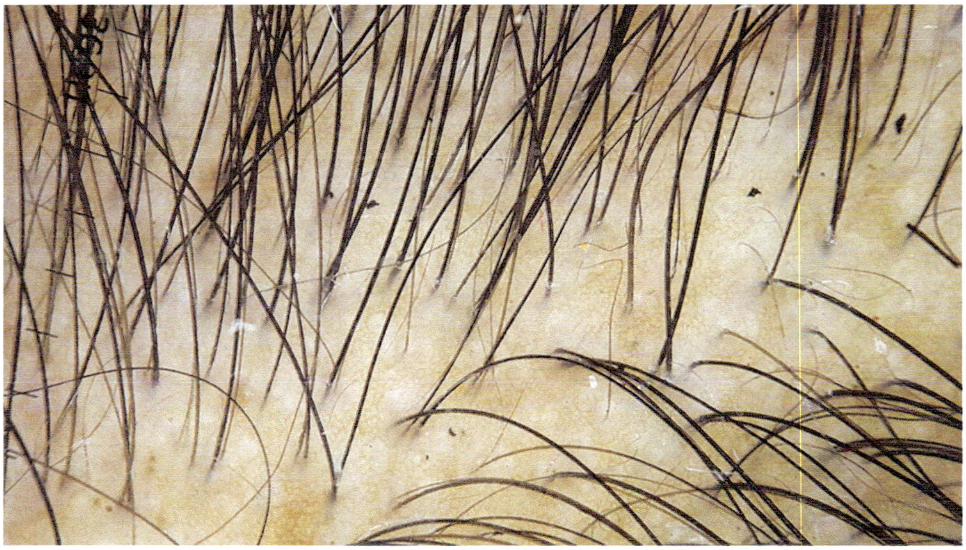

Fig. 22: Trichotillomania (TTM) 3. After 7 months, there is full recovery.

REFERENCES

1. Olszewska M, Rudnica L. Effective treatment of female androgenic alopecia with dutasteride. J Drugs Dermatol. 2005;4(5): 637-40.
2. Rakowska A, Slowinska M, Kowalska-Oledzka E, Olszewska M, Rudnicka L. Dermoscopy in female androgenic alopecia: method standardization and diagnostic criteria. Int J Trichol. 2009;1(2):123-30.
3. Gangetti G, Campanati A, Siminetti O, Cataldi I, Giuliodori K, Offidani AM. Videocapillaroscopic pattern of alopecia areata before and after diphenylciclo- propenone treatment. Int J Immunopathol Pharmacol. 2011;24(4):1087-91.

Index

Page numbers followed by *f* refer to figure, *fc* refer to flowchart.